Competency Based Questions and Answers in Microbiology

for Second MBBS Professional Examination

- 92 LONG ESSAYS
- 221 SHORT ESSAYS
- 216 SHORT ANSWERS
- 355 MCQs

Compiled and Designed as per
CBME Guidelines | Competency Based Undergraduate
Curriculum for the Indian Medical Graduate

OTHER CBS TITLES UNDER SUSHRUTHA ACADEMY

- **Competency Based Questions and Answers in Anatomy** for First MBBS Professional Examination
- **Competency Based Questions and Answers in Physiology** for First MBBS Professional Examination
- **Competency Based Questions and Answers in Biochemistry** for First MBBS Professional Examination
- **Competency Based Questions and Answers in Pathology** for Second MBBS Professional Examination
- **Competency Based Questions and Answers in Ophthalmology** for Third MBBS Professional Examination
- **Competency Based Questions and Answers in Otorhinolaryngology (ENT)** for Third MBBS Professional Examination
- **Competency Based Questions and Answers in Pharmacology** for Second MBBS Professional Examination

Competency Based Questions and Answers in Microbiology

for Second MBBS Professional Examination

- 92 LONG ESSAYS
- 221 SHORT ESSAYS
- 216 SHORT ANSWERS
- 355 MCQs

Compiled and Designed as per
CBME Guidelines | Competency Based Undergraduate
Curriculum for the Indian Medical Graduate

Pooja Rao MD
Associate Professor
Department of Microbiology
Kasturba Medical College
Managaluru, Karnataka

Sevitha Bhat MD
Associate Professor
Department of Microbiology
Kasturba Medical College
Managaluru, Karnataka

Avinash G MSc (Medical Microbiology)
Assistant Professor
Department of Microbiology
Narayana Medical College
Nellore, Andhra Pradesh

Sushrutha Academy
Bengaluru, Karnataka

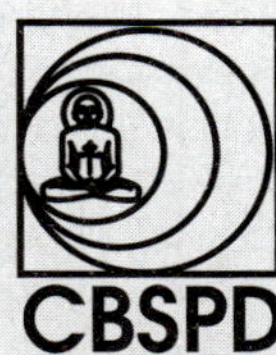

CBS Publishers & Distributors Pvt Ltd
New Delhi • Bengaluru • Chennai • Kochi • Kolkata • Lucknow • Mumbai
Hyderabad • Jharkhand • Nagpur • Patna • Pune • Uttarakhand

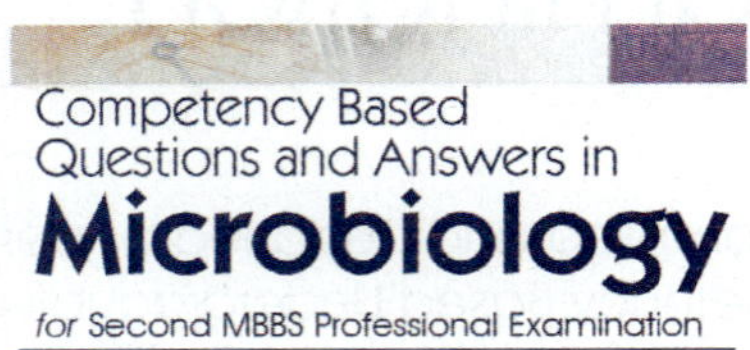

ISBN: 978-93-5466-054-2

First Edition: 2023

Reprint: 2024

Published by Satish Kumar Jain and produced by Varun Jain for

CBS Publishers and Distributors Pvt Ltd

4819/XI Prahlad Street, 24 Ansari Road, Daryaganj, New Delhi 110 002, India
Ph: 011-23289259, 23266861 Website: www.cbspd.com
e-mail: delhi@cbspd.com

Corporate Office: 204 FIE, Industrial Area, Patparganj, Delhi 110 092, India
Ph: 011-4934 4934
Fax: 011-4934 4935 e-mail: publishing@cbspd.com; publicity@cbspd.com

Branches

- **Bengaluru:** Seema House 2975, 17th Cross, KR Road, Banasankari 2nd Stage, Bengaluru 560 070, Karnataka, India
  Ph: +91-80-26771678/79 Fax: +91-80-26771680 e-mail: bangalore@cbspd.com
- **Chennai:** 7, Subbaraya Street, Shenoy Nagar, Chennai 600 030, Tamil Nadu, India
  Ph: +91-44-26680620, 26681266 Fax: +91-44-42032115 e-mail: chennai@cbspd.com
- **Kochi:** 42/1325, 36, Power House Road, Opposite KSEB, Kochi 682 018, Kerala, India
  Ph: +91-484-4059061-67 Fax: +91-484-4059065 e-mail: kochi@cbspd.com
- **Kolkata:** C/o Hind Ceramics Compound, 1st Floor, 147, Nilgunj Road, Belghoria, Kolkata 700 056, West Bengal, India
  Ph: +91-33-25633055/56 e-mail: kolkata@cbspd.com
- **Lucknow:** Basement, Khushnuma Complex, 7-Meerabai Marg (behind Jawahar Bhawan), Lucknow 226 001, Uttar Pradesh, India
  Ph: +91-522-4000032 e-mail: tiwari.lucknow@cbspd.com
- **Mumbai:** PWD Shed, Gala No. 25/26, Ramchandra Bhatt Marg, Next to JJ Hospital Gate No. 2, Opp Union Bank of India, Noorbaug, Mumbai 400 009, Maharashtra, India
  Ph: +91-22-66661880/89 e-mail: mumbai@cbspd.com

Representatives

- **Hyderabad** 0-9885175004 • **Jharkhand** 0-9811541605 • **Nagpur** 0-9421945513
- **Patna** 0-9334159340 • **Pune** 0-9923910676 • **Uttarakhand** 0-9716462459

Printed at: Tara Art Printers Pvt. Ltd., Noida, India

to

The Almighty and Our Parents

Preface

National Medical Commission (NMC), India has revamped the present MBBS curriculum to Competency Based Medical Education (CBME). The focus in CBME is on application-based learning rather than only theoretical aspects. The teaching–learning activities and the assessment methods in CBME focus on all the three domains: knowledge, attitude, and skills.

The thought of coming forward with this book is to orient the students towards the possible variety of questions under each competency. The questions are framed keeping in mind the specific learning objective under each competency. Each competency consists of case scenarios pertaining to the topic. The book focuses on the important questions and answers along with multiple choice questions under each competency to assist the students preparing for MBBS University examinations. The answers are provided in a simple language with illustrations and figures.

The recommended textbooks for MBBS students are:

1. *Textbook of Microbiology*, Dr Arora and BB Arora, 6th edition
2. Ananthanarayan and Paniker's *Textbook of Microbiology*, 12th edition
3. *Essentials of Medical Microbiology*, Apurba Sastry, 3rd edition
4. *Parasitology, Protozoology and Helminthology*, KD Chatterjee, 13th edition
5. *Review of Medical Microbiology and Immunology: A Guide to Clinical Infectious Diseases*, W. Levinson, 16th edition.

We hope that students will appreciate this book. We would request the readers to provide their valuable feedback and suggestions through e-mail. We pray that may the efforts put in by our team be beneficial to the students for preparation for exams.

Pooja Rao
Sevitha Bhat
Avinash G
Sushrutha Academy
e-mail: sushruthaacademy2020@gmail.com

Acknowledgements

We would take this opportunity to extend our sincere gratitude and appreciation to our well-wishers, whose support has been a source of inspiration for us to move ahead with this task of authoring the book.

We are deeply indebted to Sushrutha Academy for this opportunity and encouragement.

We praise and thank the Almighty God for His abundant blessings in making this work possible.

We express our sincere gratitude to Dr. Suchitra Shenoy, Professor and Head, Department of Microbiology, Kasturba Medical College, Mangaluru, Manipal Academy of Higher Education for her full support.

We are grateful to our colleagues in the Department for their support, advice and help during this project.

We would like to extend our gratitude to our parents, husband, children, brothers, relatives and well wishers who made this endeavor possible through their constant help and never-ending concern.

We would like to acknowledge all the people who are involved in the preparation of this book, especially Mr SK Jain (Chairman and Managing Director), Mr Varun Jain (Director), Mr YN Arjuna (Sr Vice President Publishing, Editorial and Publicity), Mis Ritu Chawla (GM Production), Mr Dinesh Chandra Gupta (Senior editor), Mr Parmod Kumar (DTP operator), Mr Sanju Chauhan (Graphic designer) and Ms Jassi of CBSPD for their all-time support and bringing out this book in record short time.

We hereby wish all the readers of the book all the best in their endeavors.

Pooja Rao
Sevitha Bhat

I would take this opportunity to extend my sincere thanks and gratitude to my well-wishers whose support whose support has been a prime inspiration to make a huge step forward for authoring the book amidst the tough situations of COVID-19 Pandemic.

I praise and thank the Almighty God, Goddess whom I believe for inducing immense patience in myself and always providing which I deserve and shower their blessings all through out for the successful completion of the huge work.

My sincere and indebt thanks to Sushrutha Academy without whom this book is not possible.

I extend my sincere and deep gratitude to our beloved person Dr Ponguru Narayana, Chairman, Narayana Educational Society and Narayana Group of Medical Institutions.

I express my sincere thanks, gratitude to Dr. P. Sreenivasulu Reddy, Professor and Head, Department of Microbiology, Narayana Medical College, Nellore, AP who is always with me and providing the required support and confidence.

My sincere thanks to Academic Coordinator, Administrative Officer, Librarian and other core members of the management of Narayana Medical College, who supported and extended their support all the time.

My indebt thanks to all the teaching and non-teaching members of my department.

Special thanks to my co-authors of the book Pooja Rao and Sevitha Bhat who motivated me and made me to work with immense enthusiasm.

I am deeply indebted to my father Sri GCS Rao, Mother Smt. Aruna, my better half Ms. Priya Avinash, and my children Master Skanda Virat and Kum. Srinidhi who rendered their help and support in making this academic project a momentous success.

My sincere thanks to my brother Dr. Praveen G, MS; PhD; Senior Scientist in TCS and adjunct Professor in Queensland University, Brisbane, Australia for his constant motivation and delivering his valuable suggestions in making this huge task a sweet success.

I would like to acknowledge all the people who are involved in the preparation of this book, especially Mr SK Jain (Chairman and Managing Director), Mr Varun Jain (Director), Mr YN Arjuna (Sr Vice President Publishing, Editorial and Publicity), Mis Ritu Chawla (GM Production), Mr Dinesh Chandra Gupta (Senior editor), Mr Parmod Kumar (DTP operator), Mr Sanju Chauhan (Graphic designer) and Ms Jassi of CBSPD for their all-time support and bringing out this book in record short time.

I hereby wish all the readers of the book all the best in their endeavors.

Avinash G

Contents

Details of the Number of Questions and MCQs Included as per the Competency

S. No.	Competency No.	Competency Details	Long Essays	Short Essays	Short Answers	MCQs
1. General Microbiology and Immunity						
1	MI1.1	Describe the different causative agents of infectious diseases, the methods used in their detection, and discuss the role of microbes in health and disease	06	19	15	04
2	MI1.2	Perform and identify the different causative agents of infectious diseases by Gram's stain, ZN stain and stool routine microscopy	—	03	—	01
	MI8.9	Discuss the appropriate method of collection of samples in the performance of laboratory tests in the detection of microbial agents causing infectious disease				03
	MI8.10	Demonstrate the appropriate method of collection of samples in the performance of laboratory tests in the detection of microbial agents causing infectious disease				02
3	MI1.3	Describe the epidemiological basis of common infectious diseases	—	03	05	01
4	MI1.4	Classify and describe the different methods of sterilization and disinfection. Discuss the application of the different methods in the laboratory, in clinical and surgical practice	01	05	09	01
5	MI1.5	Choose the most appropriate method of sterilization and disinfection to be used in specific situations in the laboratory, in clinical and surgical practice	01	02	02	02
6	MI1.6	Describe the mechanisms of drug resistance, and the methods of antimicrobial susceptibility testing and monitoring of antimicrobial therapy	02	06	04	01
7	MI1.7	Describe the immunological mechanisms in health	02	07	07	06
8	MI1.8	Describe the mechanisms of immunity and response of the host immune system to infections	06	06	23	01
9	MI1.9	Discuss the immunological basis of vaccines and describe the universal immunisation schedule	01	04	08	02
10	MI1.10	Describe the immunological mechanisms in immunological disorder (hypersensitivity, autoimmune disorders and immunodeficiency states) and discuss the laboratory methods used in detection.	01	08	06	03
11	MI1.11	Describe the immunological mechanisms of transplantation and tumor immunity	01	03	03	03

S. No.	Competency No.	Competency Details	Long Essays	Short Essays	Short Answers	MCQs
		2. CVS and Blood				
12	MI2.1	Describe the aetiologic agents in rheumatic fever and their diagnosis	02	03	02	03
13	MI2.2	Describe the classification aetiopathogenesis, clinical features and discuss the diagnostic modalities of infective endocarditis	02	05	05	02
14	MI2.3	Identify the microbial agents causing rheumatic heart disease and infective endocarditis	—	01	01	02
15	MI2.4	List the common microbial agents causing anemia. Describe the morphology, mode of infection and discuss the pathogenesis, clinical course, diagnosis and prevention and treatment of the common microbial agents causing anemia	03	02	06	02
16	MI2.5	Describe the aetiopathogenesis and discuss the clinical Evolution and the laboratory diagnosis of kala-azar, malaria, filariasis and other common parasites prevalent in India	05	05	06	05
17	MI2.6	Identify the causative agent of malaria and filariasis	01	03	02	04
18	MI2.7	Describe the epidemiology, the aetio- pathogenesis, evolution complications, opportunistic infections, diagnosis, prevention and the principles of management of HIV	02	07	06	07
		3. Gastrointestinal and Hepatobiliary System				
19	MI3.1	Enumerate the microbial agents causing diarrahoea and dysentery. Describe the epidemiology, morphology, pathogenesis, clinical features and diagnostic modalities of these agents	08	10	12	15
20	MI3.2	Identify the common aetiologic agents of diarrhoea and dysentery	—	01	—	06
21	MI3.3	Describe the enteric fever pathogens and discuss the evolution of the clinical course and the laboratory diagnosis of the diseases caused by them	02	04	02	09
22	MI3.4	Identify the different modalities for diagnosis of enteric fever. Choose the appropriate test related to the duration of illness	01	01	—	04
23	MI3.5	Enumerate the causative agents of food poisoning and discuss the pathogenesis, clinical course and laboratory diagnosis	01	04	04	16
24	MI3.6	Describe the aetiopathogenesis of acid peptic disease (APD) and the clinical course. Discuss the diagnosis and management of the causative agent of APD	01	01	01	10
25	MI3.7	Describe the epidemiology, the aetiopathogenesis and discuss the viral markers in the evolution of viral hepatitis. Discuss the modalities in the diagnosis and prevention of viral hepatitis	02	06	03	15
26	MI3.8	Choose the appropriate laboratory test in the diagnosis of viral hepatitis with emphasis on viral markers	—	03	01	06

S. No.	Competency No.	Competency Details	Long Essays	Short Essays	Short Answers	MCQs
		4. Musculoskeletal System Skin and Soft Tissue Infections				
27	MI4.1	Enumerate the microbial agents causing anaerobic infections. Describe the aetiopathogenesis, clinical course and discuss the laboratory diagnosis of anaerobic infections	02	03	02	19
28	MI4.2	Describe the aetiopathogenesis, clinical course and discuss the laboratory diagnosis of bone and joint infections	02	04	06	03
29	MI4.3	Describe the aetiopathogenesis of infections of skin and soft tissue and discuss the clinical course and the laboratory diagnosis	07	15	13	11
		5. Central Nervous System Infections				
30	MI5.1	Describe the aetiopathogenesis, clinical course and discuss the laboratory diagnosis of meningitis	03	03	05	16
31	MI5.2	Describe the aetiopathogenesis, clinical course and discuss the laboratory diagnosis of encephalitis	01	04	02	23
32	MI5.3	Identify the microbial agents causing meningitis	01	04	03	03
		6. Respiratory Tract Infections				
33	MI6.1	Describe the aetiopathogenesis, laboratory diagnosis and prevention of infections of upper and lower respiratory tract	08	18	16	33
34	MI6.2	Identify the common aetiologic agents of upper respiratory tract infections (Gram's stain)	—	02	—	09
35	MI6.3	Identify the common aetiologic agents of lower respiratory tract infections (Gram's stain and acid-fast stain)	—	02	—	06
		7. Genitourinary and Sexually Transmitted Infections				
36	MI7.1	Describe the aetiopathogenesis and discuss the laboratory diagnosis of infections of genitourinary system	03	05	05	10
37	MI7.2	Describe the aetiopathogenesis and discuss the laboratory diagnosis of sexually transmitted infections. Recommend preventive measures	01	01	03	10
38	MI7.3	Describe the aetiopathogenesis, clinical features, the appropriate method for specimen collection, and discuss the laboratory diagnosis of urinary tract infections	01	04	—	07
		8. Zoonotic Diseases and Miscellaneous				
39	MI8.1	Enumerate the microbial agents and their vectors causing zoonotic diseases. Describe the morphology, mode of transmission, pathogenesis and discuss the clinical course laboratory diagnosis and prevention	05	07	08	18
40	MI8.2	Describe the aetio-pathogenesis of opportunistic infections (OI) and discuss the factors contributing to the occurrence of OI, and the laboratory diagnosis	01	06	03	06

S. No.	Competency No.	Competency Details	Long Essays	Short Essays	Short Answers	MCQs
41	MI8.3	Describe the role of oncogenic viruses in the evolution of virus associated malignancy	01	02	—	05
42	MI8.4	Describe the aetiologic agents of emerging infectious diseases. Discuss the clinical course and diagnosis	02	06	02	04
43	MI8.5	Define Healthcare Associated Infections (HAI) and enumerate the types. Discuss the factors that contribute to the development of HAI and the methods for prevention	01	05	—	10
44	MI8.6	Describe the basics of Infection control	—	03	02	10
45	MI8.7	Demonstrate infection control practices and use of Personal Protective Equipments (PPE)	—	03	—	03
46	MI8.8	Describe the methods used and significance of assessing the microbial contamination of food, water and air	02	—	07	07
47	MI8.11	Demonstrate respect for patient samples sent to the laboratory for performance of laboratory tests in the detection of microbial agents causing Infectious diseases	—	—	02	03
48	MI8.12	Discuss confidentiality pertaining to patient identity in laboratory results	—	—	03	—
	MI8.14	Demonstrate confidentiality pertaining to patient identity in laboratory results				—
49	MI8.13	Choose the appropriate laboratory test in the diagnosis of the infectious disease	—	02	01	03
	MI8.15	Choose and interpret the results of the laboratory tests used in diagnosis of the infectious diseases				—
50	MI8.16	Describe the National Health Programs in the prevention of common infectious disease (for information purpose only as taught in CM)	Presented in in the form of concise content rather than Question and Answer			—
Total Content			**92**	**221**	**216**	**355**

Total Number of Fill in the Blanks: 396

CHAPTER 1

General Microbiology and Immunity

MI 1.1 DESCRIBE THE DIFFERENT CAUSATIVE AGENTS OF INFECTIOUS DISEASES, THE METHODS USED IN THEIR DETECTION, AND DISCUSS THE ROLE OF MICROBES IN HEALTH AND DISEASE

LONG ESSAYS

1. Write in detail about the infectious diseases under the following headings. (1+3+3+3 marks)

A. Definition
B. Sources of infectious diseases
C. Modes of transmission of infectious diseases with examples
D. Prevention and control of common infectious diseases

A. Definition

- Infectious diseases are defined as disorders caused by pathogenic microorganisms like bacteria, viruses, parasites or fungi that can spread directly or indirectly (vector borne) from one individual to another.

B. Sources of Infectious Diseases

1. Humans

- Patient or Carrier.
- *Carrier:* A person who harbors the pathogenic microorganism without suffering any ill effects because of it
- *Healthy carrier:* Who harbors the pathogen without suffering from the disease
- *Convalescent carrier:* Who has recovered from the disease, but continues to harbor the pathogen in his body
- *Temporary carrier:* State lasts less than six months chronic carriage may last for several years
- *Contact carrier:* Acquires the infection from patient, paradoxical carrier acquires the infection from other carrier

2. Animals

- Zoonoses are infections transmitted to human beings from animals.
- *Cattle:* Brucellosis, tuberculosis, anthrax
- *Goat:* Brucellosis
- *Sheep:* Tetanus, anthrax
- *Dog:* Rabies

3. Insects

- *Insects:* Mosquito, ticks, mite, flies, flea and lice: Vectors
- *Mechanical vectors:* Only transmit the agent
- *Biological vectors:* The pathogen undergoes a part of the life cycle in the vectors. Anopheles mosquito in malaria.

4. Soil and Water

- Spores of tetanus bacilli and parasites like roundworm, hookworm.

5. Water

- Cholera, infective hepatitis.

6. Food

- Food poisoning by *Staphylococcus aureus*, salmonellosis.

C. Modes of Transmission of Infection with Examples

Mode of transmission	*Examples*
Contact	• *Direct:* Syphilis, Gonorrhea (Contagious diseases) • *Indirect:* Fomites–inanimate objects like pencils toys
Inhalation	• Droplet nuclei (1–10 μm), e.g. influenza, tuberculosis
Ingestion	• Ingestion of contaminated food, water, e.g. cholera, food poisoning, dysentery

Contd.

Mode of transmission	*Examples*
Inoculation	• Tetanus spores implanted in deep wounds • Rabies virus by dog bite • HIV and Hepatitis B transmitted through contaminated syringes and needles
Congenital Infection	• From mother to foetus is called vertical transmission

D. Prevention and Control of Common Infectious Diseases

I. Measures: Targeting the Reservoir of Infection

1. **Human reservoirs**
   - Diagnosis and treatment of cases
   - *Isolation:* Especially in easily transmitted diseases, e.g. COVID 19, influenza
2. **Animal reservoirs**
   - Treatment of infected animals
   - Destroying the infected animal (Rabies outbreak: killing of stray dogs)

II. Measures: Targeting the Mode of Transmission

1. **Water**
   - Boiling the water, filtering, or chlorination of water
   - Protection of water sources and through proper use of latrines to prevent faecal contamination of water
2. **Food**
   - Washing and thorough cooking of food items before eating
   - Hand washing and proper use of latrines
3. **Air**
   - Isolation of cases
   - Wearing face mask in crowded places
   - Maintaining proper ventilation in rooms
   - Regular maintenance of ventilation systems
   - To keep the mouth and nose covered when coughing or sneezing
4. **Vectors**
   - Vector breeding can be prevented by proper disposal of faeces and other wastes, eradication of breeding sites, and spraying insecticides to destroy mosquitoes

III. Measures: Targeting the Susceptible Host

- *Vaccination*
- *Chemoprophylaxis:* Refers to the antimicrobials taken by the susceptible hosts to prevent them from contracting an infection, e.g. travellers going to malaria endemic area can take chemoprophylaxis
- *Maintaining a healthy lifestyle:* Proper nutrition and exercise
- *Limiting exposure to reservoirs of infection*
  1. *Safe sex:* Use of condom to prevent transmission of HIV and other sexually transmitted infections
  2. Use of nets, repellants and wearing protective clothing to prevent diseases transmitted by insect vectors
  3. Hand washing with soap and water

---

2. Discuss the methods of viral cultivation with its uses/advantages, disadvantages, and examples. (10 marks)

- Viruses are obligate intracellular parasites.
- Viruses cannot be cultivated in artificial cell free media.

Methods of Viral Cultivation

1. Animal Inoculation

- Monkeys were used for the isolation of poliovirus, yellow fever; Infant white mice for coxsackie virus; Guinea pig for rabies, herpes.
- Growth is indicated by death, disease, or visible lesions.

Use

1. To study the pathogenesis, immune response, epidemiology and oncogenesis.

Disadvantages

1. Immunity may interfere.
2. Animals harbor latent viruses.
3. Difficulty in handling animals.

2. Embryonated Eggs

- Eggs should be incubated for 5–14 days and then candled to see if germination has occurred.
- *Chorioallantoic membrane*
  - On continued incubation local lesions called as pocks/plagues appear.
  - *Uses*
    1. Titration of viruses by application of serial dilution to CAM and calculating the number of pocks
    2. Titration of antiviral sera
    3. Study of viral morphology
    4. In isolation of the virus from the infected tissue (variola, fowl pox)
    5. In production of vaccinia virus for vaccine
    6. Study of chemotherapy
- *Allantoic cavity*
  - Rich yield of influenza virus, NCD, mumps which is then recognised by chick RBC agglutination.
  - Used when large quantity of virus is required for production of vaccine, study of chemical structure and preparation of Ag.
- *Amniotic sac inoculation*
  - For primary isolation of influenza virus from throat washings.

- *Yolk sac inoculation*
  - For the primary isolation and passage of members of psittacosis—lymphogranuloma, pneumonitis group, *Chlamydia*, *Rickettsia*.

Main Applications of Egg Inoculation

1. For propagation in the laboratory of the stock strains
2. For primary isolation of strains from the pathogenic material
3. For titration of the viruses and antiviral sera
4. For yielding large quantities of the viruses for vaccine production
5. In study of viral morphology

Advantages

1. Ease of handling
2. Many sites available
3. Lack of antibody production
4. Nutritionally rich
5. Self-contained

Disadvantages

1. Narrow range of viruses
2. Age of the egg must be known
3. Contamination

3. Cell/Tissue Culture

- Based on the origin, chromosomal characters and number of generations through which they can be maintained; cell cultures are of 3 types.

1. Primary Cell Culture

- Normal cells are freshly taken from the body and cultured.
- Capable of only limited growth and cannot be maintained in serial culture, e.g. monkey kidney, human embryonic kidney, human amnion, chick embryo.

Advantages

1. Cells in the primary culture possess a diploid component of the chromosome, characteristic of the tissue cells of the donor.
2. Acid accumulation in the medium is slow because of low metabolic activity and hence cells are easily maintained.

Disadvantages

1. Cultures have to be prepared *de novo* from fresh tissue samples which may be difficult to obtain.
2. Endogenous viruses latent in animal host could be hazardous and may give difficulties with cell growth and virus isolation.
3. Primary cultures from organs of different individuals of same animal may vary in their ability to support replication of the same virus.
4. Slow metabolism, slow change in pH.
5. Cell culture from different individuals of the same species may vary in their susceptibility to viral infection.

2. Diploid Cell Lines

- Established from human diploid fibroblasts (embryonic lung/neonatal foreskin)
- Remain virus sensitive for 20–50 passages
- May undergo 50 serial doublings before senescence
- MRC-5, WI-38, HEL, FS-9
- Subculture and feeding once a week
- Maintained by freezing early passage cells in liquid nitrogen.

3. Continuous Cell Lines

- By transformation (spontaneous or engineered) of cell strains or from tumours
- Loss of contact inhibition
- Indefinite subculture
- Chromosome number is not exact multiple of haploid number.
- High plating efficiency.
- Faster growth rate; subculture twice weekly.
- Frequent pH adjustment necessary, e.g.
  1. HEp-2: sq. cell ca. of larynx, HPV16 transfected
  2. McCoy: Mouse cell line of unknown origin
  3. Vero: African green monkey kidney cells

3. Describe the role of various methods of genetic transfer in antibiotic drug resistance. (10 marks)

- The emergence and spread of antibiotic resistance are the major problem among bacteria.
- The bacteria can acquire resistance via mutation or by horizontal gene transfer (HGT) of antibiotic resistance genes among the bacteria.

Mechanism in Antibiotic Resistance in Bacteria

1. Chromosome-mediated Resistance

- Mutation in the gene that codes for either the target of the drug or the transport system in the membrane that controls the uptake of the drug.
- The frequency of spontaneous mutations is 1 in 10^7 to 10^9, cell division.
- To combat this, treatment with two or more drugs is given, e.g. drug resistance in *Mycobacterium tuberculosis.*

2. Plasmid-mediated Resistance

- Occurs in many species
- Responsible for resistance to multiple drugs
- Higher rate of transfer among the bacterial cells by conjugation
- Resistance plasmids (resistance factors, R factors).
  1. Extrachromosomal, circular, double-stranded DNA molecules that carry the genes for a variety of enzymes that can degrade antibiotics and modify membrane transport system

2. May carry one antibiotic resistance gene or may carry two or more of these genes
3. Plasmid mediated resistance
   i. Penicillins and cephalosporins β-lactamase cleavage of β-lactam ring
   ii. Aminoglycosides: Modification by acetylation, adenylylation, or phosphorylation

Structure of R factor (Fig. 1.1.1)

- Resistance transfer factor.
  - Conjugative plasmid
- R determinant
  - Resistance genes
  - Transposons

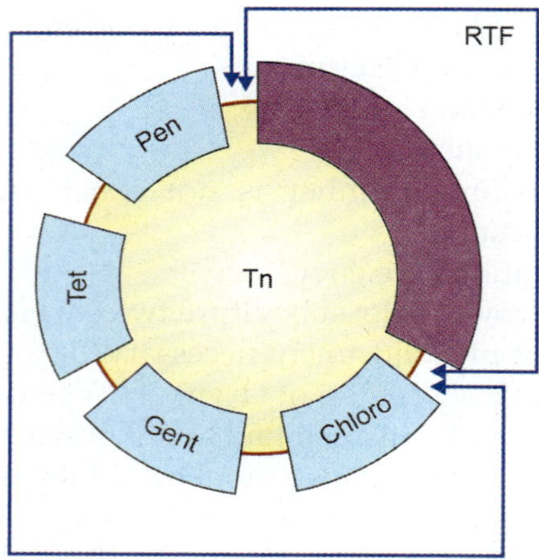

Fig. 1.1.1: Structure of R factor

3. *Transposon-mediated Resistance* (Fig. 1.1.2)

- Genes that are transferred either within or between larger pieces of DNA such as the bacterial chromosome and plasmids.
- A typical drug-resistance transposon is composed of three genes flanked on both sides by shorter DNA sequences.
- The three genes code for:
  1. Transposase, the enzyme that catalyzes excision and reintegration of the transposon
  2. A repressor that regulates synthesis of the transposase
  3. Drug resistance gene

Methods of Gene Transfer

Horizontal Gene Transfer: Conjugation, Transduction, Transformation

A. Conjugation

- Mating of two bacterial cells, during which DNA is transferred from the donor to the recipient cell.
- F (fertility) plasmid (F factor) carries the genes for the proteins required for conjugation.
- One of the most important proteins is pilin, which forms the sex pilus (conjugation tube).
- The bacteria with F plasmid are F+ and cell with no F plasmid is F^-.

Types of Conjugation

1. *F+ and F^- conjugation:* Recipient is F+ (Fig. 1.1.3).
2. Some F+ cells have their F plasmid integrated into the bacterial DNA and thereby acquire the capability of transferring the chromosome into another cell. These cells are called Hfr (Fig. 1.1.4).
3. *Hfr cells with F-:* F plasmid and a part of donor chromosome is transferred (Figs 1.1.5 and 1.1.6).

B. Transduction

- Transfer of genes (chromosomal or plasmid) among bacteria through bacteriophages.
- Types:
  1. Lytic cycle
  2. Lysogenic cycle

C. Transformation

- It is the transfer of DNA itself from one cell to another.
- Dying bacteria release their DNA which is in turn taken up by recipient cells or by the introduction of foreign DNA into bacteria in the laboratory.

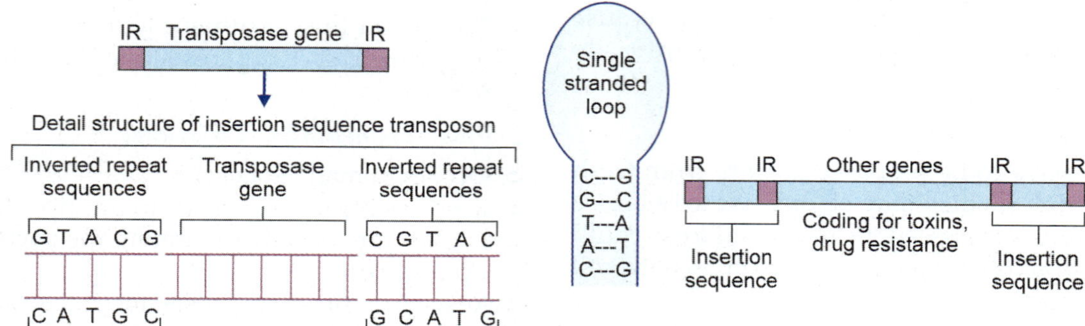

Fig. 1.1.2: Transposase

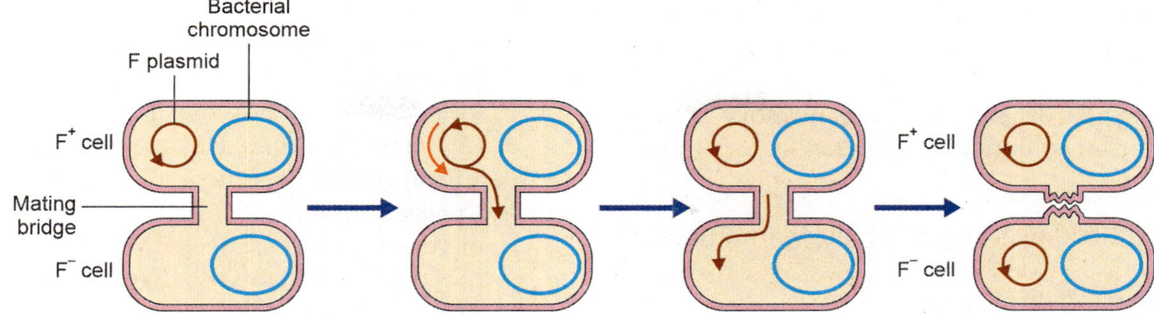

Fig. 1.1.3: Conjugation between F^+ and F^- bacteria

Fig. 1.1.4: Conversion of F^+ male into Hfr male by integration of the F plasmid into the chromosome

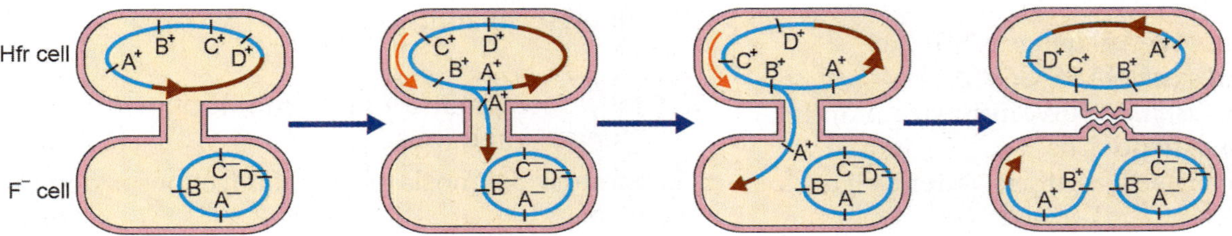

Fig. 1.1.5: *Conjugation between an Hfr and F^- bacteria*

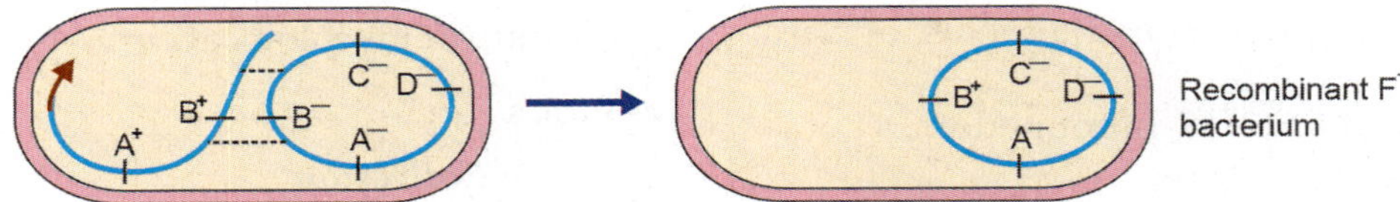

Fig. 1.1.6: *Recombination between the Hfr chromosome fragment and the F^- chromosome*

4. Describe the various methods in diagnosis of viral infections. (10 marks)

- The indications for laboratory diagnosis of viral infections are:.
  1. To confirm or diagnose the viral infection
  2. Screening in blood bank for HIV, hepatitis B and C
  3. Epidemiological surveillance of viral infections

Methods

Specimen Collection

- *Throat swab:* Influenza virus, SARS CoV 2
- *Nasopharyngeal aspirate or swab:* RSV, influenza and parainfluenza virus
- *Nasal swab:* Rhinovirus
- *Bronchial and bronchoalveolar wash:* Adenovirus and influenza virus
- *Rectal swab, stool:* Rotavirus, enterovirus, enteric adenoviruses
- *Urine:* CMV, mumps, rubella, measles, adenoviruses
- *Skin and mucous membrane lesions:* Enterovirus, HSV, VZV, rarely CMV
- *CSF:* Enterovirus, HSV
- *Blood:* CMV, HSV, VZV, enterovirus, adenoviruses

Specimen Transport

- At 2–8°C for a duration of <72 hours.
- For delay of more than 72 hours, viral specimens need to be stored at –70°C.
- Specimens should be transported in viral transport medium.

Microscopic Examination

1. Light Microscopy

- *Inclusion bodies:* The aggregates of many virus particles, seen in nucleus, cytoplasm, e.g. intranuclear inclusion in herpes, Negri body of rabies virus in the corneal smear
- Multinucleated giant cells (Tzanck smear for herpes virus), RSV, measles.

2. UV Microscopy: Direct Immunofluorescence

- Fluorescent antibody staining of virus in infected cell.
- Rabies Ag in corneal smear, respiratory viruses, adenovirus in conjunctival smears.

3. Electron Microscopy

- Virus identified by size, morphology, immune EM.
- Faeces
  - Rotavirus—wheel shaped
  - Astrovirus—star shaped

Rapid Diagnosis Based on the Detection of Viral Antigens

- By ELISA (enzyme-linked immunosorbent assay), ICT (immuno chromatography test), ELFA (Enzyme-linked fluorescent antibody assay)
- Specimens used for various viruses' identification are:
  1. *Serum:* HBsAg, HBeAg, dengue NS1 Ag
  2. *Nasopharyngeal swab:* SARS CoV 2
  3. *Nasopharyngeal aspirate:* RSV, influenza A and B, parainfluenza, Adenovirus
  4. *Faeces:* Rotaviruses, enteric adenoviruses, astrovirus
  5. *Skin:* HSV, VZV

Detection of Viral Antibodies

- Widely used method in the diagnosis of viral infections.
- By ELISA, CLIA, ELFA, ICT, Immunodot.
- IgM or 4-fold rise in IgG titre.
- Antibodies to HIV1/2, hepatitis B, hepatitis C, dengue.

Detection of Viral Nucleic Acid

- Viral genome or mRNA can be detected in patients' blood, tissue with c DNA, c RNA as probe (PCR).
- Methods.
  1. PCR
  2. Reverse transcriptase PCR (for RNA viruses)
  3. Real-time PCR
- Advantage.
  1. More sensitive and specific

Virus Cultivation

- There are three methods of cultivation.
  1. *Cell culture:* Growth is indicated by cytopathic effect (CPE) haemadsorption, immuno-fluorescence
  2. *Embryonated eggs:* Growth is indicated by pocks on CAM, haemagglutination, inclusion bodies
  3. *Animals:* Growth is indicated by disease or death

Cell Cultures

- Cell cultures are most widely used for virus isolation
- There are 3 types of cell cultures:
  1. *Primary cell lines:* Monkey kidney cell line
  2. *Semi-continuous cell lines:* Human embryonic kidney and skin fibroblasts
  3. *Continuous cell lines:* HeLa, Vero, Hep2
- Identification in cell culture
  1. *Cytopathic changes (CPE):* change in shape, size, or fusion of virus infected cell (syncytia). Time taken to produce CPE, type of cell helps in presumptive identification
  2. *Haemadsorption:* Attachment of erythrocytes to the surface of virus infected cells, e.g. mumps, influenza, parainfluenza (haemagglutinin protein)
  3. *Interference:* with formation of CPE by second virus. Rubella and ECHO virus
  4. *Decrease in acid production in infected cells detected by phenol red indicator:* Enteroviruses
  5. *Definitive identification:* CFT, HI, neutralisation, fluorescent antibody, ELISA

---

5. Briefly describe the various methods in diagnosis of fungal infections. (10 marks)

- Laboratory diagnosis of fungal infections is done to confirm.
  - Clinical suspicion
  - Choose specific antifungal therapeutic regimen
  - Monitor course of disease
  - Confirm mycological cure

Methods

Specimen Collection

- It depends on the type of infection

1. Superficial Mycoses

- Skin scraping (*Malassezia* infections, *Tinea*)
- Hair (*Piedra, Tinea capitis, Tinea barbae*)
- Nail (*Tinea unguium*)
- Mucous membrane (Candidiasis)
- Scrapings, swabs from the lesions
- *Corneal ulcers:* Corneal scrapings

2. Subcutaneous Mycoses

- Pus, aspirate from nodules
- Swab from the nodules
- Biopsy materials
- Skin scrapings from the superficial part of sub-cutaneous lesion
- Nasal washings, biopsy of polyp (Rhinosporidiosis).

3. Systemic Mycoses

- *Respiratory infections:* Sputum (early morning), tracheal aspiration, bronchial brushings, bron-choscopy specimen, percutaneous lung biopsy
- *Urinary infection:* Urine, clean–catch specimen in a sterile container

- *CNS infection:* Cerebrospinal fluid (CSF)
- *Blood:* biphasic BHIA broth or automated methods like BacT/alert

Microscopy

1. KOH mount

- *Mycotic elements seen in KOH mount:* Yeast cells, arthrospores, hyphae

Principle

- KOH digests protein debris, clears keratinised tissue, so fungi present in specimen can be seen more readily. The chitinous cell walls of fungi are somewhat resistant to action of KOH.

Procedure

- A drop of KOH (10–20%) is placed in the centre of clean glass slide. The material to be examined is added and mixed. A cover slip is placed over the preparation and slightly warmed over the flame and examined under low power (Fig. 1.1.7).

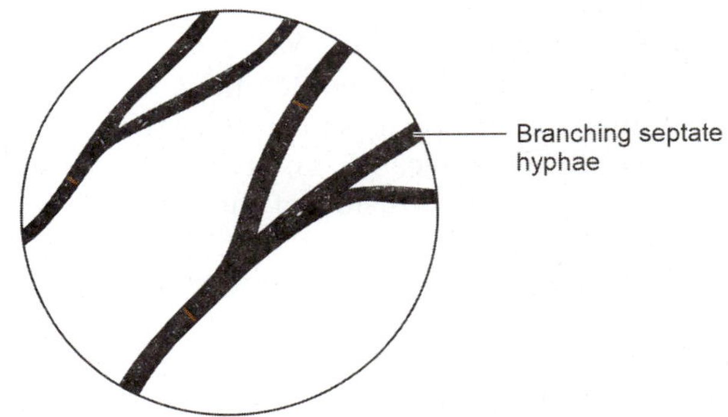

Fig. 1.1.7: KOH mount showing branching septate fungal hyphae

Other Modifications of KOH mount

1. KOH with blue black ink (2:1)
2. KOH with DMSO (dimethyl sulfoxide)
3. Calcofluor white + KOH

2. India Ink

- Detects the encapsulated yeast cells of *Cryptococcus neoformans.*
- Negative stain which creates a dark background against which yeast cells are surrounded by a clear halo (capsule which resists the stain) (Fig. 1.1.8).

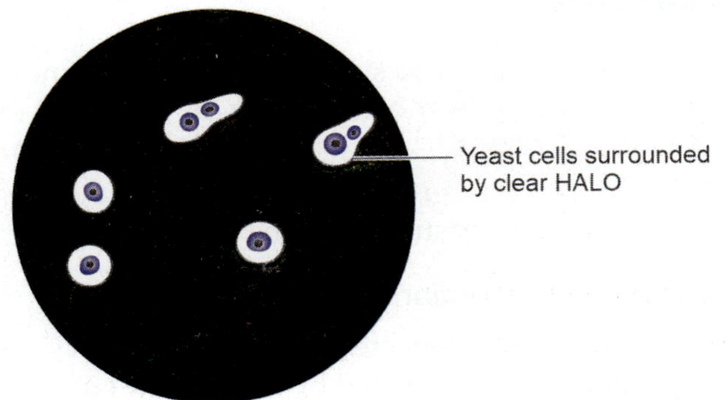

Fig. 1.1.8: India ink positive for *Cryptococcus* spp.

3. Gram's Stain

- Mainly done for the detection of yeast and yeast like budding cells which appear gram-positive.

4. Histopathology of Biopsy with Special Stains

- Haematoxylin and eosin stain
- Periodic acid-Schiff (PAS)
- Grocott's methenamine silver (GMS) stain
- Advantages:
  1. Fungus in tissue sections is almost diagnostic of mycotic infection.
  2. Tissue response of the host can also be studied.

Culture

- *Medium used:* Sabouraud dextrose agar (SDA)
- If the specimens are contaminated (sputum, antibiotics such as chloramphenicol), gentamicin (0.04 mg/ml) is added to SDA.
- Cycloheximide (0.5 mg/ml) can also be incorporated for the isolation of dermatophytes in order to get rid of saprophytic fungi.
- *Other media:* BHI agar, dermatophyte test medium, Caffeic acid agar, potato dextrose agar
- Incubated at 25–30°C for 4 weeks.
- *Identification*
  - Macroscopic features
    1. *Rate of growth*
       - Rapid growers (<5 days): Saprobes, opportunistic fungi
       - Intermediate growers (6–10 days): Dermatophytes, subcutaneous fungi
       - Slow growers (>11 days): Systemic, subcutaneous fungi
    2. *Pigment:* Surface pigmentation and pigmentation on reverse
    3. *Texture:* Glabrous (waxy), velvety, yeast like cottony, granular (powdery)
    4. *Topography:* Flat, folded, rugose, cerebriform, verrucose
       - Microscopic features
       - Lactophenol cotton blue (LPCB) teased preparation

Non-culture Approaches

- Antibody, antigen assays including detection of glucan (*Candida* spp.), mannan (*Aspergillus* spp.), enolase, proteinase by ELISA, ICT.
- *Metabolite detection assays:* mannose, arabinitol by gas-liquid chromatography
- *Molecular identification:* PCR

Examination of Fungal Growth on Primary Media–Yeast

- *Microscopic Examination:* Gram's stain, India ink
- *Biochemical Tests:* Sugar assimilation, fermentation test, urea test
- *Special tests:* Germ tube test, chlamydoconidium formation test

6. Discuss the determinants of bacterial virulence. (10 marks)

- *Pathogenicity:* It refers to the ability of the organism to cause disease.
- *Virulence:* It is the quantitative measure of pathogenicity.
- Virulence of a microbe is determined by its virulence factors.

Determinants of Bacterial Virulence

1. Transmission from an External Source into the Portal of Entry

- *Human to human:* Gonorrhea, syphilis
- *Non-human to human:* Soil, water, animals, fomites

2. Adherence to Cell Surfaces

- Pili, capsule, glycocalyx allow the bacteria to adhere to cell surfaces. These molecules are called as adhesins.

3. Invasion, Inflammation and Intracellular Survival

Invasion

i. Enzymes

- *Collagenase, hyaluronidase:* Allow the bacteria to spread through subcutaneous tissue by degrading collagen and hyaluronic acid, e.g. *Streptococcus pyogenes*
- *Coagulase:* Accelerates the formation of fibrin clot and coats the organism. *Staphylococcus aureus*
- *IgA protease:* Produced by *N. meningitidis, H. influenzae and S. pneumoniae*
- *Leukocidins:* Destroy both neutrophils and macrophages

ii. Other factors

- *Capsule:* antiphagocytic
- *Cell wall proteins of gram-positive cocci:* Antiphagocytic. M protein of *S. pyogenes* and protein A of *Staphylococcus aureus*

Inflammation

- An important host defense induced by the presence of bacteria in the body.
- *Pyogenic inflammation:* Defense against pyogenic bacteria such as *S. pyogenes*, consists of neutrophils, antibody and complement
- *Granulomatous inflammation:* the defense against intracellular granuloma producing bacteria such as *M. tuberculosis*, consists of macrophages and CD4 cells

Intracellular Survival

- *Mycobacteria, Legionella, Brucella* and *Listeria* spp.

Mechanism

- Inhibition of fusion of phagosome with lysosome.
- Inhibition of acidification of the phagosome, reducing the activity of the lysosomal degradative enzymes.
- Escape from phagosome into the cytoplasm.

4. Toxin Production

- Bacteria produces exotoxins and endotoxins.
- Mechanism of action of exotoxins.
  1. *Diphtheria toxin:* Inhibition of protein synthesis by ADP ribosylation of elongation factor 2.
  2. *Tetanus exotoxin:* Neurotoxin, prevents the release of inhibitory neurotransmitter glycine
  3. *Botulinum toxin:* Neurotoxin, blocking the release of Ach at the synapse producing flaccid paralysis
  4. *Toxic shock syndrome toxin (TSST):* Super antigen produced by *Staphylococcus aureus* causes over production of cytokines
  5. Heat labile enterotoxin of *E. coli*, cholera toxin causes watery diarrhoea by stimulating adenylate cyclase and resultant increase in the concentration of cyclic AMP
- Mechanism of action of endotoxin.
  1. Activates macrophages to produce IL 1, TNF and nitric oxide—fever (IL 1), Hypotension, shock and impaired perfusion of the internal organs (bradykinin, nitric oxide)
  2. Activates complement to produce C3a and C5a—inflammation and tissue damage
  3. Activates Hageman factor (coagulation system): DIC resulting in thrombosis, petechial rash and tissue ischaemia

5. The presence of plasmid borne, or bacteriophage borne genes coding for some virulence factor. Enterotoxin of *E. coli* and *Staphylococcus* (plasmid) and toxin of *C. diphtheriae* (bacteriophage).
6. Communicability: Ability of the organism to spread from one host to another.
7. The occurrence of an appropriate route of infection: Streptococci can establish infection whatever be the route of infection whereas *Vibrios* are effective only orally.

SHORT ESSAYS

1. Describe in brief the steps involved in diagnostic microbiology in the diagnosis of skin and soft tissue infections. (5 marks)

- The laboratory diagnostic approach to the diagnosis of skin and soft tissue infections is as follows:.

1. Specimen Collection

- Pus from wound collected by sterile swab.
- Pus from abscess collected by incision and drainage or needle aspiration.

- Subcutaneous infections: From the base of the lesion or biopsy of the deep tissues.
- Skin scrapings, plucked hair or nail clippings in suspected fungal infections.

2. Microscopy

- *Gram staining:* Gram's stain will help study the inflammatory response and morphology of the bacteria causing the infection (Fig. 1.1.9)

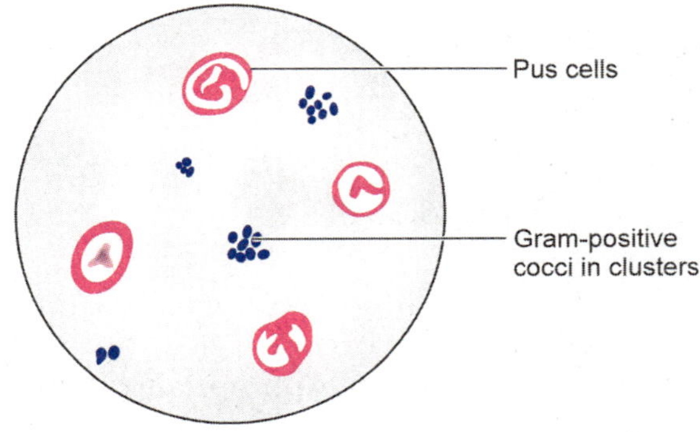

Fig. 1.1.9: Gram's stain of pus showing pus cells with gram-positive cocci arranged in clusters

- *KOH mount for suspected fungal infections:* Yeast cells or hyphae of mold
- *Tzanck smear of the vesicle fluid:* HSV, VZV

3. Culture

- *Bacteria:* Aerobic, anaerobic culture
- Fungal Culture.
- Identification of the growth based on macroscopy, microscopy, biochemical tests.
- Antimicrobial susceptibility testing.

2. Describe in brief the role of blood culture in the diagnosis of blood stream infections. (5 marks)

- Bloodstream infections are characterized by presence of bacteria in blood (bacteremia, septicemia)
- The diagnosis of bloodstream infections relies on isolation of the causative agent in the blood by performing blood culture.

Blood Culture

Specimen Collection

- Blood for culture
- Volume of blood in suspected bacteraemia
  - Ideally 2 sets of blood culture bottles (*aerobic and anaerobic*) has to be collected from two separate venipuncture sites after disinfection of the site.
  - Adults: 8–10 ml of blood per bottle.
  - Pediatrics/neonatal patient: 1–2 ml of blood per bottle.
- *Timing of collection:* Before starting antimicrobial therapy

Specimen Transport

- The inoculated blood culture bottle needs to be transported immediately to the laboratory
- In case of delay, inoculated bottles can be kept at 35°C or in the incubator

Methods of Culture

1. Conventional Medium

- BHI broth or Castaneda medium.
- *Blood:* broth is 1:5 dilution to dilute the antibacterial substances in blood
- Inoculated bottles are incubated at 35°C for 7 days with periodic subculture onto blood agar and McConkey agar.

2. Automated Systems: BACTEC, BacT/ALERT

- Growth is continuously monitored, and reading is recorded every 15–20 minutes.
- When the growth is detected (CO_2 levels), the system gives a positive signal.
- Then the bottle is removed and processed similarly as done for conventional bottles.
- *Advantages:* Faster isolation and increased sensitivity

3. Antimicrobial Susceptibility Testing

- Done by disk diffusion method or automated system.
- *For endocarditis:* Minimum inhibitory concentration (MIC) determination should be done.

3. Describe the role of microbiology in the diagnosis of respiratory tract infections. (5 marks)

- The laboratory diagnosis of respiratory infections relies on confirming the clinical diagnosis by identifying the etiological agent and performing antimicrobial susceptibility for bacterial agents.

Specimen Collection

For URTI

- *Throat swab:* 2 swabs (microscopy, culture), e.g. *Corynebacterium diphtheriae.*
- Nasopharyngeal aspirate for viral diagnosis (Influenza, RSV, SARS CoV 2 or for *B. pertussis).*

For LRTI

- Sputum, induced sputum, tracheal aspirate, broncho-alveolar lavage (BAL).

Microscopy

1. Albert Staining

- On throat swab (Fig. 1.1.10).
- *In suspected cases of Bacterial pharyngitis:* Diphtheria caused by *Corynebacterium diphtheriae*

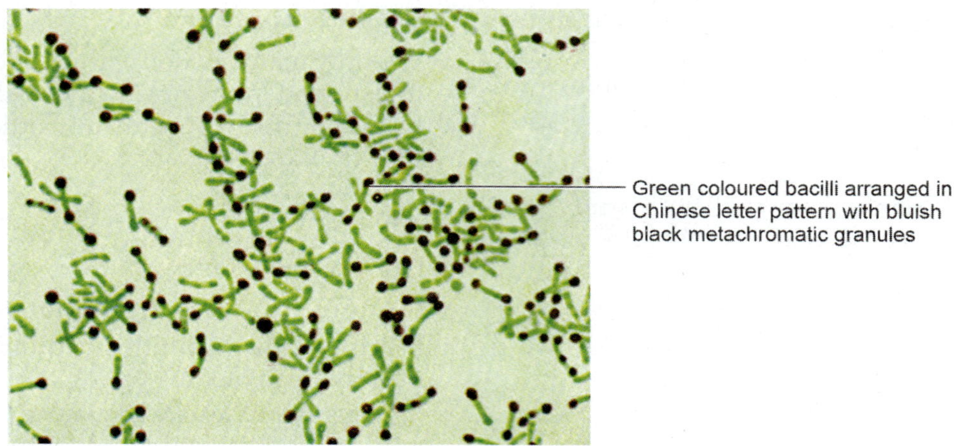

Fig. 1.1.10: Albert's stain showing *Corynebacterium diphtheriae*

2. Gram's Staining

- Of throat swab in bacterial pharyngitis due to Group A *Streptococcus*: pus cells along with gram-positive cocci in chains.

3. Gram's Stain of Sputum/BAL

- Pus cells with the causative bacteria of typical Pneumonia (Fig. 1.1.11).

4. Acid Fast Staining

M. tuberculosis

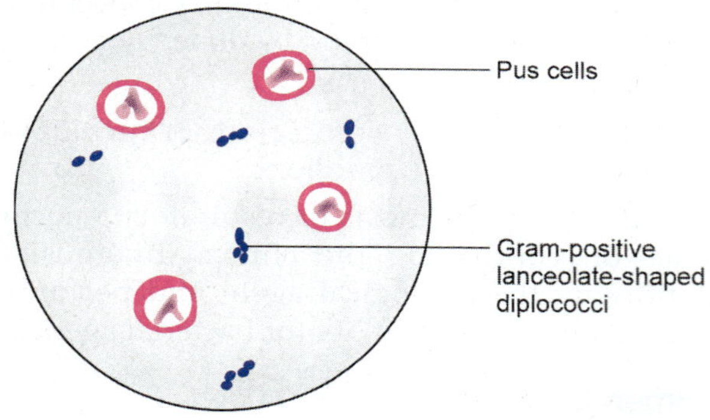

Fig.1.1.11: Gram smear of sputum with pus cells and pneumococcis

5. GMS Stain

Pneumocystis jirovecii

6. Immunofluorescence Microscopy of Nasopharyngeal Aspirate

Respiratory viruses.

Culture

1. For isolation of the bacterial agents of typical pneumonia: Blood agar, chocolate agar and MacConkey agar
2. For isolation of *C. diphtheriae*: Loeffler's serum slope and potassium tellurite agar
3. For *M. tuberculosis*: LJ medium and incubated for up to 6–8 weeks, mycobacteria growth indicator tube.
4. For isolation of fungal pathogens: Sabouraud dextrose agar
5. For isolation of viruses: Appropriate cell lines.

Serology

- Detection of antibodies
- *Mycoplasma:* Cold agglutination test, ELISA formats are available
- Chlamydial antibodies in serum: Micro-IF and CFT.

Molecular Tests

- PCR
- Biofire

---

4. Add a note on non-cultivable methods in the diagnostic microbiology (5 marks)

Non-cultivable Methods in the Diagnostic Microbiology

Rationale

These methods are useful for:

- Fastidious or slow-growing organisms
- Organisms which cannot be cultured.
- Biosafety concerns with organisms like *Mycobacterium tuberculosis* or *Coxiella burnetii.*
- *Rapid presumptive diagnosis of infections.*

Methods

Microscopy

A. Wet mount

1. *KOH mount:* For fungi.
2. *Hanging drop of stool:* For presumptive identification of *Vibrio cholerae.*
3. *Wet mount stool:* Ova, cysts of parasites.

B. Stained smears

1. *Gram's stain:* Bacteria, yeast.
2. *Auramine O stain: Mycobacterium tuberculosis.*
3. *Fluorescent antibody staining:* On clinical specimen for viruses, ANA.

Antibody Immunoassays

- For retrospective diagnosis of infections after viable microorganisms or nucleic acid have disappeared.
- Demonstration of seroconversion has higher specificity.
- Faster result and safer compared to culture methods for some organisms (e.g. *Coxiella burnetii*).
- Can also rule out acute infection based on serological evidence of previous exposure and immunity.
- Disadvantage:
  1. False-negative IgM
  2. Cross reactions
  3. Sensitivity varies with age
  4. Immunodeficiency

Serology for Antibody Detection

- HIV, hepatitis B, C, syphilis, cytomegalovirus, toxoplasmosis, dengue, chikungunya.

Antigen Detection

- Cryptococcal antigen detection in serum and cerebrospinal fluid, galactomannan antigen in invasive aspergillosis, *S. pneumoniae* antigen.
- Rapid test, results within 15 minutes.
- *Assays for both antigen and antibody:* Dengue virus NS1 antigen with IgM/IgG, or HIV antigen/antibody screening testing, offer reduced diagnostic window periods and enhanced sensitivity and specificity

Molecular Based Methods

High sensitivity and specificity

1. PCR
2. LPA
3. NASBA

5. Add a note on molecular methods available along with the principle for the diagnosis of infectious diseases. (5 marks)

Molecular Methods in Diagnostic Microbiology (Table 1.1)

6. Hanging drop of rice water stool shows actively motile bacilli with darting motility.

A. Name the appendage responsible for the motility in bacteria. (1 mark)

- Flagella is responsible for the motility in bacteria.

B. Discuss the properties, structure, functions, and demonstration of this appendage. (1+2+1+2 marks)

- Flagella are:.
  - Long, whiplike/filamentous unbranched appendages.
  - Organs of locomotion.
  - Present only in motile bacteria.

Properties

1. *Longer than bacteria:* 3–20 µm long; 12–30 nm breadth.
2. Composed of the protein flagellin.
3. Heat labile.
4. *Highly antigenic:* Flagellar antigen is called 'H' antigen.

Table 1.1.1 Molecular methods in diagnostic microbiology

Molecular method	*Principle*	*Applications*
Polymerase chain reaction	• Involves extraction of DNA from the bacteria by boiling method or commercial kits • Amplification of DNA ✦ Denaturation ✦ Primer annealing ✦ Extension ✦ Detection of the amplified product by Gel electrophoresis	• More sensitive, specific • Useful for fastidious, non-cultivable organisms • Detection of antibiotic resistance genes • Drawbacks ✦ Qualitative ✦ Detects both live and dead organisms ✦ Liable to contamination
Reverse transcriptase PCR	• RNA—reverse transcriptase forms c DNA and the rest is similar to PCR	• For detection of RNA viruses, 16S RNA of organisms
Nested PCR	• The first set of primers amplify a target sequence, and the second set of primers amplify a region within the first target sequence	• Very specific and alleviates false-positive reactions • Disadvantage: higher contamination rates
Multiplex PCR	• Two or more unique target sequences can be amplified simultaneously	• Diagnosis of respiratory infections, meningitis targeting the aetiological agents

Contd.

Table 1.1.1 Molecular methods in diagnostic microbiology

Molecular method	*Principle*	*Applications*
Real-time PCR	• The amplified target DNA is detected by fluorescently labelled probes as the hybrids are formed. The increase in fluorescence versus cycle number produces amplification plots • Amplification and product detection can be accomplished in one reaction • Quantification can be done	• Prognostic value: viral load—HIV, HBV, HCV • To detect the development of drug resistance, e.g. MRSA, VRE
LAMP (Loop Mediated Isothermal Amplification)	• At constant temperature • Auto-cycling strand displacement DNA synthesis that is performed by a DNA polymerase and a set of two inner and two outer primers	• Genotyping of HBV, HCV • Mutation in HIV, mycobacteria • Detection of HPV subtypes

Structure (Fig. 1.1.12)

- Has 3 parts.

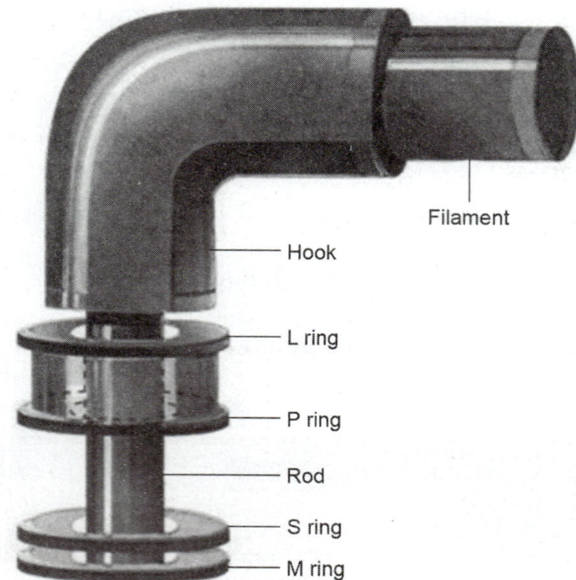

Fig. 1.1.12: Structure of flagella

1. *Filament*

- It is the part extending to exterior.
- Composed of proteins called flagellin.

2. *Hook*

- Curved sheath.
- Connects filament to cell.

3. *Basal Body*

- Anchors flagellum into cell wall and membrane.
- Flagellar arrangements (Fig. 1.1.13).
  i. *Monotrichous:* Single flagellum at one end: *Vibrio cholerae*
  ii. *Lophotrichous:* Small bunches arising from one end of cell: *Bartonella bacilliformis*

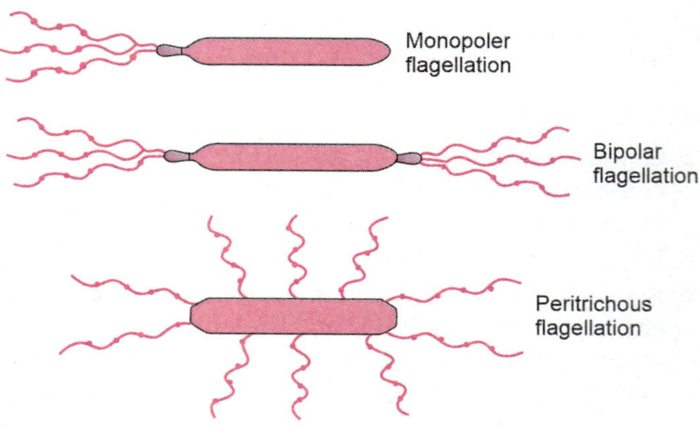

Fig. 1.1.13: Arrangement of flagella

  iii. *Amphitrichous:* Flagella at both ends of cell: *Spirillum minor*
  iv. *Peritrichous:* Flagella dispersed over surface: *Escherichia coli*

Functions

1. Organs of locomotion.
2. Locomotion helps the bacterium in the following ways:
   - To move to words the areas of better nutrition.
   - To move away from unfavourable conditions.
3. *Virulence:* Penetration and spread of infection for example: *E. coli* and *Proteus* cause UTI.
4. Antibody to H antigen is detected in Widal test for diagnosis of enteric fever.

Demonstration

Direct Method

1. Electron microscope.
2. *Special flagellar staining:* Leifson's staining (silver impregnation).

Indirect Method

1. Hanging drop Method.
2. Growth in semi-solid agar.

3. *Craigie's tube:* U-shaped tube with semisolid agar.
4. Swarming growth on solid media.
5. Dark ground illumination.
6. By demonstration of H antigen with specific antiserum (agglutination tests).

7. Describe the common vector borne infectious diseases under the following headings.

A. Define a vector and a carrier with examples (3 marks)

B. Vectors for transmission of dengue, JE, malaria (2 marks)

A. Definitions and Examples

Parameter	Definition	Examples
Vector	Living organisms that can transmit infectious pathogens between humans, or from animals to humans	1. Mosquito i. *Aedes:* Chikungunya, Dengue, Lymphatic filariasis, rift valley fever, yellow fever, Zika ii. *Anopheles:* Lymphatic filariasis, malaria iii. *Culex:* Japanese encephalitis, lymphatic filariasis, West Nile fever 2. Aquatic snails: Schistosomiasis (bilharziasis)
Carrier	Persons/animals that harbour the infectious agent in the absence of any clinical symptoms and shed the organism from the body via contact, air or secretions and risk transmission (inadequate treatment or immune response)	1. *Incubatory carriers:* Measles, mumps, polio, diphtheria, pertussis 2. *Healthy carriers:* Polio, cholera, salmonellosis, diphtheria

B. Vectors for Transmission of Dengue, Japanese B Encephalitis, Malaria

Disease	Vector
Dengue	Mosquito—*Aedes*
Japanese encephalitis (JE)	Mosquito—*Culex*
Malaria	Mosquito—*Anopheles*

8. A 20-year-old female is diagnosed with cystitis. Which cell structure of the causative bacteria is responsible for adherence to the uroepithelium? Briefly explain the significance of this cell structure. (1+4 marks)

Cell Structure of the Causative Bacteria for Adherence to the Uroepithelium

- Pili or fimbriae.

Pili

- Fine, hair-like appendages that are thinner than flagella and not involved in motility, called as fimbriae or pili (singular fimbria or pilus).
- Pili are made up of protein called pilin.
- Antigenic (but antibodies against fimbrial antigens—not protective).

Significance

- They mediate the attachment of bacteria to specific receptors on the human cell surface, which is a necessary step in the initiation of infection for some organisms, e.g. *Neisseria gonorrhoeae, P. fimbriae* in uropathogenic *E. coli.*
- Specialised kind of pilus, the sex pilus, forms the attachment between the male (donor) and the female (recipient) bacteria during conjugation.
- Transfer of virulence factors or antibiotic resistance genes among bacteria.

9. A 25-year-old man suffers from a major soft tissue injury after RTA. On examination, leg was swollen and bullae exuding. The subcutaneous crepitus extended along the limb and the skin was discoloured from knee to ankle. Extensive gas formation throughout all the muscle compartments of the right leg reaching to the level of knee joint was present. The case was diagnosed as gas gangrene. *Clostridium perfringens* was the organism isolated. What is the source of infection in this case? Explain the role of this cell structure along with the help of a diagram. (1+2+2 marks)

Source of Infection

- Spores of *Clostridium perfringens.*

Spore **(*Fig. 1.1.14*)**

Structure

- From inner to outward
  1. **Core**
     - Innermost part
     - Contains the DNA material
     - Surrounded by inner membrane

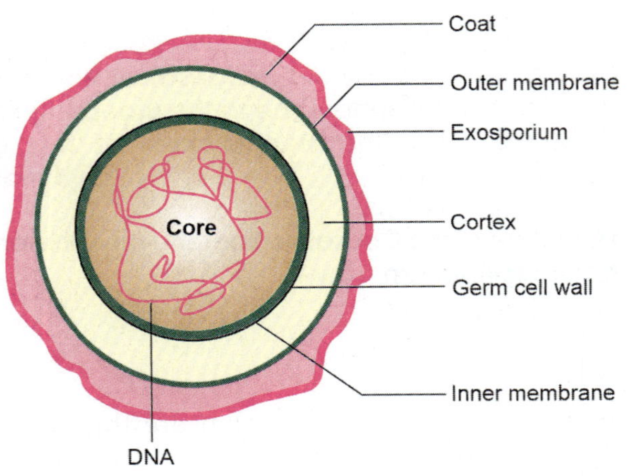

Fig. 1.1.14: Structure of spore

2. **Germ cell wall**
   - Contains normal peptidoglycan; gives rise to future cell wall of the bacterial cell
3. **Cortex**
   - Thickest layer surrounding the core, made up of a special type of peptidoglycan
4. **Spore coat**
   - Multilayered, made of a keratin like protein, impermeable—so spore is resistant to antibacterial agents
5. **Exosporium**
   - Outermost layer
   - Present in some spores

Significance

- Highly resistant to heating; spores are killed at 121°C. Medical supplies must be heated to 121°C for at least 15 minutes to be sterilised.
- Highly resistant to many chemicals, including most disinfectants, due to the thick, keratin-like coat. Only solutions designated as sporicidal will kill spores.
- It survives for many years in the soil. Wounds contaminated with soil can be infected with spores and cause diseases such as tetanus (*C. tetani*) and gas gangrene (*C. perfringens*).
- No metabolic activity, making antibiotics ineffective against spores.
- Spores are not often found at the site of infections because nutrients are not limiting.
- Spores as indicators of sterilisation.
  1. Spores of *Geobacillus stearothermophilus*: Autoclave, plasma steriliser
  2. Spores of *Bacillus atrophaeus*: Hot air oven and ethylene oxide steriliser

10. *Mycoplasma* lacks which of the cell structure component? (1 mark)

- **Give examples of antibiotics acting on this cell structure (2 marks)**
- **Draw a neat, labelled diagram of this structure (2 marks)**

Mycoplasma Lacks

- Cell wall.

Examples of Antibiotics Acting on Cell Wall

- Penicillin, cephalosporins, carbapenem, aztreonam, glycopeptides (vancomycin) inhibit the cell wall synthesis.

Diagram of ***(Fig. 1.1.15)***

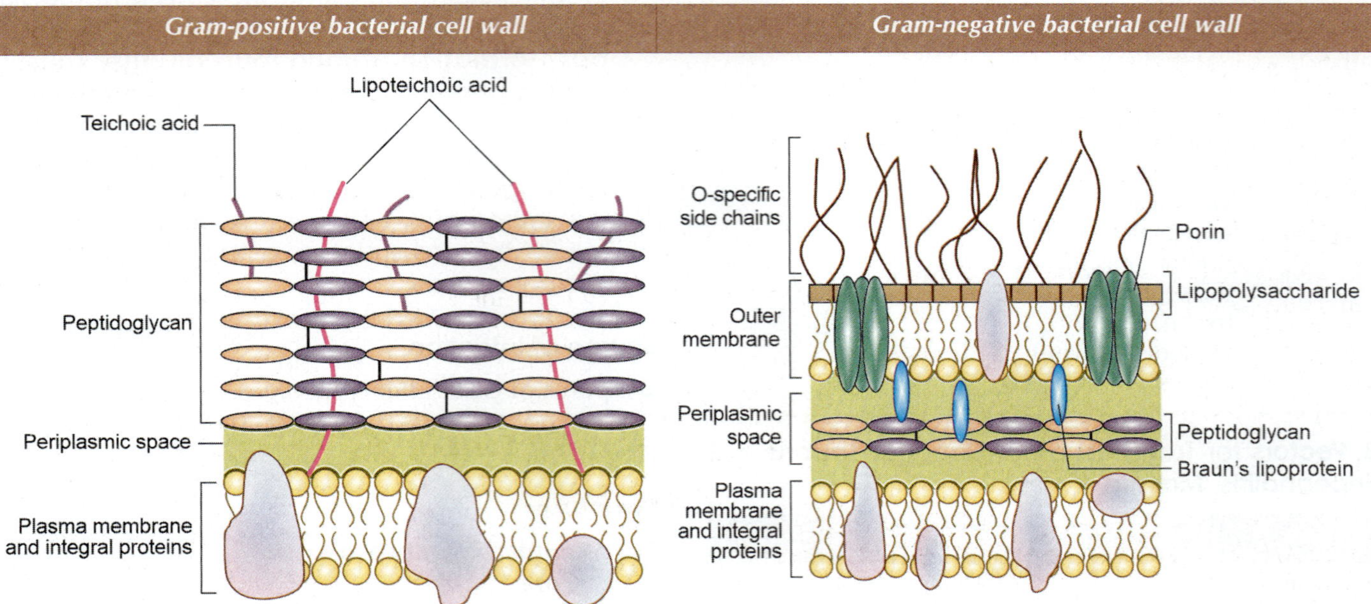

Fig. 1.1.15: Structure of gram-positive and gram-negative bacterial cell walls

11. Antibiotic resistance in *Staphylococcus aureus* is mediated by plasmids. Justify your answer explaining the properties, types, and role of plasmids. (1+1+2+2 marks)

Justification

- Antibiotic resistance in *Staphylococcus aureus* is by plasmid mediated gene blaZ encoding for beta lactamase, and mecA gene coding for altered PBP (MRSA).

Plasmids

Properties

- Extrachromosomal, double-stranded, circular DNA molecules, capable of independent replication.
- Usually extrachromosomal, but can integrate with bacterial chromosome.
- Exist in gram-positive and gram-negative bacteria.

Types

Classification 1

1. Transmissible Plasmids

- Transferred from cell to cell by conjugation.
- Large [molecular weight (MW 40–100 million)], contain genes responsible for synthesis of the sex pilus and enzymes required for transfer.
- Present in few (1–3) copies per cell.

2. Nontransmissible Plasmids

- Small (MW 3–20 million), do not contain the transfer genes; present in many (10–60) copies per cell.

Classification 2

1. Col Plasmids

- Contain genes that code for bacteriocins, proteins that can kill other bacteria.

2. F-plasmid

- Contain genes for expression of sex pili and conjugation.

3. Resistance Plasmids

- Contain genes that provide resistance against antibiotics or poison.

Role

- Plasmids carry the genes for the following functions
- and structures of medical importance.
  1. Antibiotic resistance, which is mediated by enzymes, such as the β-lactamase of *S. aureus, Escherichia coli, and Klebsiella pneumoniae.*
  2. Exotoxins: enterotoxins of *E. coli*, anthrax toxin of *Bacillus anthracis*, exfoliative toxin of *S. aureus*, and tetanus toxin of *Clostridium tetani.*
  3. Pili (fimbriae): Adherence of bacteria to epithelial cells.
  4. Resistance to heavy metals: Mercury, the active component of some antiseptics.
  5. Resistance to ultraviolet light, which is mediated by DNA repair enzymes.
  6. Bacteriocins, which are toxic proteins synthesized by certain bacteria that are lethal for other bacteria.

Plasmids are useful in molecular biology and genetics.

12. A 45-year-old man after RTA is brought to ED. O/E, a surgeon suspect's anaerobic infection of the injured leg. What is the preferred specimen to be collected? Explain the methodology of culture available in this case. (1+4 marks)

Preferred Specimen to be Collected

- Aspirate, biopsy from the lesions.
- Anaerobic bacteria are sensitive to oxygen.

Methods of Anaerobic Culture

1. Production of Vacuum

- The cultures are incubated in a vacuum desiccator.

2. Displacement of Oxygen with Other Gases

- Displacement of oxygen with gases like hydrogen, nitrogen, helium, or CO_2, e.g. Candle jar.

3. Chemical Method

- Alkaline pyrogallol absorbs oxygen.
- *Mcintosh—Fildes' Anaerobic Jar.*
  - Consists of a metal jar or glass jar with a metal lid which can be clamped airtight.
  - The lid has 2 tubes—gas inlet and gas outlet.
  - The lid has two terminals—connected to electrical supply.
  - Under the lid—small, grooved porcelain spool, wrapped with a layer of palladinised asbestos.
  - *Working.*
    - Inoculated plates are placed inside the jar and the lid clamped airtight
    - The outlet tube is connected to a vacuum pump and the air inside is evacuated
    - The outlet tap is then closed, and the inlet tube is connected to a hydrogen supply
    - After the jar is filled with hydrogen, the electric terminals are connected to a current supply, so that the palladinised asbestos is heated
    - Act as a catalyst for the combination of hydrogen with residual oxygen
- *Gaspak.*
  - Plates are kept in the jar with commercially available disposable envelope contains sodium bicarbonate and sodium borohydride which generate H_2 and CO_2 on addition of water.
  - Palladium catalyst is below the jar lid to remove traces of oxygen in the jar.

- Indicator is used—reduced methylene blue.
  - Colourless: anaerobically
  - Blue colour: on exposure to oxygen

4. Biological Method

- Absorption of oxygen by incubation with aerobic bacteria, germinating seeds or chopped vegetables.

5. Reduction of Oxygen

- By using reducing agents—1% glucose, 0.1% thioglycolate.

6. Anaerobic Glove Box and Workstation for Processing and Incubation of Culture

- Chamber for processing of the samples for anaerobic culture.

13. Briefly discuss the role of organisms in health and disease in vaginal tract and gastrointestinal tract. (2.5+2.5 marks)

Microbiome of Vaginal Tract

- Vaginal flora of adult women consists primarily of *Lactobacillus species.*
  1. Lactobacilli are responsible for the acidic pH of the adult woman's vagina
  2. The vaginal pH is high before puberty and after menopause
  3. Lactobacilli as the normal flora in vagina prevent the growth of pathogens. Antibiotics suppress the growth of lactobacilli and can lead to *Candida vaginitis*
- Due to proximity of vagina to the anus, vagina gets colonised by faecal flora. Women are susceptible to recurrent urinary tract infections by *E. coli.*
- Group B streptococci colonize vagina in 15–20% of women of child-bearing age. Associated with neonatal sepsis and meningitis, it is acquired during passage through the birth canal.
- Vaginal colonisation with *Staphylococcus aureus* in 5% of women, predisposes them to toxic shock syndrome.

Microbiome of GIT

- Colon has the complex microbial population in humans.
- *Members are anaerobic bacteria: Bacteroides* spp. and *Prevotella* spp., *Escherichia*, and *Salmonella* spp.
- Change in the microbiome plays role in:
  - Antibiotic associated colitis
  - Weight control (obesity)
  - Crohn disease and ulcerative colitis
  - Patients with IBD have significantly lower numbers of beneficial microorganisms.

14. A 48-year-old man admitted to the hospital with c/o cough and breathlessness. CXR shows left LL consolidation. Gram's stain of sputum showed numerous pus cells along with gram-positive cocci in pairs. Lanceolate shape with clearing was seen around it.

A. What is the cell structure responsible for the invasiveness of the pathogenic bacteria? (1 mark)

B. Briefly describe the role, practical and clinical significance of this cell structure (3 marks)

C. Discuss the methods of demonstration of capsule (2 marks)

A. Cell Structure Responsible

- Invasiveness in *Streptococcus pneumoniae* is attributed to its capsule.

B. Capsule

- A viscid, gelatinous extracellular polymeric substance present just external to cell and in contact with it.

Role of Bacterial Capsule

1. Protect cell wall against attack by antibacterial substances—Lysozyme, complement, bacteriocins.
2. Acts as a virulence factor—anti-phagocytic—adherence factor—attachment to host cell surfaces—loss of capsule makes the bacterium avirulent.
3. Antigenic and confers antigenic specificity on the organism.

Practical and Clinical Significance

1. Detection of capsular material in body fluids (CSF, pleural fluid, blood) helps in rapid diagnosis of infections by capsulated bacteria, e.g. in pneumococcal meningitis, detection of capsular polysaccharide of *Pneumococcus* in CSF sample.
2. Detection of capsular polysaccharide helps in identification of bacterial cultures in the lab.
3. Detection of capsular polysaccharide helps in intraspecies typing of bacteria.
4. Capsular material is antigenic: It can be used for vaccine preparation, e.g. pneumococcal vaccine contains purified polysaccharides of 23 types of pneumococci.

C. Demonstration of Capsule

1. Direct Methods

i. Stained Preparations

- *Negative staining:* Using India Ink/Nigrosin: the black particles in the stain fail to stain the capsule—the presence of a capsule is indicated by a bright halo around the bacteria against a dark background
- *Welch staining method:* Stains the capsule

- *Gram's stain or methylene blue stain:* Appear as unstained halo around the bacteria- not a good or reliable method for capsule demonstration

ii. Unstained

- Can be viewed under dark ground illumination or electron microscopy.

1. Indirect methods

i. Immunofluorescence.
ii. Serological method—Quellung reaction.

15. Which cell wall components are present in gram-negative but absent in gram-positive bacteria? Describe their structure and functions. (1+4 marks)

Cell Wall Component Present in Gram-negative but Absent in Gram-positive is

1. Lipopolysaccharide (LPS).
2. Outer membrane proteins (OMP).

Lipopolysaccharide (LPS) (Fig. 1.1.16)

- Integral part of the outer membrane (cell wall) of gram-negative bacteria, which is released only on lysis of the organism.
- It has 3 components:
  1. *Lipid A*
     - A glycolipid which is responsible for the toxicity of the LPS
  2. *Core Polysaccharide*
     - It is the backbone of the LPS molecule and linked to lipid A
     - Similar in all gram-negative bacteria
  3. *Polysaccharide Side Chain*
     - Repeating units of various sugars
     - Unique pattern in each species, therefore, forms the important "O" antigen or somatic Ag of gram-negative bacteria
     - Useful in identification of gram-negative bacteria in the laboratory.

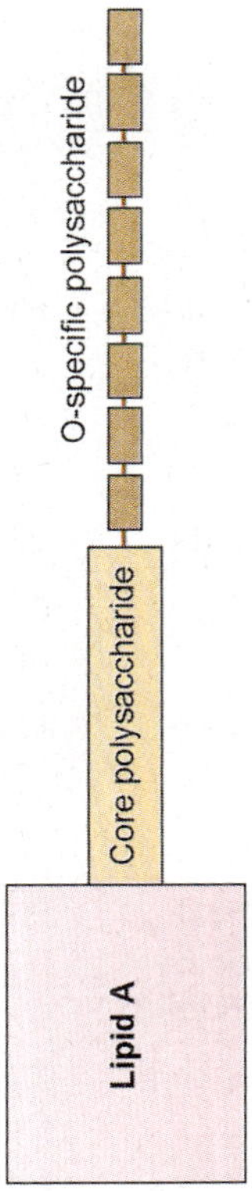

O-specific polysaccharide
Core polysaccharide
Lipid A

Fig. 1.1.16: Structure of LPS

Functions

1. Fever, hypotension, shock, DIC.
2. Activation of alternate complement pathway.
3. Activation of macrophages—increasing phagocytic action.
4. Activation of B cells, increasing antibody production.
5. The term 'endotoxin' is used to indicate LPS as it is not released into the environment but is an integral part of the cell wall.

Outer Membrane Proteins

Structure

- Protein molecules which traverse both layers of the membrane, and are called 'Porins' which form nonspecific pores or channels, e.g. OmpA, OmpC, OmpD, OmpF, LamB, Tsx.

Functions

1. These channels permit free diffusion/transport of low molecular weight solutes which are required by the cell.
2. These protein molecules may play a role in virulence.
3. Act as receptors for bacteriophages.
4. Anchor outer membrane to peptidoglycan layer.
5. Act as sex-pilus receptor in bacterial conjugation.

16. Hepatitis B vaccine is an example for recombinant vaccine. Justify your answer. What are the steps involved in recombinant DNA technology and list the applications of recombinant DNA technology? (2+2+1 marks)

Justification

- Recombinant vaccine.
  - *Viruses with large genome (Vaccinia virus):* Gene in vaccinia virus not required for the viral replication is excised and the gene for the surface antigen of hepatitis B virus is introduced into vaccinia virus. The preparation is injected leading to expression of gene of HBsAg in the infected cells

Recombinant DNA Technology (Fig. 1.1.17)

Steps

1. Isolation of genetic material.
2. Cutting the gene at the recognition sites by restriction enzymes play a major role in determining the location at which the desired gene is inserted into the vector genome.
3. Amplifying the gene copies through PCR.
4. *Ligation of DNA molecules:* Cut fragment of DNA and the vector together with the help of the enzyme DNA ligase.
5. Insertion of recombinant DNA into host.

Applications

1. *Production of vaccines, growth hormones, gene therapy:* Therapeutic purposes.
2. Production of antigens used in diagnostic kits.
3. Genetically modified (GM) vegetables, fruits, and transgenic animals.

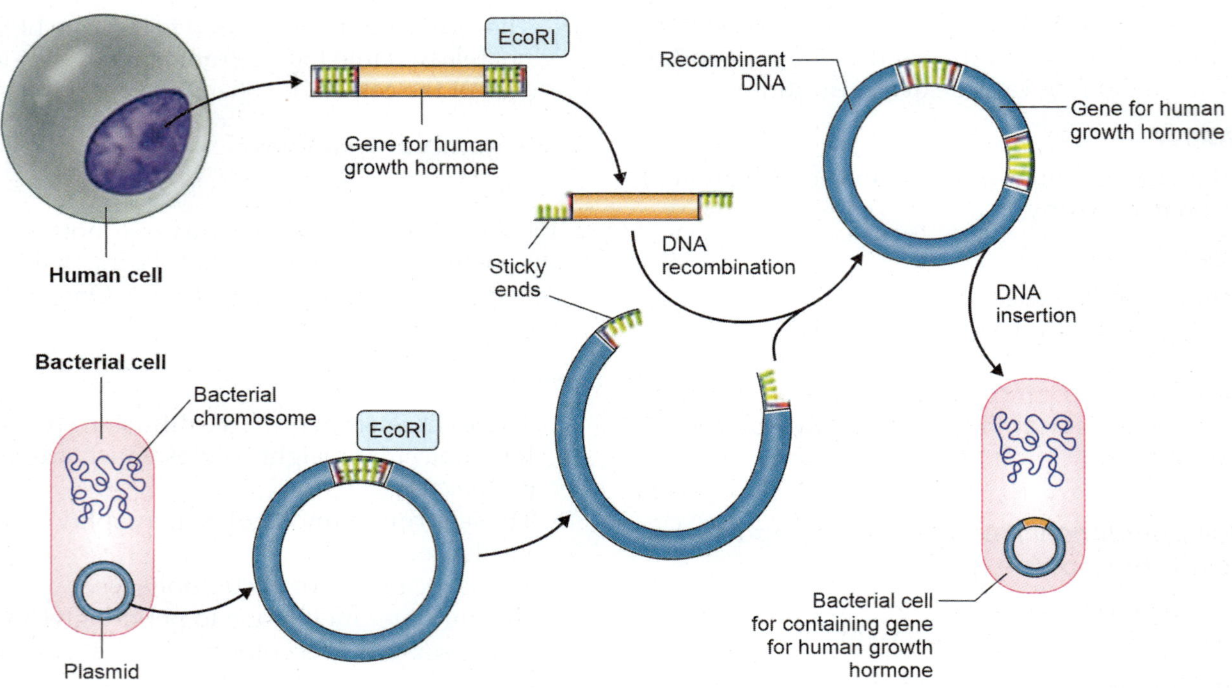

Fig. 1.1.17: Recombinant DNA technology

17. Compare Exotoxins and Endotoxins. (4 marks)

Feature	Exotoxins	Endotoxins
Definition	• Proteins secreted out of bacteria	• Lipid portion of lipopoly-saccharides (LPSs) are an integral part of outer membrane of bacteria
Source	• Mostly gram-positive bacteria and gram-negative bacteria	• Present only in gram-negative bacteria
Chemical nature	• Polypeptide	• Lipopoly-saccharide
Compo-nents	• 2 subunits 1. A (active) 2. B (binding)	• 3 components 1. O-antigen 2. Core oligo-saccharide 3. Lipid A
Location of genes	• Plasmids, bacteriophage	• Chromosome
Secreted from cell	• Yes	• No
Heat stability	• labile (60–80°C)	• Stable at 100°C
Specificity	• Specific in mode of action and host cells	• Not specific in nature
Specific receptors	• Present	• No
Immuno-genicity	• High	• Weak
Fever	• No	• Fever by IL-1 production
Toxicity	• High	• Moderate
Mode of action	• Enzyme-like mechanisms	• TNF and Interlukin-1
Potency	• *High*	• *Low*
Effects	• Cytotoxin, enterotoxin or neurotoxin	• Fever, diarrhea, vomiting
Neutrali-sation by antibodies	• Possible	• Not possible
Detection	• Detected by many tests (neutralisation, precipitation)	• Detected by Limulus lysate assay
Conversion to toxoids	• Possible (On treatment with formalin), e.g. diphtheria, botulism, and tetanus	• Not possible
Availability of vaccines	• Available	• No effective vaccines available.

Contd.

Contd.

Feature	Exotoxins	Endotoxins
Diseases caused	• Tetanus, diphtheria, botulism	• Meningococcaemia, sepsis by gram-negative rods
Examples	• Toxins produced by *Staphylococcus aureus*, *Bacillus cereus*, *Streptococcus pyogenes*	• Toxins of *E. coli*, *Salmonella typhi*

18. Enumerate the congenital viral infections. During which stage of gestation, these viruses get transmitted? (3+2 marks)

Congenital Viral Infections

1. *Rubella:* Congenital rubella
2. *CMV:* Congenital CMV
3. *HIV:* Childhood AIDS
4. *VZV:* Skin lesions, musculoskeletal, CNS abnormalities when foetus is infected <20 weeks, later childhood zoster.
5. *HSV:* Neonatal HSV.
6. *HBV:* Persistent infection.
7. *Parvo B 19:* Abortion, hydrops foetalis.

Stage of Gestation, these viruses get transmitted

Virus	Trans-placental	During birth	Shortly after birth
Rubella	+ +	–	–
Cytomegalovirus	+	+ +	+ +
Herpes simplex	+	+ +	+
Varicella zoster	+ +	+	+
Parvovirus	+ +	–	–
Enterovirus	+	+ +	+ +
HIV	+	+ +	+
Hepatitis B	+	+ +	+ +
HPV	–	+ +	–

19. Explain in brief the clinical features of any five congenital infections along with the laboratory work-up (5 marks)

See Table 1.1.2

Table 1.1.2 Clinical features of any five congenital infections

Congenital infections	Clinical features	Lab work-up
Congenital rubella syndrome	Triad of: • Patent ductus arteriosus • Microphthalmia • Sensory neuronal deafness	• HAI, ELISA—Rising titres of antibody (mainly IgG) • Presence of rubella-specific IgM—ELISA • WBCs from cord/infant blood– • PCR
Congenital Herpes	• Rare, most devastating • Skin vesicles • Chorioretinitis • Microcephaly • Micro-ophthalmia • IUGR	• Urine culture for CMV (must be in first two weeks of life to confirm congenital infection). • Cord or infant blood for CMV PCR • Serology of blood or Urine. IgM persist for 8 months • Head ultrasound
Congenital CMV infection	• Jaundice • Petechiae • Hepatosplenomegaly • IUGR (33%); Preterm • Microcephaly • Chorioretinitis • Fatal outcome	• Skin vesicles, Swabs from eyes, mouth/nasopharynx, CSF: viral culture and HSV PCR. • WBCs from cord/neonate blood for HSV PCR • CSF-cells, protein, glucose • ELISA-Subtype specific (HSV1 and 2) serology may be useful to child • Ophthalmic consultation
Congenital varicella syndrome	• Scarring of skin • Hypoplasia of limbs • Cortical atrophy, psychomotor retardation • Chorioretinitis, cataracts	• IgM—current acute infection • Immunofluorescence of vesicle fluid • Virus isolation, electron microscopy
Congenital toxoplasmosis	• Abortion, stillbirth • Neonatal disease with encephalitis • Chorioretinitis • Hepatosplenomegaly • Fever, jaundice • Intracranial calcifications • Blindness	• Microscopy: Giemsa stain- crescent-shaped trophozoite • Tissue—Cyst • IgM antibody—Immunofluorescence • IgG—rising in titre • Cell culture • Animal inoculation-mice

SHORT ANSWERS

1. Give 4 examples of organisms which are a part of normal flora and can also cause infections in the host. (4 marks)

Location	*Normal flora*	*Infections caused*
Skin	• *Staphylococcus epidermidis*	• Infections of prosthetic heart valves and prosthetic joints
Skin and nose	• *Staphylococcus aureus*	• Abscesses
Oropharynx	• *Streptococcus sanguinis* • *Streptococcus mutans*	• Subacute endocarditis
Urethra	• *Escherichia coli*	• Urinary tract infection

2. Discuss the contributions of Louis Pasteur to medical microbiology (4 marks)

Louis Pasteur

1. Father of microbiology
2. Disproved theory of spontaneous generation (or Abiogenesis).
3. Put forward theory of microbial fermentation.
4. Introduced liquid media to grow microorganisms.
5. Introduced techniques of sterilisation—Devised Steam steriliser, hot air oven, autoclave. Introduced the process of 'Pasteurisation' for milk.
6. Extensive studies on anthrax, chicken cholera, rabies virus.
7. Discovered the process of attenuation → Development of live attenuated vaccines.
8. Coined the term *'Vaccine'* in honour of Edward Jenner—against smallpox.
9. Vaccines for rabies, anthrax bacilli, chicken cholera.
10. Founder of Pasteur Institute, Paris. In India—at Coonoor, Tamil Nadu.

3. Tuberculosis disease is caused by *M. tuberculosis* and was a discovery by Robert Koch. Enumerate his postulates in the theory of disease and the exceptions. (4 marks)

Koch's Postulates

1. The bacterium should be constantly associated with lesions of the disease.
2. It should be possible to isolate the bacterium in pure culture from the lesions.
3. Inoculation of this pure culture into lab animals should reproduce the lesions of the disease.
4. It should be possible to re-isolate the bacterium in pure culture from the lesions in the lab animal.
5. *Additional criterion was added later:* Specific antibodies should be demonstrable in the serum of the patient suffering from the disease.

Molecular Koch's Postulates

- To establish that a **gene** found in a pathogenic microorganism is a virulence gene.
  1. The virulence property/phenotype under study should be associated with the pathogenic strains and not with non-pathogenic strains.
  2. Inactivation of the gene associated with the suspected virulence trait should lead to loss of pathogenicity or virulence.
  3. Replacement of mutated gene with wild type gene should restore virulence.
  4. Antibodies/immune system cells directed against the gene products should protect the host.

Exceptions to Koch's Postulates

1. Some microorganisms like Chlamydia, viruses, *Treponema pallidum*, *Mycobacterium leprae*—do not grow in artificial media.
2. *Neisseria gonorrhoeae:* No animal model.
3. *Asymptomatic carriers:* Typhoid.

4. Define true-positive, true-negative, false-positive, false-negative, sensitivity and specificity in the interpretation of test results. (4 marks)

True-positive	• An outcome where the test *correctly* predicts the *positive* result
True-negative	• An outcome where the test *correctly* predicts the *negative* result
False-positive	• An outcome where the test incorrectly predicts the *positive* result
False-negative	• An outcome where the test incorrectly predicts the *positive* result
Sensitivity	• Ability of the test to detect even very minute amounts of Ag or Ab's • Highly sensitive test false-negative results will be absent or minimal
Specificity	• Ability of the test to detect reactions between homologous antigens and antibodies only • In highly specific test, false-positive reactions are minimal or absent

5. "Not all infections are communicable". Define communicable diseases with 2 classical examples. (2+2 marks)

Definition

- Communicable diseases are illnesses caused by viruses or bacteria that people spread to one another through contact with contaminated surfaces, bodily fluids, blood products, insect bites, or through the air.

Examples

1. HIV
2. Hepatitis A, B and C
3. Measles
4. Cholera

6. Auramine O dye-stained smear for the detection of *Mycobacterium tuberculosis* is observed under which type of microscope. Discuss the principle and applications of this microscope. (2+2 marks)

Microscope Used

- Fluorescence microscope.

Principle

- Uses fluorescence property to generate an image.
- Fluorescent dye, when exposed to UV light absorb UV light and convert it to visible light.
- Source of light mercury lamp.
- Emitted rays pass through an excitation filter (allows only short wavelength UV light of about 400 nm to pass through).
- Exciting rays get reflected by a dichromatic mirror-fall on the specimen stained by fluorescent dye.
- Barrier filter—removes remaining ultraviolet light (damage the viewer's eyes), or blue and violet light (reduce contrast).

Applications

1. Auramine O stain for *Mycobacterium tuberculosis.*
2. Acridine orange (Quantitative Buffy coat) for *Plasmodium* and filarial nematodes.
3. Direct IF on clinical specimen especially for viruses.
4. *Indirect IF:* Antinuclear antibody, anti-neutrophilic cytoplasmic antibody in patients' serum.

7. The maximum growth rate of bacteria is seen in which phase of the bacterial growth. Explain the different phases in bacterial growth. (1+3 marks)

Maximum growth rate of bacteria is seen in:
- Log phase of the bacterial growth.

Phases in Bacterial Growth (Fig. 1.1.18)

Lag phase	• Period between inoculation and beginning of multiplication of bacteria • Bacteria increase in size due to accumulation of enzymes and metabolites • Bacteria reach their maximum size at the end of lag phase
Log phase	• Bacteria divide exponentially so that the growth curve takes a shape of straight line • Smaller in size • Biochemically active • Uniformly stained—It is the best time to perform the Gram's stain

Contd.

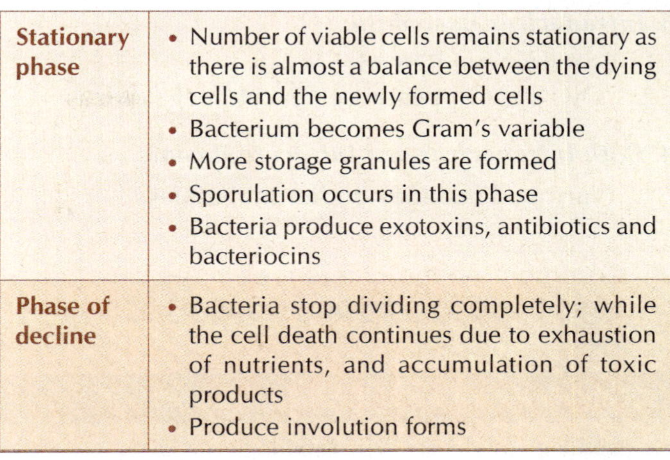

Stationary phase	• Number of viable cells remains stationary as there is almost a balance between the dying cells and the newly formed cells • Bacterium becomes Gram's variable • More storage granules are formed • Sporulation occurs in this phase • Bacteria produce exotoxins, antibiotics and bacteriocins
Phase of decline	• Bacteria stop dividing completely; while the cell death continues due to exhaustion of nutrients, and accumulation of toxic products • Produce involution forms

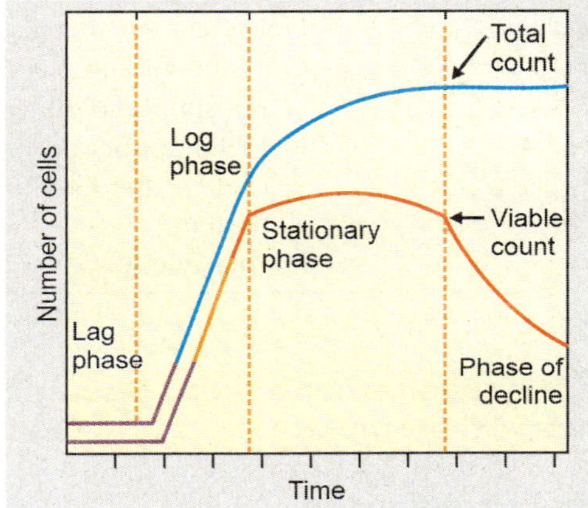

Fig. 1.1.18: Phases in bacterial growth

8. Comment on viral inclusion bodies with examples. (1+3 marks)

Viral Inclusion Bodies

- Inclusion bodies **are nuclear or cytoplasmic** aggregates of stainable substances, usually proteins.
- They typically represent sites of viral multiplication in a eukaryotic cell and usually consist of viral capsid proteins.

Examples

1. Intracytoplasmic Eosinophilic (Acidophilic)

1. Negri bodies in rabies
2. Guarnieri bodies in vaccinia, variola
3. Paschen bodies in variola or smallpox
4. Bollinger bodies in fowl pox
5. Henderson–Patterson bodies in molluscum contagiosum.

2. Intranuclear Eosinophilic (Acidophilic)

1. Cowdry type A in herpes simplex virus and varicella zoster virus.
2. Cowdry type B in polio and adenovirus.

3. Intranuclear Basophilic

1. Cowdry type B in adenovirus.
2. "Owl's eye appearance" in cytomegalovirus.

4. Both Intranuclear and Intracytoplasmic

1. Warthin–Finkeldey bodies in measles.

9. Comment on the differences in the structure of gram-positive and gram-negative bacterial cell wall (2 marks)

Gram-positive cell wall	*Gram-negative cell wall*
• Peptidoglycan layer (thick, 40 sheets)	• Peptidoglycan layer (thinner: 1–2 sheets)
• Teichoic acid	• Lipoprotein • Outer membrane ✦ Phospholipid bilayer ✦ LPS (lipopolysaccharide) ✦ OMP (outer membrane protein) • Periplasmic space

10. What is Lysogenic conversion? Discuss its significance with examples. (3+1 marks)

Lysogenic Conversion (Fig. 1.1.19)

- New properties acquired by bacterium as a result of integrated prophage genes.
- Mediated by transduction of bacterial genes from donor bacterium to the recipient bacterium via bacteriophage.
- Integration of viral DNA into bacterial cell DNA—Prophage.

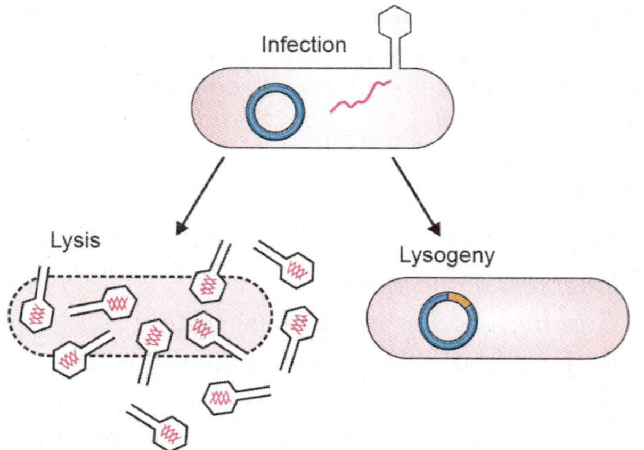

Fig. 1.1.19: Lysogenic conversion

Significance

- Exotoxins of diphtheria, botulinum, cholera and erythrogenic toxins are encoded by prophage.

11. What are L forms in bacteria and note its significance? (2+2 marks)

L-forms

- L forms are the cell wall deficient bacteria, discovered by E. Klieneberger, while studying *Streptobacillus moniliformis*.
- Named it as L form after its place of discovery i.e., Lister Institute, London (1935).
- Damage/removal of cell wall can occur by.
  - Enzymes: Lysozyme, antibiotics acting on cell wall, e.g. penicillin complement system, antibodies.
  - Cell wall damage → cell protoplasm takes up water → swells up → ruptures → cell lysis.
  - In an osmotically protective medium (isotonic solution), cell wall deficient bacteria will survive—These are called L-forms.
- Origin of L-forms.
  - *Spontaneous:* Arise spontaneously without induction, e.g. *Streptobacillus moniliformis*
  - *Induced:* Arise due to induction by certain chemicals, e.g. lysozyme (enzyme), penicillin (antibiotic)
- Classification of L-forms.
  1. *Stable L-forms*
     - Do not revert to parental forms even if cell wall inhibiting agent is removed
     - Multiply, divide and can be maintained for several generations as L- forms
     - Resemble *Mycoplasmas* (a cell wall deficient bacterium) in many properties.
  2. *Unstable L-forms*
     - Revert to parental forms once the cell wall inhibiting agent is removed.
     - Are of two types:
       i. *Protoplasts:* Originate from and revert to Gram +ve bacteria. Protoplasts have only protoplasm and cytoplasmic membrane, whole of cell wall is lost.
       ii. *Spheroplasts:* Originate from and revert to gram –ve bacteria. Spheroplasts retain outer membrane and some amount of peptidoglycan, unlike the protoplasts.

Properties of L-forms

- No regular shape- no cell wall.
- Cannot be demonstrated by ordinary staining methods.
- Resistant to antibiotics which act on cell wall.
- Can be maintained only in osmotically protective media (containing sucrose, NaCl, Mg++).
- On solid media, they grow just below the surface of the agar.
- In liquid media, they do not produce turbidity—they produce clumps.

Significance of L-forms

- Responsible for chronic infections as they are resistant to antibiotics.
- *May result in relapse of infections:* Once the antibiotics are withdrawn, they revert to parental bacterial forms—especially important in endocarditis, UTI

12. Antibiotics like penicillin and cephalosporin act on this structure of the bacterial cell. Discuss the functions and clinical and practical significance of this structure. (1+1+1+1 marks)

Antibiotics like Penicillin and Cephalosporins act on

- Bacterial cell wall.

Functions of Cell Wall

1. Gives characteristic shape, rigidity to bacterial cell.
2. Protects cell from osmotic damage.
3. Helps in cell division—formation of cross wall.
4. *Determines antigenic specificity of bacterium:* Teichoic acid in gram-positive; 'O' antigen in gram-negative bacteria.
5. Site of action for bacteriophages, antibiotics, bacteriocins.
6. *Role in virulence:* Cell wall may contain certain virulence factors (endotoxin).

Clinical Significance of Cell Wall

- Differentiating between gram-positive and gram-negative organisms is important because choice of empirical antibiotic therapy is based on it. Drugs used are different for gram-positive and gram-negative bacteria.
- Endotoxins of gram-negative bacteria are responsible for causing endotoxic shock.
- Teichoic acid of gram-positive bacteria can induce septic shock.

Practical Importance of Cell Wall

- *Due to difference in cell wall composition:* Gram's staining technique can be used to differentiate gram-positive and gram-negative bacteria—useful in identification in laboratory
- 'O" antigen of gram-negative bacteria—useful for identification and classification of bacteria, esp. *Salmonellae*
- 'O" antigen of *Salmonella* used in Widal test for diagnosis of enteric fever.

MI 1.2 PERFORM AND IDENTIFY THE DIFFERENT CAUSATIVE AGENTS OF INFECTIOUS DISEASES BY GRAM'S STAIN, ZIEHL–NEELSEN STAIN AND STOOL ROUTINE MICROSCOPY

MI 8.9 DISCUSS THE APPROPRIATE METHOD OF COLLECTION OF SAMPLES IN THE PERFORMANCE OF LABORATORY TESTS IN THE DETECTION OF MICROBIAL AGENTS CAUSING INFECTIOUS DISEASE

MI 8.10 DEMONSTRATE THE APPROPRIATE METHOD OF COLLECTION OF SAMPLES IN THE PERFORMANCE OF LABORATORY TESTS IN THE DETECTION OF MICROBIAL AGENTS CAUSING INFECTIOUS DISEASE

SHORT ESSAYS

1. An 18-year-old presents with discharge from the laparotomy site for appendicectomy. Pus is sent for culture and sensitivity. Performed Gram stain on the smear provided and reported. (Figs 1.2.1 and 1.2.2)

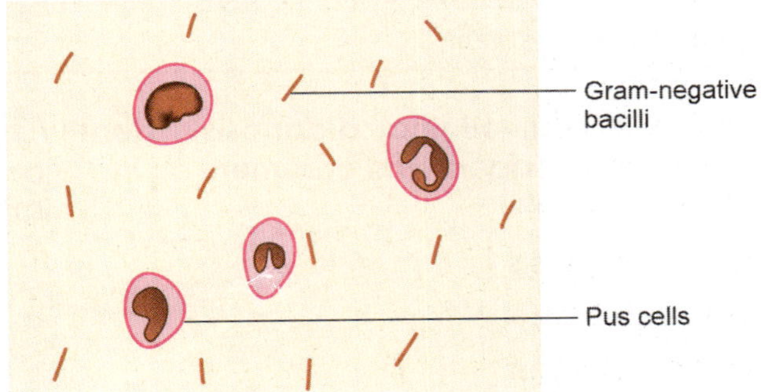

Fig. 1.2.1

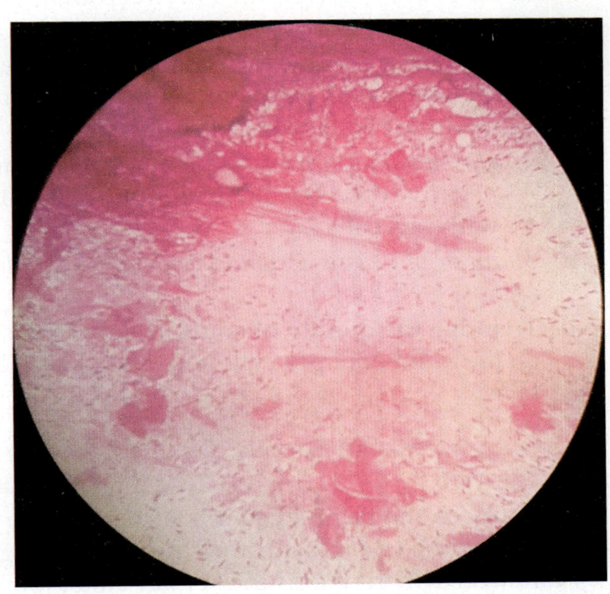

Fig. 1.2.2

Answer the questions below

A. Report on the Gram's stain and draw a neat, labelled diagram. (1 mark)

- The given smear shows the presence of polymorphonuclear leucocytes with gram-negative bacilli.

B. What is the probable diagnosis? (1 mark)

- Surgical site infection.

C. List out the probable etiological agents in this case based on the Gram's stain report. (1 mark)

1. *Escherichia coli*
2. *Klebsiella* spp.
3. *Citrobacter* spp.
4. *Pseudomonas* spp.

D. What are the further investigations required to confirm the identification of the aetiological agent? (1 mark)

- Culture and antibiotic sensitivity testing.

E. What are the clinical applications of Gram's stain? (1 mark)

1. Identification of bacteria on Gram's stain and morphology
2. To start empiric antibiotic in invasive infections: sepsis, meningitis
3. Gram's stain report helps to decide on the culture media to grow and biochemical tests required to confirm the identity of the bacteria
   a. *Clue*
      i. Gram's stain in gonorrhoea is diagnostic in symptomatic male
      ii. Bacterial vaginosis Gram's smear of vaginal swab: clue cells, few pus cells, few or absent lactobacilli, numerous gram-negative coccobacilli (*Gardnerella* spp.)
      iii. Anaerobic infection: Polymicrobial, pale organisms
      iv. Gas gangrene due to *Clostridium perfringens*: Disintegrated pus cells with thick Gram-positive bacilli without spores
      v. *Haemophilus influenzae* (pleomorphic Gram-negative coccobacilli) in sputum, CSF along with pus cells
   b. *Staining of yeasts: Cryptococcus* spp., *Candida* spp.
   c. To judge the quality of sputum sample based on the number of pus cells and epithelial cells/HPF

F. Give reasons for the Gram's staining property of the bacteria. (1 mark)

- Affinity to the basic dye (crystal violet) due to more acidic cytoplasm and thick peptidoglycan layer which retains the crystal violet iodine complex.

2. A 45-year lady presented with breast abscess to surgery OPD. The surgeon drained the abscess in minor OT and sent to microbiology laboratory for culture and sensitivity. The Gram's stain picture shows as follows (Fig. 1.2.3)

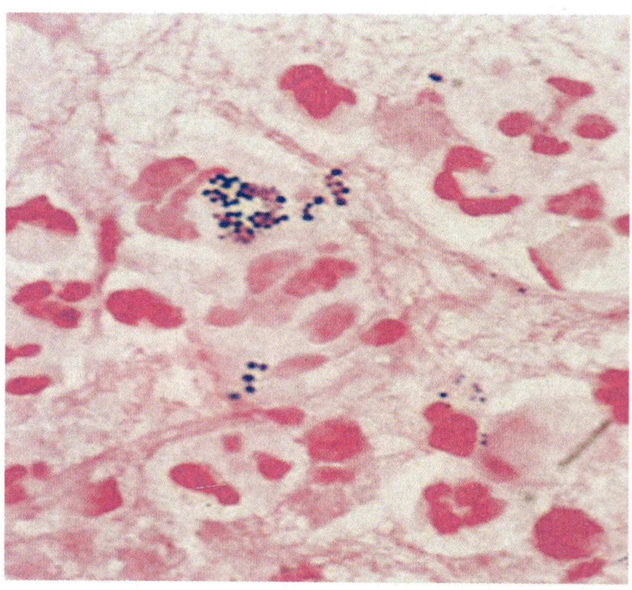

Fig. 1.2.3: Gram-positive cocci in clusters with pus cells

Sensitivity Report of the Organism Isolated

Antibiotic	*S/R*
Amoxiclav	R
Methicillin	R
Cloxacillin	R
Cefazolin	R
Clindamycin	S
Chloramphenicol	S
Erythromycin	R
Vancomycin	S
Teicoplanin	S
Linezolid	S
S: Sensitive, R: Resistant	

A. What is your clinical diagnosis? Identify the aetiological agent and comment on the Gram's stain picture? (3 marks)

Clinical Diagnosis

- Breast abscess.

Aetiological Agent

- *Staphylococcus aureus.*

Comment on the Gram's Stain Picture

- Gram-positive cocci arranged in clusters morphologically resembling *S. aureus.*

B. List the sample collection methods for skin and soft tissue infection (1 mark)

1. Pus aspirate.
2. Swab from deep wound.
3. Incision and drainage (I and D).

C. What are the recommended drugs in the above case? (1 mark)

- *Antibiotics recommended:* Linezolid, clindamycin, doxycycline, daptomycin, cotrimoxazole, Vancomycin.

3. In a village, a 25-year-old visited the primary healthcare centre (PHC) with c/o rice watery diarrhea. On eliciting history of food eaten in the past 2 days, he gives a history of having panipoori from a street shop. Stool sample was collected and investigated. Stool sample revealed the following picture. (Fig. 1.2.4)

A. Comment on the given stain. What are the preliminary investigations useful for diagnosis of this case? (2+2 marks)

The given smear of dilute carbol fuchsin shows comma-shaped bacilli morphologically resembling *V. cholera.*

- *Hanging drop:* Bacilli with darting Motility
- *Dilute Carbol Fuchsin:* Pink-comma-shaped bacilli
- To be confirmed by culture.

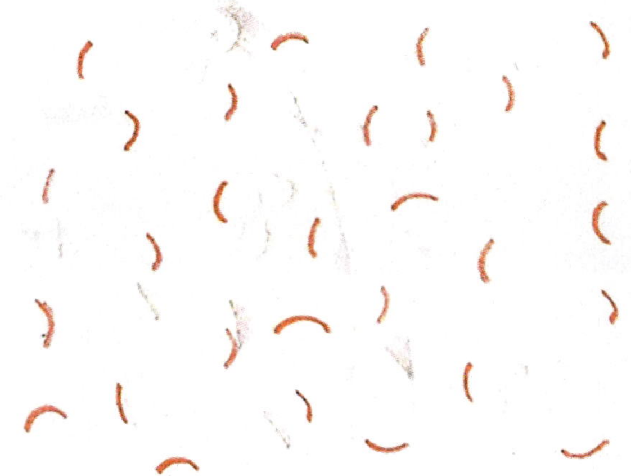

Fig. 1.2.4

B. Mention the transport media? (2 marks)

1. Alkaline Peptone water.
2. Venkatraman Ramakrishnan media.
3. Cary–Blair medium.
4. Autoclaved sea water.
5. Monsur's taurocholate tellurite peptone water (pH 9.2).

C. What are the culture media required to support your diagnosis? (2 marks)

1. Thiosulphate citrate bile salt sucrose agar (TCBS).
2. Alkaline bile salt agar (BSA, pH 8.2).
3. Monsur's gelatin taurocholate trypticase tellurite agar (GTTA).

MI 1.3 DESCRIBE THE EPIDEMIOLOGICAL BASIS OF COMMON INFECTIOUS DISEASES

SHORT ESSAYS

1. Xpert® MTB/RIF Ultra is an automated molecular assay for detection of *M. tuberculosis*. The test is highly specific and sensitive when compared to smear microscopy. Positive predictive value is 92% and negative predictive value is 99%

A. Define sensitivity and specificity in the above scenario (2 marks)

B. Define the terms PPV and NPV (2 marks)

C. What type of study is useful for evaluating a new test? (1 mark)

A. Definitions of Sensitivity and Specificity in the Above Scenario

Sensitivity

- The proportion of true-positives correctly identified by the test Xpert MTB/RIF.

Specificity

- The proportion of true negatives identified by the test method.

B. Definitions of the terms PPV and NPV

Positive Predictive Value (PPV)

- The proportion of individuals with a positive test result detected by Xpert who actually have the tuberculosis which is 92% in this case.

Negative Predictive Value (NPV)

- The proportion of individuals with a negative test result detected by Xpert who is free of tuberculosis which is 99% in this case.

C. Type of Study is Useful for Evaluating a New Test

- Cross-sectional study design is useful in evaluating a new test.

2. Classify different types of transmission with examples (5 marks)

Different Types/Modes of Transmission

Type/mode of transmission	Examples	
	Pathogen	*Disease*
Contact	• MRSA	• Wound infections
Droplet	• *C diphtheria*, • Influenza virus, SARS-CoV2, *N. meningitidis*	• Diphtheria • Influenza • Meningitis
Aerosol	• *M. tuberculosis*	• Tuberculosis
Ingestion	• *Salmonella* • *V. cholerae*	• Typhoid • Cholera
Sexual	• *N. gonorrheae*, *T. pallidum*, Herpes simplex virus 2	• Gonorrhoea, syphilis
Vertical	• *Treponema pallidum*, HSV 2, HIV, hepatitis B virus	• Syphilis, hepatitis B
Vector borne	• *Rickettsia*, *Borrelia*, Malaria	• Scrub typhus, Endemic typhus
Birth canal	• *Listeria*, group B *Streptococcus*, HSV 2	• Neonatal meningitis
Trans-placental	• TORCH (*Toxoplasma gondii*, Rubella, cytomegalovirus, HSV)	• Toxoplasmosis
Blood	• HIV, hepatitis B virus	• AIDS, hepatitis
Animal bite	• Rabies virus	• Rabies

3. A cook is positive for *S. typhi* in stool culture. He is asymptomatic. Is he a carrier or having the disease? With respect to the history briefly explain carriers and the types of carriers with examples. (5 marks)

Cook is

- A carrier of *S typhi*.

Carriers

Definition

- Are people who harbour infectious agents but are not ill.
- Carriers may present more risk for disease transmission than acute clinical cases.

Types

- Depending on the disease:
  1. Incubatory carriers
  2. In apparent infections (also called subclinical cases)
  3. Convalescent carriers
  4. Chronic carriers

Type of carrier	*Feature*	*Example*
Incubatory carriers	• Are going to become ill, but begin transmitting their infection before their symptoms start	Measles
In apparent infections	• People within apparent infections never develop an illness, but can transmit their infection to others	COVID-19
Convalescent carriers	• People who continue to be infectious during and even after their recovery from illness	*Salmonella*
Chronic carriers	• People who continue to harbour infections for a year or longer after their recovery	Hepatitis B

SHORT ANSWERS

1. Give examples for viruses causing diarrhoea and their clinical features. (3 marks)

Virus causing diarrhoea	*Clinical Features*
Rotavirus	• Fever, diarrhoea, vomiting and dehydration • There is no inflammation or loss of blood
Calicivirus	• Chills, headache, myalgia, or fever as well as nausea, abdominal pain, vomiting and diarrhoea
Astro virus **Adenovirus**	• Acute diarrhoea

2. Explain the terms infectious period, latent period and incubation period in relation to measles infection. (3 marks)

Infectious Period

- The time when a person is exposed to organism and can transmit or shedding of microorganisms to others.
- Usually for 8–13 days.

Latent Period

- The time frame when a person is exposed to a pathogen up till an infection reappears either in the same form as the primary infection or manifests with different signs and symptoms or able to transmit infection.
- Usually for 6–9 days.

Incubation Period

- The time between the person is exposed to the microbe (or toxin) and the development of symptoms.
- Usually for 6–7 days.

3. What is herd immunity in relation to polio virus? How can it be achieved? (3 marks)

Herd Immunity in Relation to Polio Virus

- Herd immunity occurs with the live polio vaccine primarily because it induces secretory IgA in the gut, which inhibits infection by virulent virus, and prevents its transmission to others.
- An individual is protected from infection by the virtue of the community being not able to transmit the virus to the individual.
- The vaccine containing the live virus replicates in the immunised person and spreads to other members of the population, thereby a greater number of people are protected.

Achieving Herd Immunity

- The important feature as far as herd immunity is concerned is the induction of IgA, which prevents transmission.
- Herd immunity can be achieved either by natural infection or vaccine.
- Here the organism is not capable of being transmitted to others who are not vaccinated.

4. Define epidemic, endemic, sporadic and pandemic diseases with examples for each. (4 marks)

Term	Definition	Example
Epidemic	• Unusual excess of expected occurrence of a disease	• Cholera
Endemic	• The constant presence of a disease or infectious agent within a given geographic area or population group without importation from outside • When conditions are favorable may burst into an epidemic	• Hepatitis A
Pandemic	• An epidemic usually affecting a large proportion of the population which can spread between two continents	• Influenza pandemics
Sporadic	• Infections occurring at irregular intervals or only in few places, scattered or isolated	• Enteric fever

5. A 7-day-old neonate develops vesicular lesions over skin. H/o vaginal herpes in the mother was elicited 15 days ago. What is the most probable mode of transmission of infection in the child? Give examples of other infections transmitted through this route. (1 + 1 marks)

Most Probable Mode of Transmission of Infection in the Child

- Maternal genital tract.

Examples of Other Infections Transmitted through this Route

1. Syphilis.
2. Varicella zoster

MI 1.4 CLASSIFY AND DESCRIBE THE METHODS OF STERILISATION AND DISINFECTION. DISCUSS THE APPLICATION OF DIFFERENT METHODS IN LABORATORY, CLINICAL AND SURGICAL PRACTICE

LONG ESSAY

1. A tertiary care hospital is used to organize its regular board meetings related to infection control on 4th Saturday of every month. Due to an increase in number of post-surgical complications and outbreak of MRSA, the chairperson of infection control committee suggested the lead microbiologist for the proper sterilisation, chemical disinfection methods to be implemented. A training programme is organised by the infection control team for the same. Assuming that one group of the training team are 2nd year UGs, answer the following questions related to sterilisation and disinfection?

A. Definitions of Sterilisation and disinfection. (1 mark)

Sterilisation

- The killing or removal of *all* microorganisms from an item, surface or medium including bacterial spores.

Disinfection

- It is a process that reduces of pathogenic organisms to a level at which they no longer constitute a risk, may or may not destroy spores.

B. Classify the methods of sterilisation, disinfection with proper examples for each. (3 marks)

Sterilisation

Method of sterilisation	Methods	Examples
Physical method	• Moist heat sterilisation	• Autoclave–Surgical instruments
	• Dry heat sterilisation	• Hot air oven–Glassware
	• Radiation	• Ionisation and non- ionising—Medical devices
Chemical method	• ETO steriliser	• Sutures, catheters, stents
	• Plasma steriliser	• Laparoscopes, arthroscopes

Disinfection

Method of disinfection	Methods	Examples
High level disinfection	• Aldehydes–Glutaraldehyde • Peracetic acid • Hydrogen peroxide	• Endoscopes • Endoscopes • Dental instruments • Wound cleaning
Intermediate level disinfection	• Alcohols—Ethyl alcohol • Phenolics—Phenol, cresol • Halogens—Iodine and chlorine	• Skin antisepsis • Skin antisepsis • Topical ointment • Skin antisepsis • Blood spill
Low level disinfection	• Quaternary ammonium compounds • Chlorhexidine	• BP cuff • Hand rub

C. Describe the principle, uses and sterilisation controls used in hospital for sterilisation of different materials used for surgery, and labware. (2+2 marks)

Principle

Autoclave

- Water boils at 100°C but when pressure inside the autoclave increases, the temperature at which water boils also increases, and steam is generated.
- The temperature used in autoclave is 121°C for 15 min at pressure of 15 psi.

Hot Air Oven

- This is dry heat method which requires temperatures in the range of 180°C for 2 hours.

Uses

Of Autoclave

1. Surgical instruments, gowns, drapes.
2. Culture media and materials which cannot withstand the higher temperature of hot air oven or media containing water which cannot be sterilised by dry heat.

Of Hot Air Oven

1. This process is used primarily for glassware like glass syringes, Petri dishes, flasks, pipettes, and test tubes.
2. Surgical instruments like scalpels, scissors, forceps, etc.
3. Chemicals such as liquid paraffin, fats, glycerol, and glove dust powder.

Sterilisation Controls

1. **Physical indicators**
   - Sterilisers have displays such as temperature, time, pressure, etc.
2. **Chemical indicators**
   - Heat or chemical sensitive materials are used to check the efficacy of sterilisation process, e.g. Bowie Dick tape, autoclave tape.
3. **Biological indicators**
   - The most reliable indicator as it uses spores of bacteria to check the efficacy of the process of sterilisation.
   - The spores are readily destroyed when the process has been effectively completed.
   - The spore vials are incubated, and result is obtained within 24 minutes to 48 hours, e.g.
     1. *Geobacillus stearothermophilus:* For steam steriliser, plasma steriliser
     2. *Bacillus atrophaeus:* Hot air oven

D. Expand CSSD. Mention various compartments of CSSD and functions of CSSD. (2 marks)

CSSD is Expanded as

- Central Sterile Supply Department.

Compartments of CSSD

1. Cleaning area.
2. Packing area.
3. Sterilisation area.
4. Sterile Storage area.

Functions of CSSD

1. Receiving and sorting soiled materials.
2. Determines whether the item should be reused or discarded.
3. The process of decontamination or disinfection is carried out prior to sterilisation.

4. Inspecting and testing instruments, equipments, and linen
5. Assembling and packing all materials for sterilisation
6. Sterilising
7. Labelling and dating materials
8. Storing
9. Issuing and distributing items to various areas in the hospital.

SHORT ESSAYS

1. Describe the chemical methods of Sterilisation under the following headings

A. Uses of commonly used alcohols, aldehydes, Chlorine as disinfectants. (2 marks)

Disinfectants	*Uses/Applications*
Alcohols—Ethyl alcohol	• Hand rub • Thermometers • Stethoscopes
Aldehydes—Formaldehyde	• Fumigation of OT • Preservation of specimens
Chlorine—Sodium hypochlorite	• Spill management

B. Spaulding's classification of medical devices and various levels of disinfectants. (2 marks)

Category	*Description*	*Level of disinfection*	*Examples*
Non-critical	• Items in contact with intact skin	• Low or Inter-mediate	• BP cuff • Crutches • Non-critical patient items/ surfaces
Semi-critical	• Items in contact with mucous membrane or body fluids	• High	• Respiratory equipment • Scopes
Critical	• Items entering sterile site of the body	• Sterilisation	• Surgical instruments • Implants • Needles

C. Plasma Sterilisation. (1 mark)

- It is a process used to create the plasma state for sterilisation.
- Gas plasma is generated when electrical field is applied which breaks H_2O_2 into free radicals that have the microbicidal action.
- *Duration of cycle:* 24–75 minutes
- *Sterilisation control:* Spores of *Geobacillus Stearothermophiluss*
- *Applications:* In CSSD for sterilisation of heat sensitive materials and devices. e.g. laparoscope, arthroscopes
- *Disadvantages*
  1. High cost of equipment
  2. Bulk items cannot be used (small chamber)
  3. Linen, paper, liquid cannot be processed.

2. The gastroenterology endoscopy room in a tertiary hospital performs 7 procedures approximately on daily basis. Briefly explain the sterilisation process for endoscopes that must be carried out in-between each patient. (5 marks)

Sterilisation Process for Endoscopes

- The endoscopes involve precleaning, manual cleaning, disinfection, and sterilisation.
  1. **Precleaning**
     - It is to remove all the debris by flushing with air and water channels along with detergent solution in-between patients.
     - Debris could include protein, fats, carbohydrates that can inactivate the detergent/ disinfectants action against the microorganisms.
  2. **Manual cleaning**
     - Fill a basin with freshly prepared medical grade detergent solution and brush with help of soft brush and cleaning tools to free the scopes from remnant debris.
  3. **Disinfection and sterilisation**
     - 2–2.4% concentration of glutaraldehyde for 20 minutes for disinfection but 10–12 hours' time to kill spores.
     - The manufacturer's recommendation must be followed for all the steps involved in cleaning and disinfection of endoscopes.

3. A pregnant lady receives blood transfusion after a post-partum haemorrhage due to very low Hb%. Meanwhile the lady is restless and disconnects the IV set and hence there is a blood spill. What are the steps necessary to be taken in management of the above blood spill? Which is the disinfectant used for this purpose. Advantages and disadvantages of the disinfectant. (2+1+1+1 marks)

Steps in Blood Spill Management

1. Wear gloves and other PPE appropriate to the task.

2. When sharps are involved use forceps to pick up sharps, and discard these items in a puncture-resistant container.
3. Cover the spill with a newspaper, blotting paper/ tissue paper.
4. Wipe the spill with a tissue paper moistened with freshly prepared hypochlorite solution (1% dilution containing minimum 500 ppm chlorine) for 20–30 minutes. Discard the paper as infected waste. Repeat until all visible soiling is removed.
5. Wipe the area with a cloth mop moistened with 1% hypochlorite solution and allow drying naturally.
6. All contaminated items used in the clean-up should be placed in a bio-hazardous bag for disposal.

Disinfectant for Blood Spill

- 1% Sodium hypochlorite.

Advantages of 1% Sodium Hypochlorite

1. Broad spectrum
2. Fast acting, non-inflammable, low cost
3. Widely available

Disadvantages of 1% Sodium Hypochlorite

1. Inactivated by organic matter
2. Unstable and toxic
3. Corrosive, carcinogenic
4. Leaves residues, offensive odour

4. Draw a neat, labelled diagram of an autoclave and enumerate its uses in a CSSD. (3+2 marks)

Diagram of an Autoclave (Fig. 1.4.1)

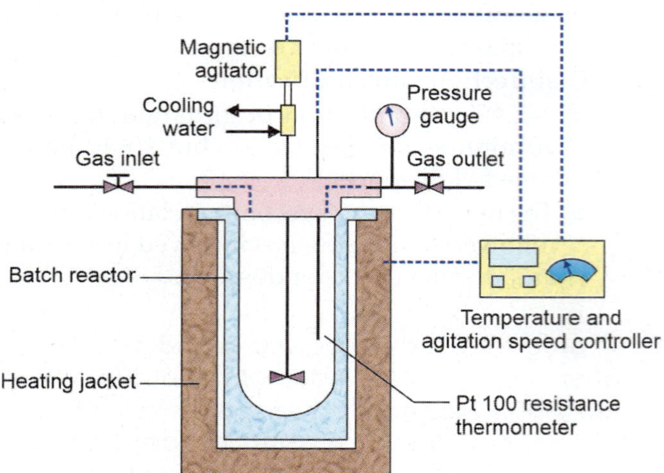

Fig. 1.4.1: *Autoclave*

Use of Autoclave in CSSD

1. Surgical instruments
2. Linen, surgical drapes and linen
3. Anaesthetic equipment
4. Dental equipment
5. Implant medical devices
6. Prosthetic devices

5. ETO steriliser. Mention its applications, advantages, disadvantages, and sterilisation control in a CSSD. (2+1+1+1 marks)

ETO Steriliser

Applications

1. Heart Lung machines
2. Sutures, catheters, and stents
3. Respirators
4. Dental equipment
5. Multi lumen tubing

Advantages

1. Large chamber
2. Suitable for heat sensitive devices
3. Non-corrosive and high penetration

Disadvantages

1. Highly inflammable, irritant, carcinogenic.
2. Long duration of cycle (12–14 hours).
3. High cost of consumables.

Sterilisation Controls

1. *Biological indicator:* Spores of *Bacillus atrophaeus.*
2. *Chemical indicator:* Bowie dick test.
3. *Physical indicator:* Temperature, time and pressure.

SHORT ANSWERS

1. Classify the moist heat methods of sterilisation at and below 100°C and their uses. (3 marks)

Heat methods of sterilisation at and below 100°C	*Uses*
Boiling at 100°C	• Surgical instruments
Steam at 100°C	• Useful for items where heating is unsuitable
Inspissation at 80–85°C for 30 minutes on 3 successive days	• Egg-based media (LJ media)
Pasteurisation (70°C for 30 minutes)	• Milk, respiratory and anaesthesia equipment

2. Applications of alcohol-based products used in a hospital set-up, its mechanisms of action (3 marks)

Alcohol-based Hand Rub

Applications

1. Non-critical item—thermometers (10–15 minutes).
2. Surface disinfection of vaccine bottles, blood culture bottles, hubs of central line.

3. Surface disinfection of stethoscope, ventilators, ultrasound machine.
4. Skin antisepsis.

Mechanisms of Action

- Act on bacteria, fungi, some enveloped virus but do not kill spores.
- Act by denaturing proteins and probably by dissolving membrane lipids.

3. A patient on ventilator support with multi-drug resistant bug gets discharged from the ICU and shifted to the ward. With respect to the case, what is meant by terminal disinfection and its applications? (2+1 marks)

Terminal Disinfection

- Preparing or disinfection of rooms or areas for subsequent patients or residents for them to be treated or cared for without the risk of acquiring an infection.

Applications

1. Subsequent to an outbreak or increased incidence of infection.
2. Following discharge, transfer or death of a patient who has had a known infection.
3. Following isolation/contact precaution nursing of a patient.

4. Add a note on disinfection of operation theatres (OT) (3 marks)

Environmental Cleaning

- Reduces the risk of transmission of infectious agents to healthcare workers and patients.

Surface Disinfection

- Cleaning must be carried out with cleansing agent like detergent followed by using aldehyde-based disinfection.

Procedure

- Disinfection should be carried out as following:

1. First before the cases begin in a day
2. In-between the cases
3. After the last case-terminal disinfection
4. Thorough wash down of the OT complex once a week
5. During any kind of renovation/construction

Note

- Fogging is not routinely recommended and done only in cases of outbreak or newly constructed or after renovation.

5. Enumerate the applications of sterilisation or disinfection process in a microbiology lab. (3 marks)

Applications of Sterilisation/Disinfection in a Microbiology Lab

1. *Sterilisation:* Autoclave-culture media, broth, biomedical waste discard (Vacutainer's culture media plates)
2. *Hot air oven:* Glass ware
3. *Surface disinfection:* 0.5% Sodium hypochlorite
4. *Blood and body fluid Spill:* 1% Sodium hypochlorite
5. *Bio safety cabinet disinfection:* Ethanol

6. Prions are resistant structures to routine methods of sterilisation. Statement is true or false. Justify your answer. (3 marks)

Statement is

- True.

Justification

- Methods used in sterilisation of prions are:
  - Autoclaving at 134°C for 1–1.5 hour.
  - Treatment with 1 N NaOH for 1 hour.
  - 0.5% sodium hypochlorite for 2 hours.

7. Alcohols are sporicidal agents. Statement is True or false. Justify your answer. (3 marks)

Statement is

- False.

Justification

- They act by denaturing proteins and possibly by dissolving membrane lipids but not sporicidal.
- Sporicidal agents are the following:
  - Ethylene oxide, formaldehyde, glutaraldehyde, hydrogen peroxide
  - Peracetic acid, O-phthalic acid, and plasma sterilisation
  - Autoclave and hot air oven.

8. Phenolic compounds can be used as antiseptic and disinfectant agent. Statement is True or False. Justify your answer.

Statement is

- True.

Justification

- Phenols such as cresols have disinfecting properties and retain its activity in the presence of organic matter but cannot be used as an antiseptic as they cause irritation of the skin.
- Phenols such as chlorhexidine, chloroxylenol can be used for skin antisepsis, the active ingredient being Savlon and Dettol, respectively.

9. Active ingredient of lysol is benzalkonium chloride. Statement is True or False. Justify your answer.

Statement is

- True.

Justification

- Quaternary ammonium compounds such as benzalkonium chloride is widely used as floor disinfectant and skin antisepsis.
- These surfactants interact with the lipid in the cell membrane through their hydrophobic chain, water and the polar group—disrupts the membrane.

MI 1.5 CHOOSE THE MOST APPROPRIATE METHOD OF STERILISATION AND DISINFECTION TO BE USED IN SPECIAL SITUATIONS IN THE LABORATORY, CLINICAL AND SURGICAL PRACTICES

LONG ESSAY

1. Describe in detassil about the physical methods of sterilisation under the following headings.

A. Classification of physical methods of sterilisation with appropriate examples. (4 marks)

Method of sterilisation		Examples
Physical	• Dry heat	• Flaming • Incineration • Hot air oven
	• Moist heat	
	• Temperature <100°C	• Pasteurisation • Water bath • Inspissation
	• Temperature at 100°C	• Boiling • Steaming • Tyndallisation
	• Temperature >100°C	• Autoclave
Filtration		• Candle filters • Asbestos filters • Membrane filters
Radiation	• Ionising radiation	• X-rays • Y-rays • Cosmic rays
	• Non-ionising radiation	• UV rays • Infrared rays

B. Uses of Cold Sterilisation (2 marks)

Type of method	Uses
Ionising radiation X-rays, gamma rays (from cobalt 60 source), and cosmic rays	1. Disposable plastics, e.g. rubber or plastic syringes, infusion sets and catheters 2. Catgut sutures, bone and tissue grafts and adhesive dressings, antibiotics, and hormones
Nonionising radiation Infrared and ultraviolet radiations	1. Sterilisation of clean surfaces in operation theatres, laminar flow hoods as well as for water treatment

C. Mention the specific surgical instruments sterilised in autoclave and hot air oven(2 marks)

Hot Air Oven

- Non sharp surgical instruments, forceps, etc.

Autoclave

- Dressings
- Metal surgical instruments
- Linens
- Glassware
- All suture materials except catgut

D. Importance of CSSD Unit in a tertiary care hospital. (2 marks)

- Bacteriological safe sterilisation
- Assurance of adequate supply of sterile products immediately and constantly available for some time and emergency use
- Conservation of trained staff
- Better quality control
- Prolonged life by proper care of equipment

SHORT ESSAYS

1. Describe the chemicals used as disinfectants in hospital practice under the following headings.

A. Disinfectants used for OT, the purpose and method of OT fogging. (2 marks)

Disinfectant used	Purpose	Method
Bacillocid • Formaldehyde-free	• Environmental decontamination	• These agents are dispersed with the aid of a foggier-like device inside the theatre environment • The contact time—1 hour
Virkon • A non-aldehyde compound • It contains oxone (potassium peroxymonosulfate), sodium dodecylbenzenesulfonate, sulphamic acid, and inorganic buffers	• For cleaning up hazardous spills disinfecting surfaces and soaking equipment	

Contd.

Disinfectant used	Purpose	Method
Formaldehyde • Pungent and harmful	• Environmental decontamination • Fumigation is obsolete in many developed nations in view of toxic nature of formalin	• During fumigation, it is tightly closed and sealed before. • The room is opened after fumigation (12–24 hours) • The room can be used once all fumes are out

B. Uses of aldehydes as disinfectants. (1 mark)

Aldehyde	Uses
Formaldehyde	1. Preservation of anatomical specimen 2. Formaldehyde gas is used for fumigation of closed areas such as operation theaters, not used anymore as it is hazardous 3. Preparation of toxoid from toxin. It is toxic, irritant, and corrosive to metals
Glutaraldehyde	1. Less toxic, less irritant, and less corrosive, hence is best used to sterilize endoscopes and cystoscopes
Ortho-phthalaldehyde (0.55%)	1. For sterilisation of endoscopes and cystoscopes 2. It does not require activation 3. Low vapour property 4. Better odour 5. More stable during storage 6. High mycobactericidal activity

C. Grading of disinfectants with examples for each. (2 marks)

Spaulding's Classification

High level disinfection	• Aldehydes—Glutaraldehyde • Peracetic acid • Hydrogen peroxide	• Endoscopes • Endoscopes, dental instruments • Wound cleaning
Intermediate level disinfection	• Alcohols—Ethyl alcohol • Phenolics—Phenol, cresol • Halogens—Iodine, chlorine	• Skin antisepsis • Skin antisepsis • Topical ointment, skin antisepsis, blood spill
Low level disinfection	• Quaternary ammonium compounds • Chlorhexidine	• BP cuff • Hand rub

2. Mention the culture media sterilised by Inspissation. Describe the method of performing inspissation. (2+3 marks)

Inspissation (Fractional sterilisation)

- It is a process of heating an article on 3 successive days at 80–85°C for 30 minutes.

Culture Media Sterilised

1. Egg based (LJ and Dorset's egg medium).
2. Serum-based media (Loeffler's serum slope).

Method of Performing Inspissation

Day	Temperature	Time	Purpose
1	85°C	60 minutes ↓ Overnight incubation	• Drying of the medium and killing the organisms in their vegetative form
			• Growth of vegetative forms from spores
2	75 to 80°C	20 minutes ↓ Overnight incubation	• Killing the organisms in their vegetative form
			• Growth of vegetative forms from any remaining spores
3	75 to 85°C	20 minutes	• Killing the organisms in their vegetative form as well as the leftover spores

SHORT ANSWERS

1. Describe the process and mention the culture media sterilised by Tyndallisation. (1+2 marks)

Tyndallisation/Intermittent Sterilisation

Process

- Involves steaming at 100°C for 20 minutes for 3 consecutive days.

Culture Media Sterilised

1. Gelatin and egg, serum or sugar containing media.
2. It kills most of the vegetative forms including spores.

2. Enumerate the testing methods of efficacy of disinfection (3 marks)

Testing Methods of Efficacy of Disinfection

1. **Phenol coefficient (Rideal–Walker) test**
   - Determined by the dilution of the disinfectant in question which sterilizes the suspension of *Salmonella typhi* in a given time divided by the

dilution of phenol which sterilizes the suspension at the same time.

2. **Chick Martin test**
   - Modified Rideal and Walker test.
   - Here the disinfectants act in the presence of organic matter (e.g. dried yeast, feces, etc.) to simulate the natural conditions.
3. **Capacity (Kelsey–Sykes) test**
   - It tests the capacity of a disinfectant to retain its activity when repeatedly used microbiologically.
4. **In-use (Kelsey and Maurer) test**
   - It determines the efficacy of chosen disinfectant in hospital practice

MI 1.6 DESCRIBE THE MECHANISMS OF DRUG RESISTANCE AND METHODS OF ANTIMICROBIAL SUSCEPTIBILITY TESTING AND MONITORING ANTIMICROBIAL THERAPY

LONG ESSAYS

1. Describe in detail about the antimicrobial drug resistance under the following headings.

A. Classify antibacterial agents and their mechanism of action. (2 marks)

B. Classify drug resistance and list out the probable reasons for acquired drug resistance. (2 marks)

C. Describe in detail the mechanism of drug resistance with suitable example. (4 marks)

D. Enumerate the various antimicrobial susceptibility testing methods (2 marks)

A. Classification of Drug Resistance (Fig. 1.6.1)

1. **Intrinsic drug resistance**
   - Resistance resulting from the normal genetic, structural, or physiological state of microorganism, e.g. vancomycin resistance among the gram-negative bacilli.
2. **Acquired drug resistance**
   - Resistance that results from altered cellular physiology and structure due to change in the usual genetic makeup of a microorganism.

B. Probable Reasons for Acquired Drug Resistance

- **Acquired drug resistance:** Resistance that result from altered cellular physiology and structure due to change in the usual genetic makeup of a microorganism
- **Mutation and selection**
  - Mutation in genes coding for drug susceptibility leads to resistant bacteria.
  - In presence of antibiotics the susceptible bacteria are eliminated whereas the resistant bacteria survive and multiply, e.g. resistance of *Mycobacterium tuberculosis* to isoniazid and rifampicin.

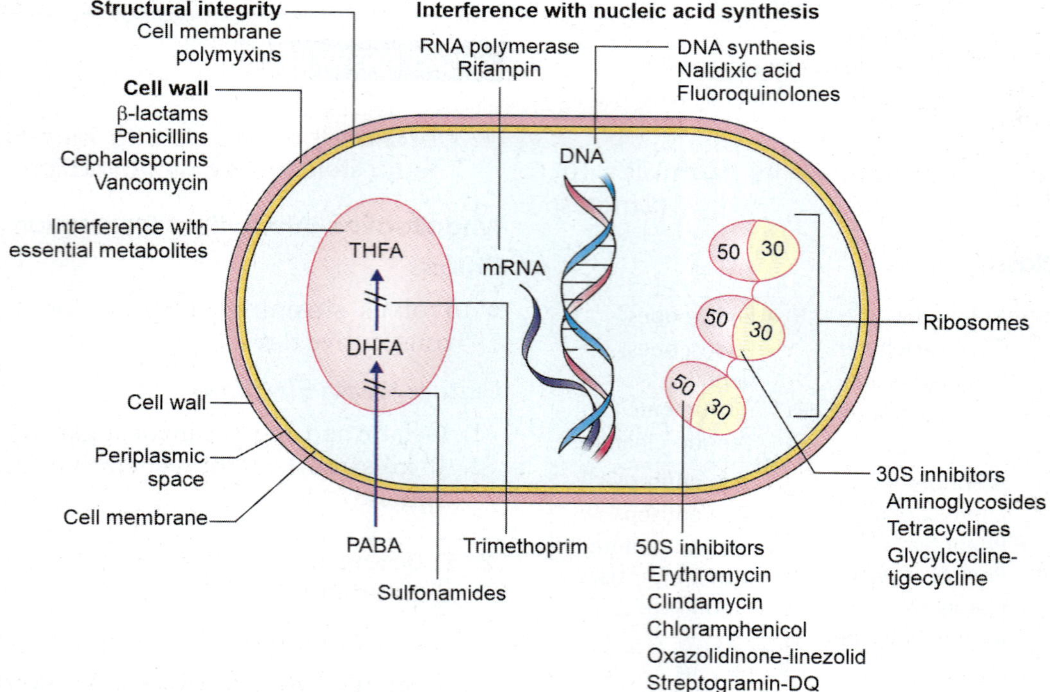

Fig. 1.6.1: Antimicrobial drug resistance

- **Acquiring drug resistant gene/transferable drug resistance**
  - Drug resistant bacteria carry genes for one and often several antimicrobial drugs.
  - The resistant gene can be transferred by transduction, transformation, and conjugation, e.g. *Salmonella typhi* may acquire R plasmid from *Escherichia coli*—conjugation.

C. Mechanisms of Drug Resistance

Mechanism	Examples
Enzymatic inactivation of the drug	• Penicillin resistance in *Staphylococcus aureus* • *N. gonorrhoeae* due to production of penicillinases
Altered target site • Resistant bacteria produce altered target for the drug, to which drug does not bind	• Altered penicillin binding protein (PBP2a) in methicillin resistant *Staphylococcus aureus* (MRSA)
Impaired membrane permeability • When the bacteria do not allow entry or influx of antibiotic inside the bacterial cell, they become resistant	• Aminoglycoside resistance in *Pseudomonas aeruginosa*
Active efflux of antibiotics • Efflux pumps remove toxic metabolites and antibiotics from the bacterial cell	• Norfloxacin resistance in *E. coli*
Alteration of metabolic pathway • An altered pathway is developed by the organism that bypasses the reaction inhibited by the drug	• Sulfonamide resistance
Altered enzyme formation • An altered enzyme is produced by the microorganism that can perform similar metabolic function without getting affected by the drug	• Trimethoprim resistance—altered dihydrofolic acid reductase enzyme is inhibited less efficiently by the drug
• Combination of different mechanism	• Carbapenem resistance in *Klebsiella* spp

D. Various Antimicrobial Susceptibility Testing Methods

1. Diffusion Method

- Kirby Bauer disc diffusion method.
- **MRSA detection:** Disk diffusion method—Cefoxitin disc method
- **ESBL detection:** Double disc test
- **E-test or diffusion:** Dilution test

2. Dilution Method

- Agar dilution method.
- Broth dilution method.
  - i. Macrodilution method
  - ii. Microdilution method

3. Detection of Antibiotic Inactivating Enzymes

i. Automated methods—Vitek 2 Systems.
ii. Molecular Methods—detection of drug resistant genes or genes encoding enzymes.

2. A 35-year-old comes to the emergency department with c/o of fever, breathlessness. On examination patient was febrile with O_2 saturation of 88%. Nasopharyngeal swab sent and positive for influenza H3N2. Oseltamivir was started. Classify the antiviral agents with examples for each type. (10 marks)

Site of action	Effective drugs	Used for
Early events (entry/uncoating)	• Amantadine • Rimantadine	• Influenza virus
Inhibition of nucleic acid synthesis Nucleoside inhibitors for herpes group	• Acyclovir • Ganciclovir • Cidofovir • Vidarabine • Iododeoxy-uridine • Trifluoro-thymidine	• HSV-1&2, VZV • CMV • CMV, HPV • HSV-Keratitis/ encephalitis • HSV-Keratitis • HSV Keratitis
Non-nucleoside inhibitors for herpes virus	• Foscarnet	• HSV, CMV • Esp. resistant to Acyclovir
Inhibition of nucleic acid synthesis Nucleoside inhibitors for HIV	• Azidothymidine • Dideoxyinosine • Dideoxycytidine • Lamivudine • Abacavir • Tenofovir • Stavudine	• HIV
• Nonnucleoside inhibitors for HIV	• Nevirapine • Delavirdine • Efavirenz	• HIV
Cleavage of precursor polypeptides	• Indinavir • Ritonavir • Nelfinavir	• HIV
Inhibition of protein synthesis	• Interferon • Methisazone • Fomivirsen	• HBV, HCV • Smallpox • CMV
Inhibition of viral release	• Zanamivir • Oseltamivir	• Influenza virus

Contd.

Site of action	Effective drugs	Used for
Antiviral	• Interferon α	• Chronic hepatitis B and C • Herpes viral infections • Malignancy: Hairy cell leukemia
Antitumor	• Interferon β	• Autoimmune disorders like multiple sclerosis
Immunoregulatory effects	• Interferon ϒ	• Chronic granulomatous diseases

SHORT ESSAYS

1. Interferons are an important part of the host defense against viral infections. Justify your answer and the role of interferons. (5 marks)

Interferons

- They host coded low molecular weight proteins produced by intact animals or cultured cells in response to viral infections or inducers.
- First line of defense
- Species specific
- Not virus specific

Classification

- Depending on the cell of origin
  1. *Leucocyte interferon:* IFN α
  2. *Fibroblast interferon:* IFN β
  3. *Lymphocyte interferon:* IFN ϒ

Inducers of IFN

- RNA viruses
- Avirulent viruses
- *Nucleic acid:* ds RNA
- Bacterial endotoxins, intracellular bacteria
- Synthetic polymers
- Inducer of IFN ϒ—mitogens like phytohaemagglutinin.

Source

- Pooled human leucocyte or lymphocyte activated by viruses or synthetic polyribonucleotides.
- DNA recombinant technology.

Actions

1. Antiviral effect.
2. Antitumour effect.
3. Immunoregulatory effects.

Uses

1. **IFN α**
   - In treatment of chronic hepatitis B and C
   - In prophylaxis and treatment of herpes viral infections
   - Localised instillation can be done in herpetic keratitis, laryngeal papillomatosis, condyloma acuminata.
   - Used in certain malignancies—lymphoma, hairy cell leukemia, CLL, Kaposi sarcoma, malignant melanoma.
2. **IFN β**
   - Used for treatment of relapsing or remitting autoimmune disorders like multiple sclerosis.
3. **IFN ϒ**
   - Used as immunostimulator in chronic granulomatous diseases and other disorders like Job's syndrome.
   - Used as an adjunct to enhance the response to DNA vaccine.
4. **Pegylated interferon**
   - Improved drug solubility.
   - Enhanced protection from proteolytic degradation.
   - Increase biological half life.
   - Reduced dosage frequency, with same efficacy and potentially decreased toxicity.

2. A 25-year-old man develops cough with blood-tinged sputum. H/o of loss of weight. Chest X ray shows right upper lobe cavity with chest infiltrates. Sputum sent for Gene Xpert® MTB report detected *M. tuberculosis* along with resistance to rifampicin.

A. What is your diagnosis? (1 mark)

- Multidrug resistant tuberculosis.

B. Briefly explain the mechanism of drug resistance in this organism. (4 marks)

- Drug resistance in *Mycobacterium tuberculosis* is chromosomal mediated.
- Drug resistance is acquired through:
  - Alteration of the drug target through mutations.
  - Overproduction of drug targets.
  - MDR occurs through accumulation of individual target genes.

Types

1. **Primary resistance:** Bacteria showing resistance in a patient, who has not received the drug in question before
2. **Acquired/Secondary resistance:** Bacteria susceptible to the drug at the beginning of the treatment but became resistant to the particular drug during the course of treatment

Mutations Conferring Drug Resistance

Drug	Gene	Gene product/ functional role	Cellular target
Rifampicin	• rpoB	• β-subunit of RNA polymerase/ transcription	• Nucleic acids
Isoniazid	• KatG • OxyR-ahpC • KasA	• Catalase-peroxidase/activation of Pro-drug • Alkyl-hydro-reductase/unknown • b-ketoacyl acyl carrier protein	• Cell wall
Ethionamide	• inhA	• Enol-ACP reductase/synthase • Mycolic acid synthesis	• Cell wall
Streptomycin	• rspl • rrs	• Ribosomal protein S12/translation • 16S rRNA/ translation	• Protein synthesis
Fluroquinolones	• gyrA	• DNA gyrase	• Nucleic acid
Pyrazinamide	• pncA	• Amidase/activation of pro-drug	• Unknown
Ethambutol	• embB	• Arabinosyl transferase/ arabinose polymerisation	• Cell wall

3. What is an antimicrobial stewardship programme and enumerate its role in a hospital? (4 marks)

Antimicrobial Stewardship

- A well-co-ordinated programme that promotes the appropriate use of antimicrobials (including antibiotics), resulting in improvement in patient outcomes, reduces microbial resistance, and decreases the spread of infections caused by multidrug-resistant organisms.

Role in a Hospital

Primary Goal

1. To optimize safe and appropriate use of antibiotics.
2. To improve clinical outcomes.
3. Minimise adverse effects of antibiotics.

Secondary Goal

1. To reduce healthcare costs without adversely impacting quality of patient care.
2. To reduce the incidence of antibiotic induced collateral damage.

4. Briefly discuss the factors a clinician should consider while prescribing any antimicrobial therapy? (5 marks)

1. **Obtaining an accurate infectious disease diagnosis**
   - Specimens are properly obtained and promptly submitted to the microbiology laboratory, preferably before the initiating of antimicrobial therapy.
2. **Timing of initiation of antimicrobial therapy**
   A. *Empiric therapy*
   - For septic shock, febrile neutropenic patients, and patients with bacterial meningitis
   - Clinicians should consider the following
     i. The site of infection and the organisms most likely to be colonizing that site
     ii. Prior knowledge of bacteria known to colonise a given patient
     iii. The local bacterial resistance patterns

   B. *Definitive therapy*
   - Once microbiology results have helped to identify the etiologic pathogen and/or antimicrobial susceptibility data are available, every attempt should be made to narrow the antibiotic spectrum
3. **In stable clinical circumstances**, antimicrobial therapy should be deliberately withheld until appropriate specimens have been collected and submitted to the microbiology laboratory like in subacute bacterial endocarditis and vertebral osteomyelitis/discitis
4. **Different AST interpretations** for different sites of infection (e.g. meningitis and non-meningitis AST results for *S. pneumoniae*)
5. **Bactericidal vs bacteriostatic therapy**
   - Bactericidal agents are preferred in the case of serious infections such as endocarditis and meningitis
6. **Use of antimicrobial combinations**
   i. When agents exhibit synergistic activity against a microorganism
   ii. When critically ill patients require empiric therapy
   iii. To prevent resistance
7. **Host factors to be considered in selection of antimicrobial agents**
   i. Renal hepatic function
   ii. Age
   iii. Pregnancy/lactation
   iv. H/o allergy
   v. H/o recent antibiotic use

5. The reason why methicillin-resistant *Staphylococcus aureus* (MRSA) strains are resistant to methicillin and nafcillin. Justify your answer. (4 marks)

Methicillin-resistant *Staphylococcus aureus* (MRSA)

- Staphylococcus aureus strains emerged that were resistant to the β-lactamase-stable penicillins. These strains were termed "methicillin resistant S. aureus" (MRSA), because methicillin was initially used to detect their resistance to β-lactamase-stable penicillins (oxacillin, methicillin, nafcillin).

Sources

1. Asymptomatically colonised patients and health-care workers.
2. The most common site of MRSA carriage is the anterior nares.
3. A significant risk factor for acquisition of MRSA is the duration of hospital stay.

Mechanism

- Primarily mediated by the *mec*A gene, which codes for the modified penicillin-binding protein 2a (PBP 2a or PBP 2′).
- PBP2a is in the bacterial cell wall and has a low binding affinity for β-lactams.

Detection

A. Phenotypic Detection Systems

1. Dilution Methods

i. *Agar dilution.*
   - Tests on MH with 2% NaCl and an inoculum of 10^4 cfu/ml will distinguish most resistant from susceptible strains.
   - The method require incubation for 24 hours at 33–35°C.
   - In both methods an oxacillin MIC of ≤2 mg/L indicates that the strain is susceptible and >2 mg/L resistant.

ii. *Broth microdilution.*
   - The CLSI method, which requires the use of MH broth with 2% NaCl, an inoculum of 5×10^5 cfu/ml and incubation at 33–35°C for 24 hours.

2. E-test Method

- MIC value.

3. Agar Screening Method

- Requires suspending the test organism to the density of a 0.5 McFarland standard and inoculating MH agar containing 4% NaCl and 6 mg/L oxacillin with a spot or a streak of the organism. Plates are incubated at 35°C or less for 24 hours and any growth other than a single colony is indicative of resistance.

4. Cefoxitin Disc Diffusion Test

- Cefoxitin, which is a potent inducer of the *mecA*.
- An inhibition zone diameter of ≤21 mm is reported as methicillin resistant and ≥22 mm is considered as methicillin susceptible.

5. Automated System

- Vitek system.
- Phoenix system.

B. Genotypic Detection System

- PCR for the detection of *mecA* gene.

Treatment

- Vancomycin or daptomycin are the agents of choice for treatment of invasive MRSA infections. Alternative agents that may be used for second-line therapy include ceftaroline, linezolid, cotrimoxazole, clindamycin.

6. A patient with UTI whose urine culture and sensitivity report revealed *E. coli* resistant to all the antibiotics tested under the panel. Briefly discuss the possible types of mechanism of antibiotic resistance prevailing in this case scenario. (4 marks)

Antibiotic Resistance in Uropathogenic *Escherichia coli*

1. **Resistance to β-lactams**
   - Production of different types of β-lactamase enzymes (penicillin, cephalosporin, monobactams, and carbapenems).
   - ESBL are enzymes that confer resistance to β-lactam antibiotics (all penicillins, cephalosporins, and monobactams), except for carbapenems, cephamycins, and β-lactamase inhibitors. Result of mutations in the genes coding for ancestral enzymes responsible are blaTEM-1, blaTEM-2, and blaSHV-1.
2. **Quinolone resistance**
   - Mutation in the genes *gyrA* and *gyrB* that catalyze DNA supercoiling.
   - Presence of efflux pumps.
   - Decreased uptake of the antibiotics due to changes in the outer membrane porin proteins .
3. **Fosfomycin resistance**
   - Fosfomycin uptake is reduced by the bacterial cells due to mutations in the genes related to the inactivation of fosfomycin by enzymatic cleavage.
4. **Nitrofurantoin resistance**
   - Mutations in genes *nsfA* and *nfsB* encoding the oxygen-insensitive nitroreductases.
5. **Resistance to sulphonamides, aminoglycosides**
   - Associated with the presence of specific plasmids. Resistance to sulphonamides is determined

by three genes (*sul1*, *sul2* and *sul3*) and *aadB*, *aac(3)-II* and *aac(3)-IV* genes are related to the gentamicin, tobramycin, neomycin resistance.

SHORT ANSWERS

1. Amphotericin B is noted for both its antifungal efficacy and side effects when administered to humans. Statement is true or false. Classify antifungal agents and their mechanism of action with appropriate examples. (3 marks)

Statement is

- True.

Classification of Antifungal Agents

Mechanism of action	*Examples*	
• Inhibit lanosterol 14α-demethylase—the enzyme required to convert lanosterol into ergosterol	**Imidazoles**	
	1. Clotrimazole 2. Oxiconazole 3. Miconazole	4. Econazole 5. Tioconazole 6. Ketoconazole
	Triazoles	
	1. Fluconazole 2. Itraconazole 3. Terconazole	4. Voriconazole 5. Isavuconazole 6. Posaconazole
• Inhibits mitosis in dermatophytes	• Griseofulvin	
• Pyrimidine analogue—converted into S-fluorouracil by the fungal enzyme cytosine deaminase	• Flucytosine	
• Inhibit cell wall synthesis by targeting glucans—inhibit 1,3-β-glucan synthase	• Micafungin • Anidulafungin • Caspofungin	
• Inhibits squalene epoxidase	• Amorolfine • Naftifine • Terbinafine	

2. Define intrinsic resistance in bacteria. Give 4 examples. (1+2 marks)

Intrinsic Resistance

Definition

- Drug resistance resulting from normal genetic, structural, or physiologic state of the bacteria.

Examples

1. Penicillin resistance in cell wall deficient bacteria like *Mycoplasma*.
2. *Enterococci* are resistant to cotrimoxazole and cephalosporins.
3. Vancomycin resistance in gram-negative bacilli.
4. Tigecycline in *Pseudomonas aeruginosa*.

3. Some bacteria become resistant to penicillin. Which are the different mechanisms for development its resistance? (3 marks)

1. Plasmid-encoded penicillinase .
2. Inactivation of the antibiotic by production of penicillinase.
3. Antibiotic efflux.
4. Modification of target Penicillin binding protein (PBP).
5. Impaired penetration of the drug to the target PBP.

4. Lower the MIC of an antimicrobial agent better is the therapeutic efficacy. Justify your answer. (3 marks)

- MIC is a reasonable approximate order of magnitude of concentration of free drug needed at the site of infection.
- Minimal concentration of an antimicrobial needed to inhibit bacterial growth.
- A lower MIC is an indication of a better antimicrobial agent.
- An MIC number for one antibiotic CANNOT be compared to the MIC number for another antibiotic.
- Minimum inhibitory concentrations (MICs)—useful in selecting the best antimicrobial agent for a given patient with known culture and susceptibility results.
- Antibiotics with high MICs may still be effective if it concentrates at the site of infection (e.g. treatment of UTI with gentamicin, which concentrates in the urine).

MI 1.7 DESCRIBE THE IMMUNOLOGICAL MECHANISMS IN HEALTH

LONG ESSAY

1. Describe in detail about immunity and immunological mechanisms under the following headings.

A. Define and classify immunity. (1+1 marks)

Definition

- Resistance of the individual to the damage done by microbe or the microbial product.

Classification of immunity (Fig. 1.7.1)

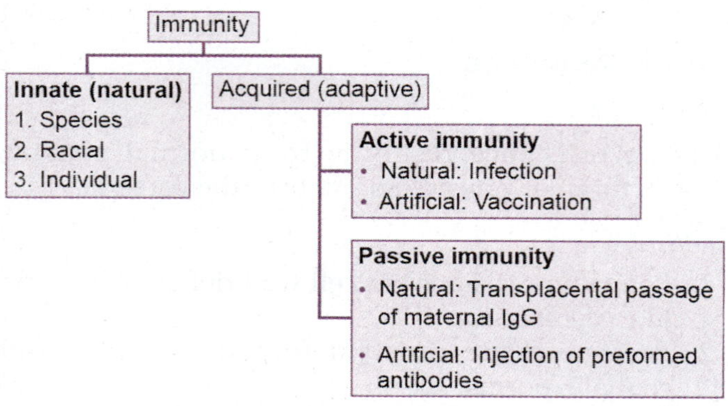

Fig. 1.7.1: Classification of immunity

B. Cilia present in the respiratory tract helps in clearance of microorganisms and provides immunity. Discuss the components and mechanism of this type of immunity. (1+7 marks)

- Innate immunity is the inborn resistance against infections that an individual possesses right from the birth, due to his genetic or constitutional makeup.

Components

1. **Mechanisms defined at body surface.**
   - Physiological factors, mechanical barriers and surface secretions.
2. **Systemic natural immunity.**
   - Cellular factors.
   - Other body defense mechanisms of systemic natural immunity.

Mechanisms of Innate Immunity (Fig. 1.7.2)

Barriers

Skin

- Protective integument prevents entry of microorganisms.
- Skin secretions-antibacterial activity of sweat and sebaceous secretions—acidic pH, high salt content, long chain saturated fatty acids.
- Epithelial shedding.
- Normal flora—prevents adherence, colonisation.

GIT

- Hydrolytic enzymes in saliva, gastric acidity kill the bacteria.
- Mucous membrane, mucus entraps the organism.
- Proteolytic enzymes, bile: Antibacterial activity.
- Peristaltic movement expelling the organism.
- Normal intestinal flora (microbial antagonism): Block the receptors, produce bacteriocins, compete for nutrition.
- Gut-associated lymphoid tissue, mucosa associated lymphoid tissue.

Respiratory System

- Architecture of nose prevents entry of organisms.
- Mucus entraps the organism.
- Antibacterial and antiviral substances—lysozyme, secretary IgA.
- Cilia, sneezing, cough reflex, help to remove the organisms out.
- Alveolar macrophages—phagocytosis.

Genitourinary Tract

- Flushing action of urine
- Uromucoid—entraps the bacteria.
- High acidic pH of vagina.
- Antibacterial secretions of glands (prostatic).

Conjunctivae

- Lacrimal secretions
- Lysozyme
- Shedding of microorganisms: Salivation, urination, defaecation, desquamation of skin, lacrimal secretions.

Lysozyme

- Present in tears, saliva, respiratory and cervical secretion. Hydrolytic enzyme breaks the cell wall.

Systemic Mechanisms

1. **Cellular systemic immunity**
   - Natural defense against tissue and blood invasion. Immune cells as a part of Innate immunity come into play when the integrity of the barrier (first line of defence) has been breached.
   - Phagocytosis—intracellular killing by neutrophils, macrophages.
   - Reticuloendothelial system present in liver, spleen and bone marrow.
   - Fixed macrophages clear organisms from circulation.

Attachment: binding of the surface molecules of microorganisms (MAMP) to the receptors of cells of innate immunity (Toll like receptors) → Signals are generated → activate transcription factors → stimulate expression of genes → Cytokines: Antimicrobial activity

Fig. 1.7.2: Mechanism of innate immunity

- *Eosinophils:* Line of defense against the migratory larvae of parasites: *Trichinella* and *Strongyloides*
- *Natural killer cells:* Virus infected and cancer cells

2. **Inflammation**
   - Response of the body to the damage done by pathogen.
   - Vasoconstriction → vasodilatation → migration of PMNLs → phagocytosis.
   - There is accumulation of phagocytes at the site of infection with outpouring of natural antibacterial substances, fibrin deposition and localisation of infection.
3. **Fever**
   - Endotoxin, antigen antibody complex activate macrophages, which produces interleukin-1.
   - IL-1 acts on thermoregulatory centre of hypothalamus → Fever.
   - Elevated temperature retards bacterial growth.
4. **Acute phase proteins**
   - C-reactive protein (CRP), mannose binding protein, alpha-1-acid glycoprotein, serum amyloid P component.
   - *Action:* activation of complement system, prevent tissue injury, promote repair of inflammatory lesions
5. **Interferons:** Antiviral activity.
6. **Complement system**
   - Alternate pathway (bacterial endotoxin), mannose binding pathway (mannose residue on bacterial surface).
   - Destroys pathogenic organisms by various biological activities (lysis, opsonisation).
7. **Antibacterial substances in blood and tissues**
   - β-lysin-active against many bacteria like *Bacillus anthracis.*
   - Basic polypeptides—leukins.
   - Acidic substances like lactic acid seen in inflammatory tissue.
   - Lactoperoxidase in milk.
8. **Toll-like receptors (pathogen-associated molecular pattern PAMP)**
   - 13 TLRs on the macrophages, dendritic cells, mast cells recognise pathogens, enhance phagocytosis led to inflammation at the site.
9. **Defensins**
   - Positively charged (cationic) peptides, produced in the gastrointestinal and lower respiratory tracts.
   - Create pores in lipid membranes of bacteria, fungi, and viruses.
   - *Neutrophils and Paneth cells in the intestinal crypts:* α-defensins (antiviral activity)
   - *Respiratory tract:* β-defensins (antibacterial)
10. **Apolipoprotein B RNA editing enzyme**
    - Antiretroviral activity.
    - Causes hypermutation in retroviral DNA and mRNA.

---

2. Discuss the type of immunity acquired by an individual during life under the following headings.

A. Definition. (1 mark)

- Immunity acquired by an individual during life is Acquired Immunity or Adaptive Immunity.
- It is the resistance acquired by an individual during life.

B. Characteristics. (3 marks)

- It has two components.
  1. Cell-mediated immunity (T cells)
  2. Humoral or antibody mediated.
- Features—diversity, memory, specificity.
- Mediators.
  - T cells and B cells
  - Classical complement pathway
  - Antigen presenting cells
  - Cytokines (IL-2, IL-4, IL-5)
- Immunity acquired through effective prior contact with antigen.
- Effective contact of immunogen with immune system → Leads to immune response against the immunogens → Resulting in specific immunity against antigen.
- Immunity—both humoral and cellular immunity.
- Associated with immunological memory (improves upon repeated exposure).
- Duration of immunity.
  1. Lifelong as in mumps, measles.
  2. Short as in influenza.

C. Types with examples. (6 marks)

1. Active Immunity

- Protection based on exposure to the organism in the form of overt disease, subclinical infection, or a vaccine.

Characteristics

- Active involvement of the host in mounting an immune response consisting of antibodies and activated T lymphocytes.
- Develops slowly and persists for long time
- Specific
- Negative phase
- Lag phase
- Primary and secondary immune response
- Booster effect observed during subsequent injection.

A. Natural Active Immunity

- Resistance developed by the host in response to infection
- Immunity is long lasting—measles, chickenpox or short-live (influenza).
- Premunition or concomitant immunity—Immunity may last as long as the microbe is present. Once the disease is cured, the patient becomes susceptible to the microbe again (*Spirochaetes* and *Plasmodium*).

B. Artificial Active Immunity

- Produced by vaccination.

2. Passive Immunity

Characteristics

- Specific immunity
- No active immune response in the host
- Gives immediate protection
- Short lived or temporary protection.

A. Natural Passive Immunity

- Placental transfer of antibodies (IgG) from mother to faetus gives protection up to 3–6 months
- Through milk and colostrum
  - Secretary IgA antibodies
  - Protection against enteric infection

B. Artificial Passive Immunity

- Preformed antibodies acquired artificially through immune serum (antisera) and immunoglobulins.
- Given for immediate protection of non-immune host.
- Antisera-obtained by hyperimmunisation of horses ARS for rabies, ADS for diphtheria, ATS for tetanus.
- Advantage: Immediate protection.
- Disadvantages.
  1. Risk of hypersensitivity (foreign protein)
  2. Large doses required
  3. Immunity short lived.

SHORT ESSAYS

1. What are macrophages and classify macrophages based on their location? Discuss the functions of different types of macrophages. (3+2 marks)

Macrophages

They are:

- A type of white blood cell of the immune system that engulfs and digests cancer cells, microbes, cellular debris, foreign substances by phagocytosis.
- *Function:* To defend the host against infection and injury
- Derived from bone marrow histiocytes.

Classification of Macrophages

1. Free macrophages (Monocytes).
2. Fixed macrophages.
   i. Kupffer cells in liver.
   ii. Alveolar macrophages in lungs.
   iii. Microglial cells in brain.

Functions

1. **Phagocytosis**
   - Ingestion of bacteria, viruses, and other foreign particles
   - Fusion of phagosome containing microbe with lysosome
   - Killing of the microbe within the phago-lysosome
     - Reactive metabolites such as H_2O_2, superoxide anions
     - Reactive N_2 metabolite—nitric oxide
     - Lysosomal enzymes—proteases, nucleases, and lysozyme
2. **Antigen presentation**
   - Capture and process antigen.
   - Present antigen in association with class II MHC protein.
   - Display B7 protein which acts as co-stimulatory signal for T cells activation.
3. **Production of cytokines**
   - IL-1 (Endogenous pyrogen).
   - TNF (Inflammatory mediator).
   - IL-8 (Chemoattractant).

2. Describe the barriers of innate immunity with appropriate examples. (5 marks)

Anatomic site	Mechanical barriers	Chemical barriers	Biological barriers
Skin	• Keratinised squamous epidermis cells	• Fatty acids • Defensins	• Normal Skin flora
Gastro-intestinal tract	• Mucins: A sticky mixture of glycoproteins produced by secretory epithelial cells • Peristalsis • Normal shedding of epithelial cells	• Gastric acid • Digestive enzymes • Defensins lysozyme • Iron-binding protein	• Gut flora • IgA
Genito-urinary tract	• Urine flow	• Low pH	• Vaginal flora • IgA

Contd.

Anatomic site	*Mechanical barriers*	*Chemical barriers*	*Biological barriers*
Respiratory tract	• Airflow • Ciliated airway cells • Coughing	• Surfactant proteins: lipoproteins produced in the lung alveoli that bind to the surface of microbes, which can facilitate their phagocytosis (i.e. opsonin function) or can be directly bactericidal	• Nose, mouth, and pharyngeal flora • IgA

3. Define herd immunity. Discuss the role of herd immunity in a community/city with respect to COVID-19 infection (2+3 marks)

Herd Immunity

Definition

- Overall immunity of persons in a community against infectious disease or
- Indirect protection from an infectious disease that happens when a population is immune either through vaccination or immunity developed through previous infection, e.g. in OPV, MMR.

Role of herd immunity in a community/city with respect to COVID-19 infection

- Herd immunity against COVID-19 can be achieved by vaccinating all the individuals in the community and ideally not by exposing the individuals to infection.
- To achieve herd immunity against COVID-19, a substantial proportion of a population would need to be vaccinated.
- This reduces the amount of virus spread in the community.

4. An elderly gets a pneumococcal vaccine. Which type of specific immunity plays a significant role in this case scenario? Define vaccine. List the different types of vaccines. (1+1+3 marks)

Type of specific immunity plays a significant role in this case

- Artificial active immunity attained by vaccination.

Vaccine Definition

- Preparation of live, attenuated or killed microorganisms or their antigens or active materials derived from them (toxoids) used for immunisation.

Types of Vaccines

They are:

1. Live attenuated vaccines
2. Killed vaccines
3. Toxoids
4. Subunit vaccines
5. Recombinant vaccines
6. Synthetic peptides
7. DNA vaccines
8. Edible vaccines
9. Anti-idiotype vaccines.

5. Compare and contrast active and passive immunity. (1+4 marks)

Active Immunity

- Protection based on exposure to the organism in the form of overt disease, subclinical infection, or a vaccine.

Passive Immunity

- Protection based on the transfer of preformed antibody from one person (or animal) to another person.

Differences between Active Immunity and Passive Immunity

Feature	*Active immunity*	*Passive immunity*
Method of acquisition	• Effective contact with antigen	• Preformed antibodies
Immune response	• Present	• Absent
Duration of immunity	• Long lived months to years	• Short lived
Immunological memory	• Present	• Absent
Lag phase	• Present	• Absent
Utility in immunocompromised	• No	• Yes

6. Enumerate the systemic mechanisms of innate immunity and their mode of action. (5 marks)

Systemic mechanisms of innate immunity	*Mode of action*
Cellular systemic immunity • Natural defense against tissue and blood invasion	• *Phagocytosis:* Intracellular killing by neutrophils, macrophages • *Reticuloendothelial system:* Present in liver, spleen and bone marrow • *Fixed macrophages:* Clear organisms from circulation • *Eosinophils* (defense against parasites) and *natural killer cells* (virus infected and cancer cells)
Inflammation	• Vasoconstriction → vasodilatation → migration of PMNLs → phagocytosis • Accumulation of phagocytes at site of infection with outpouring of natural antibacterial substances, fibrin deposition and localisation of infection
Fever	• Endotoxin, antigen antibody complex → Activate macrophages → which produces interleukin-1 • IL-1 acts on thermoregulatory centre of hypothalamus • Fever increases rate of phagocytosis and antibody production
Acute phase proteins	• C-reactive protein (CRP), mannose binding protein, alpha-1-acid glycoprotein, serum amyloid P component • Activate complement, prevent tissue injury, promote repair of inflammatory lesions
Interferons	• Antiviral activity
Complement system	• Alternate pathway (activated by bacterial endotoxin), mannose-binding pathway (activated by mannose residue on bacterial surface) • Destroys pathogenic organisms by various biological activities (lysis, opsonisation
Antibacterial substances in blood and tissues	• β-lysin-active against many bacteria like *Bacillus anthracis* • Basic polypeptides-leukins • Acidic substances like lactic acid seen in inflammatory tissue • Lactoperoxidase in milk
Toll like receptors (pathogen associated molecular pattern PAMP)	• TLRs on the macrophages, dendritic cells, mast cells recognise pathogens • TLR stimulate expression of genes encoding cytokines and enzymes → antimicrobial activity
Defensins	• Highly positively charged (cationic) peptides that create pores in the membranes of bacteria, which kills them. • Neutrophils and Paneth cells in the intestinal crypts contain α-defensins • Respiratory tract produces β-defensins
Apolipoprotein B RNA editing enzyme	• Antiretroviral activity

Contd.

7. Enumerate the proteins that either increase or decrease exponentially during acute inflammatory conditions. Justify your answer. Elaborate on two such important proteins. (1+1+2 marks)

Proteins that either increase or decrease exponentially during acute inflammatory conditions are:

- Acute phase reactants (APR)
- The positive acute phase proteins include procalcitonin, C-reactive protein, ferritin, fibrinogen, hepcidin, and serum amyloid A.
- Synthesized by endothelial cells, fibroblasts, monocytes, and adipocytes.

Justification

- These markers show significant changes in serum concentration during inflammation.
- Produced in the liver during acute and chronic inflammatory states.

Examples of APR

1. CRP

- *Normal range for CRP:* 2–10 mg/L.
- CRP levels can increase 100–1000-fold during acute inflammation.
- Levels of CRP increase in:
  - Malignancies, pancreatitis, myocardial infarction.
  - *Marked increase* (>10 mg/dl)—acute bacterial infections, major trauma, and systemic vasculitis.
  - hs (high sensitivity) CRP is used to determine the risk for cardiovascular diseases.
- *Function:* Promote phagocytosis and facilitate the innate immune response against infectious pathogens
- Measured by latex agglutination or on automated platforms by nephelometry and turbidometry.

2. Procalcitonin

- LPS, microbial toxins, or inflammatory mediators can activate the procalcitonin gene in the liver,

kidney, adipocytes, pancreas, colon, and brain during inflammation.
- Sensitive marker for following the progression of infections, especially for pneumonia and sepsis. Levels of procalcitonin are used to guide antibiotic therapy.
- Measured by ELFA, ECLIA.

SHORT ANSWERS

1. Mention two examples for live attenuated vaccines and killed vaccines (2 marks)

Examples of Live Attenuated Vaccines

1. BCG vaccine for tuberculosis.
2. Measles, mumps, rubella (MMR) vaccine.

Examples of Killed Vaccines

1. TA vaccines for enteric fever.
2. Polio vaccine (Salk vaccine).

2. An intern has an accidental needle stick injury while drawing blood from hepatitis B patient. She is not vaccinated against hepatitis B. Which approach must be taken to prevent hepatitis B for the intern? (2 marks)

- In passive–active immunity (combined immunisation) the intern gets both preformed antibodies to provide immediate protection and a vaccine to provide long-term protection. These preparations are given at different sites in the body to prevent the antibodies from neutralising the vaccine. This approach is used to prevent hepatitis B.

3. Mr XYZ must travel 3 days from now to a country where hepatitis A is endemic. She knows that both vaccine and serum globulin preparation are available for prophylaxis. She asks which you would recommend? Justify your answer and which type of immunity does it confer? (2 marks)

- In this scenario, the serum globulin preparation containing antibodies against the virus is best because it provides immunity in the shortest time. The type of immunity provided by preformed antibodies is artificial passive immunity.

4. Describe in detail about Pattern Recognition Receptors with appropriate examples. (3 marks)

- Components of the innate immune arm have receptors, called pattern recognition receptors (PRRs) that recognise a molecular pattern, called a pathogen-associated molecular pattern (PAMP), that is present on the surface of many microbes.
- Two classes of receptors (Toll-like receptors and C-type lectin receptors)—recognise microbes that are outside the cells or within the cells' vesicles.
- Two classes of receptors in the cytoplasm of cells (NOD-like receptors and RIG-I helicase receptors) recognise microbes in the cells cytoplasm.
- Any mutations in the genes encoding these pattern receptors result in a failure to recognise pathogens and predispose to severe bacterial, viral, and fungal infections.
- Immune response is shaped by the combination of PRRs activated during the initial encounter with innate immunity.

5. Live viral polio vaccine induces what type of immunity. Define this type of immunity. Mention the significance of this type of Immunity. (1+2 marks)

Type of Immunity Induced by Live Viral Polio Vaccine

- Local or mucosal immunity.

Local Immunity Definition

- Immunity at the site of entry of infectious agents provided by secretory IgA which is produced by plasma cells present in submucosa.

Significance of Mucosal Immunity

1. To protect the mucous membranes from the colonisation and invasion by pathogens.
2. *To prevent antigen uptake:* Foreign proteins derived from ingested food, air-borne matter, and commensal microorganism.
3. To prevent the development of harmful immune responses to these antigens if they do reach the body interior.

6. Enumerate the bridges between Innate and Acquired Immunity and discuss their role clinically. (4 marks)

Feature	*In Innate Immunity*	*In Acquired Immunity*
Macrophages	• Engulfs and kills many classes of microbes, removal of debris, tissue repair	• Have surface IgG receptors that facilitate phagocytosis (opsonisation) • activated by IFN-γ, TNF-α from T cells • Professional APC expressing class II MHC

Contd.

Feature	In Innate Immunity	In Acquired Immunity
Dendritic cells	• Antigen uptake and presentation	• Professional APC expressing class II MHC
Neutrophils	• Engulfs and kills bacteria and fungi, digests cellular debris	• Attracted into tissues by chemokines, which are increased by T cell-derived IL-17
Eosinophils	• Granule proteins are toxic to cells • Involved in asthma and allergic diseases • Protective against helminth infections	• Surface IgE receptors; maturation and survival supported by IL-5 from T cells
Mast cells and basophils	• Release histamine, proteases, chemokines, and cytokines; contribute to allergic disease and anaphylaxis	• IgE receptors hold IgE molecules that survey for antigen
Complement system	• Alternate and mannose binding pathways activated by Endotoxin, mannose residue on the bacteria	• Classic pathway activated by Ag Ab complex
Cytokines	• Released by cells of innate immunity	• Activate cells of acquired immunity, e.g. IL1 by macrophages activate T cells
Antibody dependent cell-mediated cytotoxicity	• Cells of innate immunity such as NK cell, eosinophils, and neutrophils destroy (by cytotoxic effect) the target cells coated with specific antibodies	

7. Compare and contrast Innate and Acquired Immunity. (4 marks)

Feature	Innate Immunity	Acquired Immunity
Presence	• Since birth	• Acquired later in life
Specificity	• Nonspecific • No exposure to antigen required	• Specific response developing after exposure to foreign antigen
Response	• Rapid	• Slower (1-2 weeks)
Specificity of response	• Response not specific to some microbe, rather shared by many microbes (called as microbes-associated molecular patterns)	• Response is targeted to specific Antigens
Immunological memory	• Absent	• Present
Components	• Barrier • Phagocytes • NK cells, Mast cells, Dendritic cells • Alternate and mannose binding pathways • Fever and inflammatory responses • Normal resident flora • Cytokines: TNF-α, certain interleukin (IL-1, IL-6, IL-8, IL-12, IL-16, IL-18), IFN-α, β and TGF- β • Acute phase reactant proteins (APRs)	• T cell • B cell • Classical complement pathway • Antigen presenting cells • Cytokines (IL-2, IL-4, IL-5, IFN-γ) • Types • Active and passive immunity • Artificial and natural immunity

MI 1.8 DESCRIBE THE MECHANISMS OF IMMUNITY AND RESPONSE OF THE HOST IMMUNE SYSTEM TO INFECTIONS

LONG ESSAYS

1. Discuss the principle, types, and applications of agglutination reactions. (2+6+2 marks)

Agglutination Reactions

Principle

- When a particulate Ag reacts with Ab in the presence of electrolytes at suitable temperature and pH, the particulate Ag is clumped or agglutinated.

- *Marrack's hypothesis:* Zone phenomenon in agglutination occurs when Ag and Ab are present in optimal proportions
- Agglutination is more sensitive than precipitation for the detection of antibodies, better with IgM.
- For agglutination the Abs should be at least bivalent.
- Incomplete or monovalent Abs do not cause agglutination, though they combine with Ag. They act as blocking antibodies and are responsible for false-negative results.

Types Based on Principle

1. Active/direct agglutination tests.
2. Passive agglutination tests.
3. Reverse passive agglutination.

Active/Direct Agglutination Tests

- Particulate Ag is directly agglutinated by the Ab.
  1. **Slide agglutination test**
     - Smooth suspension of the particulate Ag on the slide + a drop of antiserum
     - Clumping of the Ag within seconds
     - *Uses*
       1. To identify unknown bacteria using known antisera.
       2. ABO grouping of blood.
  2. **Tube agglutination test**
     - Convenient method to detect Ab in the patient serum
     - Can be done to quantitate antibodies
     - Patient's serum is diluted in physiological saline 2 folds and fixed amount of Ag is added to each of the dilution
     - Highest dilution of the patient's serum which shows agglutination is the endpoint. The reciprocal of endpoint is the titre
     - Examples
       1. *Widal test:* Tube agglutination test to demonstrate O and H agglutinins against typhoid and paratyphoid bacilli in patient serum.
       2. *Standard agglutination test:* for brucellosis
       3. *Weil-Felix test:* Heterophile agglutination test for the serodiagnosis of typhus fever.
       4. *Streptococcal MG agglutination test:* Heterophile agglutination test used in the diagnosis of primary atypical pneumonia.
       5. *Paul Bunnell test:* Based on the presence of sheep cell agglutinins in the sera of infectious mononucleosis patients, which are adsorbed by ox RBCs, not by Guinea pig kidney extract.
       6. *Cold agglutination test:* Positive in mycoplasmal primary atypical pneumonia. Patient's sera agglutinate human O group erythrocytes at 4°C, being reversible at 37°C.
  3. **Coombs' test (Antiglobulin test)**
     - Used to detect anti Rh antibody.
     - Performed to diagnose Rh incompatibility by detecting Rh antibody from mother's and baby's serum.
     - This Ab is incomplete.
     - It binds on the surface of Rh + erythrocytes but does not agglutinate.
     - Such sensitized erythrocytes agglutinate when antiglobulin (Rabbit antibody to human globulin–antiglobulin/Coombs' serum) is added.

Passive Agglutination Tests

- Ag coated inert carrier particles are agglutinated by Abs.
- It is possible to label carrier particle with soluble Ag.
- It is possible to use soluble Ag in agglutination by binding the Ag to an inert carrier particle.
- More convenient and sensitive for Ab detection.
- Characters of the inert particle.
  - Should be coloured.
  - Should be antigenically inert.
  - Must be stable and preservable.
  - Must be easy to label the carrier particle with the Ag.
- Carrier particles.
  - RBCs (not stable, susceptible to hemolysis)
  - Latex particles
  - Bentonite

1. Passive Haemagglutination Test

- *Uses.*
  1. *Streptozyme test:* to detect Abs against enzymes and toxins of Streptococcus pyogenes
  2. *TPHA (Treponema Pallidum Haemagglutination Test):* Used to detect specific antitreponemal Abs in syphilis

2. Passive Latex Agglutination Test

- Polystyrene latex are uniform spherical particles.
- 0.8–1 μm in diameter.
- Latex particles labelled with the Ag are used to detect specific Ab.
- *Use:* Detection of ASO, CRP, RA, hCG
- *Advantages*
  1. Easy to perform
  2. Rapid
  3. Highly sensitive
  4. Relative stability of the reagents
- *Disadvantages*
  1. False-positive results due to cross reacting antibodies.
  2. False-negative results due to presence of Ab's in low titre.

Reverse Passive Agglutination

- Carrier particles are labelled with Ab and the Ab labelled carrier particles are used to detect the Ag.
- *Uses.*
  1. In the diagnosis of cryptococcal meningitis, acute bacterial meningitis.
  2. Detection of *Streptococcus pyogenes* Ag in the throat swab.
  3. Detection of Vi Ag of *Salmonella typhi* in serum, urine.
  4. *In virology:* detection of Rotavirus Ag in the stool, HbsAg in serum

2. Which is the serological test method used to detect dengue IgM antibodies in the patient serum employing enzyme substrate complex? Describe in detail the principle, types, applications, advantages and disadvantages of the above test method. (1+3+4+2 marks)

- The test used to detect the presence of dengue IgM is ELISA.

ELISA

Principle

- Enzyme-linked immunosorbent assay is a plate-based assay technique designed for the detection and quantification of peptides, proteins, antibodies, and hormones.
- Antigen must be immobilised to a solid surface and then complexed with an antibody that is linked to an enzyme.
- Detection is done by assessing the conjugated enzyme activity via incubation with a substrate to produce a measurable product.
- Colour is detected by spectrophotometer.
- Substrates are specific for each enzyme (o-phenyl-diamine-dihydrochloride for Horse radish peroxidase).

Types ***(Fig. 1.8.1)***

1. Noncompetitive Binding Assay

i. **Direct**
   - Antigen measuring system (well + serum (Ag) + primary antibody labeled with enzyme + substrate → Colour)

ii. **Indirect**
   - Antibody measuring system (Titre wells coated with antigens + serum (Ab) + Enzyme labelled antiantibodies + substrate → Colour)

2. Sandwich ELISA

- Well is coated with capture antibody + Serum (for Ag detection) + Antibody specific for Ag + substrate → Colour.
- Indirect Sandwich ELISA.
  - Primary antibody and the capture antibody belong to different species.
  - Another enzyme-labelled secondary antibody targeted against the primary antibody is added.
  - More specific than direct sandwich ELISA.

3. Competitive ELISA

- Unlabelled antibody is incubated with the serum to be tested for antigen.
- The antibody/antigen complexes are then added to the antigen coated well.
- Free antibody will bind to the well, more the test Ag in serum, less amount of free Ab will bind to the well.
- The plate is washed to remove unbound antibody.
- Antiglobulin specific to the primary antibody, coupled to enzyme is added.
- A substrate is added, and remaining enzymes elicit a chromogenic signal.
- For competitive ELISA, the higher the original antigen concentration, the weaker the eventual signal.

4. IgM capture ELISA

- Microtitre wells coated with anti IgM + Patient's serum (IgM) + Ag + Enzyme labelled secondary antibody + Substrate → Colour.

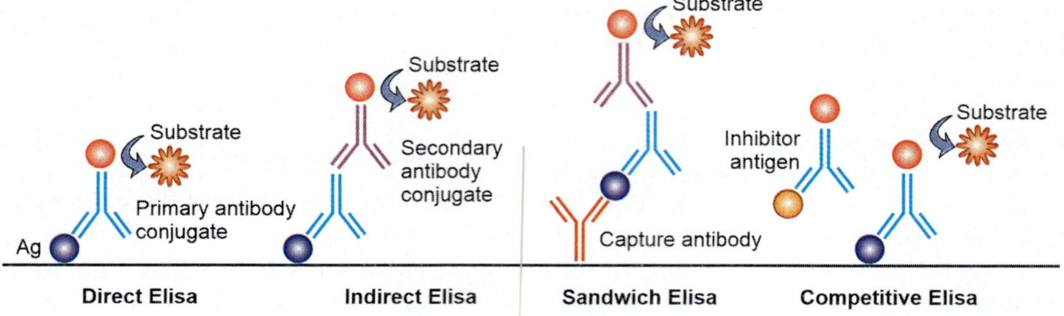

Fig. 1.8.1: Types of ELISA

5. Modifications of ELISA—Cassette ELISA. (Fig. 1.8.1)

- Ag is fixed on solid phase which is porous.
- Underneath the solid phase absorbing material is kept.
- The test sample where the Ab has to be detected is put on the solid phase.
- If the sample has Ab it will bind to the solid surface and then enzyme labelled antiglobulin is added, followed by substrate.
- Colour change occurs if the sample has Ab.

Applications of ELISA

1. *For antigen detection:* HBsAg, HBeAg, Dengue NS1 Ag.
2. *For antibody detection:* Hepatitis B, Hepatitis C, Toxoplasmosis, Dengue Leptospirosis.
3. Measuring hormone levels HCG (as a test for pregnancy), LH (determining the time of ovulation) TSH, T3 and T4 (for thyroid function).
4. For the detection of allergens in food and house dust.
5. Measuring rheumatoid factor and other auto-antibodies in autoimmune diseases: Anti CCP, anti-dsDNA
6. Measuring toxins in contaminated food.
7. Therapeutic drug monitoring—barbiturates, morphine, digoxin.

Advantages of ELISA

1. Economical.
2. 2–3 hours.
3. *High sensitivity:* Screening for HIV, Hepatitis B and C in blood bank.

Disadvantages of ELISA

1. More time compared to rapid tests.
2. Not preferred when sample load is low.

---

3. Discuss immune response under the following headings.

A. Define and classify the immune response with main functions (3 marks)

Immune Response

Definition

- Specific reactivity induced in the host by an antigenic stimulus.

Types

1. Humoral (antibody mediated).
2. Cellular (cell mediated).

Functions

Humoral immunity	• Directed primarily against toxin-induced diseases • Infections with capsulated bacteria (Pneumococci, Meningococci, *Haemophilus influenzae*) • Viral infections • Participates in the pathogenesis of immediate (1,2,3) hypersensitivity and certain autoimmune disorders
Cellular immunity	• Responsible for • Resistance to intracellular pathogens bacterial infections—tuberculosis, leprosy, listeriosis, brucellosis, viruses—measles, mumps • Resistance to fungal and protozoal infections • Resistance to tumours

B. What type of immunity is activated in toxin-mediated diseases? Explain the basis of this type of immune response. (1+6 marks)

- Humoral Immunity is active against toxin-mediated diseases.

Basis of Humoral Immune Response

- Humoral immunity is mediated by antibodies.
- Antibodies provide resistance through the following mechanisms.
  1. Antitoxin neutralises bacterial toxins (diphtheria, tetanus).
     - Antitoxins are formed by previous infection or through artificial immunisation
     - Neutralisation of toxin with antitoxin nullifies the effect of toxin
  2. Antibodies attach to the surface of bacteria and.
     - Act as opsonins and enhance phagocytosis
     - Prevent the adherence of microorganisms to their target cells, e.g. IgA in the gut
     - Activate the complement and that leads to bacterial lysis
     - Clump bacteria (agglutination) leading to phagocytosis

Three Steps in Antibody Production

1. Entry of antigen, its distribution in the tissue and contact with the appropriate immunocompetent cell (afferent limb).
2. Antigen processing by the cell and control of antibody production (Central limb).
3. Secretion of antibody, its distribution in the tissue and its effects (Efferent limb).

T-cell Independent Response

- *T cell independent Ag:* These are large multivalent structures, mostly polysaccharides that cross-link many IgM receptors—Signal 1

- Signal 2 has complement C3b derivatives bound to the bacterial cell or pathogen-associated molecular patterns.
- Short-lived responses dominated by IgM plasma cells, although some IgG is also generated.

T-cell Dependent Response

- T-cell–dependent antigen has some protein component.
- Ag is recognised followed by binding to the B-cell receptor (BCR) and the Ag is then endocytosed by the B cell.
- peptides are processed and complexed with class II MHC proteins.
- B cells present antigen to peptide-specific T follicular helper (Tfh) cells that had been previously activated by dendritic cells presenting the same peptide fragment of the antigen.
- Activated T cells now produce IL2,4,5 that stimulate the growth and differentiation of B cell.
- In the germinal center, the B-cell clones that receive more CD40 ligand (CD40L) and cytokines are able to proliferate, class switch, and become long-lived memory B cells and plasma cells.

Primary vs Secondary Immune Response ***(Fig. 1.8.2)***

Feature	Primary immune response	Secondary immune response
Occurrence	• The immune response developing to the first exposure to any antigen	• Occurs following re-exposure to the same Ag
Responding cells	• B and T cells	• Memory cells
Lag phase duration	• 4–7 days	• 1–4 days
Time taken for immune establishment	• Longer time	• Quick
First antibody produced during response	• IgM	• IgG
Level of antibodies	• Declines quickly	• Remains for a long period

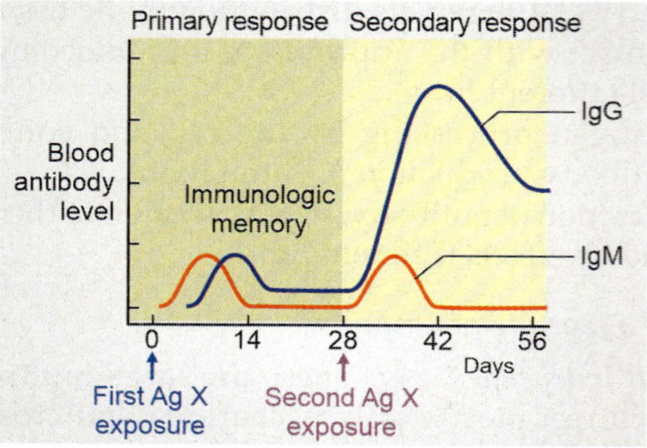

Fig. 1.8.2: Primary response vs secondary response

Tests for Evaluation of Humoral Immunity

1. Measuring the immunoglobulins (i.e., IgG, IgM, and IgA) in the patient's serum by nephelometry or by enumeration of B-cell numbers by flow cytometry.
2. *B-cell function in vivo:* absence of a normal rise in the concentration of IgM and IgG following immunisation points to either an intrinsic defect in the B cells or an extrinsic defect that inhibits T cells' capacity to provide help in activating B cells.

---

4. Which type of immunity plays a role in resistance against tuberculosis infection? Explain the different types of cells involved with the mechanism of this type of immune response. Add a note on evaluation of this type of immunity.
(1+6+3 marks)

- Cell-mediated immune response plays a role in resistance against *Mycobacterium tuberculosis*.

Cell-mediated Immunity

- Immune response that does not involve antibodies, but rather is mediated by cytotoxic T-lymphocytes, NK cells, macrophages and granulocytes and cytokines in response to an antigen.
- Exist in two forms.
  1. Delayed type hypersensitivity mediated by CD4+ Th1 cells.
  2. Cell-mediated lysis mediated by CD8+ cytotoxic T lymphocytes.

Mechanism of Cell-mediated Immunity ***(Figs 1.8.3 and 1.8.4)***

Activation of Cytotoxic T Cells

1. **Ag processing and presentation**
   - Cytosolic pathway.
   - Endogenous (intracellular) antigens (viral antigens and tumour antigens) are processed.
   - Presented along with MHC class I molecules to CD8 T cells.
2. **Activation of T-cells**
   - Activation of T cells requires 3 signals.
     - Ag specific signal is by binding MHC I + Ag to TCR
     - Co-stimulatory signal CD28(CTL)/B7 (APC)
     - IL-2 signaling inducing proliferation (CTL-P do not express IL-2 R)
       - IL-2 is provided by T_{H1} or CTL-P itself
       - IL-2R is expressed only after activation
   - Activated CD8 TC-cells proliferate and differentiate into a clone of effectors cells CTLs.
3. **Killing of the target cells by cytotoxic T cells**
   - Effectors CTLs kill target cells, i.e., nucleated cells (expressing MHC-I) infected with viruses, tumour cells or graft cells.

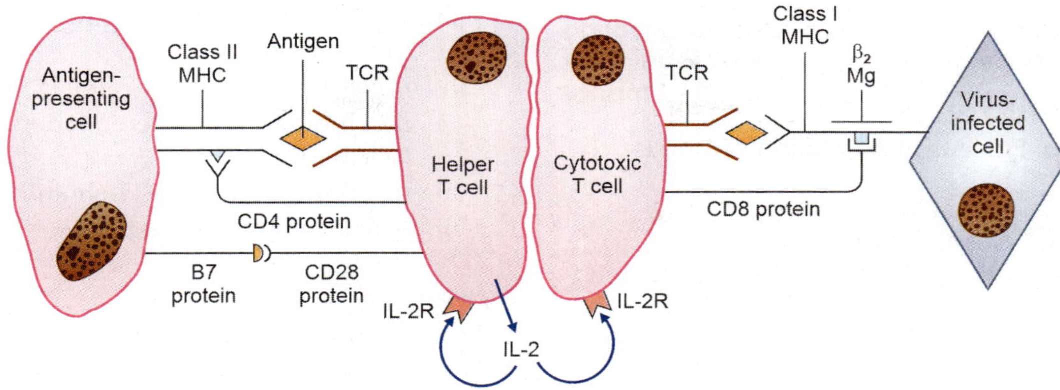

Fig. 1.8.3: Activation of T cells

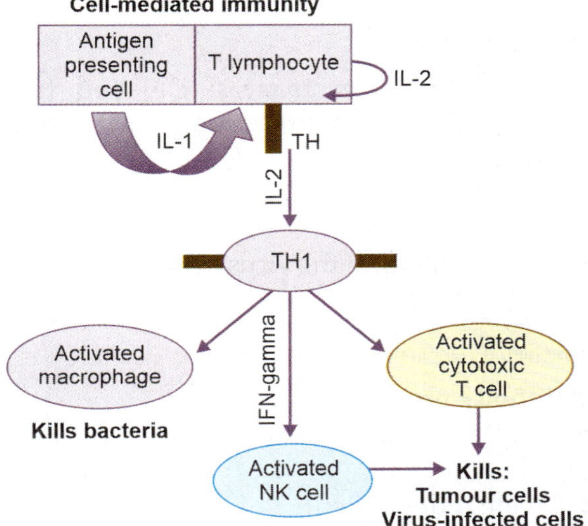

Fig. 1.8.4: Th1 immune response

- Perforins produce pores in the target cell membrane; through which granzymes are released inside.
- Granzymes are serine proteases; they induce cell death by apoptosis through caspase pathway.

Activation of Macrophages and delayed Type Hypersensitivity (DTH)

- Activated macrophages can also kill abnormal host cells (tumour cells).
- Cytotoxicity is nonspecific and stimulated by TNF, nitric oxide, enzymes, and oxygen metabolites.
- If infection is not fully resolved, activated macrophages cause tissue injury and fibrosis, i.e. DTH reaction.

Natural Killer Cells

- Play two important roles in immunity.
  1. Kill virus-infected cells and tumour cells.
  2. Produce gamma interferon that activate macrophages to kill the ingested bacteria.

Antibody-mediated Cell Cytotoxicity

- Antibodies bound to the infected cells are recognised by IgG receptors on the surface of macrophages, NK cells and the infected cell is killed.
- Antibody provides the specificity, e.g. macrophages, NK cells, neutrophils, eosinophils.
- Killing of target cell is accomplished.
  - Through perforin, granzyme (NK, Eosinophils).
  - Through TNF (Macrophages, NK).
  - Through lytic enzymes (macrophages, neutrophils, eosinophils, NK).

Delayed Type Hypersensitivity

- *Induction phase:* Memory T cells recognise their MHC plus peptide complex presented by APC and are activated
- TH1 cells secrete cytokines that activate local macrophages and recruit more macrophages and TH1 cells to area.
- If chronic antigen is present, a large mass of activated macrophages and TH1 cells may form a granuloma.
- *Granuloma:* Walled off portions of tissue within which microbes are trapped causing tissue damage

Evaluation of Cell-mediated Immunity

In Vivo Tests for Lymphoid Cell Competence

1. *Skin tests for the presence of delayed type of hypersensitivity:* Normal persons respond with delayed type of reactions to skin test antigen – *Candida*, streptokinase- streptodornase or mumps.
2. *Skin tests for the ability to develop delayed type hypersensitivity* to simple chemicals—DNCB.

In Vitro Tests for Lymphoid Cell Competence

1. *Lymphocyte blast transformation test:* When sensitized T lymphocytes are exposed to specific antigen, they transform into large blast cells with greatly enhanced DNA synthesis as measured by incorporation of tritiated thymidine.
2. Macrophage migration inhibitory factor is elaborated by cultured T cells when exposed to the Ag to which they are sensitized. Its effect can be measured by observing the reduced migration of macrophages in the presence of the factor compared with the levels in the controls.
3. Enumeration of T and B cell, subpopulations by flow cytometry.

5. Explain the immunological process of activation of T cells. Mention its effector and regulatory functions (8+2 marks)

Immunological Process of Activation of T cells

T cells

- Constitutes 65–80% of lymphocytes.
- Present in inner and subcortical region of lymphocytes.

Types of T cells

- T helper (CD4) cells.
  - Th1 cells
  - Th 2 cells
  - Th17 cells: produce IL17---Maintains mucosal barrier, recruit neutrophils
- Cytotoxic T cells (CD8 cells)
- Regulatory T cells (Suppressor T cells) CD4, CD 25

Activation of T Cells

Ag Presentation

- Cells present antigenic peptides (endogenous) with MHC Class I to cytotoxic T cells (CD8).
- Antigen presenting cells (dendritic cells, macrophages) present Ag with MHC Class II to helper T cells (CD4).

Antigen Processing

- *Cytosolic pathway:* For endogenous antigens (viruses, tumor)
- *Endocytic pathway:* For exogenous antigens (extracellular bacteria, toxins)

Activation of Helper T Cells (Figs 1.8.2 and 1.8.3)

- Two signals are required to activate T cells.
  - Interaction of antigen and the MHC protein with the T cell receptor specific for that antigen.
  - Second co-stimulatory signal is the B7 protein on APC must interact with CD28 protein on the helper T cell.
  - Interleukin-1 (IL-1) produced by the macrophage.
- T cell now produces IL-2 which is also known as T-cell growth factor.
- This stimulates the T cell to multiply into a clone of antigen specific helper cells capable of performing regulatory, effector and memory functions.

Effector T Cells

- Are of two subsets.
  1. Th1 cells.
     i. *IL2:* Activation of T cells, NK cells.
     ii. *IFN:* Activates macrophages, inflammation in delayed type of hypersensitivity, inhibits Th2 proliferation.
     iii. *TNF:* Enhances phagocytic activity of macrophages.
  2. Th2 cells.
     i. *IL4:* Inhibits Th1 differentiation, stimulates B cells to produce IgE.
     ii. *IL5:* Protection against helminths.
     iii. *IL 6:* B cell proliferation.

Memory T Cells

- Derived from activated helper T cells.
- Get activated on subsequent antigenic stimulus into effector cells.

Functions of T Cells

Effector Functions

1. *Th1 cells and macrophages:* Delayed type of hypersensitivity that protects against intracellular organisms.
2. *Th2 cells:* protection against helminths by IL 4, IL5.
3. *CD 8 cells:* killing of the virus infected cells, tumour cells, graft cells.

Regulatory Functions

1. **Antibody production**
   - T cell dependent: all classes of Ig, memory cells
   - T cell Independent: Polysaccharide Ag, only IgM, no memory
2. **Cell mediated immunity**

6. Discuss the activation and biological effects of complement system. (6+4 marks)

Complement System

- Components.
  - C1-C9, C1 has 3 subunits C1q, C1 r, C1 s.
  - Properdin system: factor B.
- Synthesised in the liver.
- Heat labile (inactivated at 56°C—1 hour).
- Complement plays a role in inflammatory responses of both the innate and adaptive immune responses.
- Present as proenzymes, which must be cleaved to active form.
- Activation of complement system is by either by.
  - Ag-Ab complex: Classic pathway.
  - Endotoxin: Lectin and alternative pathway.
- All the 3 pathways result in formation of C3b and Membrane attack complex (C5b,6,7,8,9).
- In the pathway, b fragment continues in the main pathway and a fragment is split off and has other functions.

Pathways of Complement Activation (Fig. 1.8.5)

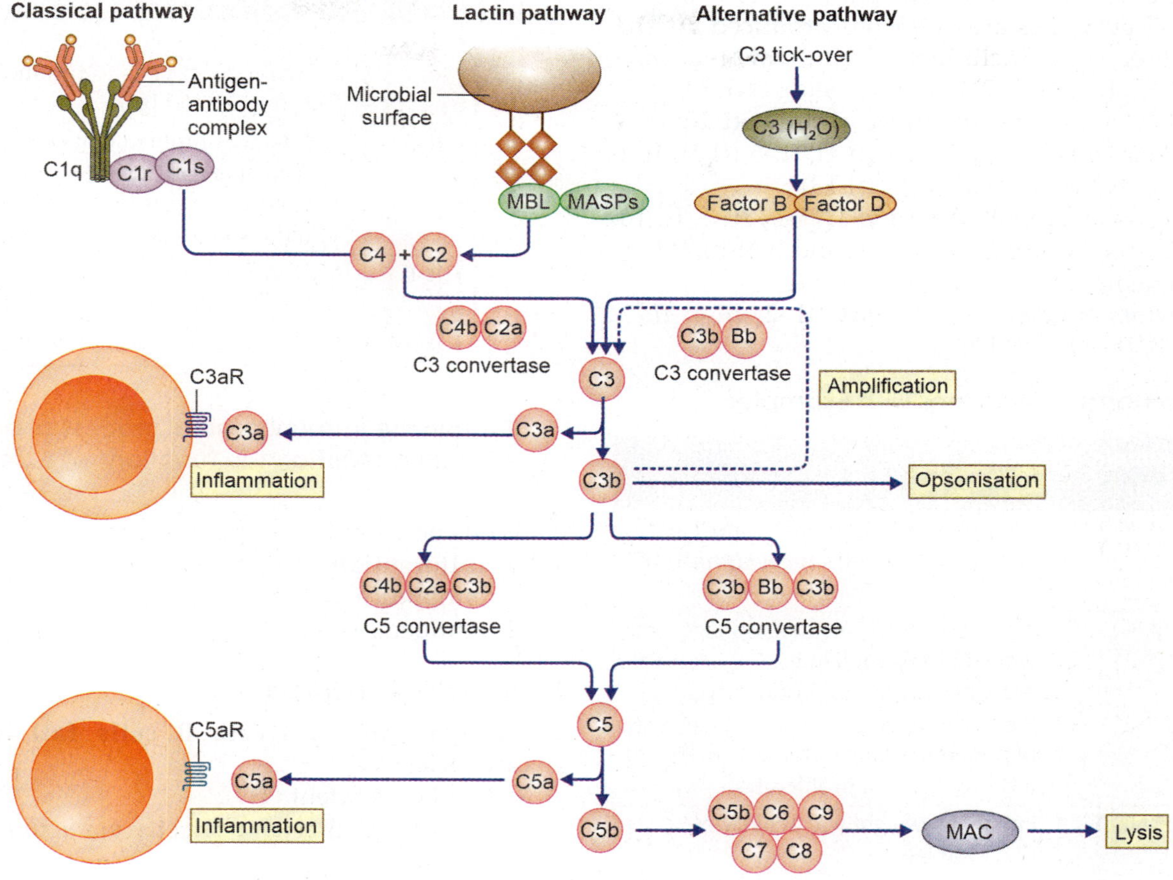

Fig. 1.8.5: Pathways of complement activation

Biological Functions of Complement

1. **Opsonisation:** Bacteria and viruses are phagocytized better in the presence of C3b due to the presence of C3b receptors on the surface of phagocytes.
2. **Chemotaxis**
   - C5a and the C5,6,7 complex attract neutrophils to the area.
   - C5a also enhances the adhesiveness of neutrophils to the endothelium.
3. **Anaphylatoxin:** C3a, C4a, and C5a—mast cell degranulation with release of mediators (e.g., histamine), leading to effects like increased vascular permeability and smooth muscle contraction, especially contraction of the bronchioles, leading to bronchospasm.
4. **Cytolysis**
   - Insertion of the C5b,6,7,8,9 membrane attack complex into the cell membrane forms a "pore" in the membrane.
   - *Results in lysis of cell:* Erythrocytes, bacteria, and tumour cells
5. **Enhancement of antibody production:** The binding of C3b derivatives to its receptors on the surface of activated B cells (complement receptor 2 [CR2]) provides the signal 2, which greatly enhances antibody production.

SHORT ESSAYS

1. Cytokine storm syndrome is one of the host responses post viral infections. Classify and enumerate the role of important cytokines with examples (2+3 marks)

Cytokines

- Low molecular weight biologically active proteins/glycoproteins produced by cells (lymphocytes, macrophages, platelets, and fibroblasts) that are activated by some stimulus.
- Peptide mediators, intracellular messengers, who regulate immunological, inflammatory, and reparative host cell responses.

Classification of Cytokines

1. *Lymphokines:* Biologically active substance released by activated T Lymphocytes.
2. *Monokines:* Substances secreted by monocytes and macrophages.

3. *Interleukins:* Produced by lymphocytes which exert a regulatory effect on other cells.
4. Type-1 cytokines are cytokines produced by Th1 T-helper cells. Include IL-2 (IL2), IFN-gamma (IFN-G), IL-12 (IL12) and TNF beta (TNF-b).
5. Type-2 cytokines are those produced by Th2 T-helper cells. Include IL-4 (IL4), IL-5 (IL5), IL-6 (IL6), IL-10(IL10), and IL-13 (IL13).
6. *Mediators of natural immunity:* TNF-α, IL-1, IL-10, IL-12, type I interferons (IFN-α and IFN-β), IFN-γ, and chemokines.
7. *Mediators of adaptive immunity:* IL-2, IL-4, IL-5, TGF-β, IL-10 and IFN-γ.

Role of Important Cytokines with Examples

Cyto-kines	*Example*	*Functions*
T_H1	• IL-2	1. Promotes activation of T_H and T_C cells 2. Activates NK cells to become LAK* cells
	• IFN-γ	1. Activates the resting macrophages into activated macrophage 2. Activates B cells to produce IgG 3. Promotes inflammation of delayed type of hypersensitivity (along with TNF-β) 4. Inhibits T_H2 cell proliferation
	• TNF-β	1. Enhances phagocytic activity of macrophage

Cyto-kines	*Example*	*Functions*
T_H2	• IL-4	1. Inhibits T_H1 cell differentiation 2. Stimulates B cells to produce IgE and also IgG4 and IgG1
	• IL-5	1. Enhances proliferation of eosinophils 2. Both IL-4 and IL-5 together provide protection against helminthic infections and also mediate allergic reaction
	• IL-6	1. Promotes B cell proliferation and antibody production
	• IL-10	1. Inhibits T_H1 cell differentiation

2. Explain the immunological process of activation of B cells. Mention the functions of B cells (4+2 marks)

- B cells perform two important functions.
  1. differentiate into plasma cells and produce antibodies.
  2. Antigen presentation to helper T cells.

B Cell Activation (Fig. 1.8.6)

- **Antigens that activate B cells fall into two categories:**
  - T cell dependent (TD).
    - Activate B cells indirectly via activation of T cells

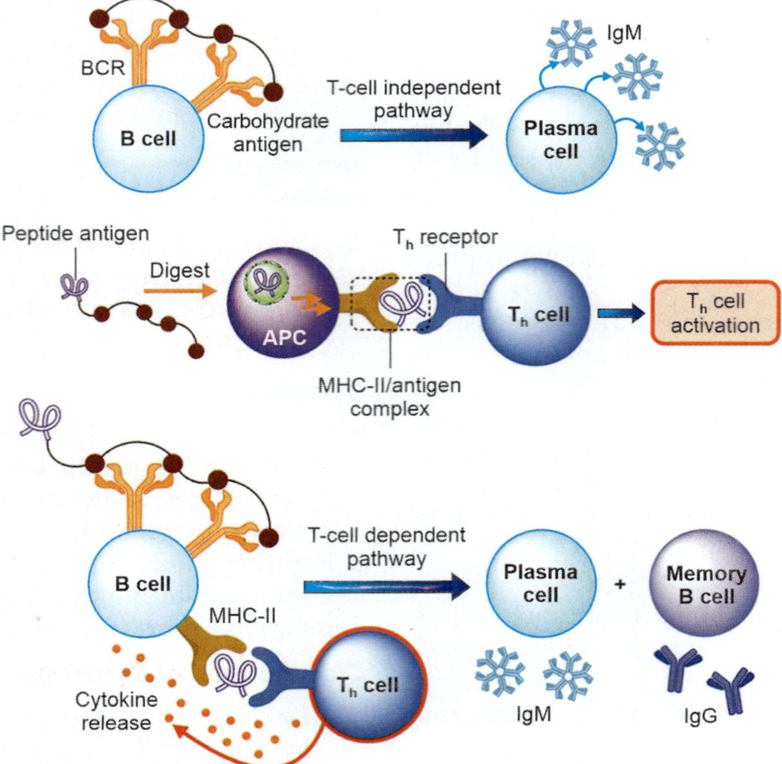

Fig. 1.8.6: Activation of B cells

- TD antigens are processed by APCs → presented to T_H cells following which the activated T_H cells → cytokines that in turn activate the B cells
- T cell independent (TI) antigens (e.g. bacterial capsule) are not processed by APC. They can directly activate B cells without the help of T cell induced cytokines.

- IL-2, IL-4 and IL-5 stimulate the growth and differentiation of the B cell.
- The activated B cells get converted to plasma cells and produce large amounts of immunoglobulins.
- Some activated B cells form memory cells which can remain quiescent for long periods but are capable of being activated rapidly on re-exposure to antigen.
- Effector function.
  - Secreted antibodies by plasma cells which in turn counter act with the microbes in many ways such as neutralisation, opsonisation, complement activation, etc.
  - Mediates mucosal immunity.

3. Discuss the biological effects of complement. (5 marks)

1. **Opsonisation**
   - Bacteria and viruses are phagocytized better in the presence of C3b due to the presence of C3b receptors on the surface of many phagocytes.
2. **Chemotaxis**
   - C5a and the C5,6,7 complex attract neutrophils.
   - C5a also enhances the adhesiveness of neutrophils to the endothelium.
3. **Anaphylatoxin**
   - C3a, C4a, and C5a cause mast cell degranulation with release of mediators (histamine), leading to the effects of increased vascular permeability and smooth muscle contraction, especially contraction of the bronchioles, leading to bronchospasm.
4. **Cytolysis**
   - Insertion of the C5b,6,7,8,9 membrane attack complex into the cell membrane forms a "pore" in the membrane.
   - results in the killing (lysis) of many types of cells, including erythrocytes, bacteria, and tumour cells.
5. **Enhancement of antibody production**
   - The binding of C3b derivatives to its receptors on the surface of activated B cells (complement receptor 2 [CR2]) provides the signal 2, which greatly enhances antibody production compared with that by B cells that are activated by antigen alone.

4. Define monoclonal antibodies. Write their applications. (1+4 marks)

Monoclonal Antibodies

- These are the antibodies produced by a single clone of cells or cell line and consisting of identical antibody molecules.

Applications

1. **Diagnostic uses**
   i. Identification of leucocytes.
   ii. HLA typing.
   iii. Identification of microorganisms.
   iv. Preparation of serological kits used for serodiagnosis of infection.
2. **Therapeutic uses (Table 1.8.1)**

5. In DPT vaccine, which component acts as an adjuvant. Write the mechanism of action of an adjuvant with 2 examples. (1+3+1 marks)

- In DPT vaccine, killed *Bordetella pertussis* component acts as Adjuvant.

Adjuvant

- A substance which enhances immunogenicity of an Ag

Mechanisms of Action

1. Depot action (slow release of Ag).
2. Modulation of immune system
3. Increase uptake by macrophage.
4. Enhance T cell activation.
5. Increase T cell proliferation.

Table 1.8.1 Therapeutic uses

Function	*Name*	*Target*	*Uses*
Transplant related immunosuppression	• Basiliximab • Daclizumab	• IL 2 receptor • CD 3 on T cell	• Prevent or treat allograft rejection and GVH
Treatment of autoimmune diseases	• Infliximab	• TNF—alpha	• Treatment of rheumatoid arthritis, Crohn's disease
Prevention of infectious diseases	• Palivizumab	• Fusion protein for RSV	• Prevents pneumonia in susceptible neonates
Treatment of cancer	• Rituximab	• CD 20 on B cell • Epidermal growth factor receptor	• Treatment of non-Hodgkin lymphoma, breast cancer.

Examples

1. Alum—used in vaccines (depot action).
2. Mineral oil.
3. Freund's incomplete adjuvant (water in oil emulsion + protein).
4. Freund's complete Adjuvant (water + protein with killed Tubercle bacilli + oil).

6. Detection of antinuclear antibody (ANA) by IF is suggested for the diagnosis of systemic lupus erythematosus (SLE). Discuss the principle, types, and applications of Immunofluorescence. (1+3+1 marks)

Immunofluorescence

Principle

- Ag–Ab reaction which involves antibody labelled with fluorochromes.
- Fluorescence is defined as the property of absorbing light rays of one wavelength and emitting light rays with a different wavelength.
- Fluorochromes are substances which get excited after absorption of UV light. After excitation the fluorochrome returns to normal level and while doing so emits visible light.
- Fluorochromes used.
  - *Fluorescein isothiocyanate*
    - Absorbs light of wavelength 490–495 nm and emits light of wavelength of 470 nm
    - It produces apple green colour
  - *Lissamine rhodamine*
    - Absorbs light of wavelength 460 nm and emits light of 480 nm
    - It produces orange red colour

Classification/Types of Immunofluorescence or Fluorescent Antibody Technique (Fig. 1.8.7)

1. Direct immunofluorescence

- Clinical sample for the detection of Ag is smeared on the slide.

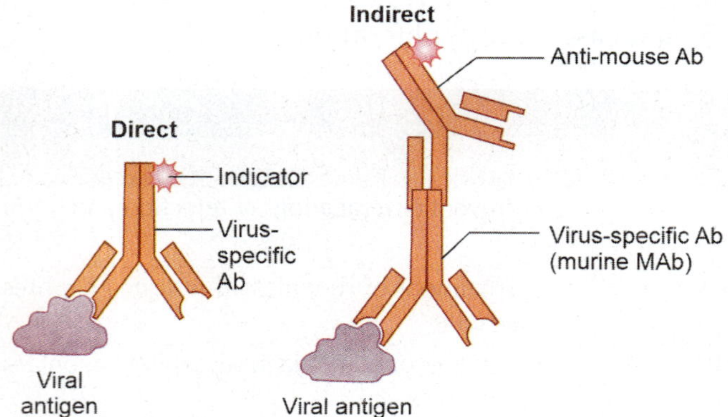

Fig. 1.8.7: Types of immunofluorescence or fluorescent antibody technique

- It is stained using specific Ab which is labelled with fluorochrome.
- If Ag is present, fluorescence is seen.

Use/Application

1. Detection of microbial Ag in the clinical samples.
   - Rabies Ag in the corneal smears
   - Herpes virus Ag in skin scraping

Advantages

1. Rapid diagnosis.
2. More specific than indirect IF.

Disadvantages

1. Requires labelling of each specific Ab.
2. Less sensitive than indirect IF.

2. Indirect Immunofluorescence

- Two-step procedure.
- Detection of either Ag or Ab.
- Ag is fixed onto the solid phase and unlabeled Ab is made to react with it.
- Free Abs are removed by washing.
- Fluorescent labelled antiglobulin is added and after the reaction free antiglobulin is washed.
- If Ag –Ab reaction has taken place, fluorescent labelled antiglobulin binds to the complex.

Uses/Application

1. Detection of specific Abs in *Chlamydia* infection, *Legionella* infection viral infections, extra-intestinal amoebiasis toxoplasmosis, kala azar.
2. Detection of antinuclear antibodies (ANA) in patients' serum.
3. Detection of antineutrophilic cytoplasmic antibody (ANCA) in patients' serum.

Advantages

1. More sensitive.
2. Requires only 1 Ab labelled with the fluorescent compound.
3. Possible to differentiate between IgM and IgG Ab in the clinical sample.

Disadvantages

1. Nonspecific fluorescence.
2. Longer procedure.

SHORT ANSWERS

1. Describe in brief about antigenic determinants of immunoglobulins with a neat labelled diagram. (2+2 marks)

Immunoglobulin Structure

- Glycoprotein made up of 2 light (L) and 2 heavy (H) polypeptide chains.
- Y shape.
- 4 chains are linked by disulfide bonds.

- L and H chains are subdivided into variable and constant regions. Regions are composed of 3 dimensionally, folded repeating segments called domains.
- L chain has 1 VL and 1 CL domain.
- H chain has 1 VH and 3 CH domains.
- *Variable region:* Antigen binding sites
- Within the variable region, there are some zones (hot spots) that show relatively higher variability in the amino acid sequences. Called as hypervariable regions or complementarity determining regions (CDRs). Form the antigen-binding site.
- *Constant region of H chain:* Biological functions (complement activation, binding to cell surface receptors)
- L chain 2 types—Kappa and lambda. Both occur in all the types, but 1 Ig has only 1 type of L chain.
- H chains are specific for each class.

Labelled Diagram of Immunoglobulin (Fig. 1.8.8)

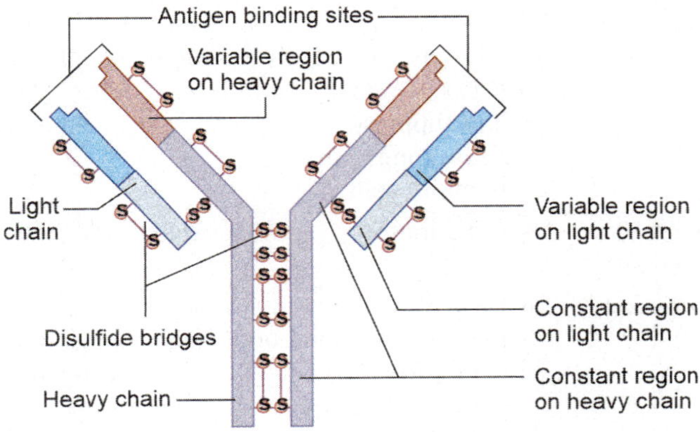

Fig. 1.8.8: Structure of immunoglobulin

2. Draw a neat, labelled diagram of Immunoglobulin M molecule. Enumerate its few properties and clinical significance. (2+2 marks)

Labelled Diagram of Immunoglobulin M (Fig. 1.8.9)

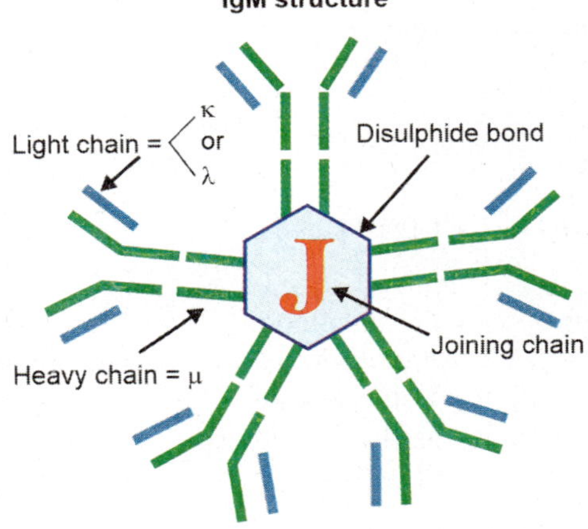

Fig. 1.8.9: Structure of immunoglobulin M

Properties of IgM

- Pentamer with 5 subunits and J chain.
- Highest molecular weight among all immunoglobulins.
- 5–10% of serum proteins.
- Distributed intravascularly.
- 2 forms.
  - *Monomeric:* Bound on the surface of B cells
  - *Pentameric:* Secreted form

Clinical Significance of IgM

1. Demonstration of IgM used in diagnosis of acute infections and congenital infections.
2. Protection against intravascular organisms.
3. Very efficient in agglutination opsonisation, complement fixation.

3. A nurse caring for a patient with varicella-zoster infection in an isolation ward. Which immunoglobulin titre measurement is required for nurse and patient to be tested? Briefly discuss the clinical significance of both these antibodies. (1+2 marks)

- IgM has to be detected in the patient for acute infection and IgG in the nurse for the antibody titre.

Clinical Significance of IgM

- Demonstration of IgM used in diagnosis of acute infections and congenital infections.
- Very efficient in agglutination opsonisation, complement fixation.
- *Protection against intravascular organisms:* Deficiency of IgM predisposes to septicaemia

Clinical Significance of IgG

- Predominant antibody in secondary response and defense against bacteria and viruses.
- Only antibody that can cross placenta—passive immunity to the newborn.
- Activates complement.
- Opsonisation and enhances phagocytosis.
- Participates in precipitation.
- Major role in neutralisation of toxins.

4. A 45-year-old man, alcoholic and h/o IV drug abuse for 15 years comes with severe jaundice. He has raised AST and ALT levels and has hepatitis B, due to which complement components are reduced. Briefly describe the clinical significance of complement deficiency. (3 marks)

Clinical Significance of Complement Deficiency

• Inherited (or acquired) deficiency of some complement components, especially C5–C8	• Neisseria bacteraemia

Contd.

• C3 deficiency	• Recurrent pyogenic sinus and respiratory tract infections.
• C1 esterase inhibitor deficiency	• Angioedema (acquired or genetic disease called hereditary angioedema
• Acquired or inherited deficiency of decay-accelerating factor (DAF)	• Paroxysmal nocturnal haemoglobinuria (increased complement mediated hemolysis)
• Complement levels: low	• Immune complex diseases (acute glomerulonephritis and systemic lupus erythematosus)
	• Severe liver disease (alcoholic cirrhosis or chronic hepatitis B) → predisposed to pyogenic infections

5. A 1-year-old baby admitted for recurrent *Staphylococcus* furuncles and fungal diaper rash. On examination, the paediatrician noticed mild hepatosplenomegaly with chronic lymphadenopathy and suspected as chronic granulomatous disease (CGD). Which cell type is affected in this case? Role of this type of cell in innate immunity. (1+2 marks)

- CGD is due to a defect in the intracellular microbicidal activity of phagocytes as a result of a lack of NADPH oxidase activity (or similar enzymes).
- Neutrophils are affected in this condition.

Role of Neutrophils in Innate Immunity

- Abundant, 50–60% of the circulating WBC.
- White blood cells, subgroup called granulocytes, named for their cytoplasmic granules.
- Phagocyte of innate immunity and is the first cell to respond in inflamed or necrotic tissue.
- Engulfs and kills bacteria and fungi, digests cellular debris.
- severe bacterial and fungal infections occur if they are too few in number (neutropenia) or are deficient in function.
- Neutrophils have surface receptors for IgG, making it easier for them to phagocytize opsonised microbes.
- "Two-edged" sword. The positive edge of the sword is their powerful microbicidal activity, but the negative edge is the tissue damage caused by the release of degradative enzymes.

6. Compare and contrast T lymphocytes and B lymphocytes (3 marks)

Feature	T lymphocytes	B lymphocytes
Percentage in peripheral blood	• 80% of circulating lymphocytes	• 20% of circulating lymphocytes
Life span	• Longer	• Shorter
Origin and maturity	• Originate in thymus and mature in bone marrow	• Bone marrow
Location	• Outside the lymph node	• Inside the lymph node
Distribution	• Parafollicular areas of cortex in lymph nodes, periarteriolar in the spleen	• Germinal centers of lymph nodes, spleen, gut, respiratory tract; also, subcapsular and medullary cords of lymph nodes
Surface receptor	• Immunoglobulin surface receptors	• T cell receptors
Cell surface marker	• CD3 in T cells	• CD19 in B cells
Types	• T cells: Cytotoxic T cells (CD8+ T cells), helper T cells (CD4+ T cells) and suppressors cells along with memory cells	• B cells: Plasma cells and memory cells
Secretory product	• Cytokines	• Antibodies
Functions	• Help lyse virus-infected cells tumour cells and intra-cellular bacterial pathogens	• Provide immunity against most foreign antigens and bacteria

7. Compare MHC 1 and MHC class II proteins. What is meant by MHC restriction? (3+1)

Feature	MHC Class I	MHC Class II
Nomenclature	• HLA-A, HLA-B, HLA-C	• HLA-DP, HLA-DQ, HLA-DR
Found on	• All nucleated somatic cells	• Macrophages, B-cells, Dendritic cells, Langerhans cells of skin and activated T cells
Recognised by	• CD8 TC cells	• CD4 TH cells
Functions	• Presentation of Ag to cytotoxic T cells leading to elimination of tumour or infected host cell	• Presentation of Ag to helper T cells which secrete cytokines

Contd.

MHC Restriction

- Means that different T cells are restricted to either Class I or Class II MHC antigens.
- Cytotoxic T cells are activated only by antigens presented in association with Class I MHC protein present on nucleated body cells, thus play a role in protecting against virus-infected cells or tumour cells.
- Helper CD4 cells are activated only by antigens presented along with Class II MHC proteins on the Antigen presenting cells, thus play a role in increasing the humoural immune response.

8. Comment on the principle of conjugate vaccine with one example. (3 marks)

- The immunogenicity of polysaccharide capsule vaccine is enhanced by coupling it with a carrier protein resulting in a stronger immunological response.
- T cell dependent response occurs, characterised by antibody class switching from IgM to IgG, memory cells and longer response, e.g. pneumococcal 'conjugate' vaccine.
- Conjugation of capsular polysaccharides on common serotypes of *Streptococcus pneumoniae* with a highly immunogenic protein, i.e. diphtheria toxoid, induces a B- and T-cell response resulting in mucosal immunity and thus protects against vaccine serotypes and also reduces vaccine serotype carrier rates.

9. Write about.

A. Class Switch over (2 marks)

B. Paratope (1 mark)

A. Class Switching

- Also called as Isotype switching.
- Mechanism that changes B cell production of antibodies from one type to another (IgM to IgG).
- In immune response, IgM is the first class of Ig to be formed, followed by other types—IgG, IgA.
- The new antibodies formed uses the same VH but different CH chains. Since the variable region does not change, class switching does not affect antigen specificity.
- *Significance of this phenomenon:* 4 isotypes have specialised functions. IgG is the major antibody in interstitial fluids, whereas IgA is the protective antibody of mucosal surfaces

B. Paratope

- The site on the hypervariable regions that make actual contact with the epitope of an antigen is called as paratope.

10. Describe in brief the mechanisms of "antibody diversity". (2 marks)

- 10^{11} possible heavy chain–light chain combinations.
- Antibody diversity depends on:
  - Multiple gene segments.
  - rearrangement into different sequences.
  - The combining of different l and h chains in the assembly of immunoglobulin molecules.
  - Mutations.
  - Junctional diversity applies primarily to the antibody heavy chain. Junctional diversity occurs by the addition of new nucleotides at the splice junctions between the V–D and D–J gene segments.
- The resulting antibodies have the potential to recognise the three-dimensional structure of a wide range of proteins, carbohydrates, nucleic acids, and lipids.

11. A clinician suspects parasitic infection in his patient. Blood tests reveal raised eosinophil counts. Which is the immunoglobulin raised in this condition? Enumerate the importance of this immunoglobulin. (1 + 3 marks)

- IgE levels in the serum is increased in parasitic infections.

Importance of IgE

- Produced in the linings of the respiratory tract and GIT.
- Least abundant serum Ig.
- Shortest half life.
- heat labile antibody (inactivated at 56°C in one hour).
- Has affinity for the surface of tissue cells (mainly mast cells) of the same species (homocytotropism).
- Extravascular in distribution.
- Mediates immediate hypersensitivity and participates in host defenses against certain parasites.

12. Compare T cell dependent and T cell independent antigens. (4 marks)

Feature	*T cell dependent antigen*	*T cell independent antigen*
Nature	Proteins	Lipopolysaccharide Capsular polysaccharide
Antigen processing and presentation	By APC to helper T cells is required	Ag directly stimulate B cells for production of antibodies without the assistance of T cells
Immunogenicity	Immunogenic over wide range of dose	Dose dependent immunogenicity

Contd.

Feature	*T cell dependent antigen*	*T cell independent antigen*
Polyclonal activation	No	Polyclonal activation of B cells occurs in high doses
Immunologic memory	Present	No immunologic memory
Affinity maturation	Yes	No
Isotype switching	Occurs (*i.e., antibodies of all classes are produced)*	No isotype switching

13. Write about the determinants of antigenicity. (3 marks)

Determinants of Antigenicity

1. Size
   - >100,000 Daltons. Molecules of lesser size are weakly immunogenic.
2. Foreignness.
   - Self-antigens are non-immunogenic because of self-tolerance.
   - To be immunogenic, molecules must be recognised as non self or foreign.
3. Chemical nature.
   - Proteins are highly immunogenic, then carbohydrates, lipid, nucleic acid.
4. Chemical complexity.
   - Amino acid homopolymers are less immunogenic than heteropolymers containing 2 or 3 different amino acids.
5. Susceptible to tissue enzyme digestion.
   - Latex particles are less immunogenic.
6. Dosage, route and timing of antigen administration.
7. Genetic constitution of the host (HLA genes) determines whether a molecule is an immunogen.

14. Describe Superantigens with examples. (2+1 marks)

Superantigens

- Superantigens are a subclass of antigens that cause overstimulation of the immune system.
- non-specific activation of T-cells which ends with polyclonal activation of T cells and massive cytokine release (IL-2 from the T cells and IL-1 and TNF from macrophages).
- Superantigens bind to the outside of MHC Class II protein and TCR of T cell without any specificity, resulting binding and activation of large numbers of T cells.
- **Cytokines:** IL2, TNF alpha, IL8 are responsible for nausea, vomiting, fever, endothelial damage, acute respiratory distress syndrome, DIC, shock, and multiple organ failure, e.g. staphylococcal enterotoxins, and toxic shock syndrome toxin
- Responsible for the effects seen in toxic shock syndrome, scalded skin syndrome, food poisoning.

15. Define antigen/immunogen, hapten, epitope/paratope. (1+1+1 marks)

Antigen

- Any substance which when introduced parenterally into the body stimulates production of antibody and reacts with it in a specific and observable manner.

Immunogen

- It is a substance which can induce immune response.
- Two attributes of complete antigen.
  - Ability to induce antibody production (immunogenicity).
  - Ability to react specifically with antibody (immunologic reaction).

Hapten

- A low molecular weight substance that cannot induce immune response by itself but can react with the specific antibody.
- Are not immunogenic.

Epitope/Paratope

- Small chemical groups on the antigen that can elicit and react with antibody.

16. Enumerate various abnormal immunoglobulins in different diseases conditions. (3 marks)

Abnormal Immunoglobulins

1. **Bence Jones proteins**
   - Monoclonal light chain excreted in urine of people suffering from multiple myeloma.
   - L chain made up of kappa or lambda.
   - Precipitates when heated to 60°C but dissolves at 70°C.
2. **Macroglobulinaemia (Waldenstorm's)**
   - Myeloma of IgM producing cells.
3. **Heavy chain disease**
   - Fc portion of heavy chain is excessively produced and excreted in urine in association with myeloma.

17. Discuss immunochromatography: Principle and applications. (2+2 marks)

Immunochromatography Assay (ICA)/Lateral Flow Test

- *Principle:* Combination of chromatography (separation of components of a sample based on differences in their movement through a sorbent) and immunochemical reactions

- Device to detect the presence of Ag or Ab.
- Cassette or strip format.
  - *Test band:* At the test line, the Ag-labelled Ab complex is immobilised by binding to the monoclonal Ab in the test line to form a Coloured band.
  - *Control band:* The free colloidal gold labelled Ab can move further and binds to the anti-human Ig to form a colour control band. Control band should be positive for the test to be valid.

Types

1. Sandwich assay
2. Competitive assay
3. Multiplex assay

Applications

1. Detection of HIV, hepatitis B antibodies in patient's serum.
2. Detection of dengue NS 1 Ag, IgG, IgM in patient serum.
3. Urine pregnancy test by detection of hCG.

18. Write about the principle and applications of Immunoblot. (3 marks)

Immunoblotting (Western Blotting)

- Is sensitive assay for the detection and characterisation of proteins based on the specificity of antigen-antibody recognition.

Principle

1. Involves the solubilisation and electrophoretic separation of proteins, glycoproteins, or lipopolysaccharides by gel electrophoresis (separates the proteins by size, charge).
2. Quantitative transfer of proteins and irreversible binding to nitrocellulose.
3. Immunoprobing, and visualisation using chromogenic or chemiluminescent substrates.

Applications

1. Identification of a specific protein in a complex mixture of proteins.
2. Estimation of the size and amount of protein in the mixture.
3. Supplemental test for HIV diagnosis.
4. To detect antibody in Lyme's disease, herpes simplex virus infection, cysticercosis, hydatid disease and toxoplasmosis.

19. Enzyme-linked fluorescent assay: Describe the principle and applications. (2+2 marks)

Enzyme-linked Fluorescent Assay (ELFA)

- Automated system.
- Single test format.
- 10 different analytes can be tested simultaneously.

Principle

- Based on the principle of detection of Ag–Ab enzyme complex by fluorescence.

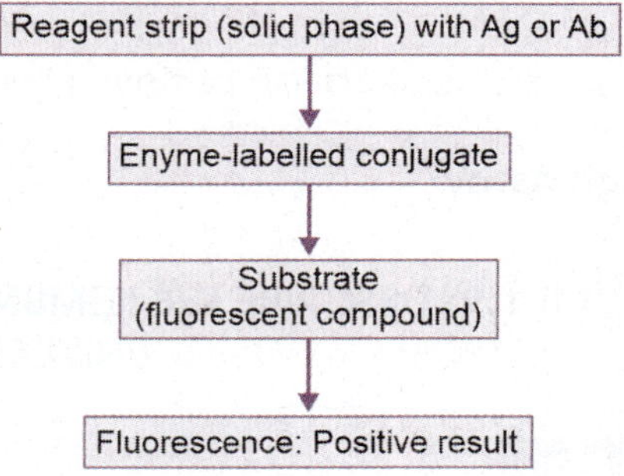

Applications

1. Detection of IgM and IgG of TORCH panel, hepatitis markers, measles, IgG, varicella IgG, Toxin of *Clostridium difficile*.
2. *Biomarker:* Procalcitonin.

20. Chemiluminescent-linked immunassay (CLIA). Describe the principle and applications. (2+2 marks)

Chemiluminescent-linked Immunassay (CLIA)

Principle

- Chemiluminescence (CL) is defined as the emission of electromagnetic radiation caused by a chemical reaction to produce light.
- An assay that combines chemiluminescence technique with immunochemical reactions.
- **CLIA utilize chemical probes:** Luminol, acridinium ester which could generate light emission through chemical reaction to label the antibody
- Detected by Luminometer.

Applications

1. Detection of antigens or antibodies to HIV, Hepatitis B, Hepatitis C, SARS CoV2.
2. *Biomarker:* PCT Q.

21. What are the major functions of T cells and B cells? (2+2 marks)

T cells

Regulatory Functions

1. Help B cells to develop into antibody producing plasma cells.
2. Help CD8 T cells to become activated cytotoxic T cells.

Effector Functions

1. Help macrophages effect delayed hypersensitivity.
2. CD8 cells perform cytotoxic functions; that is, they kill virus-infected, tumour and allograft cells.

B cells Functions

1. Differentiate into plasma cells and produce antibodies.
2. Antigen presentation to helper T cells.

22. Principle and application of flow through assay. (1+1 marks)

Flow Through Assay

Principle

- Sample flows *vertically* through the nitrocellulose membrane (NCM) as compared to lateral flow in ICT.

Application

- Flow-through tests can be used for both antigen and antibody detection, e.g. HIV TRIDOT test.

MI 1.9: DESCRIBE THE IMMUNOLOGICAL BASIS OF VACCINES AND DESCRIBE THE UNIVERSAL IMMUNISATION SCHEDULE

LONG ESSAY

1. Discuss in detail about methods of preparation of Vaccine under the following headings.

A. Define Vaccine and classify the types of Vaccines with examples (3 marks)

Definition of Vaccine

- A vaccine is a preparation that consist of either live, live attenuated or killed microorganisms, or microbial products or its genetic elements, used to induce active immunity in an individual, against that specific microorganism or infection caused by the same.

Type of Vaccines

Type of vaccine	*Examples*
Live vaccines (Historic)	• Smallpox vaccine
Attenuated live vaccines	• BCG vaccine
Inactivated (killed vaccines)	• DPT vaccine
Subunit vaccines and toxoids	• Hepatitis B virus vaccine • DPT vaccine
Conjugate vaccines	• *H. influenzae* b conjugate vaccine
Recombinant (Surface antigen) vaccines	• Hepatitis B Virus (HBV) vaccine
DNA vaccines	• H5N1 DNA vaccine
Anti-idiotypic vaccines	• HBV vaccine in animals
Edible vaccines	• Norwalk virus vaccine

B. Describe in brief different types of vaccines and its active component and their role. (4 marks)

Type of vaccine	*Active component and their role*
Live attenuated vaccines	• Virulent pathogenic organisms are treated to become attenuated and avirulent but retain antigenicity and immunogenicity
Inactivated vaccines	• Vaccine strain stimulates immunity, but microorganism cannot multiply

Contd.

Type of vaccine	*Active component and their role*
Subunit vaccines and	• A particular antigenic determinant induces a good protective immune response
Toxoids	• Modified bacterial toxin made nontoxic but retains immunogenicity
Conjugate vaccine	• Covalent coupling of polysaccharide antigen to a carrier protein can improve the T cell mediated immune response
Recombinant (Surface antigen) vaccines	• Produced using recombinant DNA technology or genetic engineering where genes for desired protective antigens are inserted into a plasmid vector and introduced into an expression system and protein is expressed in large quantities and then purified which induces humoural immunity
DNA vaccines	• DNA that codes protein antigen of the pathogen and inserted into a plasmid vector which induced both humoural and cellular immunity
Anti-idiotypic vaccines	• Antibodies (anti-idiotypes) can be raised against the idiotype in the antibody by injecting the antibody into another animal that has the potential to neutralise the virus
Edible vaccine	• Antigenic proteins that are genetically engineered into a consumable crop. When the crop is digested, some of the protein makes its way into the blood stream causing an immune response

C. Distinguish between a Vaccine and a toxoid. (2 marks)

Vaccine	*Toxoid*
• Live, live attenuated or killed microorganisms or their products • Made nontoxic by heating, disinfectant • Retains the capacity to stimulate active immunity, e.g. BCG, HBV vaccine	• Modified bacterial toxin • Made nontoxic but retains immunogenicity • Retain the capacity to stimulate the formation of antitoxin, e.g. tetanus toxoid

D. Give 2 examples for bacterial live attenuated vaccines (1 mark)

1. Bacillus Calmette–Guérin (BCG).
2. Typhoid vaccine.

SHORT ESSAYS

1. With respect to N-COVID 19, describe the available vaccines, the type, dose, schedule, efficacy and adverse effects. (5 marks)

- Refer Table 1.9.1

2. Describe the vaccines given for children included in Universal Immunisation schedule (from neonate to 9 years of age under the following headings.

A. BCG (Type of Vaccine, age of administration, route of administration, dose). (2 marks)

- *Type of vaccine:* Bacilli, Calmette Guerin—live attenuated vaccine—Danish strain
- *Age of administration:* Given at birth
- *Route of administration:* Intradermal
- *Dose:* 0.05 ml diluted with saline

B. MR (Type of Vaccine, age of administration, route of administration, dose). (2 marks)

- *Type of vaccine:* Measles, rubella—live attenuated vaccine
- *Age of administration:* 1st dose—9 months; 2nd dose—16–24 months
- *Route of administration:* Subcutaneous
- *Dose:* 0.05 ml

C. HBV Vaccine (age of administration, Site of administration). (1 mark)

- *Type of vaccine:* Hepatitis B vaccine—recombinant, subunit vaccine
- *Age of administration:* 0, 1, 6 months or at birth or 6, 10, 14 weeks
- *Route of administration:* Intramuscular
- *Dose:* 0.05 ml

3. Define "cold chain". Discuss various compartments of cold chain with examples. (1+4 marks)

Cold Chain Definition

- Refers to maintaining an optimum temperature required for manufacturing storage, transport, and handling of vaccines.

Various Compartments of Cold Chain

- The optimum temperature for refrigerated vaccines between 2°C and 8°C.
- *For frozen vaccines:* –15°C or lower
- Improper temperature maintenance leads to vaccine failure especially vaccines such as oral polio vaccine.
- *Vaccine storage in freezer compartment:* Polio and measles vaccines
- *Vaccine storage in cold part but not allowed to freeze:* DPT, *H influenzae* type B, hepatitis B vaccine

Vaccine Vial Monitor (VVM)

- A tool to monitor the potency of vaccine
- To check the efficiency of vaccines

Table 1.9.1 Available vaccines, the type, dose, schedule, efficacy and adverse effects

Vaccine Brand	Type	Dose	Schedule	Efficacy	Adverse Effects
Covishield (AstraZeneca)	Viral vector vaccine	2	12 weeks apart	90%	• Fever • Pain at the site of injection • Myalgia • Thrombosis • Thrombocytopenia
Covaxin	Inactivated virus vaccine	2	4 weeks apart	82%	• Fever • Pain at the site of injection • Myalgia
Moderna	mRNA vaccine	2	4 weeks apart	94.5%	• Anaphylaxis (<0.01)
Pfizer BioNTech	mRNA vaccine	2	3 weeks apart	95%	• Anaphylaxis (<0.01)
Johnson and Johnson's Janssen	Viral vector vaccine	1	—	66%	• Anaphylaxis (<0.01) • Thrombosis • Thrombocytopenia
Sinopharm-BBIBP	Inactivated virus vaccine	2	3 weeks apart	79%	• Fever • Pain at the site of injection • Myalgia
	Viral vector vaccine	2	3 weeks apart	90%	• None
	Inactivated virus vaccine	2	2 weeks apart	50%	• None

Features

- Heat sensitive label lining the vaccine vial.
- Outer blue circle, inner white square.
- Temperature, time affects inner square.

Staging of VVM

Stage 1

- **Inner square:** White → can be used

Stage 2

- **Inner square:** Pale blue → can be used

Stage 3

- **Inner square:** Blue → discard the vial

Stage 4

- **Inner square:** Dark blue → discard

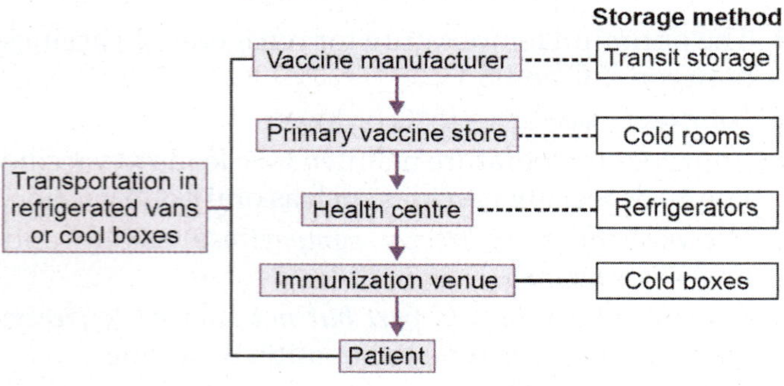

4. **Enumerate live attenuated and killed vaccines. (4 marks)**

Bacterial	
Live attenuated	*Killed*
BCG	• Typhoid
Typhoral	• Cholera
	• Pertussis
	• Plague
	• Diphtheria, pertussis, tetanus (DPT)

Viral	
Live attenuated	*Killed*
OPV (Sabin)	• IPV(Salk)
Live attenuated Influenza	• Killed influenza vaccine
Japanese B encephalitis (14–14-2 strain)	• Japanese B encephalitis
MMR	• (Nakayama strain)
Yellow fever 17 D vaccine	• Rabies
Hepatitis A	• Hepatitis A
Rotavirus	

SHORT ANSWERS

1. **Compare and contrast the features in OPV and IPV (3 marks)**

Feature	*Inactivated polio vaccine*	*Oral polio vaccine*
Type	Killed formalised vaccine	Live attenuated vaccine
Route of administration	Intramuscular	Orally
Type of immunity induces	Humoural immunity only	Humoural and local immunity quickly
Paralysis	Prevents paralysis	Prevents paralysis and reinfection
Herd immunity	No	Herd immunity is produced
Epidemic control	Not useful	Useful in epidemics control
Storage requirement	Does not require stringent storage and transport conditions	Requires stringent storage and transport conditions
Shelf life	Longer	Shorter
Price	Costlier	Cheaper

2. **Mention the complete schedule of DPT vaccine. What is the role of adjuvant in it? (1+2 marks)**

Diphtheria, Pertussis, Tetanus Toxoid Vaccine (DPT Vaccine)

Schedule

- At 6, 10, 14 weeks.
- Booster dose DPT → 1st: 16–24 months DT-I 2nd: 5–6 years, TT-3rd: 10 years and 16 years.
- *Dose:* 0.5 ml
- *Route of administration:* Intramuscular

Role of Adjuvant

- Adjuvants have a component which increase the immunogenicity of the vaccine antigen.
- Alum and pertussis component acts as adjuvant in DPT vaccine.

3. **Enumerate the diseases treated with hyper-immune human immunoglobulins and its indications. (3 marks)**

Immunoglobulin preparation	*Indications*
Diphtheria	• Respiratory Diphtheria
Tetanus Ig	• Post exposure prophylaxis (PEP) of tetanus for inadequately immunised individuals

Contd.

Immunoglobulin preparation	*Indications*
Botulinum antitoxin	• Botulism
Varicella zoster Ig	• PEP for immunosuppressed contacts of acute cases or newborn contacts
Rabies Ig	• Treatment of rabies and PEP in previously unimmunised individuals
Hepatitis B Ig	• PEP as percutaneous/mucosal/sexual exposure, newborn of HBsAg positive mothers
Rubella	• Women exposed in early pregnancy

4. Mention the properties of live attenuated vaccines and give 2 examples. (3 marks)

Properties

1. Induces long-lasting immunity.
2. Induces herd-immunity.
3. Induces good cell-mediated immunity as well as local immunity.
4. Multiple booster doses may not be required.
5. Mimics natural infection.
6. Immunoglobulins IgA and IgG produced.

Examples

1. Bacillus-Calmette Guérin (BCG vaccine).
2. Sabin polio vaccine.

5. Conjugate vaccines. Give 2 examples. Write advantages and disadvantages. (1 + 1 + 1 marks)

Conjugate Vaccines

- Covalent coupling of polysaccharide antigen to a carrier protein can improve the immune response elicited.

Examples

1. *H. influenzae* b conjugate vaccine.
2. Typhoid Vi conjugate vaccine.

Advantages

- Conjugation of a polysaccharide antigen to a carrier protein brings about a T-cell dependent immune response, and thereby memory.

Disadvantages

- Infants/young children have immature immune systems, may not recognising certain antigens.

6. Subunit vaccine. Give 2 examples, the merits and demerits. (1 + 1 + 1 marks)

Subunit Vaccine

- Contains only a particular antigenic determinant which induces a good protective immune response.

Examples

1. Influenza vaccines.
2. Herpes simplex vaccines.
3. Hepatitis B vaccine.
4. Typhoid Vi polysaccharide vaccine.

Advantages

1. Safe.
2. Induces specific immune response.

Disadvantage

1. Expensive.

7. A 3-year-old c/o of severe diarrhoea with dehydration. Stool sample was positive for capsid antigens of the virus. Briefly explain the prophylaxis available for this condition for this child (3 marks)

Prophylaxis Required

- Rotavirus vaccine.
- Rotavac—live attenuated G9P(10) strain and Rotarix-G1P(8) stain.
  - *Dose:* 5 drops
  - *Schedule:* At 6,10, 14 weeks
  - *Route of administration:* Oral
  - *Efficacy:* 55%
  - *Side effects:* Crying, irritability, fever, diarrhoea

8. A 28-year-old woman who had tested positive for hepatitis B surface antigen delivered a child. Explain in detail the recommended therapy to minimise the transmission to the neonate. (3 marks)

- **Hepatitis B vaccination.**
  - *Route of administration:* Intramuscular
  - *Dose:* 0.5 ml dose
  - *Schedule:* Within 12 hours of birth, 2nd dose: 1 month, 3rd dose: 6 months
- **Hepatitis B Immunoglobulin.**
  - *Route of administration:* Intramuscular
  - *Dose:* 300–500 IU
  - *Schedule:* Immediately within 12 hours of birth.

MI 1.10 DESCRIBE THE IMMUNOLOGICAL MECHANISMS IN IMMUNOLOGICAL DISORDERS (HYPERSENSITIVITY, AUTOIMMUNITY, IMMUNODEFICIENCY DISORDERS) AND THE LABORATORY METHODS USED IN THE DETECTION

LONG ESSAY

1. A 32-year-old business executive at the department of emergency medicine and critical care developed breathlessness, repeated hitting sensation in the head and chest tightness followed by an intramuscular injection of penicillin for treatment of cellulitis. IV antihistamines and IM adrenaline was given. O_2 therapy also administered. Patient recovered on the same day.

A. Define and classify hypersensitivity reactions (2 marks)

Hypersensitivity

Definition

- Hypersensitivity is an augmented immune response in a sensitised host, following subsequent contact with specific antigen which is harmful to the host.

Classification (Combs and Gell)

A. **Immediate hypersensitivity reaction**
   1. Type I hypersensitivity
   2. Type II hypersensitivity
   3. Type III hypersensitivity

B. **Delayed hypersensitivity reaction**
   1. Type IV hypersensitivity.

B. Mechanism, mediators and manifestations of hypersensitivity in this case. (7 marks)

- Type I Hypersensitivity is mediated in this case.

Mechanism

1. **Sensitisation phase**
   - The allergen induces IgE antibody which binds to mast cells and basophils when exposed to the allergen the first time (priming dose).
2. **Effector phase**
   - The allergen crosslinks the bound IgE when exposed to allergen again and induces degranulation and release of mediators (shocking dose).

Mediators

1. **Primary mediators (preformed)**

Histamine	• The most important vasoactive amine in human anaphylaxis • Formed by decarboxylation of histidine found in granules of mast cells, basophils, and platelets • It causes vasodilatation, increased capillary permeability and smooth muscle contraction

Contd.

Serotonin (s-hydroxy tryptamine)	• Base derived from decarboxylation of tryptophan • Found in intestinal mucosa, brain tissue and platelets • It causes smooth muscle contraction, increased capillary permeability and vasoconstriction
Chemotactic factor	• Accumulate at the site of injury • Eosinophilic chemotactic factor—chemotaxis • Neutrophilic chemotactic factor—chemotaxis
Enzymatic mediators	• Proteases and hydrolases—bronchial mucous secretion, degradation of blood vessel basement membrane

2. **Secondary mediators**
   - These are either synthesized after target cell activation or released by the breakdown of membrane phospholipids during degranulation.

Slow reacting substance of anaphylaxis (SRS-A)	• Contraction of smooth muscles in lungs and cause increased vascular permeability
Prostaglandins and thromboxane A2	• Prostaglandins cause dilatation and increase vascular permeability of capillaries and bronchoconstriction • Thromboxane aggregates platelets and cause vasodilatation and increased mucous secretion
Platelet activating factor (PAF)	• Released from basophils which cause aggregation of platelets and release of their vasoactive amines

Manifestations (Table 1.10.1)

C. Common allergens associated with this type of hypersensitivity. (2 marks)

1. *Drugs:* Aspirin, antibiotics (penicillin, streptomycin), vitamins (thiamine, folic acid).
2. *Insect venom:* Honeybees, wasps, hornets.
3. Fish.
4. *Legumes:* Peanut beans.
5. *Seeds:* Sesame, mustard.
6. Nuts, berries.
7. *Hormones:* Insulin.
8. *Crustaceans:* Lobster, crab.

Table 1.10.1 Manifestations

Main Organ Affected	*Disease*	*Allergens*	*Clinical System*	*Route of Exposure*
Lung	• Asthma	• Egg • Feather • Grass pollen • House dust mite	• Wheezing • Dyspnoea • Tachypnoea	• Inhalation
Eye	• Rhinitis • Conjunctivitis • Hay fever	• Pollen	• Running nose, • Redness and itching of eye	—
Skin	• Eczema (atopic dermatitis) • itching	• food	• Pruritic vascular lesions • Pruritic bullous lesions	• Ingestion
Intestinal tract	• Allergic • Gastroenteropathy	• Foods	• Vomiting and diarrhoea	• Ingestion
Systemic	• Anaphylaxis	• Insect venom • Drugs • Nuts	• Shock • Hypotension • Wheezing	• Sting • Various • Ingestion

D. How do you detect and treat this type of hypersensitivity? (2+2 marks)

Detection

History

- Type, duration, season.

Allergy skin testing

- Cutaneous test, patch test, scratch test.
- **Advantages**
  1. Allows screening of a large number of allergens at one time.
  2. Results are available with no delay.
- **Disadvantages**
  1. May sensitize to new allergens.
  2. May rarely induce systemic anaphylaxis.
  3. Principle disadvantage is the need to discontinue certain inhibitory drugs.

Tests for IgE levels

- Radioallergosorbant test (RAST).

Treatment

- Drugs to counteract the action of mediators.
- Ensuring a protected airway.
- Support of respiratory and cardiac function.
- Single or in combination epinephrine, antihistamines, corticosteroids, or cromolyn sodium, should be given. Cromolyn sodium prevents release of mediators (e.g., histamine) from mast cell granules.
- Prevention by identifing the allergen by a skin test and avoidance of that allergen.

SHORT ESSAYS

1. Define atopy and its mechanism with examples. (1+4 marks)

Atopy

Definition

- Refers to an inheritance propensity to respond immunologically to common naturally occurring inhaled or ingested allergens with the continual production of IgE antibodies.

Mechanism

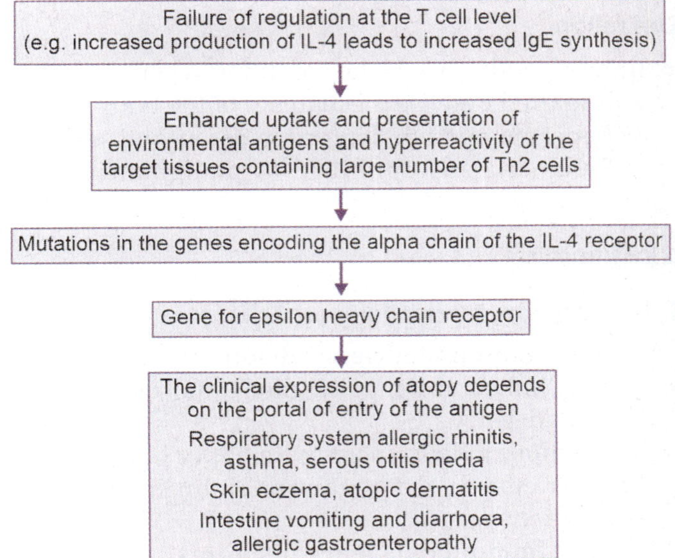

Examples

1. Pollen allergens.
2. House dust mite.
3. *Mould allergens:* Fungal spores.
4. *Arthropod allergens: Dermatophagoides pteronyssinus.*
5. *Animal allergens:* Household pets like cats and dogs.
6. *Food allergens:* Legume, cow's milk, egg white.

2. A 9-month-old child with h/o diarrhoea, several episodes of respiratory tract infections. O/E paediatrician noticed gingivostomatitis due to HSV along with oral thrush. X-ray revealed absence of thymic shadow and blood picture showed absence of T lymphocytes. Mother gives a h/o rash after birth.

A. What is the most likely diagnosis of this case? (1 mark)

- DiGeorge syndrome.

B. Briefly describe about this condition and its treatment. (2 marks)

DiGeorge Syndrome

- Absence of T cells and suppressed antibody responses.
- Defective development of pharyngeal pouches, associated with chromosome 22 deletions, congenital defect in development of thymus.
- Viral, fungal, and protozoal infections; tetany caused by hypoparathyroidism.
- *Treatment:* Thymus transplant.

C. Define and classify immunodeficiency disorders. (2 marks)

Definition

- Immunodeficiency is the condition where
  - Impaired defense mechanism of the body.
  - Repeated microbial infection of varying severity.
  - Enhanced susceptibility to malignancies and autoimmune diseases.

Classification

I. Primary/Congenital Immunodeficiency

1. **B cell immunodeficiency disorders.**
   i. X linked gammaglobulinaemia selective IgA deficiency.
   ii. Immunodeficiencies with hyper IgM.
   iii. Transient hypogammaglobulinaemia of infancy.
2. **T cell immunodeficiency disorders.**
   i. Thymic aplasia (DiGeorge's).
   ii. Chronic mucocutaneous candidiasis.
3. **Combined B cell and T cell deficiencies.**
   i. Severe combined immunodeficiency (SCID).
   ii. Wiskott-Aldrich syndrome.
   iii. Ataxia–Telangiectasia.
4. **Disorders of phagocytosis.**
   i. Chronic granulomatous disease.
   ii. Chediak–Higashi syndrome.
   iii. Job's syndrome.
5. **Disorders of complements.**
   i. Hereditary angioedema.
   ii. Paroxysmal nocturnal Haemoglobinuria.
   iii. Recurrent pyogenic infections.
   iv. Autoimmune disorders.

II. Secondary/Acquired Immunodeficiency

i. *Viral infections:* HIV, measles.
ii. *Bacterial infections:* Lepromatous leprosy.

3. Describe the immunodeficiency disorders and their molecular defect with clinical manifestations. (5 marks)

See Table 1.10.2

4. A 36-year-old auditor comes to the hospital, he shows signs of excessive nervousness, irritability, and complaints it's too hot in the room. O/E he has goitre and exophthalmia. Laboratory analysis of his blood reveals high antibody titres against the thyroid-stimulating hormone (TSH) receptor.

A. What is the most likely diagnosis? (1 mark)

- Graves' disease.

B. Define Autoimmunity. Classify auto-Immune diseases with examples. (1 + 3 marks)

Definition

- Autoimmunity is a condition in which the body's own immunologically competent cells or antibodies act against its self-antigens resulting in structural or functional damage.

Classification

I. Local/Single Organ Autoimmune Diseases

1. **Addison's disease**
   - Characterized by lymphocytic infiltration of adrenal glands and the presence of circulating antibodies directed against the cells of zona glomerulosa.
2. **Graves' disease**
   - Auto antibodies that the receptor for TSH, activating adenylate cyclase and resulting in over production of hormones.
   - Low TSH levels.

Table 1.10.2 Manifestations

Deficient component and name of disease	*Specific deficiency*	*Molecular defect*	*Clinical features*
B cell			
• X-linked (Bruton's)	• Absence of B cells; very low Ig levels	• Mutant tyrosine kinase	• Pyogenic infections (*S. aureus, H, influenza, S. peumoniae)*
• Selective IgA	• Very low IgA levels	• Failure of heavy-chain gene switching	• Sinus and lung infections
T cell			
• Thymic aplasia (DiGeorge's)	• Absence of T cells	• Defective development of pharyngeal pouches; not a genetic disease	• Viral, fungal, and protozoal infections • Tetany
• Chronic mucocutaneous candidiasis	• Deficient T-cell response to *Candida*	• Unknown	• Skin and mucous membrane infections with *Candida*
Combined			
• Severe combined immunodeficiency (SCID)	• Both B-cell and T-cell function deficiency	• Either defective IL-2 receptor, defective recombinases, defective kinases, absence of class II MHC proteins, or ADA or PNP deficiency	• Bacterial, viral, fungal, and protozoal infections
Complement deficiencies			
• Hereditary angioedema	• Deficiency of C1 protease inhibitor	• Too much C3a, C4a, and C5a generated	• Edema, especially laryngeal edema
• C3b	• Insufficient C3	• Unknown	• Pyogenic infections, especially with *S. aureus*
• C6,7,8	• Insufficient C6,7,8	• Unknown	• *Neisseria* infections
Phagocyte deficiencies			
• Chronic granulomatous disease	• Defective bactericidal activity because no oxidative burst	• Deficient NADPH oxidase activity	• Pyogenic infections, especially with *S. aureus*

3. **Myasthenia gravis**
   - Autoantibodies that bind the acetylcholine receptors on the motor end plates of muscles.

II. Systemic Type

1. **Rheumatoid arthritis**
   - Chronic inflammatory response ultimately destroys cartilage and bone, rendering the affected joints immobile.
   - The rheumatoid factors are an IgM antibody that binds to circulatory IgG forming. IgM-IgG complexes that are deposited in the joints.
2. **Sjogren's syndrome**
   - Triad of keratoconjunctivitis sicca (dry eyes), xerostomia (dryness of mouth) with or without salivary gland enlargement and rheumatoid arthritis.
3. **SLE**
   - Affected individual produces autoantibodies to vast array of tissue antigen such as DNA, histones, RBCs, platelets, leucocytes, and clotting factors.

5. Briefly describe type 2 hypersensitivity with examples. (5 marks)

Type 2 Hypersensitivity

- These reactions involve a combination of IgG (rarely IgM) antibodies with the antigenic determinants on the surface of cells leading to cytotoxic or cytolytic effects.

Mechanism **(*Fig. 1.10.1*)**

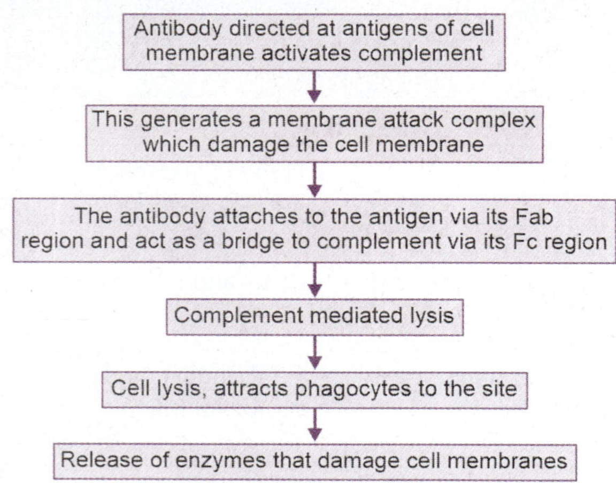

Examples

I. **Hypersensitivity reactions against erythrocytes**
   1. Non compatible blood transfusion -mismatch of ABO blood group, severely destroy RBCs.
   2. Rh incompatibility—Hemolytic disease of newborn.
   3. Autoimmune haemolytic anaemia—Conversion of a hapten to a full antigen by drug induce self-antibody.
   4. Drug induced haemolytic anemia—Penicillin, quinidine.

II. **Hypersensitivity reactions due to infections**
   1. Rheumatic fever after group A *Streptococcus* infection.
   2. Haemolytic anaemia after *Mycoplasma pneumoniae* infection.

III. **Superacute rejection** in allogenic organ transplantation—due to prior sensitisation

IV. **Hypersensitivity against solid organs**
   1. *Good pasture syndrome:* Antibody to basement membrane of kidneys and lungs.
   2. *Graves' disease:* Antibody to TSH receptors.
   3. *Myasthenia gravis:* Antibody to acetylcholine receptors.

6. Briefly describe type 3 hypersensitivity with examples. (5 marks)

Type 3 Hypersensitivity

- An inflammatory response in tissues caused by the deposition of antigen-antibody complexes.
- There is inflammation of blood vessels, kidney glomerular membranes, joints and skin.

Mechanism **(*Fig. 1.10.2*)**

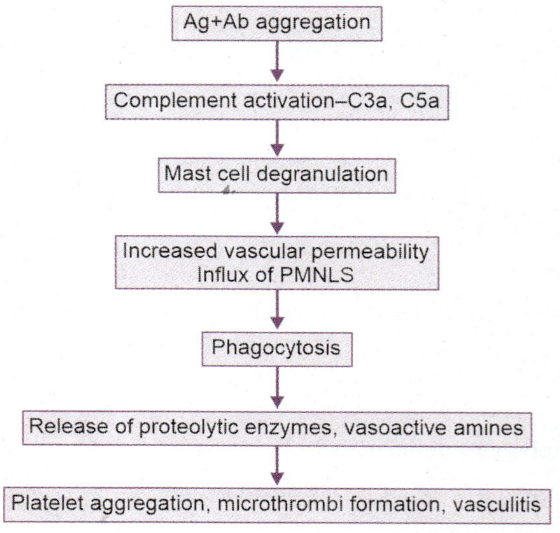

Reactions

1. Cutaneous Arthus Reaction

- It is the inflammation caused by the deposition of immune complexes at a localised site.
- Arthus response are slow and more persistent.
- **Clinical manifestations**
  i. Farmer's lung.
    - Hypersensitivity pneumonitis or allergic alveolitis
    - Associated with the repeated inhalation of thermophilic actinomycetes growing in plant material (hay)

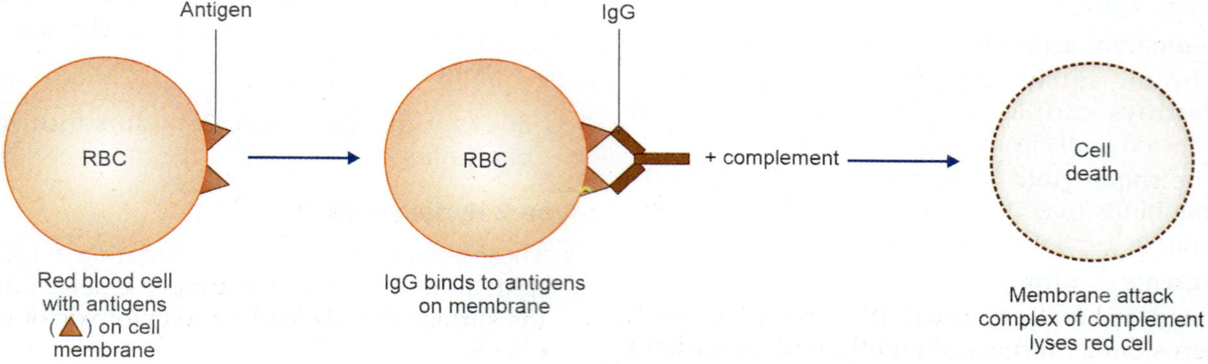

Fig. 1.10.1: Mechanism of type 3 hypersensitivity

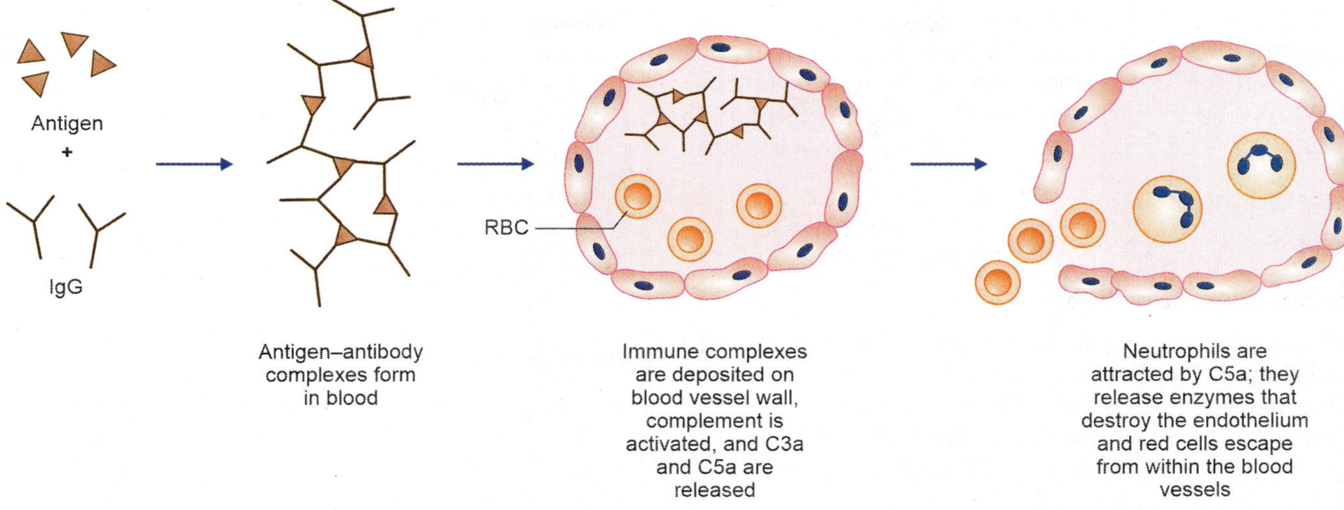

Fig. 1.10.2: Mechanism of type 3 hypersensitivity

ii. Cheese worker's lung.
   - Extrinsic allergic alveolitis caused by the inhalation of spores of *Penicillium casei* from moldy cheese

iii. Wood worker's lung.
   - Inhalation of wood particles in an occupational setting can cause various lung symptoms

iv. Mushroom worker's lung.
   - Inhalation of thermophile actinomycetes in the compost

2. *Systemic Serum Sickness*

- Systemic inflammatory response due to the presence of immune complexes deposited in many areas of the body.
- This condition occurs after administration of a large dose of foreign antigen (antiserum or certain drugs).
- **Clinical manifestations**
  - First sign is often a pruritic rash, which may be urticarial, maculopapular, or erythematous.
  - Fever, arthralgia, lymphadenopathy, splenomegaly and eosinophilia complete the clinical features.
  - Occasionally there are headache, nausea and vomiting.
  - Recovery takes 7–10 days.

Examples

1. Glomerulonephritis.
2. Rheumatoid arthritis.
3. Systemic lupus erythematosus.

---

7. "AutoImmunity results due to breakdown of immunological tolerance". Describe the mechanism of autoimmunity in support of the statement given. (5 marks)

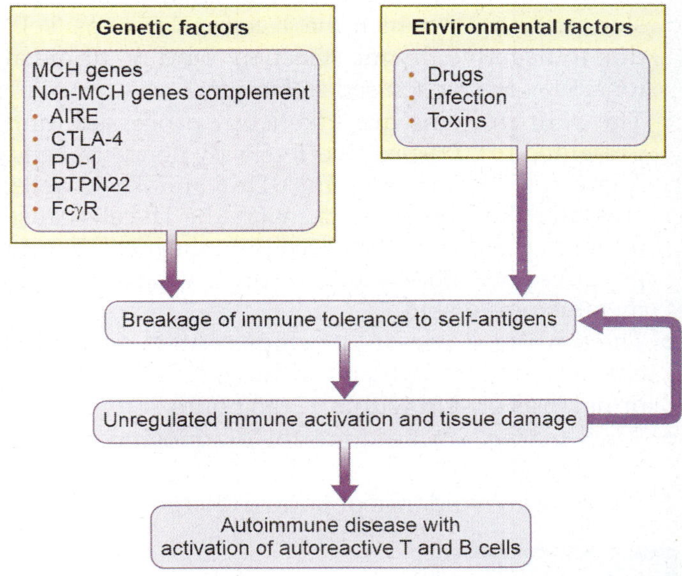

Release of Sequestered Antigens

- Sperm, central nervous system, lens, and uveal tract of eye are sequestered so that the antigens are not exposed to immune system.
- Immunologically privileged sites.
- Bacterial and viral infections → damage cells cause release of sequestered antigens → elicit immune response, e.g. lens antigen of eye.
- Lens protein is enclosed in its capsule and does not circulate in the blood.
- Hence immunological tolerance against this antigen is not established during fetal life.
- When antigen leaks out, following injury, it may induce an immune response causing damage to lens of other eye.

8. An 18-year-old student gets a new watch with metal strap. Next day he notices rash over his wrist in the area where he has worn his watch. What is your likely diagnosis? Briefly describe this type of reaction. (1+4 marks)

Likely Diagnosis

- Contact hypersensitivity.

Contact Hypersensitivity

- It is an eczematous skin disease caused by cell mediated hypersensitivity to an environment allergen.
- It occurs in people sensitized to chemicals, plant materials, topically applied drugs, some cosmetics, soaps and other substances.
- The small molecules acting as haptens enter the skin, attach to body proteins, and modify those proteins enough to 'break tolerance.' For example, normal skin proteins, to which the T cells tolerate as 'self' due to negative thymic selection, binding to metal ions, they are recognised as foreign.
- The skin proteins are taken up, processed, and presented to CD4-positive T cells by dendritic cells. The T cells differentiate into Th-1 and Th-17 cells, and later skin contact with metal, the Th cells cause inflammation when they recognise the metal bound peptides presented by antigen-presenting cells in the metal-exposed skin.
- The sensitized person develops contact dermatitis characterized by erythema, itching, vesicles, eczema, or necrosis of skin within 12–48 hours.
- *Patch testing* can be done for diagnosing contact hypersensitivity.
- *Prevention:* Avoidance of known allergen.

SHORT ANSWERS

1. Briefly describe the Laboratory diagnosis of SLE. (3 marks)

Laboratory Diagnosis of SLE

1. **Immunofluorescence**
   - Direct immunofluorescence.
   - LE factor antibody detection.
2. **Antinuclear antibodies tests**
   - Antibodies to DNA, histones, non-histones bound to RNA, nucleolar antigens.
3. **ELISA**
   - Antibodies to dsDNA.
4. **Immunoblot assay**
   - Antibodies to dsDNA.
5. **Other tests**
   - Platelets, RBC`s, WBC count.

2. Enumerate the serological/laboratory tests applicable for the diagnosis of Rheumatoid Arthritis. (3 marks)

1. RA factor for rheumatoid arthritis.
2. Antibodies to cyclic citrullinated peptide.
3. Low complement levels.

3. Define 'molecular mimicry' with an example. (3 marks)

Definition

- Infectious agents possess antigen or similar amino acid sequence that elicit an immune response that cross reacts with components of human cells because of the similarity in the structure with the host.

Examples

- Antibodies against M proteins cross react with cardiac myosin, leading to rheumatic fever *Streptococcus pyogenes*—Rheumatic fever.

4. Give examples for intracellular microbes inducing delayed type of hypersensitivity and its mechanism. (1+2 marks)

Examples

1. *M. tuberculosis*.
2. *Coccidioides immitis*.

Mechanism (Fig. 1.10.3)

- CD4 T cells and macrophages are the immune cells involved in granuloma formation when exposed to components of intracellular microbes.

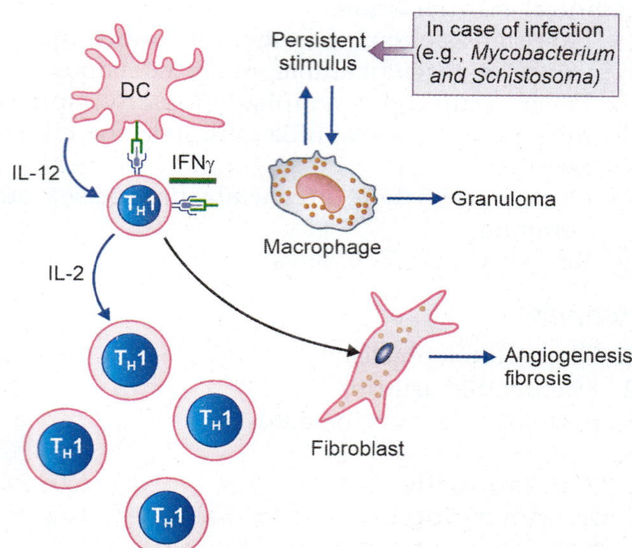

Fig. 1.10.3: Mechanism of delayed hypersensitivity

5. List out the drugs used in the treatment of Type-I Hypersensitivity (3 marks)

Anaphylaxis

- Single or in combination—Epinephrine, antihistamines, corticosteroids, or cromolyn sodium, should be given.
- Cromolyn sodium prevents release of mediators (e.g. histamine) from mast cell granules.

Asthma

- Inhaled β-adrenergic bronchodilators.
- Corticosteroids, such as prednisone, are also effective but carry significant toxicity if used chronically.
- *A monoclonal anti-IgE antibody:* Omalizumab
- *Leukotriene antagonist:* Montelukast

6. Briefly describe X-linked disorders leading to immunodeficiency. (3 marks)

1. **Bruton Disease (X-linked Agammaglobulinaemia).**
   - Failure of pre-B-cells to differentiate into immature B-cells in the bone marrow.
   - Absence of an enzyme tyrosine kinase leading to total absence of B-cells, plasma cells and all classes of Ig.
   - The B-cell maturation stops at pre B cell stage; after the synthesis of heavy-chain without forming the light chains, leading to incomplete immunoglobulins synthesis.
   - Seen primarily in males; rarely in females.
   - *Onset:* after 6 months of life
   - *Secondary infection:* Recurrent bacterial infections, viruses (enteroviruses) and parasites (*Giardia lamblia*)
   - Autoimmune diseases (such as SLE and dermatomyositis) also occur in up to 20% of cases.
3. **X-linked Severe Combined Immunodeficiency (SCID)**
   - Defect in IL2 receptor on T cells with lack of gamma chain of IL2 receptor which is essential for the development of T cells.
4. **Wiskott–Aldrich syndrome**
   - Decreased IgM and elevated IgA and IgE level.
   - Decreased T-cell function with increased susceptibility to autoimmunity and malignancy.
   - Syndrome of eczema, recurrent pyogenic infections, and thrombocytopenia.

MI 1.11 DESCRIBE THE IMMUNOLOGICAL MECHANISMS OF TRANSPLANTATION AND TUMOUR IMMUNITY

LONG ESSAY

1. A 65-year-old male patient with chronic kidney disease underwent renal transplantation donated by an unrelated donor. Patient developed rejection reaction within 1 month. With respect to this case/transplantation answer the following questions.

A. Define a graft. Classify the types of graft. (2 marks)

Graft

- A tissue or an organ transplanted surgically in the same or genetically different individual is termed as graft.
- The organ/tissue is called 'transplant'.

Classification of Grafts

Based on Genetic Relation

1. *Autograft:* is an organ or tissue taken from an individual and grafted in the same individual.
2. *Isograft:* is a graft/ tissue taken from an individual and placed on another individual of the same genetic constitution.
3. *Allograft:* is tissue transferred between genetically non identical members of the same species.
4. *Xenograft:* is tissue transferred between members of different species.

Based on Anatomical Site

1. *Orthotopic graft:* when tissues/organs are transplanted in their same anatomical position Examples: Skin graft.
2. *Heterotopic graft:* when tissues/organs are placed at abnormal sites Examples: thyroid tissue is placed in subcutaneous pocket.

Based on Organ Transplanted

1. *Vital graft:* Live grafts.
2. *Static grafts:* Nonliving graft.

B. Define Transplantation Antigens. (1 mark)

- Types of tumour antigens.
  1. **Tumour specific transplantation antigen.**
     - An antigen that induces the immune response against the transplant cells that are transformed by virus
  2. **Tumour associated transplantation antigen.**
     - Antigens which develop on the cells surface during the process of neoplastic transformation and are considered as "nonself"

C. Enumerate the types of graft rejection and distinguish between each other. (5 marks)

Types of Graft Rejection (Table 1.11.1)

1. Acute graft rejection
2. Chronic rejection
3. Hyperacute rejection (White graft rejection).

D. Add a note on immunosuppressive therapy. (2 marks)

- Immunosuppression of the recipient—by administration of.
  1. **Immunosuppressive drugs**
     - *Cyclosporine:* Prevents activation of T cells
     - *Azathioprine:* Disrupt the synthesis of DNA and RNA and cell division
     - *Tacrolimus:* Calcineurin inhibitor
  2. **Corticosteroids**
     - Inhibit cytokine production and hence inflammation
  3. **Monoclonal antibodies**
     - Block IL-2 receptors
     - To suppress the activity of subpopulation of T-cells
     - To block co-stimulatory signals
     - Examples: Daclizumab
  4. **Antilymphocyte serum**
     - Selectively destroys mature T cells (in GVH)

SHORT ESSAYS

1. Discuss in brief about Immunosurveillance theory. (5 marks)

- Refers to the policing or monitoring function of immune system cells to recognise and destroy clones of transformed cells prior to their development into neoplasms and to destroy tumours after they develop.
- It is mediated by the cellular limb of immune response.
- T cells surveillance system detects and eliminate newly arising clones of neoplastic cells.
  - Less expression of major histocompatibility complex (MHC) class I–complexed TAAs.
  - Release of soluble factors that promote the activity of immunosuppressive leukocytes, including T regulatory (Treg) cells.
  - Expression of cell surface molecules that inhibit the function of cytotoxic T cells and NK cells.

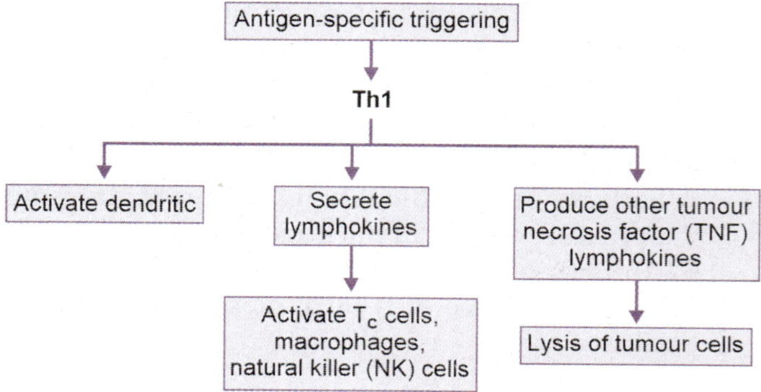

- Immune system kills and induces changes in the tumour resulting in tumour escape and recurrence-Cancer Immuno-editing by.
  - Elimination: Innate and adaptive immunity.
  - Equilibrium: Cancer persistence-genetic instability and immune selection.
  - Escape-cancer progression—chronic inflammation.

Table 1.11.1 Types of graft rejection

Feature	Acute graft rejection	Chronic rejection	Hyperacute rejection (White graft rejection)
Duration	• Occurs after one week	• Occurs after months to years	• Occurs in min to hours
Cells involved	• Cytotoxic T-cell, macrophage and antibody mediated, • myocyte and endothelial damage,	• T cells react with the graft alloantigens secrete cytokines resulting in proliferation of fibroblasts in the vascular intima	• Due to preformed anti-ABO antibodies the graft will be immediately rejected
Aetiology	• Inflammation: damage the graft	• Due to atherosclerosis of endothelium of blood vessels	• Vasospasm of blood vessels
Factors	• Current immunosuppressive drugs prevent the acute rejection by blocking the activation of alloreactive T cells	• Appears due to side effects of immunosuppressive therapy/alterations in minor MHC antigens • Occurs in most solid organ transplants, e.g. heart, kidney • Mostly refractory to therapy	• Exposure to foreign HLA antigens due to previous blood transfusion, transplants, or pregnancy • This type is uncommon as it avoided by prior matching of donor and recipient

2. A 15-year-old with acute lymphocytic leukaemia fails all standard therapy. A transplant was carried out before which he received antibiotics and immunosuppressive agents. After 21 days duration, he developed sever rash, diarrhoea and jaundice.

A. What is the most likely diagnosis? (1 mark)

- Acute allograft rejection.

B. Explain the immunological process of this condition. (2 marks)

- Rapidity of rejection depends on:
  1. Degree of dissimilarity between donor and recipient HLA Ags.
  2. Immunocompetency of the recipient.
  3. Prior sensitisation of the recipient to donor tissues/blood.
     - Recognition of transplanted cells that are self or foreign is determined by polymorphic genes (MHC) that are inherited from both parents and are expressed co-dominantly
     - Alloantigens elicit both cell-mediated and humoral immune responses

Direct Pathway

- Direct presentation.
- Recognition of an intact MHC molecule displayed by donor APC in the graft.
- Basically, self MHC molecule recognises the structure of an intact allogeneic MHC molecule.
- Involves both $CD8^+$ and $CD4^+$ T cells.
- CD4 T cells—damages the graft by delayed type of hypersensitivity and CD8 T cell kill nucleated cells of graft.

Indirect Pathway

- Indirect presentation
- Donor MHC is processed and presented by recipient APC
- Basically, donor MHC molecule is handled like any other foreign antigen
- Involve only CD4+ T cells
- Antigen presentation by class II MHC molecules
- Donor APCs migrate to regional lymph nodes and are recognised by the recipient's T_H cells.
- Alloreactive T_H cells in the recipient induce generation of CTLs, delayed type of hypersensitivity and B cell activation (by complement mediated lysis and Antibody dependent cell cytotoxicity) then migrate into the graft and cause graft rejection.

C. Mention the pre-transplantation workup and prevention for such case. (2 marks)

1. Blood group matching.
2. HLA matching of donor and recipient: Micro-cytotoxicity, mixed lymphocyte reaction, PCR.
3. Immunosuppression of the recipient—by administration of.
   - *Cyclosporine:* Prevents activation of T cells
   - *Corticosteroids:* Inhibit cytokine production
   - *Monoclonal antibodies:* Block IL-2 receptors
   - Antilymphocyte serum selectively destroys mature T cells (in GVH).
   - Chronic rejection is considered irreversible.

3. Explain the structure of MHC with the help of diagram and its clinical significance. (2+2+1 marks)

Structure of MHC (Fig. 1.11.1)

- MHC molecules or human leukocyte antigens (HLA) serve as a unique identification marker for every individual as the genetic sequence of MHC genes differs for every individual.
- In humans, HLA complex coding for MHC proteins is located in short arm of chromosome 6.
- The genes are clustered in three regions named as MHC region-I, II and III.
- MHC I and II help in antigen presentation to T-cells.
  - MHC I present intracellular antigen on viral/tumor cells to cytotoxic T-cells.

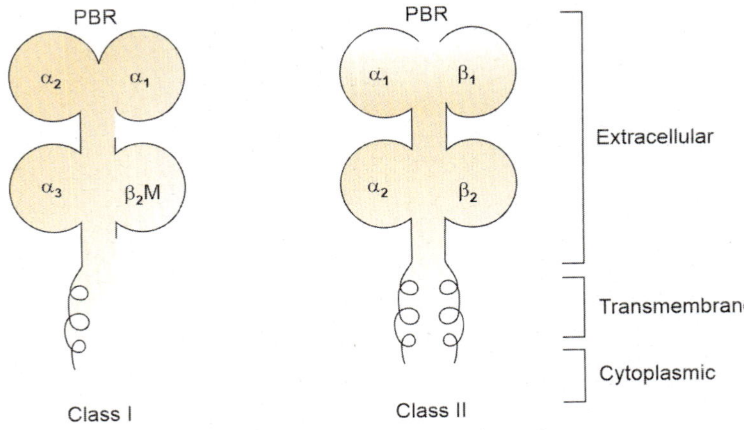

Fig. 1.11.1: Structure of MHC

  - MHC II presents extracellular antigen on APCs to helper T-cells.
  - MHC III does not help in Ag presentation, but code for various proteins such as complement factors (C2, C4, C3 convertase, factor B and properdin), heat shock protein.
- TNF-α and β and steroid 21-hydroxylases.

Clinical Significance

- It determines the histocompatibility between the donor graft and the recipient.

SHORT ANSWERS

1. A 50-year-old businessman c/o of vague abdominal pain and notices blood in stool. The gastroenterologist performs a sigmoidoscopy and notices a mass in the colon. Which is the tumour marker the clinician should order for? Give examples of tumour-associated transplantation antigens. (1+2 marks)

Tumor Marker the Clinician should Order for is

- Carcinoembryonic antigen—Tumour marker for carcinoma colon.

Examples of Tumour Associated Transplantation Antigens

1. *Alfa fetoprotein:* Hepatoma, testicular cancer.
2. *Carcinoembryonic antigen:* Ovarian, lung, GIT cancers.
3. *CA125:* Ovarian cancer.
4. *Prostatic specific antigens:* Prostate cancer.

2. Write in brief about GVH Reaction. (3 marks)

- The disease produced by the reaction of immunocompetent T lymphocytes of the donor graft that are histoincompatible with the tissues of the recipient.
- The recipient must be either immunologically immature, immunosuppressed by irradiation or drug therapy, or tolerant to the administered cells, and the grafted cells must also be immunocompetent.
- The recipient must express antigens foreign to the donor cells.
- The donor`s cytotoxic T cells play a key role in destroying the recipient's cells.
- GVH is usually seen in.
  - Bone Marrow transplant cases.
  - After random blood transfusion in neonates.
  - Patients with congenital immunodeficiencies.
  - Cancer (leukaemia) patients.

3. Define cancer immunotherapy. Explain the role of monoclonal antibodies and cytokine therapy in the treatment of cancers. (1+2 marks)

Cancer Immunotherapy

- It is the artificial stimulation of the immune system to treat cancer, improving on the immune system's natural ability to fight the disease.

Role of Monoclonal Antibodies

- Most successful with targeted therapy.
- *Rituximab (anti CD20 Ab):* treatment of relapsed low-grade NHL and follicular NHL
- *Daclizumab:* treatment of human T lymphotropic virus (HTLV)
- *Trastuzumab—ErbB2:* treatment of breast cancer

Role of Cytokine Therapy

- Increased class I MHC expression on tumour cells, thereby increasing CTLs activity against tumours.
- Inhibits angiogenesis—TNF.
  - IFN α: in Hairy cell leukaemia, Kaposi sarcoma.
  - IL-2: Malignant melanoma, renal cell carcinoma

CHAPTER 2

CVS and Blood

MI 2.1 DESCRIBE THE ETIOLOGICAL AGENTS OF RHEUMATIC FEVER AND THEIR DIAGNOSIS

LONG ESSAYS

1. A 11-year-old girl presented to the hospital with c/o fever, difficulty in breathing, migratory joint pain in the last 4 weeks. His parents give h/o sore throat 5 weeks ago. Blood investigations: haemoglobin of 12.1 g%, total leucocyte count of 10,800 mm³, ESR of 50 mm/h, positive ASO (>400 IU/ml), CRP (6.89 mg/dL). ECG showed prolongation of PR interval.

A. What is the probable diagnosis and the bacteria associated with the condition? (2 marks)

Probable Diagnosis

- Acute rheumatic fever.

Bacteria Associated

- Post-streptococcal infection associated with *Streptococcus pyogenes.*

B. Pathogenesis and the clinical manifestations of this condition. (3+3 marks)

Pathogenesis of Acute Rheumatic Fever (ARF)

- Multisystem, immunologically mediated inflammatory disease, occurring as a delayed sequel to group A streptococcal (GAS) infection.
- Episodes of recurrent ARF culminates in chronic rheumatic heart disease (RHD).

Predisposing Factors

- Common in females.
- *Genetic predisposition:* HLA –DR7 AND HLA DR4 more susceptible

Sequence of Events (Fig. 2.1.1)

Theories

1. **Autoimmune theory:** Molecular mimicry.
   - Following repeated attacks of Group A *Streptococcus* (GAS) pharyngeal infection, there

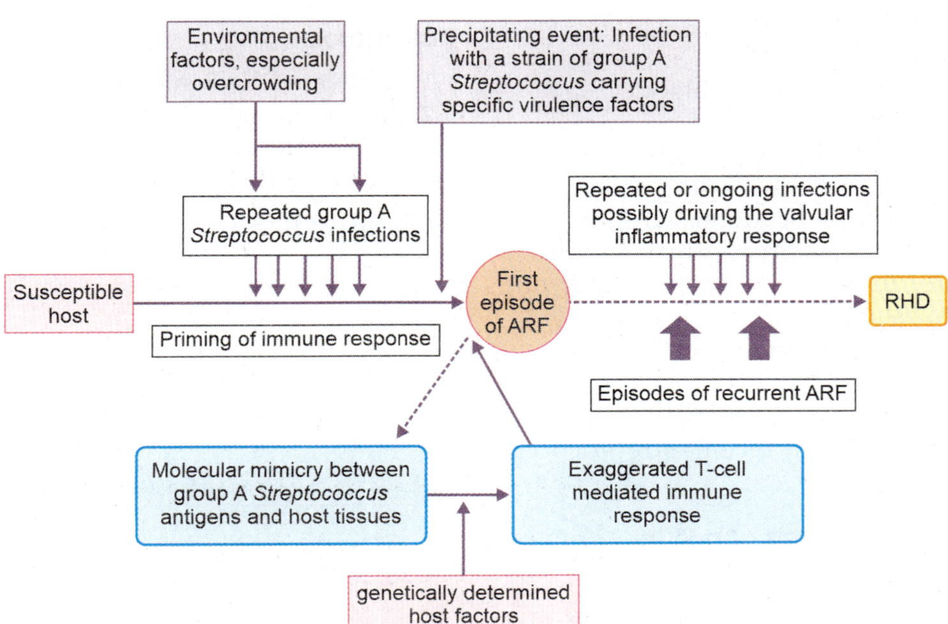

Fig. 2.1.1: Sequence of events in the pathogenesis of ARF

is production of IgG and IgM antibody and activation of CD4+ T cells.
- Structural similarity between the cardiac tissue and Streptococcal antigens results in cross reactive immune response.
- Antibodies cross react with cardiac tissue and joints causing damage.
- Damage induced accounts for the manifestations of rheumatic fever: Transient arthritis, chorea due to binding of antibody to basal ganglia, and carditis due to antibody binding and infiltration of T cells

2. **Cytotoxic theory**
   - Streptococcal toxins (SPE), enzymes (Streptolysin O) are directly toxic to the human cardiac cells.

Clinical Manifestations

- *Onset:* 2–3 weeks after streptococcal pharyngitis
- Infection may be either subclinical or presents as sore throat.
- Updated Jones clinical criteria.
  - *Major criteria:* 5 Criteria
    1. Pancarditis (pericarditis, endocarditis, myocarditis).
    2. Migratory polyarthritis.
    3. Sydenham's chorea (rheumatic chorea).
    4. Subcutaneous nodules.
    5. Erythema marginatum.
  - *Minor criteria*
    1. Fever (≥38°C).
    2. Arthralgia.
    3. Elevated acute phase reactants (C-reactive proteins).
    4. Prolonged P-R interval in ECG.
    5. Previous rheumatic fever.
    6. Leucocytosis.
    7. First-degree atrioventricular block.
  - *Plus*
    - Supporting evidence of preceding streptococcal infection: recent scarlet fever, raised antistreptolysin O or other streptococcal antibody titre, positive throat culture (particularly important if there is only one major manifestation)
  - To diagnose rheumatic fever.
    - 2 major criteria
    - One major + Two minor criteria
    - Plus, evidence of a recent streptococcal infection for both

C. Laboratory diagnosis of this condition. (2 marks)

Evidence of a Systemic Illness

- Elevated leucocyte count, raised erythrocyte sedimentation rate and increased C-reactive protein.

Evidence of Preceding Streptococcal Infection

- *Throat swab culture:* Group A β-haemolytic streptococci
- *Antistreptolysin O antibodies (ASO titres):* Rising titres, or levels of >200 IU/ml (adults) or >100 IU/ml (children)

Evidence of Carditis

- *Chest X-ray:* Cardiomegaly; pulmonary congestion
- *ECG:* Features of pericarditis, T-wave inversion, reduction in QRS voltages
- *Echocardiography:* Cardiac dilatation and valve abnormalities

---

2. An 18-year-old female presents to the medicine OPD with h/o fever and joint pain. She also gives h/o sore throat 3 weeks back. On examination, she was febrile. CRP was 54 mg/L, ESR was 90 mm/hr, ASO titre was 750 IU/ml. Transoesophageal echocardiography revealed severe mitral stenosis and regurgitation. Thickening of the mitral with restricted motion of posterior mitral valve leaflet were observed. Severe aortic regurgitation was also present. There was dilation of the LA and LV. Blood cultures were negative.

Answer the following questions related to the case.

A. Most probable diagnosis of the condition discussed. (2 marks)

- Acute rheumatic fever by modified Jones criteria.
  - *1 major criteria:* Carditis
  - *2 minor criteria:* Fever, elevated CRP, plus evidence of post-streptococcal infection (ASO: >200 IU/ml).

B. Immunopathogenesis of the condition. (3 marks)

Risk Factors

1. Untreated GAS infection.
2. *Environmental factors:* Poor nutrition, low SE status, overcrowding.
3. Genetic predisposition.

Sequence of Events

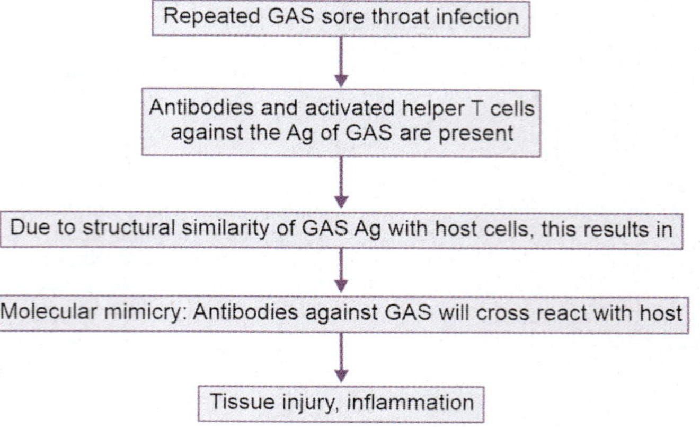

- *Tissue injury:* Fever, arthralgia, increased CRP and ESR, erythema marginatum, subcutaneous nodules
- Antibodies and lymphocytes attach to myosin and cardiac proteins → Pancarditis and valvular injury.
- *Antibodies target neuronal cells:* Sydenham chorea

C. Clinical manifestations of the condition (3 marks)

- Acute rheumatic fever is diagnosed by modified Jones criteria.
  - Two major or one major and two minor criteria plus evidence of past streptococcal infection.

Criteria	Manifestations
Major manifestations	• Subcutaneous nodules
	• Pancarditis
	• Arthritis (migrating polyarthritis)
	• Chorea (CNS manifestation)
	• Erythema marginatum (skin lesion)
Minor manifestations	• *Clinical:* Fever, arthralgia • *Laboratory:* Elevated ESR and C-reactive protein • *ECG:* Prolonged P-R interval

D. Microbiological investigations required for the diagnosis of the case. Discuss the prevention of this condition. (1 + 1 marks)

Microbiological Investigations Required

- ASO titre.
  - *Specimen:* Serum
  - *Methods:* Latex agglutination test/Turbidometry/Nephelometry
  - >200 IU/ml in adults and children above 5 years, > 100 IU/ml in children below 5 years of age is suggestive of ARF.
  - A sharp rise in the titre may occur at 2–3 weeks after the sore throat and persist up to 6 weeks during the disease.
- Elevated CRP levels.
- Throat swab culture-negative for GAS.
- Blood culture –negative.

Prevention of ARF

- *Primary prevention:* Prompt treatment of group A streptococcal sore throat with antibiotics (Penicillin)
- *Secondary prevention*
  - Antibiotic prophylaxis to prevent recurrent attacks of acute RF in documented cases of ARF.
  - Given long term penicillin prophylaxis to prevent recurrence.
  - Intramuscular benzathine penicillin IM given every 4 weeks depending upon the severity of the disease.

SHORT ESSAYS

1. Discuss in detail about non-suppurative complications of group-A beta haemolytic streptococci. (5 marks)

- Non-suppurative disorders are the disorders in which the local infection, with group A *Streptococcus* is followed weeks later by infection in an organ not affected by *streptococci*.
- Mediated by the immune response to streptococcal M protein cross reacting with human tissue.
- They are:
  1. **Acute Rheumatic Fever**
     - 2 weeks after the attack of streptococcal sore throat, characterised by fever, migratory arthritis, carditis (vegetations in mitral, aortic valves), chorea, elevated ASO and ESR.
     - Occurs in 5–15 years age group.
     - Damage is due to cross reaction between antibodies against M protein of *S. pyogenes* and proteins on the surface of joint, heart and brain.
     - Diagnosed by modified Jones criteria.
     - Prevented by prompt treatment of group A streptococcal sore throat and reinfection in Rheumatic fever is prevented by long-term penicillin prophylaxis.
  2. **Post-streptococcal Glomerulonephritis (PSGN).**
     - Occurs 2–3 weeks after skin infections with certain group A streptococcal types in children.
     - Clinical features include hypertension, oedema of face (periorbital) and ankle, smoky urine.
     - Recurrence is rare.
     - Due to deposition of antigen antibody complexes in the glomerular basement membrane.
     - Titres of anti-DNase B are high in group A streptococcal skin infections in patients with suspected PSGN.

2. Describe in detail the diagnostic criteria for rheumatic fever (5 marks)

- Acute rheumatic fever (ARF) presents within one to five weeks (usually 2–3 weeks) of a group A streptococcal (GAS) pharyngitis.

Diagnostic Criteria (Updated Jones Criteria)

Major Criteria: 5 Criteria

1. Pancarditis (pericarditis, endocarditis, myocarditis).
2. Migratory polyarthritis.
3. Sydenham's chorea (rheumatic chorea).
4. Subcutaneous nodules.
5. Erythema marginatum.

Minor Criteria

1. Fever
2. Arthralgia
3. Elevated acute phase reactants (C-reactive proteins)
4. Prolonged P-R interval in ECG
5. Previous rheumatic fever
6. Leukocytosis
7. First-degree atrioventricular block.

Plus

- *Supporting evidence of preceding streptococcal infection:* Recent scarlet fever, raised antistreptolysin O or other streptococcal antibody titre, positive throat culture (particularly important if there is only one major manifestation)

To Diagnose Rheumatic Fever

- Two major criteria.
- One major + two minor criteria.
- Plus, evidence of a recent streptococcal infection for both.

3. Acute rheumatic fever is characterised by inflammatory lesions of the small synovial joints of the body. Justify the statement given by describing the mechanism of involvement of joints in rheumatic fever by group-A beta haemolytic streptococci. (4 marks)

Arthritis in ARF

- Present in 60–80% of patients of ARF
- Usually affects the peripheral large joints—Knees, ankles, elbows, and wrists
- Involved joints are red, warm, and swollen
- Asymmetrical, migratory, and painful, though few patients may present with mild symptoms
- Resolves spontaneously in 2 or 3 weeks

Pathogenesis (Fig 2.1.2)

- Following group A *Streptococcus* (GAS) infection of the pharyngeal epithelium, GAS antigens activate both B and T cells.
- Molecular mimicry between GAS group A carbohydrate or serotype-specific M protein and the host heart, brain or joint tissues can lead to an autoimmune response.
- Arthritis might be a result of the formation of immune complexes that bind to the synovial membrane and/or collagen in joints, which leads to recruitment of inflammatory cells in Acute Rheumatic fever.

SHORT ANSWERS

1. Write the clinical significance of ASO test. (2 marks)

- An elevated ASO titre usually indicates recent infection with a group A β-hemolytic *Streptococcus*.
- Used for the diagnosis and management of acute rheumatic fever.
- ASO titre increases a week following infection peaks at 3–5 weeks, begins to fall at 8 weeks, and returns to pre-infection levels at around 8 months.

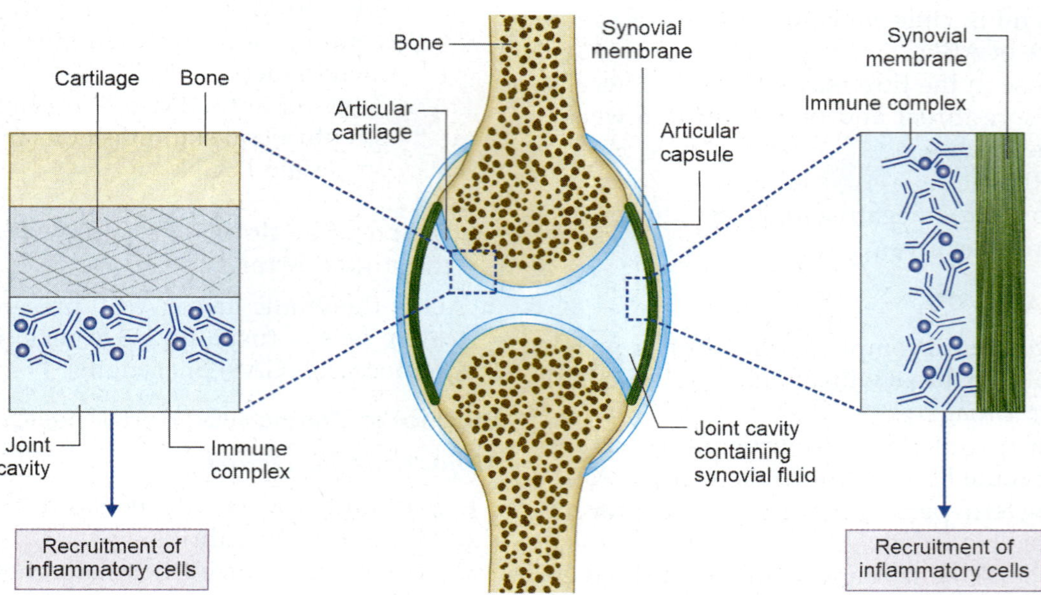

Fig. 2.1.2: Pathogenesis of arthritis in ARF

- 80–85% of individuals, with a current streptococcal infection or their sequelae, have an elevated ASO titre.
- **Interpretation.**
  - Less than 200 IU/mL (adults, children above 5 years).
  - Less than 100 IU/mL (children <5 years).
  - Rise in titre (≥2-fold) in paired sera (acute and convalescent) is suggestive of prior infection with group A *Streptococcus*. Single high titre is diagnostic in endemic area.
- **Limitations.**
  1. ASO titre may decrease by the time a patient present with acute rheumatic fever; therefore, a previous streptococcal infection cannot be ruled out due to a negative ASO result.
  2. *False-negative ASO:* In hyperlipidaemia.
  3. *False-positive ASO results:* Myeloma, hypergammaglobulinaemia, liver disease, and autoimmune disease with elevated rheumatoid factor.

2. Write about the prevention of acute rheumatic fever (ARF). (3 marks)

Prevention of ARF

Primary Prevention

- Prompt treatment of group A streptococcal sore throat with antibiotics (Penicillin).

Secondary Prevention

- Antibiotic prophylaxis.
- To prevent recurrent attacks of acute RF and is recommended for patients with well-documented RF.
- Given long-term penicillin prophylaxis to prevent recurrence.
- Intramuscular benzathine penicillin IM given every 4 weeks depending upon the severity of the disease.

MI 2.2 DESCRIBE THE CLASSIFICATION, ETIOPATHOGENESIS, CLINICAL FEATURES AND DISCUSS THE DIAGNOSTIC MODALITIES OF INFECTIVE ENDOCARDITIS

LONG ESSAYS

1. A 68-year-old male was hospitalised with history of fever of 102°F, weakness of lower limbs, and backache. On physical examination, small, non-tender, erythematous nodular lesions were observed on soles. With the advice given by cardiologist, Echocardiography was performed, which revealed vegetations on the bicuspid valve. Past medical history of the patient revealed cardiac valvular lesions few years back. All the required haematological tests were performed. CRP: 7 mg/dl; ESR: 70 mm/hr; Creatinine: 4.8 mg/dl. Two blood cultures grew viridans streptococci. The patient was kept on benzyl penicillin.

A. What is the probable clinical diagnosis? (2 marks)

- Infective endocarditis.

B. What are the typical causative agents associated with the above condition? (1 mark)

1. *Staphylococcus aureus*
2. Viridans streptococci
3. Coagulase-negative staphylococci
4. *Enterococcus* spp
5. Gram-negative bacilli: *Enterobacteriaceae, Pseudomonas spp*
6. HACEK group
7. Fungi (*Candida* spp.)
8. *Diphtheroids*

C. Describe the diagnostic criteria used for this condition. (5 marks)

Duke's Criteria for Infective Endocarditis

- Duke's criteria are a set of clinical criteria set forward for the diagnosis of infective endocarditis
- For diagnosis the requirement is
  - 2 major and 1 minor criterion, or
  - 1 major and 3 minor criteria, or
  - 5 minor criteria.

Major Criteria

1. *Positive blood culture:* Any one of the following.
   - Typical IE organism isolated from two separate sets of blood cultures, or
   - Persistently positive blood culture with agents other than typical IE organisms: Blood culture sets drawn >12 h apart; or All of 3 or a majority of ≥4 separate sets of blood culture, with first and last drawn at least 1 h apart
   - Single positive blood culture for *Coxiella burnetii* or phase I IgG antibody titer of >1:800
2. *Positive echocardiogram:* Any one of the following:
   - Oscillating intracardiac mass on valve *or.*
   - Abscess, *or*
   - New partial dehiscence of prosthetic valve.
3. *New valvular regurgitation.*

Minor Criteria

1. *Predisposition:* Predisposing heart condition or IV drug use.

2. *Fever:* ≥38.0°C (≥100.4°F).
3. *Vascular phenomena:* Major arterial emboli, septic pulmonary infarcts, mycotic aneurysm, intracranial haemorrhage, conjunctival haemorrhages or Janeway lesions.
4. *Immunologic phenomena:* Glomerulonephritis, Osler's nodes, Roth's spots, or rheumatoid factor.
5. *Microbiologic evidence:* Positive blood culture but not meeting major criterion as noted previously or serologic evidence of active infection with organism consistent with infective endocarditis.

Definite Diagnosis

- Two major criteria, or
- One major and three minor criteria, or
- Five minor criteria.

Possible Diagnosis

- One major and one minor criteria, or
- Three minor criteria.

D. How will you collect specimen for the laboratory diagnosis of the above condition. (3 marks)

Specimen Collection of Blood for Culture

Site

- From two different sites.
- If a central line is present, then one sample from central line and one from peripheral line.

Preparation of Site

- *Antiseptics:* 70% isopropyl alcohol → second antiseptic solution (tincture iodine or chlorhexidine)

Timing of Collection

- Before starting antimicrobial therapy or just before the next dose of antimicrobial agent.

Blood Volume to be Collected

- 8–10 ml per bottle for adult.
- 1–3 ml per bottle for children.

Number of Blood Cultures

- *2–3 blood culture sets (each set consists of two bottles:* 1 aerobic and 1 anaerobic) are required to have good isolation chance

In Suspected Case of Infective Endocarditis

- 2 sets collected at an interval >12 hours between the two OR 3 sets collected over one hour with 30 min gap between each.

E. Discuss the treatment in the above case. (1 mark)

- For viridans streptococci: Penicillin or ceftriaxone for 4 weeks

2. A 72-year-old male with history of smoking and alcoholism underwent valve replacement surgery in a superspeciality hospital. But after 9 months, he developed mild chest pain, dyspnoea, fever and is hospitalised. Blood sample is collected for culture. Serum creatinine is also elevated. Blood culture beeps positive and Gram's staining of the positive blood culture broth showed the presence of gram-positive cocci in grape like clusters. Answer the following questions related to the case discussed above:

A. Most probable diagnosis of the case discussed. 2 marks)

- Prosthetic valve endocarditis caused by *Staphylococcus* spp.

B. The probable etiological agent in this case and 2 tests to identify the species in this case. (2 marks)

Probable Aetiological Agent

- *Staphylococcus epidermidis* or *Staphylococcus aureus.*

Two Tests to Identify the Species

- *Coagulase test and DNase test* to differentiate *Staphylococcus aureus* from *Staphylococcus epidermidis.*

C. Pathogenesis of Infective Endocarditis. (4 marks)

Risk Factors

1. Prosthetic valves and a prior history of endocarditis.
2. Rheumatic valvular disease, cyanotic congenital heart disease, and degenerative valve lesions.
3. Bacteraemia.
   - Dental manipulation.
   - Procedures—cannula, colonoscopy, endoscopy.
   - Infection in other organs—abscess, pneumonia.
   - IV drug abuse.

Sequence of Events

1. **Injury to valvular endothelium.**
   - The intact endothelial lining of the heart and its valves are resistant to infection with bacteria and fungi.
   - Endothelial injury can occur by:
     - Turbulent blood flow attributed to congenital or acquired intracardiac abnormality.
     - Intravascular catheter or another device.
     - In injection drug users, direct injection of contaminating debris may damage the tricuspid valve surface.
2. **Adherence of platelets and fibrin.**
   - Deposition of platelets and fibrin due to clotting of blood.

3. **Secondary infection of the nidus.**
   - Can occur by distant infection or transient bacteraemia.
   - Further activation of the coagulation system via the extrinsic clotting pathway, adherent monocytes release a variety of cytokines, and activated endothelial cells continue to lead to further local deposition of fibronectin.
4. **Vegetation.**
   - Bacterial growth occurs within cells and within the matrix of fibronectin inside vegetations, making it difficult for host immune responses to control or eradicate the ongoing infection.

D. Which antibiotic is preferred in this scenario? (1 mark)

- Cloxacillin or vancomycin for 6 weeks with Rifampicin (4 weeks) and gentamicin (2 weeks) for prosthetic valve endocarditis caused by *Staphylococcus* spp.

SHORT ESSAYS

1. Discuss in detail about the "modified Duke's criteria" for the clinical diagnosis of infective endocarditis (5 marks)

- *Refer to Page No. 81, Q. No. 1 of Long Essays.*

2. Classify Infective Endocarditis. (4 marks)

Based on the Onset and Progress

1. **Acute endocarditis.**
   - Days up to 6 weeks.
   - Bacteria of greater virulence.
   - Metastatic lesions.
2. **Subacute endocarditis.**
   - 6 weeks to 3 months.
   - Low virulence.
3. **Chronic endocarditis.**
   - >3 months.

Based on the Source of Infection

1. Nosocomial endocarditis.
2. Community acquired endocarditis.

Based on the Mature of the Valve

1. Native valve endocarditis.
   i. Acute bacterial endocarditis.
   ii. Subacute bacterial endocarditis.
2. Prosthetic valve endocarditis.

Based on Location of Valves Involved

1. Right-sided endocarditis
2. Left-sided endocarditis

3. Discuss in detail the HACEK group. (4 marks)

HACEK Group

- The name "HACEK" is an acronym of the first letters of the genera of the following bacteria: *Haemophilus aphrophilus and Haemophilus paraphrophilus, Actinobacillus (Aggregatibacter) actinomycetem comitans, Cardiobacterium hominis, Eikenella corrodens,* and *Kingella kingae*

Characteristics

- Heterogeneous group of small gram-negative rods that have in common the following.
  - Frequently colonize the oropharynx.
  - Slow growth in culture.
  - Requirement for high CO_2 levels to grow in culture.

Clinical Significance

- Have the ability to cause endocarditis
- Count for 5–10% of cases of infective endocarditis involving native valves and are the most common gram-negative cause of endocarditis among people who do not use drugs intravenously and a cause of culture-negative endocarditis.

4. Compare and contrast bacteraemia and septicaemia. Enumerate the types of Bacteraemia. (3+2 marks)

Feature	*Bacteraemia*	*Septicaemia*
Presence of bacteria	• Viable bacteria in blood	• Presence and multiplication of bacteria
Toxin production	• No	• Yes
Number of bacteria present	• Less number	• Large amounts
Origin	• Trauma, infection, or through a surgical procedure	• Can arise from infections in the lungs, abdomen, and urinary tract
Symptoms	• Usually, no symptoms or mild fever	• Associated with fever, chills, tachycardia
Seriousness of the condition	• Not dangerous	• Life threatening
Treatment	• Resolves without treatment	• Untreated cases progress to sepsis

Types of Bacteraemia

Transient bacteraemia	*Intermittent bacteraemia*	*Persistent bacteraemia*
Bacteraemia lasting for minutes or a few hours	• Bacteraemia due to the same microorganism that is detected intermittently in the same patient because of a cycle of clearance and recurrence	• At least two positive blood cultures obtained on different calendar days during the same infectious episode
Dental procedures, after gastrointestinal biopsy; catheterisation of the vascular system, bladder, or common bile duct; and following surgical debridement or drainage	• Undrained closed-space infections (intra-abdominal or soft-tissue abscesses) liver abscesses, cholangitis • Focal infections (Pneumonia, osteomyelitis, spondylodiscitis)	• Infective Endocarditis (IE) • Intravascular infections: vascular-graft infection, infected thrombus • Systemic bacterial infections, brucellosis, and typhoid fever

5. Discuss manual blood culture versus automated blood culture. (4 marks)

Manual Blood Culture

- *Blood culture medium:* Tryptic soy broth, also known as soybean-casein digest broth, supplemented peptone broth and brain heart infusion broth
- 10 ml of blood is inoculated into 100 ml of blood culture broth in the bottle.
- Incubated at 37°C aerobically in presence of 5–10% CO_2.
- Subcultures are done on to solid media every 3 days for 8 weeks.
- Risk of contamination.

Castaneda Biphasic Medium

- The need for frequent subcultures can be avoided by use of two-phase system in which both solid and liquid media are contained in the same bottle.
- Less contamination, less risk of infection to the laboratory workers.

Automated System for Blood Culture

- Carbon dioxide production by microorganisms in the bottles is continuously monitored, either by colorimetric or fluorescent detection. During incubation, the bottles are continuously agitated in the automated equipment.
- Advantages:
  1. Better yield and speed of growth.
  2. Less contamination compared to conventional blood culture.
- Disadvantages:
  1. Costly.
  2. Require regular maintenance and are not adapted to tropical, dusty environments.

BacT/Alert

- Based on the colorimetric detection of CO_2 in the bottle as the microorganisms grow.
- Sensed by CO_2 sensitive chemical located at the bottom of the tube which is separated from the blood broth mixture by CO_2 permeable membrane.
- As the CO_2 levels increase, the bottle is flagged off as positive.

BACTEC system

- Uses fluorescence to detect the CO_2 levels in the blood culture bottle.

SHORT ANSWERS

1. List out the causative agents of endocarditis in IV drug abusers. (2 marks)

1. *Staphylococcus aureus*.
2. Coagulase-negative staphylococci.
3. Group A streptococci.
4. *Pseudomonas aeruginosa*.
5. HACEK organisms (*Haemophilus aphrophilus*, *Actinobacillus actinomycetemcomitans*, *Cardiobacterium hominis*, *Eikenella corrodens*, and *Kingella kingae*).

2. Differentiate primary bacteraemia and secondary bacteraemia. (2 marks)

- Bacteraemia is defined as either a primary or secondary process.

Primary bacteraemia	*Secondary bacteraemia*
Majority of hospital acquired blood stream infections	• Accounts for majority of community acquired bloodstream infections
Use of intravascular catheters contaminated with bacteria	• Occurs following entry of bacteria through the cuts in the skin, or the mucous membranes of respiratory, GI or urinary tract

3. Enumerate the causative agents for culture negative Endocarditis. What antibody titre level can be considered as significant to be included under major criteria. (2 + 1 marks)

Causative Agents for Culture Negative Endocarditis (CNE)

1. True bacterial endocarditis with negative blood cultures owing to prior receipt of antimicrobials.
2. CNE caused by fastidious organisms: "HACEK" group, nutritionally deficient *Streptococci*, *Pasteurella* spp., *Helicobacter* spp., mycobacteria, and fungi.
3. Intracellular organisms that are detectable via serology or polymerase chain reaction (PCR) of valvular tissue, e.g. *Bartonella quintana*, *Coxiella burnetii* and *Tropheryma whipplei*.

Antibody Detection in CNE

- Serology is indicated when the suspected aetiological agent is difficult to cultivate, e.g. *Brucella*, *Bartonella*, *Legionella*, *Coxiella* spp.

4. List the investigations in a suspected case of Infective endocarditis. (2 marks)

Investigations

- Three sets of blood culture was sent at an interval of 30 minutes from different peripheral venepuncture sites.
- Transthoracic echocardiography to study the vegetations.
- Complete blood count.
- CRP
- ESR

5. What are the indications for blood culture? (2 marks)

Indications for Blood Culture

1. Sepsis
2. Infective endocarditis
3. Pyrexia of unknown origin
4. Enteric fever
5. Brucellosis
6. Suspected fungaemia in immunocompromised.

MI 2.3 IDENTIFY THE MICROBIAL AGENTS CAUSING RHEUMATIC HEART DISEASE AND INFECTIVE ENDOCARDITIS

SHORT ESSAY

1. A 19-year-old female with fixed orthodontic appliance for one year presented with fever, migratory joint pain for the past 2 months. Blood cultures were positive for *S viridians*. CRP 20 mg/dl and ESR 40 mm/hr. Transoesophageal echocardiography revealed a vegetation of 8 mm attached to the anterior mitral valve leaf. Smear from the blood culture broth is focussed.

A. Comment on Gram's stain from the broth of the positive blood culture. (1 mark)

- The given smear shows the presence of gram-positive cocci in pairs and chains.

B. How are the bacteria further identified? (1 mark)

- Subculture of blood culture broth onto blood agar and chocolate agar and identification based on cultural and biochemical characteristics.

C. Comment on the growth on blood agar. (1 mark)

- Alpha haemolytic colonies on blood agar, resistant to Optochin.

D. What is the probable diagnosis in this case, justify? (2 marks)

Probable Diagnosis

- Infective endocarditis caused by viridans streptococci.

Justification

- Duke criteria—2 major criteria, 2 positive blood cultures with *S viridans* and the identification of the vegetation echographically.

E. What is the protocol for specimen collection for blood culture in a suspected case of IE? (1 mark)

- 3 Sets of Blood culture was sent at an interval of 30 minutes from different peripheral venepuncture sites.

SHORT ANSWER

1. A 10-year-old girl presented with complaints of progressive breathlessness, fever, and migratory joint pain (bilateral knee) for 10 days. On examination, child was febrile with a pulse of 110/min, respiratory rate 48/min, BP-130/50. Cardiovascular examination revealed pan systolic murmur in the mitral area. Investigations revealed haemoglobin of 12.1g%, total leucocyte count of 10,800 mm^3, ESR of 50 mm/h, positive ASO (>400 IU/ml), CRP (6.89 mg/dL). Prolongation of PR interval (0.18 sec) and left axis deviation was seen in ECG. Throat swab and blood culture showed no growth. She gives h/o sore throat one month back.

A. Interpret the test shown. (1 mark)

- Latex agglutination test for the detection of Antistreptolysin O antibodies.
- Titre >400 IU/ml is significant for ASO antibodies.

B. What is the probable diagnosis? (1 mark)

- Acute rheumatic fever and the agent associated with this condition is *Streptococcus pyogenes* (modified Jones criteria 1 major criteria: Migratory polyarthritis 2 minor: Elevated CRP and prolongation of PR interval)

C. What is the justification for negative blood culture in this case? (1 mark)

- The manifestations in acute rheumatic fever are not directly related to group A *Streptococcus*. The manifestations are a result of antibodies to streptolysin O which cross react with cardiac tissue and joints and cause the damage.

MI 2.4 LIST THE COMMON MICROBIAL AGENTS CAUSING ANAEMIA. DESCRIBE THE MORPHOLOGY, MODE OF INFECTION AND DISCUSS THE PATHOGENESIS, CLINICAL COURSE, DIAGNOSIS AND TREATMENT OF MICROBIAL AGENTS CAUSING ANAEMIA

LONG ESSAYS

1. A 7-year-old child came to a PHC for her routine school health check-up. On examination, she had pallor. Peripheral blood smear showed microcytic hypochromic anaemia. Stool wet mount revealed non-bile-stained egg with segmented ovum.

A. What is your diagnosis and the causative agent? (2 marks)

Diagnosis

- Hookworm infection.

Causative Agent

- *Ancylostoma duodenale* or *Necator americanus*.

B. Briefly describe the life cycle of the causative agent (3 marks)

Life Cycle (Fig. 2.4.1)

- *Host:* Involves only one host (man)
- *Infective stage:* Third stage filariform (L3) larva

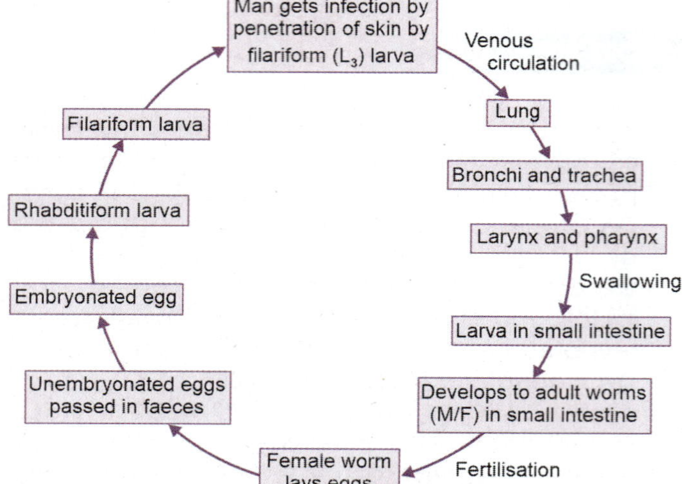

Fig. 2.4.1: Life cycle of *Ancylostoma duodenale*

- *Mode of transmission:* Skin penetration by the third stage larva

C. Pathogenesis and clinical features. (3 marks)

Pathogenesis

Effects Due to Migrating Larvae

- Ancylostoma dermatitis or ground itch.
- Creeping eruptions/cutaneous larva migrans.
- Lesions in lungs.

Effects Due to Adult Worm

- Attach to the mucosa of small intestine.
- Sucks blood.
- *Worm secretions:* Anticoagulant activity
- Leads to Iron deficiency anaemia.

Clinical Features

- Weakness and pallor attributed to microcytic anaemia caused by blood loss.
- 'Ground itch,' a pruritic papule or vesicle at the site of entry of the larvae into the skin.
- Cutaneous larva migrans.
- Pneumonia with eosinophilia during larval migration through the lungs.

D. Laboratory investigations useful in the diagnosis of this condition. (2 marks)

- *Stool wet mount:* Demonstration of non-bile-stained eggs with segmented ovum (Fig. 2.4.2)
- Occult blood in the stool.
- Elevated eosinophil count.

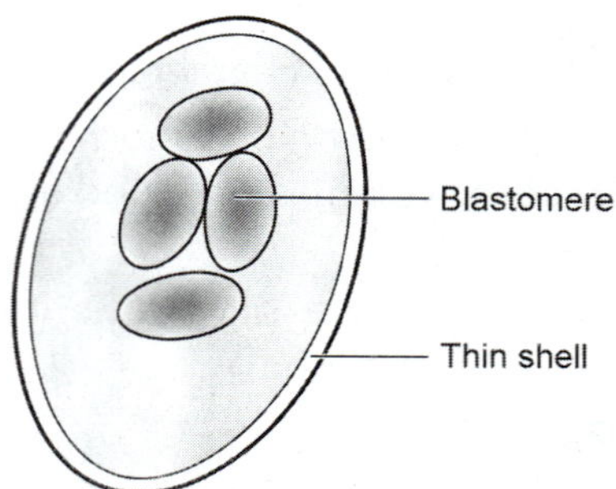

Fig. 2.4.2: Egg of hookworm

2. An 8-year-old child presents with an acute abdominal pain and nausea. He was malnourished. On stool microscopy, abundant bile-stained oval eggs with thick outer wall coat were observed.

A. Identify the disease condition and the aetiological agent. (2 marks)

Disease Condition

- Whipworm infection (Trichuriasis).

Aetiological Agent

- *Trichuris trichiura.*

B. Draw a neat, labelled diagram of the ova seen on microscopy. (2 marks)

- *See* Figure 2.4.3.

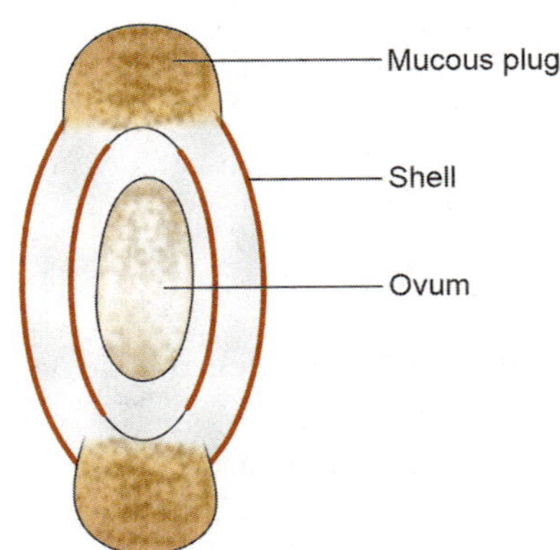

Fig. 2.4.3: Egg of *Trichuris trichiura*

C. Briefly discuss the pathogenesis, clinical features and complications of this disease. (3+2+1 marks)

Pathogenesis

- *Reservoir:* Man
- *Mode of transmission:* Ingestion of embryonated eggs from contaminated drinking water and food
- *Risk factors*
  1. Low socioeconomic status
  2. Low levels of education
  3. Poor sanitation
  4. Proximity to water sources.
- *Sequence of events*
  - Eggs following ingestion hatch in the small intestine and the larvae enter the intestinal crypts.
  - The larvae migrate to the proximal colon and mature into adult worms.
  - The adult worms live in the cecum and ascending colon and attach themselves to the colonic mucosa with their anterior portions threaded into the mucosa.
  - The females begin to oviposit 60–70 days after infection.
  - Whipworm causes disease by colonic mucosal invasion of the adult worms, resulting in inflammation of the colonic mucosa.

Clinical Features

- Abdominal pain, painful passage of stools, and mucus discharge.
- Nocturnal passage of stools.

Complications

1. Rectal prolapse in a heavy infestation.
2. Children may develop anaemia, growth retardation, and even impaired cognitive development.

3. Mention platyhelminthes parasites causing anaemia. Describe in detail about "fish tapeworm" under the following headings.

Platyhelminthes Parasite Causing Anaemia

- *Diphyllobothrium latum.*

A. Morphology of Fish Tapeworm and its Scientific name. (1 mark)

Morphology of Fish Tapeworm

- Pseudophyllidean cestode
- Longest tapeworm infecting man
- Head or scolex, neck and strobila
- Head has 2 bothria for attachment to the small intestine.
- Strobila has 3,000 segments divided into immature, mature and gravid segments.

Scientific Name

- *Diphyllobothrium latum.*

B. Life cycle. (4 marks)

- *Definitive host:* Humans
- *First intermediate hosts:* Fresh water copepods mainly of the genera *Cyclops* and *Diaptomus*
- *Second intermediate hosts:* Fresh water fishes
- *Infective form:* Third stage plerocercoid larvae in predator fish
- *Modes of transmission:* Ingestion of undercooked fresh water fish containing third stage plerocercoid larva
- *Life cycle of Diphyllobothrium latum* (Fig. 2.4.4).

C. Clinical features. (2 marks)

- Mostly asymptomatic, but abdominal discomfort and diarrhoea can occur.
- Causes little damage in the small intestine.
- Megaloblastic anaemia as a result of vitamin B_{12} deficiency caused by preferential uptake of the vitamin by the worm. The adult worm causes dissociation of vitamin B_{12} intrinsic factor complex leading to vitamin B_{12} deficiency and megaloblastic anaemia.

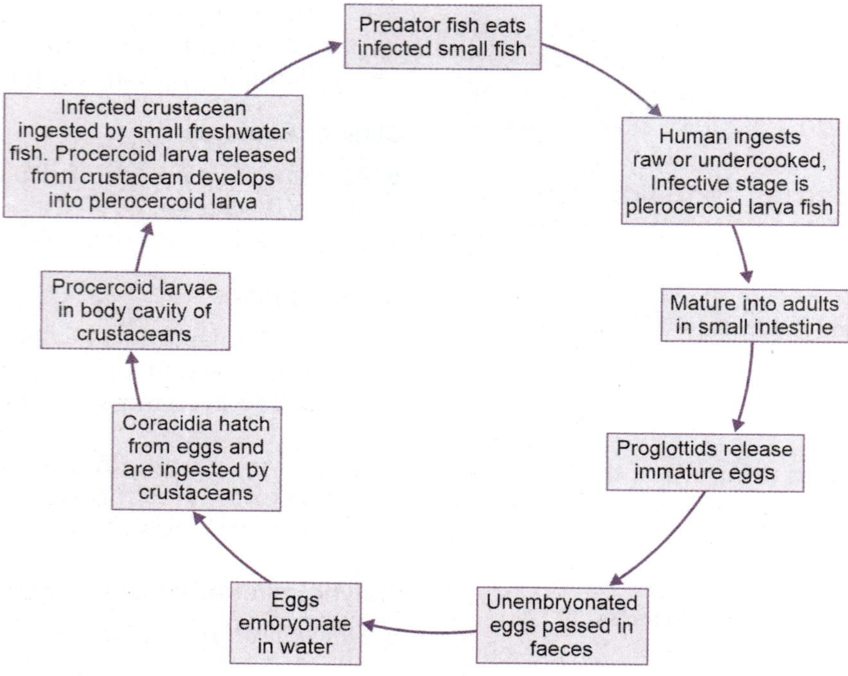

Fig. 2.4.4: Life cycle of *Diphyllobothrium latum*

D. Laboratory diagnostic modalities (2 marks)

- Diagnosis depends on finding the typical eggs, i.e. oval, yellow brown eggs with an operculum at one end) in the stool.
- There is no serologic test.

SHORT ESSAYS

1. Mention the protozoan parasites causing anaemia. Describe in detail the pathogenesis, clinical features, diagnosis, and treatment of babesiosis. (1+1+1+1+1 marks)

Protozoan Parasites Causing Anaemia

1. *Plasmodium* spp.
2. *Babesia* spp.

Babesiosis

Etiological Agent

- *Babesia microti.*

Pathogenesis

- *Reservoir host:* Rodents
- *Transmission:* Bite of the tick *Ixodes dammini* (renamed *I. scapularis*)
- *Effect:* Infects red blood cells, resulting in lysis. no exoerythrocytic phase

Clinical Features

- Influenza like symptoms begin gradually and may last for several weeks
- Hepatosplenomegaly and anaemia.

Diagnosis

- *Microscopy:* Giemsa stain—intraerythrocytic ring-shaped parasites
- The intraerythrocytic ring-shaped trophozoites are often in tetrads in the form of a Maltese cross.

Treatment

- *For mild to moderate disease:* Combination of atovaquone and azithromycin
- *For severe disease:* Combination of quinidine and clindamycin
- Exchange transfusion in severe disease.

2. Mention the viruses causing anaemia. Discuss the mechanism involved in causing anaemia by any one virus in brief. (2+3 marks)

Viruses Causing Anaemia

1. Cytomegalovirus
2. Epstein-Barr virus
3. Varicella zoster virus
4. Parvovirus B19
5. HIV
6. Hepatitis C virus.

Anaemia in Human Parvovirus B19

1. **Transient aplastic crisis**
   - Bone marrow failure, by affecting erythroid-lineage cells.
   - Anaemia is critical in those afflicted with haemolytic diseases. This condition is called transient aplastic crisis that may complicate chronic haemolytic anaemia, such as in patients with sickle cell disease, thalassaemia, and acquired haemolytic anaemia in adults.
2. **B19 infection in immunodeficient patients**
   - Persistent infections cause chronic suppression of bone marrow and chronic anaemia in immunocompromised patients.
   - Called pure red cell aplasia.
   - Anaemia is severe, and patients are dependent on blood transfusions.
3. **B19 infection in pregnancy.**
   - Resulting in hydrops foetalis and fetal death due to severe anaemia.
   - The overall risk of human parvovirus infection during pregnancy is low; fetal loss occurs in fewer than 10% of primary maternal infections. Foetal death occurs most commonly before the 20th week of pregnancy.

SHORT ANSWERS

1. With the help of a neat, labelled diagram, describe the morphology of Egg of old-world hookworm. (3 marks)

Morphology of Egg of Old-World Hook Worm (See Fig. 2.4.2)

- Oval-shaped
- Measures 60 × 40 μm
- Non-bile stained, appear colourless in saline mount.
- Hyaline egg shell
- Ovum (embryo) is segmented; comprises of 4 to 32 blastomeres
- Floats on saturated salt solution
- Eggs of both *A. duodenale and N. americanus are* morphologically indistinguishable.

2. List out the examples of bacteria causing Anaemia. (2 marks)

I. Haemolytic Anaemia

1. *Escherichia coli (haemolytic uremic syndrome).*
2. *Clostridium perfringens.*
3. *Rickettsia* species.
4. *Mycoplasma pneumoniae*

II. Aplastic Anaemia (Impaired RBC Production)

1. *Mycobacterium tuberculosis*
2. *Helicobacter pylori.*

3. Discuss the pathogenesis and clinical features of Anaemia caused by Bartonella bacilliformis. (2+1 marks)

Anaemia Caused by *Bartonella bacilliformis*

Pathogenesis

- *B. bacilliformis* produces an extracellular protein called deformin that promotes deformity (indentation) of red blood cell membranes, and flagella provide the organisms with the mechanical force to invade red blood cells.
- Replication of the organism occurs within an endocytic vacuole facilitated by outer membrane proteins and erythrocyte membrane fragments created at the time of attachment and membrane deformity.

Clinical Features

- *Oroya fever:* rapid development of severe anaemia caused by red blood cell destruction, enlargement of the spleen and liver, and haemorrhage into the lymph nodes
- *Mortality rate:* 85%
- Weeks to months following acute infection, a second stage of infection called verruga peruana, characterised by vascular nodular skin lesions occurring in successive crops.
- This infection lasts for about 1 year and produces little systemic reaction and no fatalities.
- Mucosal and internal lesions have been described.

4. Mention the type of anaemia caused by human blood fluke. Mention the factors explaining the association. (1+2 marks)

Type of Anaemia Caused by Human Blood Fluke

- Iron deficiency anaemia is associated with schistosomiasis.

Factors Explaining the Association

- The mechanisms implicated are extra-corporeal loss of iron, splenomegaly leading to red blood cell sequestration, autoimmune haemolysis and anaemia of inflammation.

3. Describe in detail the causes for anaemia in malaria. (3 marks)

- After a few paroxysms of fever, patient develops normocytic normochromic anaemia.
- Causes for anaemia in malaria.
  1. Parasite-induced lysis of RBC.
  2. Removal of infected and uninfected RBC coated with immune complexes by spleen.
  3. Bone marrow suppression leading to decreased RBC production.
  4. Increased fragility of RBC.
  5. Autoimmune lysis of coated RBC.

4. Individuals with sickle cell anaemia are resistant to malaria. Justify the statement with relevant explanation. (3 marks)

Individuals with Sickle Cell Anaemia are Resistant to Malaria—Justification

- The sickle cell gene is caused by a single amino acid mutation in the beta chain of the haemoglobin gene. Inheritance of this mutated gene from both parents leads to sickle cell disease and people with this disease have shorter life expectancy. On the other hand, individuals who are carriers for the sickle cell disease (with one sickle gene and one normal haemoglobin gene, also known as sickle cell trait) have some protective advantage against malaria.
- The prevalence of sickle cell carriers is high in malaria-endemic areas. The sickle RBC s have stretched membranes owing to their unusual shape. The membrane become porous, and nutrients leak out. The parasites cannot survive, and the faulty cells get eliminated quite fast by the organisms, destroying the parasite along the way.

MI 2.5 DESCRIBE THE AETIOPATHOGENESIS AND DISCUSS THE CLINICAL EVOLUTION AND LABORATORY DIAGNOSIS OF MALARIA, KALA-AZAR, FILARIASIS AND OTHER COMMON PARASITES PREVALENT IN INDIA

LONG ESSAYS

1. A 65-year-old male presented with history of fever, chills, mild myalgia, and occasional sweating. As a part of routine evaluation, complete blood count, rapid screening test for dengue and peripheral blood smear examination were ordered. The peripheral blood smear revealed crescent shaped gametocytes and multiple ring forms in the RBCs.

A. What is the aetiological agent in the above case. (1 mark)

- Malaria caused by *Plasmodium falciparum*.

B. Briefly discuss life cycle of this aetiological agent. (4 marks)

Definitive Host

- Female Anopheles mosquito in which the sexual cycle (sporogony) of the parasite takes place.

Intermediate Host

- Humans, in whom the asexual cycle (schizogony) takes place.

Life Cycle (Fig. 2.5.1)

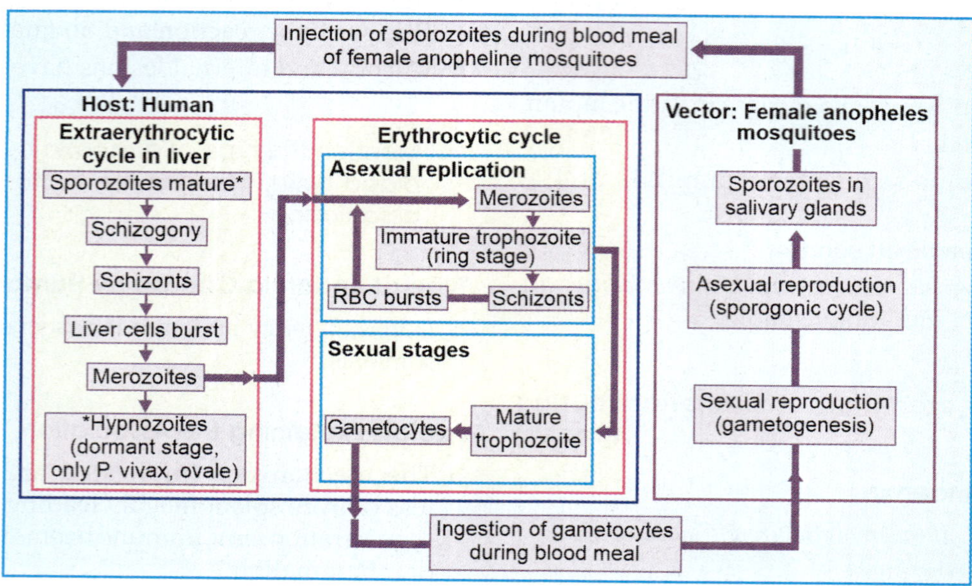

Fig. 2.5.1: Life cycle of *Plasmodium falciparum*

C. Pathogenesis and Clinical manifestations of this disease. (5 marks)

Pathogenesis

- *Mode of infection:* By bite of infected female anopheles mosquito
- *Incubation period:*
  - 10–14 days: *P. falciparum, P. vivax, P. ovale.*
  - 28–30 days: *P. malariae.*
- *Sequence of events.*
  1. *Sporozoites.*
     - In blood, cause no apparent harm.
     - In liver, destroy hepatocytes but as only few hepatocytes are involved, no noticeable damage.
  2. *Merozoites.*
     - Once merozoites are formed, they enter the erythrocytic cycle and cause significant pathogenic effects.

Clinical Manifestations

1. **Malarial Paroxysms**
   i. *Cold stage.*
   - Characterised by initial chills which last for 15–60 minutes.
   - RBCs rupture → release red cell fragments, merozoites and pigments → act on macrophages/polymorphs → release endogenous pyrogen → act on thermoregulatory centre → fever.

   ii. *Hot (pyrexial) stage.*
   - Spiking fever (39–40.5°C).
   - Headache.
   - Bone and joint pains.
   - Often vomiting and diarrhoea.
   - Lasts for 2–6 hours.
   - Parasites invade fresh RBCs.

   iii. *Sweating stage.*
   - Patient perspires and is drenched with profuse sweat
   - Temperature falls
   - Patient falls asleep to wake up refreshed until the next paroxysm.
2. **Anaemia Normocytic, Normochromic Haemolytic anaemia**
   - *Caused by:*
     - Destruction of parasitised RBCs.
     - Destruction of non-parasitised RBCs due to autoimmune reaction.
     - Decreased erythropoiesis.
3. **Splenomegaly**
   - Enlarged by second week of disease due to accumulation of macrophages.
   - Early stages, it is soft, congested with distended capsule.
   - Later stages, becomes dark due to accumulation of malaria pigment, cellular hyperplasia.
   - Finally, becomes hard due to fibrosis.

D. Mention the laboratory tests available in the diagnosis of the above case. (5 marks)

- Clinical diagnosis must be confirmed by laboratory evidence of malarial infection.
- *Gold standard for diagnosis:* Demonstration of the malarial parasite in peripheral blood of the patient

Specimen Collection

Blood

- Best collected a few hours after the peak of fever, as parasites are abundant within the RBCs at that time.
- Common practice is to collect sample on presentation and a second one after a few hours of fever.
- Repeated samples have to be examined before considering a case as negative for malaria.
- *Thick blood smear:* Thick films help in detection as there are 20–30 layers of blood cells in a small area
- Thin blood smear as morphology of RBCs is preserved, thin smears are useful in identifying the species of plasmodia causing infection.
- Which are stained by Romanowsky's stains such as Leishman's, Giemsa and Field's, Wright's or JSB stain.

Microscopy

I. Peripheral Blood Examination

Stages seen in peripheral blood smear (Fig. 2.5.2)

1. All asexual stages (ring forms, trophozoites, schizonts) and gametocytes are seen in *P. vivax, P. malariae* and *P. ovale.*
2. Rings forms and crescent-shaped gametocytes are seen in *P. falciparum.*
3. Multiple ring forms and accole forms in *P. falciparum.*
4. RBC are enlarged in *P. vivax;* no enlargement is seen in *P. falciparum.*

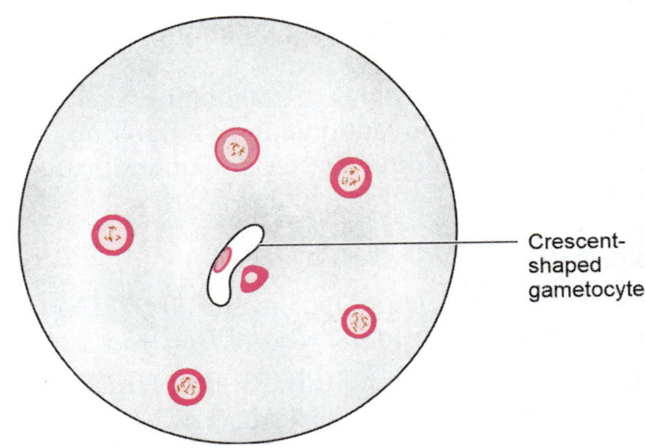

Fig. 2.5.2A: Gametocyte

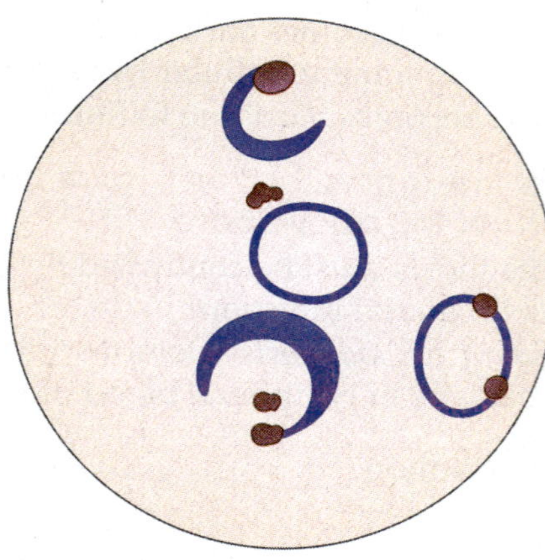

Fig. 2.5.2B: Stages of *Plasmodium falciparum* in the peripheral blood smear

Advantages

1. Peripheral smear is simple, rapid, and cheap.
2. *Thick smear:* useful in detecting the parasites, can detect as low as 5–10 parasites per μl of blood.
3. Quantification of parasitaemia
4. Demonstrating the malaria pigments
5. Thin smear is useful in speciation of malaria parasite.

Disadvantages

1. Labour intensive and requires experienced microscopist.
2. *Low sensitivity:* The detection limit of thin smear is more than 200 parasites per μl of blood.

II. QBC (Quantitative Buffy Coat) Test (BD)

- 50–100 μl of blood is taken into a capillary tube whose inner surface is coated with the fluorescent dye—Acridine orange.
- Now, tube is centrifuged at high speed
- The parasites get concentrated in the tip of the RBC column and are stained by the fluorescent dye.

Advantage

1. Rapid and sensitive test.

Limitations

1. Reduced specificity due to staining of leucocyte DNA
2. Requires specialised instrumentation.
3. Costlier than conventional light microscopy.
4. Poor at determining species and quantification of parasites.

Rapid Tests

1. Detection of P. falciparum specific circulating proteins in the whole blood (Rapid Diagnostic Test).

- Histidine-rich protein II (PfHRP-II or HRP-II).
  - Histidine rich protein II (HRP-II) antigen is produced by blood stages of *Plasmodium falciparum.*
  - Detected by ELISA antigen test and dipstick Becton Dickinson ParaSight ®-F test.

Advantages

1. Highly sensitive and specific
2. Fast and simple.

Limitations

1. Circulating antigens can be detected up to 2–4 weeks after treatment.
2. Quantification of parasite load is not possible.
3. Stage identification is not possible.
4. Costly.

2. Parasite-specific Lactic Dehydrogenase (LDH)

- In patients with *P. falciparum* and *P. vivax* parasitaemia (pLDH optiMAL).
- *Blood levels of parasite-specific lactate dehydrogenase (pLDH):* Method of quantifying parasitaemia and drug resistance

Advantages

1. Simple and rapid.
2. Superior to HRP-II because of its shorter shelf life in blood.

Disadvantages

1. Lack of sensitivity at low levels of parasitaemia.
2. Inability to quantify parasite density.
3. Inability to differentiate between *P. vivax, P. ovale* and *P. malariae.*
4. Inability to differentiate between the sexual and asexual stages of the parasite.
5. Persistently positive tests (for some antigens) despite parasite clearance following chemotherapy.
6. Relatively high cost per test.

Serology

- Based on the detection of antibodies against asexual blood stage malaria parasites.
  1. IFAT.
     - Indirect immunofluorescent antibody test (sensitive and specific, but time consuming).
  2. ELISA.
     - Only measures exposure and antibodies persist after clinical cure.

Molecular Methods

- PCR
- DNA probes
- Sensitive assay and drug resistance genes can be studied.

2. A 50-year-old man presented with unilateral swelling of the leg. He had h/o of on and off fever for 6 months. His peripheral blood picture showed microfilaria, tail tip free of nuclei.

A. What is your diagnosis and the aetiological agent? (2 marks)

Diagnosis

- Lymphatic filariasis.

Aetiological Agent

- *Wuchereria bancrofti.*

B. Briefly write the life cycle, pathogenesis, clinical features of this disease condition. (4 marks)

Life Cycle (Fig. 2.5.3)

- *Host:* Mosquitoes (intermediate host), Human (final host)
- *Location:* Lymphatics and lymph nodes
- *Infective stage:* Infective larvae
- *Transmission stage:* Microfilariae
- *Diagnostic stage:* Microfilariae

Pathogenesis

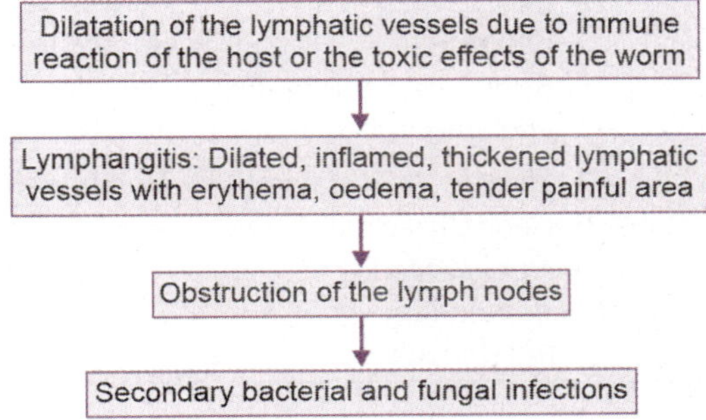

Clinical Features

Endemic Normal

- No clinical features
- No microfilariae

Asymptomatic

- Have microfilariae in the blood no clinical features.

Acute Filariasis

- Inflammatory phase.
- *Filarial fever:* Low grade, with chills, general malaise, headache, and pain
- *Lymphoedema:* Presence of adult worms in the lymphatic vessels
- *Lymphadenitis:* Inflammation of the lymph nodes
- *Lymphangitis:* Inflammation of the lymphatic channels. Results in epididymoorchitis, funiculitis, retroperitoneal lymphangitis

Chronic Filariasis

- Obstructive phase.
- Takes 10–15 years to develop.
- *Lymph varices:* varicose lymph ducts
- *Hydrocoele:* Obstruction of the lymphatic vessels of the spermatic cord and exudation from the inflamed testis, epididymis
- *Elephantiasis:* Complex immune reaction of the long duration and repeated superinfection over years. Scrotum, legs, arms are involved. Seen in highly endemic areas

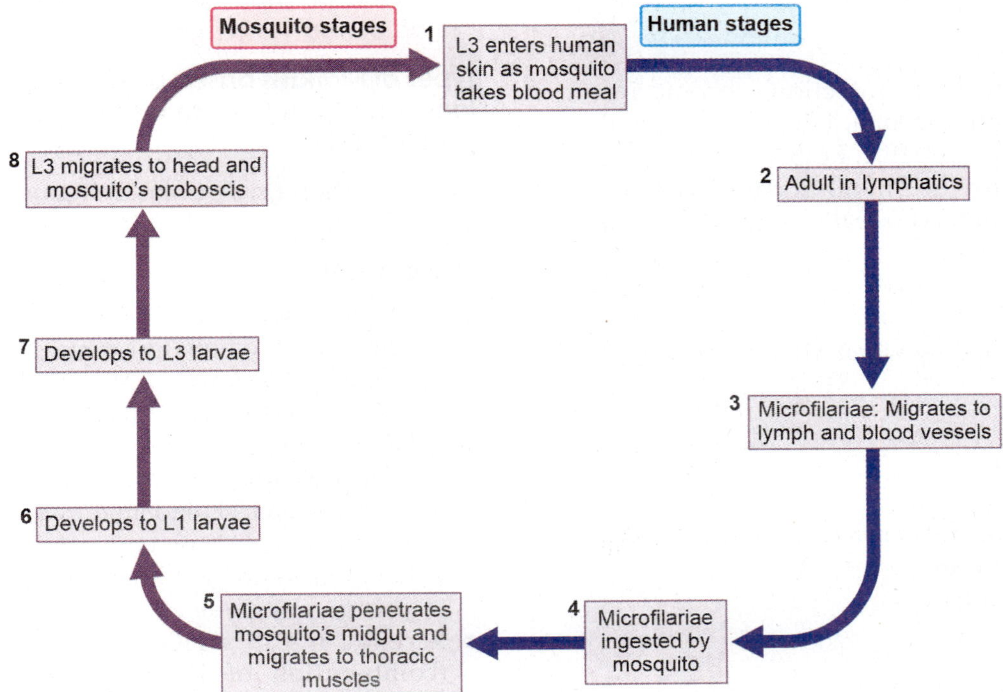

Fig. 2.5.3: Life cycle of *Wuchereria bancrofti*

- *Chyluria:* Urine with chyle mixed with blood. Caused by obstruction of the lymphatic vessels of kidney, abdomen

Occult Filariasis

- Hypersensitivity reaction of the host to microfilarial Ag.
- Lymphatic vessels, lung, liver, spleen affected.
- Tropical pulmonary eosinophilia common. Also, arthritis, glomerulonephritis, thrombophlebitis, dermatoses.
- Mf in peripheral blood absent.
- High titre of filarial Abs is diagnostic.

C. Laboratory workup and treatment for the above case. (3 + 1 marks)

Laboratory Workup

Specimen Collection

- Blood, chylous urine, hydrocoele fluid.

Blood Microscopy

- *Direct wet mount:* Live Mf with serpentine movement
- *Stained thick blood smear with Giemsa, Leishman:* Sheathed Mf with absence of nuclei at the tail tip
- *Concentration of blood:* Knott method of sedimentation, membrane filtration with millipore membrane filter to increase the sensitivity of direct microscopic examination to detect Mf.
- *DEC provocation test:* Single dose of Hetrazan 100 mg orally induces the appearance of nocturnal Mf during daytime. After 30 minutes blood is collected and examined for Mf.

Immunodiagnosis

- Useful in prepatent infection, chronic infection without microfilariaemia, TPE, filarial granuloma.
- *Demonstration of Ab:* IFA, ELISA
- *Demonstration of Ag:* 2 monoclonal Abs based ELISA
- *ICT filariasis card test (rapid):* for the detection of Ag in patient's serum

Molecular Methods

- PCR is positive only when Mf are found in blood.

Imaging Methods

- X-ray, USG.

Others

- *Biopsy of the enlarged lymph nodes:* shows cross section of the adult worms
- *CBC:* Eosinophilia

Treatment

- *Diethylcarbamazine (DEC):* 12-day treatment of DEC (6 mg/kg/day)
- *Doxycycline (200mg/day for 4–6 weeks).*
  - Kills adult worm.
  - First-line ant filarial therapy for nonpregnant adults and children >8 years of age with lymphatic filariasis.

---

3. *Wuchereria bancrofti* differs from other filarial forms in many aspects. Supporting the statement discuss the following.

A. Compare the microfilaria of *Wuchereria bancrofti* and *Brugia malayi* (2 marks)

- See Table 2.5.1

Table 2.5.1 Comparison of microfilaria of hdhgdhhgdh Wuchereria bancrofti and Brugia malayi

	Head end	*Tail end*
Wuchereria bancrofti	• *Sheath:* Faintly stained • Length and breadth are equal • Cephalic space (1:1) • *Coarse nuclei:* Discrete • *Body curves:* Regular and smooth	• Terminal nuclei elongated • No nuclei in the tail tip • Pointed tail tip • *Body curves:* Irregular and kinky
Brugia malayi	• *Sheath:* Well stained • Cephalic space (2:1) • *Nuclei:* Darkly stained large coarse not discrete	• Two widely spaced round nuclei in tail tip

B. Compare and contrast the types of Filariasis based on their aetiological agents, location of adult worm and microfilaria and vector. (4 marks)

Types of Filariasis based on their aetiological agents, location of adult worm and microfilaria and vector (Table 2.5.2)

C. Prevention and control measures of Filariasis. (2 marks)

Vector Control

- *Antilarval measures:* Mosquito larvicidal oil, pyrethrum-based oil (Pyrosene oil-E)
- *Anti-adult measures:* DDT and hexachlorocyclohexane (HCH) are not effective
- WHO recommends yearly single dose of DEC + Albendazole in all endemic areas except,.
  - In onchocerciasis endemic areas where Ivermectin + Albendazole is given.
  - In *Loa loa* endemic area (albendazole twice per year given).
- Recently in 2018, WHO recommended IDA regimen (combination of ivermectin, DEC and albendazole) under elimination program. It is yet to be implemented.

Table 2.5.2 Types of Filariasis based on their aetiological agents, location of adult worm and microfilaria and vector

Etiological agents	*Location of adult worm*	*Location of microfilaria*	*Features*	*Vector*
Lymphatic Filariasis				
Wuchereria bancrofti	Lymphatics	Blood	Sheathed, pointed tip free of nuclei	Culex
Brugia malayi	Lymphatics	Blood	Sheathed, blunt tip with 2 terminal nuclei	Mansonia
Brugia timori	Lymphatics	Blood	Longer than *Mf malayi*	Anopheles
Subcutaneous Filariasis				
Loa loa	Connective tissue, conjunctiva	Blood	Sheathed nuclei up to pointed tail tip	*Chrysops* spp.
Onchocerca volvulus	Subcutaneous nodules	Skin, eyes	Unsheathed, blunt tail free of nuclei	*Simulium* spp.
Mansonella streptocerca	Subcutaneous	Skin	Unsheathed, blunt tail with nuclei	Culicoides
Serous Cavity Filariasis				
Mansonella ozzardi	Peritoneum, pleura	Blood	Unsheathed, pointed tail tip without nuclei	Culicoides
Mansonella perstans	Peritoneum, pleura	Blood	Unsheathed, pointed tail tip with nuclei	Culicoides

Elimination of Lymphatic Filariasis in India

- Transmission control through mass drug administration (MDA) and disease control through individual patient management.

4. A 24-year-old male, resident of Africa presents with chief complaints of haematuria, dysuria, and fever. His skin appears pale. He has a habit of swimming in lake. His haemoglobin levels and RBC count are low. Urine analysis shows reddish coloured erythrocytes and crystals. Microscopic examination of urine detects eggs of a trematode.

A. Which is the probable aetiological agent of this condition? (1 mark)

- *Schistosoma haematobium.*

B. Explain the life cycle of this trematode. (3 marks)

- *Definitive host:* Man
- *Intermediate host:* Freshwater snails of genus *Bulinus*
- *Mode of transmission:* Penetration of skin by the infective form (cercariae) present in contaminated water
- *See* Figure 2.5.4.

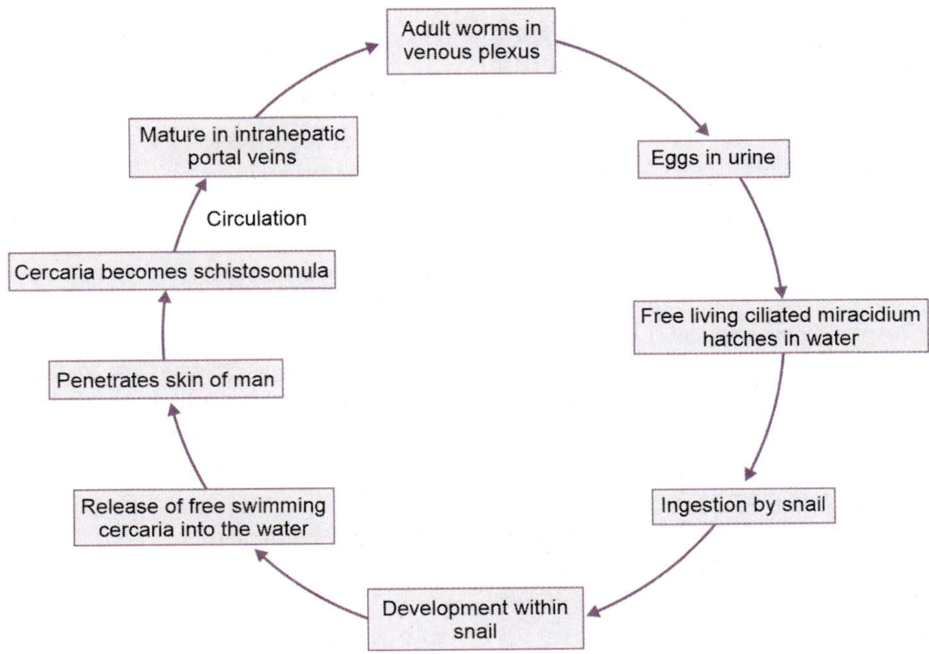

Fig. 2.5.4: Life cycle of *Schistosoma haematobium*

C. Discuss the pathogenesis and clinical features of this trematode. (4 marks)

Pathogenesis

Due to the Cercaria

- Skin penetration by human schistosome cercaria results in type I allergy.
- Cercarial dermatitis with petechiae and rashes.
- Localised pneumonitis and urticaria.

Due to Adults

- The mechanical effect and toxic effect of adults and their metabolites cause mesenteric phlebitis, hepatitis, and abdominal pain; the immune complex may cause the damage to the kidney, schistosome nephritis results from type III allergy.

Due to Eggs

- Egg induces strong inflammatory and granulomatous reaction leading to development of granulomas. Granuloma consists of eosinophils, macrophages and T cells which is delayed type of hypersensitivity.
- Degenerated or calcified eggs at centre surrounded by fibroblast proliferation and fibrosis is the main pathology.
- Eggs during its passage from venules into the lumen of urinary bladder cause traumatic lesions.
- Continuous toxic and mechanical irritation is responsible for malignant tumours.

Clinical Features

- Urinary schistosomiasis.
- *Acute schistosomiasis:* Cercarial dermatitis: itching and pruritic papular lesion in the skin within 24 hrs by the invasion of cercariae. Fever, malaise, right upper quadrant pain are the symptoms of serum sickness like illness
- *Chronic schistosomiasis:* Painless terminal haematuria dysuria and frequent urination
- Complications—hydroureter, hydronephrosis, secondary microbial infection. Frequent UTI by Salmonella, urinary bladder carcinoma usually squamous cell type.

D. How is the infection diagnosed and treated? (2 marks)

Parasitic Diagnosis

- *Specimens:* Urine, faeces, rectal biopsy, aspiration obtained by proctoscopy or cystoscopy
- *Urine:* Collected between 10 am to 2 pm, examined after centrifugation or membrane filtration. Presence of terminal spined eggs of *S. haematobium* (Fig. 2.5.5)

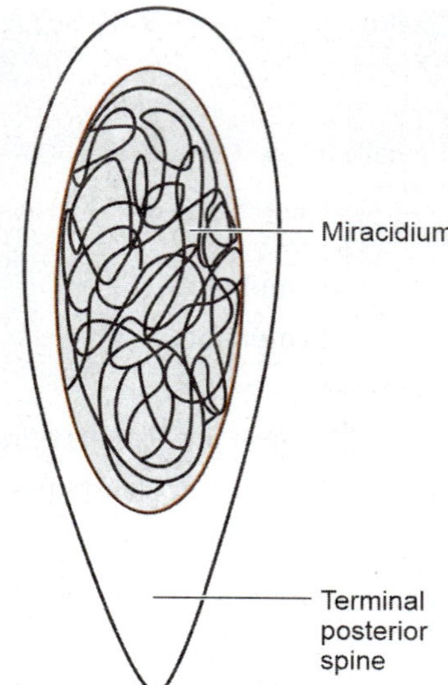

Fig. 2.5.5: Egg of *Schistosoma haematobium* with terminal spine

- *Urine egg count* in 24 hr collection to quantitate the severity of the infection (>50 eggs/ 10 ml is heavy infection).
- *Egg viability test* to assess the effectiveness of treatment. Done by mixing urine with distilled water and observe for hatching miracidium.

Serodiagnosis

- *Detection of antibodies:* IHA, Indirect IF, ELISA, RIA. Diagnosis of infection in prepatent period, chronic and ectopic cases
- *Detection of antigen:* In serum, urine by CIEP, ELISA, RIA. Helps to detect acute infection and of prognostic value

Histological Diagnosis

- Detection of parasitic eggs in the biopsy specimens.

Other Tests

1. Eosinophilia
2. Haematuria
3. Proteinuria

SHORT ESSAYS

1. With respect to the various visceral organs affected, describe in detail the pathogenesis and clinical features of kala-azar. Add a note on complications of kala-azar. (3+2+1 marks)

Aetiological Agent

- *Leishmania donovani.*

Pathogenesis

- *Reservoir host:* Man

- *Mode of transmission.*
  - Bite of an infected female phlebotomine sand fly.
  - Rarely by transfusions, contaminated needles, and from pregnant mother to her child.
- *Infective stage.*
  - Promastigotes.
- *Incubation period:* Months and as long as years
- *Sequence of events.*
  - After being bitten by an infected sand fly, the promastigotes are phagocytised by host macrophages.
  - Amastigotes is the tissue stage.
  - Proliferate to infect other mononuclear phagocytic cells in different tissues.
  - *Organs infected:* Spleen, liver, and bone marrow.
  - If left untreated it is a life-threatening disease.

Clinical Features

- *Incubation period:* 2–6 months
- The hallmark of VL is a pentad of fever, progressive weight loss, hepatosplenomegaly, pancytopenia and hypergammaglobulinaemia
- Fever and hyperpigmentation
- Splenomegaly
- Lymphadenopathy
- Pedal edema and ascites
- Haematological abnormalities.
  - *Pancytopenia: Anaemia*, leukopenia and thrombocytopenia.
  - Hypergammaglobulinaemia.
- Leishmanoma.

Complications

1. Secondary bacterial infections including pneumonia and tuberculosis
2. Septicaemia
3. Disfigurement of nose, lips, and palate (Cancrum oris)
4. Uncontrolled bleeding
5. Splenic rupture
6. *Late stages:* Oedema, cachexia, and hyperpigmentation.
7. *Post-kala-azar dermal leishmaniasis (PKDL).*
   - Macular, papular, or nodular rash or a combination of the three.
   - Starting from the face or any other part of the body typically, after being treated for visceral leishmaniasis.
   - Ocular lesions can be seen in some patients.

2. *Plasmodium falciparum* escapes immune surveillance mechanism and is having multiple virulence factors. Supporting this statement, describe the factors and complications of *falciparum malaria*. (2+3 marks)

Reasons for Complications

- The parasite infects RBCs of all ages, thus causing hyperparasitaemia.
- Infected RBC's show morphological changes.
  - "knobs" on their surfaces which contain adhesive proteins at their tips.
  - Adherence proteins mediate adhesion of such RBCs to capillary and venous endothelial surfaces.
  - Leads to sequestration of such RBCs in capillary beds of deep organs (disappear from peripheral circulation).
  - Infected RBCs may also adhere to uninfected RBCs to form "rosettes".
- Cytoadherence, sequestration and rosette formation of RBCs result in anoxic damage to vital organs.

Complications seen in Falciparum Malaria (Non-immune, immunosuppressed, pregnancy)

1. **Cerebral malaria**
   - Referred to as a complex of life-threatening complications that sometimes supervenes acute infection by *P. falciparum.*
   - Characterised by.
     - Congestion of meninges and brain
     - Occlusion of capillaries of brain
     - Petechial, perivascular haemorrhages
     - Necrotic lesions in midzonal brain tissue
     - Peripheral glial reaction (malarial granuloma).
     - *Features:* Hyperpyrexia, coma, paralysis.
2. **Pernicious malaria**
   1. *Black water fever.*
      - Sudden intravascular haemolysis followed by fever, haemoglobinuria, and dark urine.
      - It occurs following quinine treatment to subjects previously infected with *P. falciparum.*
      - Antibodies develop against parasitised and quininised RBCs. With subsequent infection and quinine treatment, there is immunocomplex formation followed by complement mediated massive destruction of both parasitised and nonparasitised RBCs.
   2. *Algid malaria.*
      - Cold clammy skin, hypotension, peripheral circulatory failure, and profound shock.

iii. *Septicemic malaria.*
- High degree of prostration, high grade fever with dissemination of the parasite to various organs leading to multiorgan failure.

3. **Pulmonary oedema and adult respiratory distress syndrome:** Mortality rate is >80%.
4. **Hypoglycaemia:** It is associated with a poor prognosis; specially in children and pregnant women and following quinine therapy.
5. **Renal failure:** It occurs due to erythrocyte sequestration in renal microvasculature leading to acute tubular necrosis.
6. **Bleeding/disseminated intravascular coagulation:** Patient presents with significant bleeding and haemorrhages from the gums, nose, and GIT with or without evidence of DIC.
7. **Severe jaundice:** It results from haemolysis, hepatocyte injury and cholestasis.
8. **Severe normochromic, normocytic anaemia:** Characterised by haematocrit of less than 15% or haemoglobin level of less than 5 g/dl with parasitaemia level of more than 100,000/µl (>2%).
9. **Acidosis:** Results from accumulation of organic acids like lactic acid.

3. Mention the hosts required for the completion of life cycle of *Leishmania donovani*. Describe the life cycle of *L. donovani* with diagrammatic illustrations wherever required. (1 + 4 marks)

Hosts Required for the Completion of Life Cycle of *Leishmania donovani*

- **Reservoir (source) of infection**
  - *India:* Only humans
  - *Other regions:* Humans, dogs, rodents
- **Definitive host:** Humans
- **Intermediate host (Vector):** Sandfly (*Phlebotomus argentipes*)

Life cycle of *Leishmania donovani* (Fig. 2.5.6)

4. Describe in brief about.

A. Tropical splenomegaly syndrome. (2 marks)

B. Cerebral malaria. (3 marks)

Tropical Splenomegaly Syndrome

- *Hyperreactive Malarial Splenomegaly.*
- Occurs as a result of immunological over-stimulation to repeated attacks of malarial infection over a long period of time.
- Occurs in people of malaria endemic areas in tropical Africa and Asia (including India).
- Characterised by elevated IgM, massive splenomegaly, hepatic sinusoidal lymphocytosis, peripheral B cell lymphocytosis (in Africa).

Cerebral Malaria

- Occurs due to plugging of brain capillaries by the rosettes of sequestered parasitised RBCs leading to vascular occlusion and cerebral anoxia.
- It manifests as diffuse symmetric encephalopathy characterised by generalised convulsion in 10% of adults and up to 50% of children.

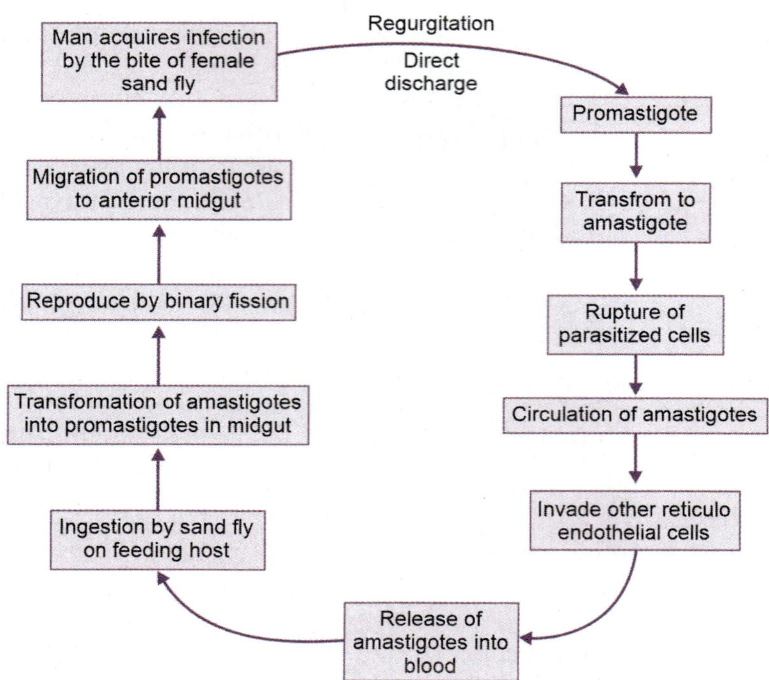

Fig. 2.5.6: Life cycle of *Leishmania donovani*

- Muscle tone and tendon reflexes are reduced, retinal haemorrhages, neurologic sequelae, repeated seizures, and rarely deep coma.
- Signs of focal neurologic and meningeal irritations are absent.
- *High mortality rate:* 20% among adults and >15% among children

5. A 24-year-old man in Bihar presents with h/o recurrent fever with chills for six months, progressive generalised weakness for five months and loss of appetite for one month. On general examination the patient had moderate pallor, no icterus, cyanosis, and lymphadenopathy. On abdominal examination, the liver was palpable about 2 cm right below costal margin and spleen was palpable up to 7 cm below the left costal margin. Routine haematological investigations revealed pancytopenia with haemoglobin level of 7 g/dl. Blood cultures were negative. Bone marrow smears revealed abundance of amastigote forms of *Leishmania donovani* (also known as LD bodies) both intracellularly within the macrophages as well as extracellularly.

A. What is the diagnosis?

- Kala azar (Visceral leishmaniasis).

B. Explain the tests available to diagnose this infection.

Specimen Collection

- Splenic aspirate (98% sensitivity, danger of bleeding/rupture).
- Bone marrow aspirate (80–85% sensitivity).
- Peripheral blood.
- Lymph node aspirate.

Microscopy—Demonstration of parasite

- Smears of specimen stained with Leishman/Giemsa.
  - Amastigote forms within macrophages or monocytes are seen as.
    - Oval bodies of 2–4 µm with,
    - Pale blue cytoplasm
    - Nucleus appears red
    - Kinetoplast appears purple
    - Vacuole remains unstained

Culture

- *Culture media:* Novy-Mc'Neal-Nicolle (NNN) medium
- Specimen inoculated into water of condensation and incubated at 24°C for 7 days.
- *Observation:* Motile promastigotes are observed microscopically, which sometime form large rosettes with their flagella entangled

Antibody Detection

- ELISA, IFA, direct agglutination test, ICT (rk 39, rke16).

Ag Detection

- Carbohydrate Ag in urine by latex agglutination .

Molecular Methods

- PCR.

Others

- Nonspecific serum test for hypergammaglobulinaemia.
  1. Napier's aldehyde test.
  2. Chopra's antimony test.
- Others.
  1. Pancytopenia.

SHORT ANSWERS

1. Write briefly on clinical features of cutaneous leishmaniasis. (1+2 marks)

Cutaneous Leishmaniasis

- Typically occurs at the site of inoculation by infected sandfly bite.

Clinical Features

- Solitary lesions are typical, but multiple lesions do occur
- Starts as a small red papule, which enlarges up to 2 cm in diameter
- Central ulceration
- Moist ulcers with pus or dry with a crusted scab
- Sores usually appear on exposed areas of the skin, especially the face and extremities.
- **The incubation time:** 2 weeks to 6 months
- Lesions are painless, and resolve spontaneously leaving residual atrophic scarring.
- Resolution of the lesions take 2 months to more than a year.
- Sporotrichoid spread with lymphocutaneous nodules may occur.
- Chronic disease and dissemination in immunodeficient patients can occur.

2. Post-kala-azar dermal Leishmaniasis. (3 marks)

Post Kala-azar Dermal Leishmaniasis (PKDL)

- Mucocutaneous disease is seen in cured, inadequately treated or untreated cases of visceral leishmaniasis.

- Endemic to many parts of India, Nepal, Bangladesh, and eastern Africa (Sudan, Ethiopia, Kenya).
- *Clinical manifestations:* Combination of hypopigmented patches, erythematous succulent papuloplaques, and nodular lesions on the face and upper body and at times extending to the extremities, genitalia, and tongue
- *Atypical morphology (especially in endemic areas):* photosensitivity, verrucous, hypertrophic, xanthomatous, and ulcerative lesions.
- Recognition of spectrum of mucocutaneous changes helps in early initiation of treatment and in reducing disease transmission in the community.
- No significant morbidity, but the affected patients continue to act as a reservoir of the disease, active case detection is required to identify cases early to control the disease transmission in the community.

Diagnosis is based on

- Detection of Amastigote in the skin in >80% of cases. easily detected from nodular lesions.
- **Serological tests:** Direct agglutination test (DAT) and antibodies to rK39 antigen are positive

3. Based on the involvement of spleen, classify the endemicity of Malaria. (3 marks)

Malaria Endemicity

1. *Hypoendemic:* Very intermittent transmission.
2. *Mesoendemic:* Regular seasonal transmission.
3. *Hyperendemic:* Intense, but with periods of no transmission during dry season.
4. *Holoendemic:* Transmission occurs all year long.

WHO Criteria for Classification of Endemicity by Spleen Rates

- **Spleen rate:** Number of palpable enlarged spleens per 100 individuals of similar ages

Endemicity	*Children aged 2–9 years (%)*	*Adults 9 (> 16 years)*
Hypoendemic	0–10	No measure
Mesoendemic	11–50	No measure
Hyperendemic	>50	High (⩾25%)
Holoendemic	>75	Low (⩽25%)

4. Compare and contrast relapse and recrudescence in malaria. (3 marks)

Relapse	*Recrudescence*
Seen in *Plasmodium vivax and P. ovale infections*	*Although seen in all species, more common in P. falciparum* followed by *P. malariae*
Few sporozoites do not develop into pre-erythrocytic schizont, but remain dormant (known as *hypnozoites)* for 3 weeks to 1 year	Falciparum malaria—recrudescence is due to persistence of drug resistant parasites, even after completion of treatment
Reactivation of hypnozoites leads to initiation of erythrocytic cycle and relapse of malaria	In *P. malariae infection, long-term recrudescence for up to* 60 years can be seen, due to long-term survival of erythrocytic stages at a low undetectable level in blood

5. Describe in brief.

A. Exflagellation. (1 marks)

B. Stages of malarial parasite. (2 marks)

A. Exflagellation

- Release of mature flagellated male sex cells by the microgametocytes of the malarial parasite.
- It is completed in 10–15 minutes.
- Occurs after the microgametocytes have been transferred from a human to the stomach of a mosquito.

B. Stages of Malarial Parasite

- All asexual stages (ring forms, trophozoites, schizonts) and gametocytes are seen in *P. vivax, P. malariae and P. ovale.*
- Rings forms and crescent shaped gametocytes are seen in *P. falciparum.*
- Multiple ring forms and accole forms in *P. falciparum.*
- RBC are enlarged in *P. vivax,* no enlargement is seen in *P. falciparum.*

6. *Plasmodium* exhibits: "Alteration of generations with alteration of hosts". Discuss. (3 marks)

- Plasmodium is considered from the sporozoan parasites that parasites on both the human and female Anopheles mosquito.
- In the life cycle of *Plasmodium*, there is a generation that reproduces sexually by gametes (in mosquito) and alternates with generations that reproduce asexually by sporogony (in mosquito) and by schizogony (in human).

MI 2.6 IDENTIFY THE CAUSATIVE AGENT OF MALARIA AND FILARIASIS

LONG ESSAY

1. A peripheral blood smear is prepared from a 40-year-old female patient with h/o fever, myalgia, chills. Focus the slide and answer the following questions.

A. Mention the stains useful to demonstrate the common morphological forms of *Plasmodium falciparum*. (2 marks)

- Peripheral blood smears are stained with Romanowsky's stains like
  1. Leishman's stain
  2. Giemsa stain
  3. Field's Wright's stain
  4. JSB stain.

B. Blood collection for microscopy. (3 marks)

- Best collected a few hours after the peak of fever, as parasites are abundant within the RBCs at that time.
- Common practice is to collect sample on presentation and a second one after a few hours of fever.
- Repeated samples must be examined before considering a case as negative for malaria.
- Difficulties faced in detection of malarial parasite in blood.
  - Early stages of infection.
  - Sample collected during apyrexial periods between paroxysms—especially with *P. falciparum*.
  - Samples collected after administration of antimalarials.

C. Compare and contrast thick and thin smears. (3 marks)

Feature	Thick smear	Thin smear
Preparation of smear	Tip of the ring finger is pricked. 2–3 drops of blood placed on a clean glass slide. Second slide (spreader slide) at an angle of 30–45°. Spread over area of approximately 2 cm in diameter	1 drop of blood taken spread over large area. Thick at one edge and thin at the other
Preparation of smear	Fixed with methanol, de-haemoglobinised and stained	Fixed with methanol and stained
Thickness of smear	Help in detection as there are 20–30 layers of blood cells in a small area	A single layer thick
Sensitivity	5–10 parasites per µl of blood.	More than 200 parasites per µl of blood
Speciation	Speciation not possible as parasites may be distorted and free	As morphology of RBCs is preserved, thin smears are useful in identifying the species of plasmodia causing infection

Contd.

D. Draw the various stages of *Plasmodium falciparum* seen in the peripheral blood smear examination. (2 marks)

- *See* Figure 2.5.2.

SHORT ESSAYS

1. Discuss with the help of a diagram the microfilariae larvae of *Wuchereria bancrofti* and *Brugia malayi*. (5 marks)

Feature	Microfilaria larvae of *Wuchereria bancrofti*	Microfilaria larvae of *Brugia malayi*
Length of microfilaria	• 250–300 µm	• 175–230 µm
Appearance	• Graceful sweeping curves	• Kinky with secondary curves
Cephalic space	• Length and breadth equal	• Length is twice the breadth
Stylet at anterior end	• Single	• Double
Excretory pore	• Not prominent	• Prominent
Nuclear column	• Discrete	• Blurred
Tail tip	• Pointed free of nuclei	• 2 distinct nuclei at the tip
Sheath	• Faintly stained	• Well stained

2. A 25-year-old lady presents to the medicine OPD with h/o fever, chills, and rigor in the last 3 days. Her blood is collected. The peripheral blood smear is focussed/shown (Fig. 2.6.1).

A. Identify the diagnostic stage. (1 mark)

Diagnostic Stage

- Crescent-shaped gametocyte of *Plasmodium falciparum*

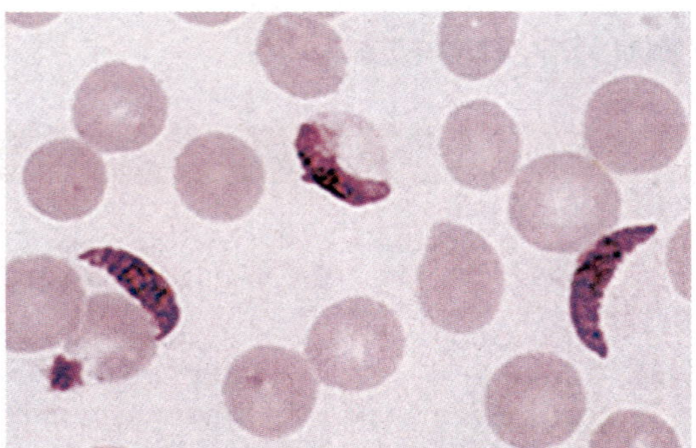

Fig. 2.6.1: Peripheral blood smear

B. What is the time for blood collection? (1 mark)

- Blood is collected few hours after the febrile paroxysm before administering antimalarial drugs.

C. What are the advantages of thick and thin smear in the diagnosis of this condition? (1 mark)

- Thick smears are more sensitive than thin smear (5–10 parasites/µl).
- Thin smears help in speciation of the malarial parasites.

D. What are the stains used for the peripheral blood smear examination in malaria? (1 mark)

- Romanowsky stain.
  1. Leishman.
  2. Giemsa.
  3. Wright.

E. What are the different diagnostic stages of this parasite seen in the peripheral blood smear? (1 mark)

- *Plasmodium falciparum:* Trophozoites (ring form), Gametocytes

3. A 35-year-old man presents with fever, malaise and swelling of the lower limb. Peripheral blood smear is focussed/shown (Fig. 2.6.2).

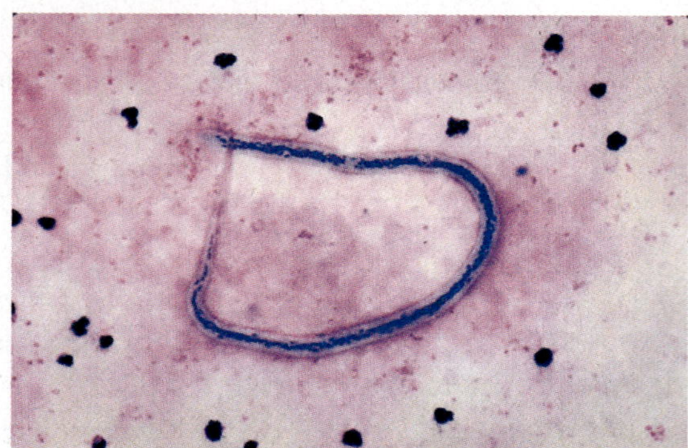

Fig. 2.6.2: Peripheral blood smear

A. Identify the structure and draw a neat, labelled diagram. (2 marks)

- Microfilaria of *Wuchereria bancrofti* (Fig. 2.6.3).

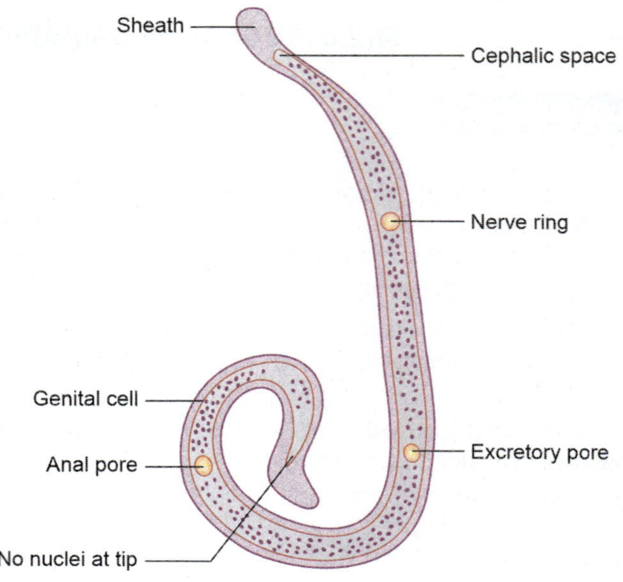

Fig. 2.6.3: Microfilaria of *Wuchereria bancrofti*

B. Name the 2 nematodes which can cause similar condition. (1 mark)

1. *Wuchereria bancrofti.*
2. *Brugia malayi.*

C. Compare and contrast the larval stages of the above 2 nematodes. (2 marks)

Feature	*Mf. bancrofti*	*Mf. malayi*
Length	• 250–300 µm	• 175–230 µm
Appearance	• Graceful sweeping curves	• Kinky with secondary curves
Cephalic space	• Length and breadth equal	• Twice as long as broad
Stylet at anterior end	• Single	• Double
Excretory pore	• Not prominent	• Prominent
Nuclear column	• Discrete	• blurred
Tail tip	• Pointed free of nuclei	• 2 distinct nuclei at the tip
Sheath	• Faintly stained	• Well stained

SHORT ANSWERS

1. Name the stains useful to demonstrate the microfilaria larva of *Wuchereria bancrofti*. (2 marks)

- Microfilariae of *Wuchereria bancrofti* are demonstrated in the thin and thick blood smears after staining with Giemsa, Leishman, or polychrome methylene blue smear.

2. Enumerate the blood concentration methods to demonstrate Microfilaria larva of *Wuchereria bancrofti*. (3 marks)

- Concentration methods for improved detection of microfilariae in blood or other body fluids.
  1. *Knott concentration:* 10 ml of 2% formalin in 15 ml centrifuge tube + 1 ml venous blood and centrifuged at 200 G for 2 minutes. The sediment is examined for microfilariae.
  2. *Membrane filtration:* 5 ml of heparinised blood in the syringe is fitted to nucleopore membrane and the blood is filtered. The membrane is then dried and the microfilariae sticking to the membrane are examined microscopically.
- The Knott's technique is more sensitive to pick up the Mf when their load is low. The use of quantitative buffy coat has been reported to be acceptable for the diagnosis of microfilariae, with a sensitivity similar to that of a thick film.

MI 2.7 DESCRIBE THE EPIDEMIOLOGY, AETIOPATHOGENESIS, CLINICAL EVOLUTION, COMPLICATIONS, OPPORTUNISTIC INFECTIONS, AND PRINCIPLES IN THE MANAGEMENT OF HIV

LONG ESSAYS

1. A 60-year-old truck driver presented with history of fever, cough, weakness for the last 3–4 weeks is visited the clinician. The patient gives h/o high risk behaviour. He was found to be reactive for antibodies to HIV 1.

A. Draw a neat, labelled diagram of HIV and describe in brief the structure of HIV. (2 marks)

Neat, Labelled Diagram of HIV (Fig. 2.7.1)

Structure of HIV

- HIV—Lentivirus subgroup of retroviruses.
- Spherical, enveloped virus.
- Inner cylindric core-two copies of ss RNA, enzymes reverse transcriptase, integrase, protease, and capsid protein-p 24.
- Double layered lipid envelope with gp120, gp41 glycoproteins.
- *Genome:* Virus has 3 structural genes—gag, pol, env and 6 regulatory genes—vif, vpr, vpu, tat, rev, nef

B. Various modes of transmission of HIV. (2 marks)

1. By transfer of infected blood (90–95% risk of transmission).
2. Perinatal transmission from infected mother to neonate also occurs, either across the placenta, at birth, or via breast milk (40–50% risk of transmission).
3. Sexual contact (0.1–1% risk of transmission).

C. Describe in brief the clinical manifestations of AIDS. (3 marks)

WHO Clinical Staging

Clinical Stage 1	• Asymptomatic HIV infection • Persistent generalised lymphadenopathy

Contd.

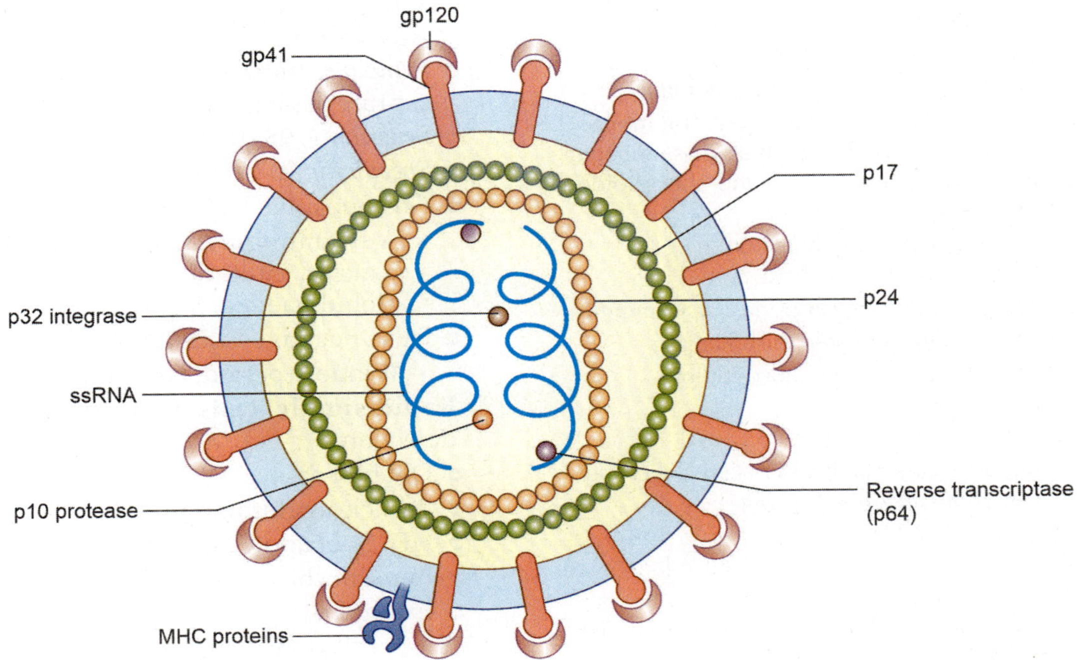

Fig. 2.7.1: Structure of HIV

Clinical Stage 2	• Unexplained moderate weight loss (<10%) • Recurrent respiratory tract infection (sinusitis, tonsillitis, otitis media, pharyngitis) • Herpes zoster • Angular cheilitis • Recurrent oral ulcers • Papular pruritic eruptions • Seborrheic dermatitis • Fungal nail infection
Clinical Stage 3	• Unexplained severe weight loss (>10%) • Unexplained chronic diarrhoea—>1 month • Unexplained persistent fever—1month • Oral candidiasis • Oral hairy leucoplakia • Pulmonary tuberculosis • Severe bacterial infection • Acute necrotizing ulcerative stomatitis, gingivitis, and periodontitis
	• Unexplained anaemia • HIV wasting syndrome (Slim disease)—Characterised by profound weight loss (>10%), chronic diarrhoea (>1 month), prolonged unexplained fever (1 month) • Bacterial opportunistic infections ✦ Recurrent severe bacterial infections ✦ Extrapulmonary tuberculosis ✦ Disseminated nontubercular mycobacterial infection ✦ Recurrent septicaemia (including non-typhoidal salmonellosis) • Viral opportunistic infections ✦ Chronic HSV infection ✦ Progressive multifocal leukoencephalopathy ✦ CMV (retinitis, or other organ infection excluding liver, spleen, and lymph node) • Fungal opportunistic infections ✦ Pneumocystis jirovecii pneumonia ✦ Oesophageal candidiasis, extrapulmonary cryptococcosis (meningitis), disseminated mycoses (histoplasmosis and coccidioido-mycoses) • Parasitic opportunistic infections ✦ Toxoplasma encephalitis ✦ Chronic intestinal isosporiasis (>1 month) ✦ Atypical disseminated leishmaniasis ✦ Chronic intestinal cryptosporidiosis (>1 month) • Neoplasia ✦ Kaposi's sarcoma, Invasive cervical cancer ✦ Lymphoma (cerebral, B cell and non-Hodgkin) • Other conditions (direct HIV induced) ✦ HIV encephalopathy ✦ Symptomatic HIV associated nephropathy or cardiomyopathy

D. Briefly describe the screening and confirmatory tests done for the diagnosis of HIV infection (3 marks)

Screening Tests

1. ELISA.
2. Rapid/simple tests.

- Advantages are:
  - High sensitivity
  - Cheaper
  - Easily available
  - Easy to perform

Supplemental Tests

1. Western blot
2. Indirect IF

Confirmatory Tests

1. P24 Ag detection
2. HIV RNA PCR
3. HIV DNA PCR (paediatric AIDS)
4. Real time PCR (prognosis)
5. NASBA
6. Viral culture

1. **ELISA (2–3 hours)**
   - For the detection of antibodies to HIV1, 2
   - 1st generation ELISA—Antigens from cultured virus.
   - 2nd generation ELISA—Recombinant antigen.
   - 3rd generation ELISA—Synthetic peptide antigen.
   - 4th generation ELISA—Recombinant antigen and synthetic peptide antigen can detect both Ag and Ab
   - *Principle:* Indirect, competitive, sandwich and capture assays available
   - *Sensitivity:* 98–100%
   - *Specificity:* 90–100%
   - False-positive ELISA.
     - Autoimmune disorders, multiple pregnancies, multiple transfusion, hypergammaglobulinaemia, hepatitis.
   - False-negative ELISA.
     - Window period, late stage, technical error.
2. **Rapid/simple tests (<30 minutes):** Antibody detection
   - Dot blot assay
   - Particle agglutination tests
   - HIV Spot and Comb test
   - Immunochromatography
   - Examples
     1. Capillus HIV-1, HIV-2 assay
     2. HIV tridot.

3. **Western blot.**
   - Detects individual antibodies in serum separately against various antigenic fragments of HIV.
   - The antigen antibody complexes appear as distinct bands on nitrocellulose strip.
   - *WHO criteria:* Presence of at least two envelope bands (out of gp120, gp160 or gp41) with or without gag or pol bands
   - *CDC criteria:* Presence of any two out of p24, gp120, gp160, gp41 bands
4. **p24 Ag detection:** ELISA.
   - Detectable as early as 2 weeks after infection.
   - Not detectable when p24 Abs are formed.
   - Useful in HIV infected neonates.
   - To diagnose late stage of HIV/AIDS (immune collapse) or CNS disease.
5. **Viral RNA detection**
   - Reverse transcriptase polymerase chain reaction (RT-PCR)
   - Branched DNA assay
   - NASBA—Nucleic acid sequence-based amplification
   - Real time RT-PCR- for estimating viral load.
   - Most sensitive and specific method for confirmation, diagnosis in window period.

---

2. Serological assays and molecular tests are the main stay in diagnosis of HIV/AIDS. Supporting the statement.

A. Discuss in detail the available molecular assays for the diagnosis of HIV/ AIDS. (5 marks)

I. Viral RNA Detection

Methods

1. Reverse transcriptase polymerase chain reaction (RT-PCR)
2. Branched DNA assay
3. NASBA—Nucleic acid sequence-based amplification
4. Real time RT-PCR for estimating viral load.

Advantages

1. Sensitive and specific method for confirmation of HIV.
2. Diagnosis of HIV infection in window period.
3. To monitor the patients on antiretroviral therapy and to study the progression of disease in the patients.
4. HIV RNA viral load is an indicator to start and adjust anti-retroviral therapy.

II. HIV Proviral DNA Detection: PCR

- Diagnosis of HIV infection in the neonate
- Supplemental test to determine the significance of an indeterminate HIV Western Blot report

III. HIV-1 Genotypic Resistance Assay

- Sequencing of the HIV pol gene to study the mutations in the gene associated with resistance to antiretroviral drugs.

B. Discuss the precautions, safety measures to be taken during sample collection and performing of tests regarding a suspected seropositive case of HIV. (3 marks)

- The diagnosis and monitoring of HIV infection is done by detection of antibody or antigen in serum/ plasma/whole blood.
- Precautions for sample collection from a suspected HIV positive case are:
  1. Pre-test counselling and informed consent has to be obtained.
  2. Hands are disinfected with an alcohol-based hand sanitizer.
  3. Gloves has to be worn to comply with standard precautions.
  4. Masks and protective eyewear should be worn if mucous membrane contact with blood or body fluids is anticipated. Gloves should be changed, and hands washed after completion of specimen processing.
  5. Preventing needle stick injury by avoiding recapping of needles and ensuring safety disposal of sharps in puncture proof container.
  6. Appropriate disposal of biomedical waste generated.

C. Discuss the precautions to prevent transmission of HIV in health-care settings (2 marks)

- Hand hygiene
- Use of personal protective equipment to prevent exposures
- Safe disposal of sharps and waste
- Safe cleaning and disinfection of the environment and equipment
- Preventing needle stick injuries and occupational exposure to blood includes
  - Eliminating unnecessary injections and sharps use
  - Applying standard precautions procedures (such as prohibiting recapping of needles and ensuring safety disposal immediately after use of the sharp)
- Start of post-exposure prophylaxis in case of accidental needle stick injury
- Screening of blood and blood products for HIV for donation safety.

SHORT ESSAYS

1. Define opportunistic infections. Based on the WHO clinical staging, classify different types of opportunistic infections in HIV patients. (1 + 4 marks)

Definition of Opportunistic Infections

- Defined as those infections occurring due to bacteria, fungi, viruses, or commensal organisms that normally inhabit the human body and do not cause a disease in healthy people, but become pathogenic when the body's defense system is impaired.

Types of Opportunistic Infections in HIV Patients

Bacterial opportunistic infections	• Recurrent severe bacterial infections • Extrapulmonary tuberculosis • Disseminated non tubercular mycobacterial infection • Recurrent septicaemia (including non-typhoidal salmonellosis)
Viral opportunistic infections	• Chronic HSV infection • Progressive multifocal leukoencephalopathy • CMV (retinitis, or other organ infection excluding liver, spleen, and lymph node)
Fungal opportunistic infections	• *Pneumocystis jirovecii* pneumonia • Oesophageal candidiasis • Extrapulmonary cryptococcosis (meningitis) • Disseminated mycoses (histoplasmosis and coccidioidomycoses)
Parasitic opportunistic infections	• *Toxoplasma* encephalitis • Chronic intestinal isosporiasis (>1 month) • Atypical disseminated leishmaniasis • Chronic intestinal cryptosporidiosis (>1 month)

2. Describe in detail the NACO strategies for the diagnosis of HIV infection (5 marks)

Strategy 1 (for Blood Transfusion/Transplant Safety)

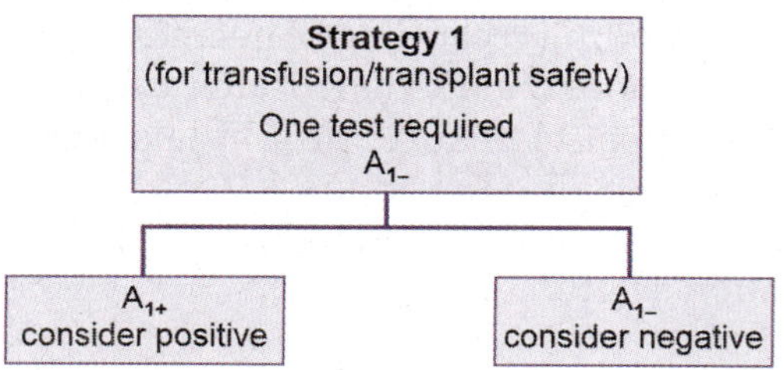

Strategy 2A (Used in Sentinel Surveillance)

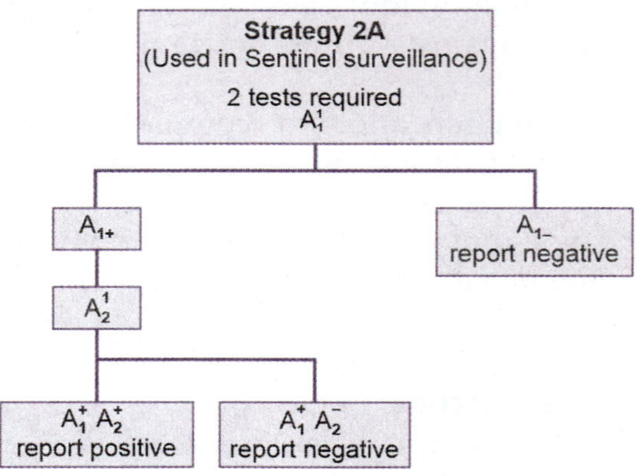

Strategy 2B (Used for Diagnosis in Symptomatic Patients)

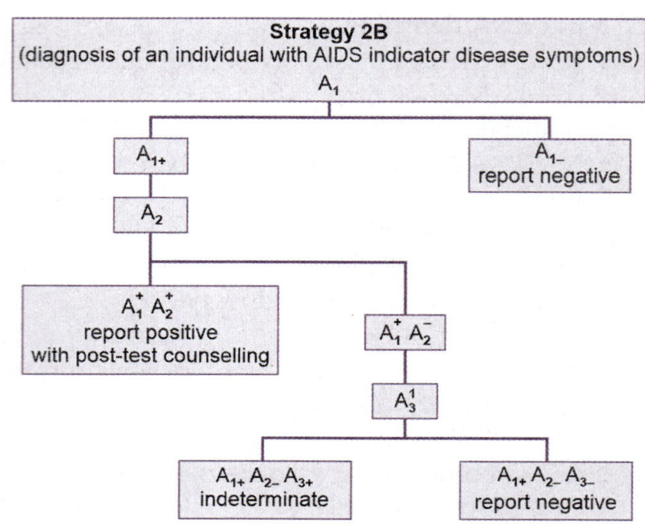

Strategy 3 (Used for Diagnosis in Asymptomatic Patients) (Fig. 2.7.2)

- Assays A1, A2, A3 represent 3 different assays based on different principles or different antigenic compositions. Assay A1 should be of high sensitivity and A2 and A3 should be of high specificity. A2 and A3 should also be able to differentiate between HIV 1 and 2 infection. Such a result is not adequate for diagnostic purposes: use strategies 2B or 3.

3. Describe in detail the immunological mechanisms (Immunopathogenesis) in HIV. Discuss the progress of HIV infection. (2 + 3 marks)

Immunopathogenesis in HIV Infection

- Human immunodeficiency virus primarily targets CD_4 T cells and cells of the macrophage lineage (e.g. monocytes, macrophages, alveolar macrophages of the lung, dendritic cells of the skin, and microglial cells of the brain).

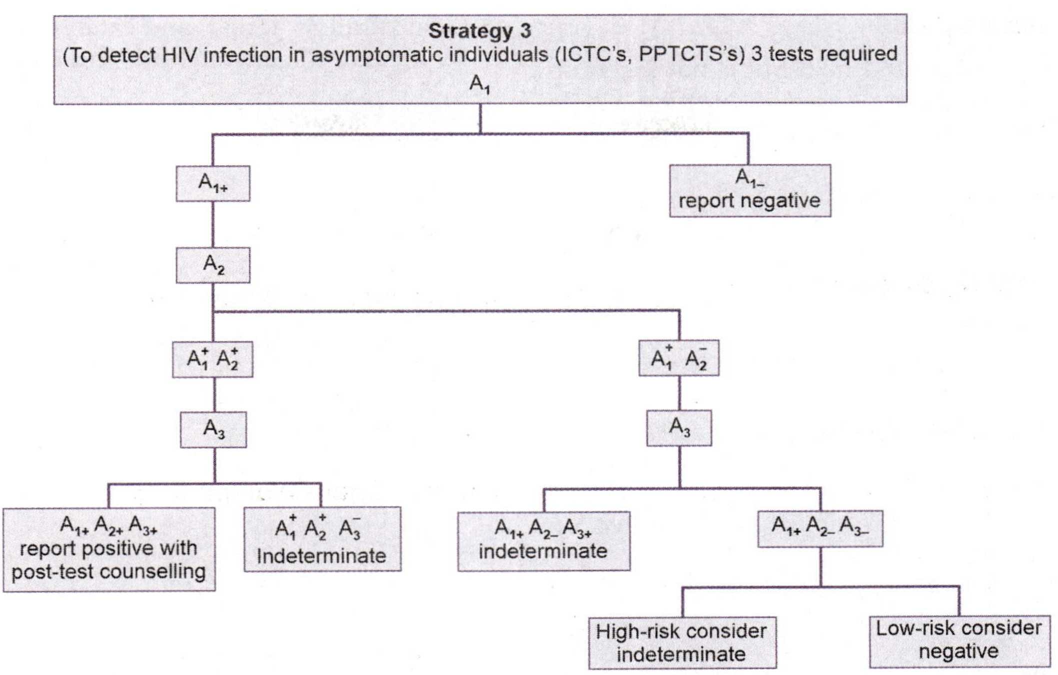

Fig. 2.7.2: Diagnosis of HIV is asymptomatic patient

- CD 4 cell depletion.
  - CD4 cell count decreases in HIV disease (in the absence of treatment) leading to continuous viral replication and increased opportunistic infections.
  - Mechanism of CD_4 cell depletion.
    - Direct damage by virus by accumulation of unintegrated viral DNA and inhibition of cellular protein synthesis
    - CD4 infected cells expressing viral antigens on surface attract CD4 uninfected cell-fusion—Syncytium formation
    - Autoimmune mechanisms
    - Superantigens
    - Apoptosis
- Other immunological changes in HIV infection.
  - Polyclonal B cell activation—High Ig—Autoimmune disorders, thrombocytopenia.
  - Monocyte macrophage function affected.
  - CD_8 cells count increases in primary infection.
  - Loss of DTH function—intracellular pathogens.

Progress of HIV Infection

- Based on kinetics of virologic and immunologic events, three dominant patterns of HIV disease are described.

1. *80–90% of HIV infected:* Typical progressors with 11 years survival.
2. *5–10 %:* Rapid progressors with median survival time of 3–4 years.
3. *7–10%:* "long-term nonprogressors" (LTNPs).

4. Mention the opportunistic pathogens causing diarrhoea in immunocompromised hosts.

Describe the laboratory diagnostic steps for diarrhoea causing agents in immunocompromised host. (2+3 marks)

Opportunistic Pathogens Causing Diarrhoea

- Enteric bacteria including *Shigella flexneri*, *Salmonella enteritidis*, and *Campylobacter jejuni.*
- *Mycobacterium avium*-complex (MAC).
- Parasites *Cryptosporidium parvum, Microsporidia, Isospora belli, Giardia lamblia.*
- *Viruses:* Cytomegalovirus, astrovirus, rotavirus, herpes virus, adenovirus

Laboratory Diagnostic Steps for Diarrhoea Causing Agents

- Stool cultures (*Salmonella* spp., *Shigella* spp., *Campylobacter* spp.).
- Toxin (*Clostridium difficile*).
- Stool for ova and parasites.
  - *Giardia lamblia, Entamoeba histolytica:* using saline, iodine, trichrome stain.
  - *Stool stains:* Modified Kinyoun acid-fast stain (for *Cryptosporidium parvum and Isospora belli).*
  - *Concentrated stool:* Zinc sulphate, sheather sucrose flotation.

5. CSF sample collected from a 50-year-old male truck driver (HIV positive) with history of headache, fever, confusion, neck stiffness.

A. Discuss the relevant investigations useful for the case discussed. (3 marks)

The investigations required in this case:

1. India Ink Staining: CSF

- Stain fills the background field but is not taken up by the thick *Cryptococcus* capsule, forming a halo of light by which it can be visualised using a light microscope.
- Quick, low-resource method.
- Sensitivity is 60–80%.

2. Cryptococcal Ag detection

- By latex agglutination.
  - Sensitivity and specificity of >99% in blood and CSF.
  - Detects polysaccharide antigens of the *Cryptococcus* capsule.
- By Lateral flow assay.
  - Immunochromatographic dipstick assay on serum, plasma, CSF.
  - Sensitivity of 99.3% and specificity of 99.1% for CSF.

3. CSF Culture

- Gold standard for diagnosis of cryptococcal meningitis.
- Disadvantages.
  1. 7–10 days for a reliable quantitative count.
  2. False negative results when the fungal burden is low.

4. Molecular Method

- *PCR:* Multiplex platform for the meningitis group

B. What could be the probable diagnosis of the above case considering the seropositivity for HIV. (2 marks)

- Cryptococcal meningitis caused by *Cryptococcus neoformans.*

---

6. What is the most common screening test performed for HIV at blood banks and at tertiary care centres? Discuss its principle. (1+4 marks)

Common Screening Test Performed for HIV at Blood Banks and at Tertiary Care Centres

- ELISA (high sensitivity).

Principle of Indirect ELISA

- Serum is diluted and added to a plate to which HIV antigens are immobilised.
- HIV antibodies if present in the serum bind to HIV antigens.
- The plate is then washed to remove all unbound components.
- Secondary antibody linked to the enzyme—is then applied to the plate, followed by another wash.
- A substrate is added, and catalysis of the substrate by the bound enzyme leads to a change in colour.

SHORT ANSWERS

---

1. Classify Retroviruses. In brief describe the major antigens/proteins in HIV. (1+2 marks)

Classification of Retroviruses

1. Genus *Lentivirus* —Human Immunodeficiency Virus (HIV)—1 and 2.
2. Genus *Delta retrovirus*—Human T cell lymphotropic virus-1 (HTLV-1).

Major Antigens/Proteins in HIV

Envelope

1. *Glycoprotein-120 (gp120):* Knob-like spikes on the surface.
2. *Glycoprotein-41 (gp41):* Form anchoring trans-membrane pedicles.

Core

1. *p18:* Constitutes the matrix or shell antigen.
2. *p24 and p15:* Constitute the core antigens.

---

2. Which stage of HIV is considered as the "stage of clinical latency, but not microbiological latency"? Discuss in brief. (3 marks)

- HIV infected patients pass through a phase of symptomless infection (clinical latency), lasting for several years
- Cell-mediated immune response (HIV specific CD8 T cells) and humoral response (HIV specific neutralising antibodies) develop within 1 month of exposure
- Viraemia drops down and CD4 T cell count becomes normal
- Immune response cannot clear the virus completely, virus continues to replicate
- Positive antibody tests during this phase
- No symptoms but contagious
- After this phase of latency, there is rapid progression of disease leading to death within 2 years if left untreated. The median time between primary HIV infection and development of AIDS is approximately 10 years.

---

3. Enumerate the non-specific tests useful in the diagnosis of HIV. (3 marks)

1. Complete blood count.
2. CD4 T cell count—by flow cytometry method.
   - Assessing the risk of opportunistic infections.

- Initiation of antiviral therapy—if CD4 T cell count falls below 350/mm^3.
- Monitoring the response to antiviral therapy.

3. Abnormal proteins such as neopterin, beta 2-microglobulin and soluble IL-2 receptor.

4. Discuss the post-exposure prophylaxis for HIV. (3 marks)

- PEP (post-exposure prophylaxis) means taking medicine to prevent HIV after a possible exposure. PEP should be used only in emergency situations after occupational exposures such as needle stick or sharp injury or mucocutaneous exposure.
- PEP should be started immediately—ideally within 2 hours of an exposure but no later than 72 hours after an exposure—because the effectiveness of PEP decreases over time after 2 hours.
- Assessment of exposure, HIV and other baseline testing, and other related activities can proceed after the first dose of PEP is administered.
- There should be a designated centre for PEP management in the hospital.
- *Regimen (TLE):* Single daily dose of Tenofovir (300 mg) + Lamivudine (300 mg) + Efavirenz (600 mg) is given for 28 days.

5. List the 4 opportunistic mycotic infections in HIV positive cases. (3 marks)

1. *Pneumocystis jirovecii* (pneumocystosis).
2. *Cryptococcus neoformans* (cryptococcosis).
3. *Candida* spp. (Candidiasis).
4. *Talaromyces (Penicillium) marneffei* (talaromycosis).

6. Define window period in HIV infection. List the methods available for the diagnosis of HIV infection in window period. (1+2 marks)

Window Period

- Refers to the time interval between the exposure and appearance of detectable levels of antibodies in the serum.
- Antibodies are detectable after 3–12 weeks with the assays available presently.

Methods Available for the Diagnosis of HIV Infection in Window Period

1. p24 antigen detection (30% sensitivity).
2. HIV RNA detection (PCR).

CHAPTER 3

Gastrointestinal and Hepatobiliary System

MI 3.1 ENUMERATE THE MICROBIAL AGENTS CAUSING DIARRHOEA AND DYSENTERY. DESCRIBE THE MORPHOLOGY, EPIDEMIOLOGY, PATHOGENESIS, CLINICAL FEATURES AND DIAGNOSIS OF THE CAUSATIVE AGENTS

LONG ESSAYS

1. A 50-year-old traveller consumed road-side food during his visit to a seashore. After 3 days he suffered from mild pyrexia, weakness, vomiting and passed mucopurulent stools with blood. He was admitted to hospital and stool sample is sent for microscopy and culture. Stool microscopy revealed plenty of pus cells and RBCs. Culture grew typical non-lactose fermenting colonies, which were non-motile gram-negative bacilli. Patient is kept on symptomatic treatment with plenty of electrolyte substitution. Patient recovered after 1 week.

A. What could be the most probable diagnosis of the above case and enumerate the causative agents of the above case and modes of transmission. (3 marks)

Probable Diagnosis

- Bacillary dysentery caused by *Shigella* spp.

Causative Agents

- The causative agent is *Shigella* spp.
- Consisting of four serogroups:
  1. *Shigella sonnei*
  2. *Shigella boydii*
  3. *Shigella flexneri*
  4. *Shigella dysenteriae*.

Mode of Transmission

- Exclusively a human disease.
- Faecal–oral route.
- 5 Fs—Fingers, Flies, Food, Fomites and Faeces aid in transmission.
- *Minimum infective dose:* 10–100 bacilli

B. Pathogenesis, clinical features seen in this infection. (3 marks)

Pathogenesis

Virulence Factors

- *Direct invasion of intestine:* Entry via M cells, invasion into submucosa and direct cell to cell spread with release of inflammatory cytokines such as IL-1 and IL-18 which results in intestinal inflammation and subsequent activation of the innate immune system.
- *Toxins.*
  - *Shigella enterotoxins:* Enterotoxic effect: blocks the intestinal absorption of glucose, amino acids and electrolytes
  - *Shiga toxin:* neurotoxic, cytotoxic
  - *Cytotoxic effect:* by inhibition of protein synthesis, cell death and damage to microvasculature in intestine and haemorrhage
  - *Neurotoxic effect:* Fever, abdominal cramps
  - Cause enterocolitis and HUS

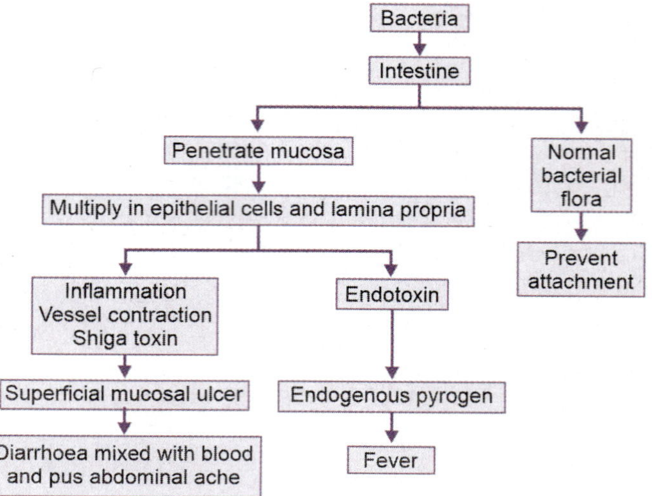

Clinical Features

- *Dysentery:* Frequent passage of bloody mucopurulent stools with increased tenesmus and abdominal cramps
- Complications.
  1. Dehydration
  2. Seizures
  3. Rectal prolapse
  4. Haemolytic uremic syndrome—low red blood cell count (haemolytic anaemia), low platelet count (thrombocytopenia) and acute kidney failure
  5. Toxic megacolon
  6. Reactive arthritis
  7. Bloodstream infections (bacteraemia).

C. Describe the approach to laboratory diagnosis in the above case. (3 marks)

Specimen Collection

- Fresh stool (Rectal swabs are not satisfactory).

Transport Media

- Sach's buffered glycerol saline.

Microscopy

- *Wet mount of the stool:* large number of pus cells, erythrocytes and macrophages

Culture

- *On enrichment broth:* Selenite F broth, tetrathionate broth
- On selective media.

Plating media	*Colony morphology*
• Mildly selective media • MacConkey's agar	• NLF; *S sonnei* late lactose fermenter
• Highly selective media • DCA (Deoxycholate citrate agar)	• NLF; slightly smaller
• XLD (Xylose lysine deoxycholate)	• Red without black center
• Hektoen enteric agar	• Green
• Salmonella–*Shigella* agar	• Colourless

- *Culture smear and motility testing:* Short, gram-negative bacilli non-motile

Biochemical Identification

1. *Catalase:* Catalase positive except *S. dysenteriae serotype-1.*
2. *Oxidase test:* Negative.
3. *Mannitol fermentation:* All species ferment mannitol except *S. dysenteriae and other biochemical tests.*

Slide Agglutination Test

- Confirmation using group specific and species-specific antisera.

D. Discuss the treatment of the above condition. (1 mark)

- *Antibiotic:* Ciprofloxacin
- *Alternative drugs:* Ceftriaxone, azithromycin
- *Duration:* 3 days except for *S. dysenteriae type 1 infection—5 days*
- Oral rehydration solution (ORS).

---

2. An 8-year-old girl presents with complaints of abdominal pain and upset stomach. Routine stool examination was ordered, and the following egg was observed in the wet mount (Fig. 3.1.1).

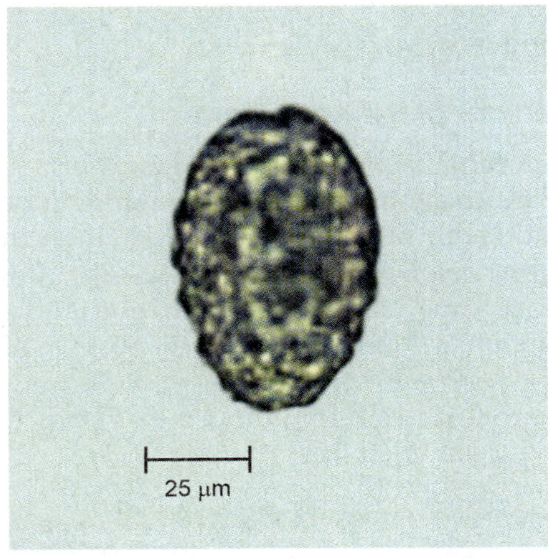

Fig. 3.1.1: Egg of *Ascaris lumbricoides*

A. What is the most likely cause of this infection? (1 mark)

- *Ascaris lumbricoides.*

B. Briefly explain the life cycle of this parasite. (4 marks)

- *Infective form:* Embryonated eggs
- *Site of inhabitation:* Small intestine
- *Route of infection:* By mouth
- *Host:* Man is the only host; No intermediate hosts
- *Life span of the adult:* About 1 year
- *Chief source of infection:* Human faeces
- *Transmission:* By faeco-oral route
- *Transmitted by:* Eating raw vegetables contaminated with the infective eggs
- *Sequence of events:*
  - Digestive juices dissolve the eggshell and larva is released in small intestine
  - Larvae penetrate the intestinal mucosa and enter lymphatics and mesenteric vessels
  - Carried by circulation—liver, right heart—lungs where they penetrate the capillaries into the

alveoli in which they molt twice and stay for 10–14 days and then they are carried, or migrate, up the bronchioles, bronchi, and trachea to the epiglottis
- When swallowed, the larvae pass down into the small intestine where they develop into adults
- *Life Cycle (Fig. 3.1.2).*

C. Briefly explain the pathogenesis of the disease. (3 marks)

Pathogenicity of the Larvae

- Migrating larvae in persons repeatedly infected with *Ascaris*, produce inflammatory and hypersensitive reactions in the lung and liver.
- Associated with the formation of granulomas and eosinophilic infiltrates—Pneumonitis (Loeffler's syndrome).

Pathogenicity of the Adult Worm

- *Mechanical action:* Adult worm in the late stages cause trauma, obstruction and inflammation of the appendix, bile duct, pancreatic duct, intestine
- *Spoliative action:* Worm takes the nutrition from the host. This leads to malnutrition and growth retardation in young children with heavy worm load
- *Allergic reaction:* Metabolites of living and dead adult are toxic and immunogenic. It leads to fever, urticaria, conjunctivitis

D. Describe the clinical findings. (2 marks)

Intestinal Disease

- Increased numbers of the worm produce abdominal pain, nausea, vomiting, fever, weight loss and diarrhoea.
- Heavy infection—malabsorption of nutrients, growth retardation. May lead to intussusception, partial or total intestinal obstruction.

Pulmonary Disease

- Seen during initial stage of the infection.
- Caused by migrating larvae in the lung tissue.
- Cough and wheezing are the symptoms in newly infected patients.
- In persons already infected, eosinophilic pneumonia—Loeffler's syndrome. Allergic reaction caused by hypersensitivity of host to the allergens of the migrating larvae.
- Characterised by fever, cough, dyspnoea, rales and pulmonary infiltrates. Eosinophilia, urticaria are common.

Ectopic Ascariasis (Wander Lust)

- They probe into any apertures.
- May enter the opening of biliary and pancreatic duct causing acute biliary obstruction/pancreatitis.
- Liver abscess.
- The worm can crawl up the oesophagus and come out through the mouth or nose.

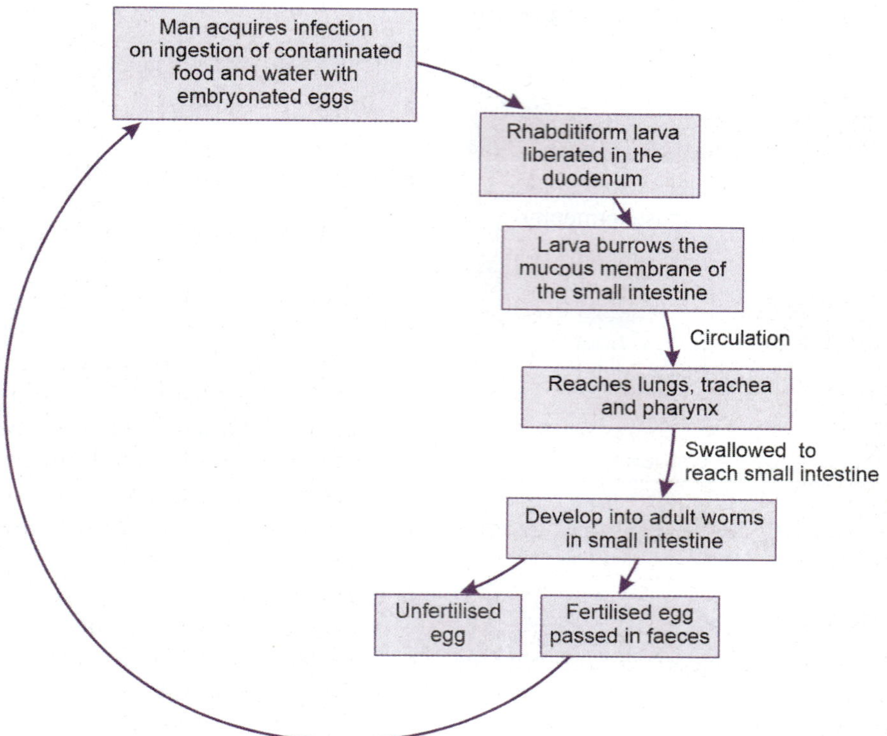

Fig. 3.1.2: Life cycle of *Ascaris lumbricoides*

- It may move into the trachea and lung causing respiratory obstruction or lung abscess.
- Migrate down → obstructive appendicitis.
- Perforated intestine → peritonitis.

Complications

1. Intestinal obstruction
2. Appendicitis
3. Biliary ascariasis
4. Perforation of the intestine, cholecystitis.
5. Pancreatitis and peritonitis may occur, in which biliary ascariasis is the most common complication.

E. Discuss the laboratory diagnosis of this condition. (3 marks)

Laboratory Diagnosis

1. **Demonstration of eggs (Figs 3.1.3 and 3.1.4).**
   - In faeces—Concentration of faeces by salt floatation or formalin ether method to detect light infection.
   - Eggs are not found in the stool in infection with only male worms, prepatent infection, extra-intestinal infection.

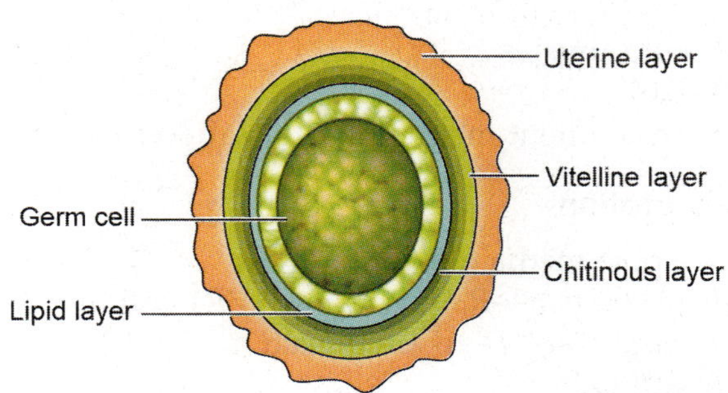

Fig 3.1.3: Fertilised egg of *Ascaris lumbricoides*

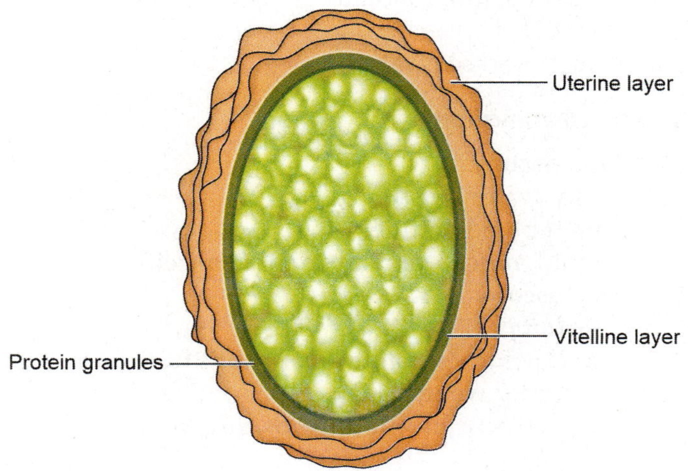

Fig. 3.1.4: Unfertilised egg of *Ascaris lumbricoides*

   - Eggs can be demonstrated in bile obtained by duodenal intubation.
   - In pulmonary infections, larvae are found in gastric aspiration, sputum, or bronchial aspirates.
2. **Serodiagnosis**
   - Antibody detection by IHA, IFA
   - Useful in extraintestinal ascariasis
3. **Complete blood count.**
   - Peripheral eosinophilia
   - Serum levels of IgG and IgE are elevated.
4. **Imaging methods**
   - X ray, USG, CT scan
   - In heavily infested individuals, particularly children, large collection of worms may be detected on plain film of the abdomen. The mass of worms' contrasts against the gas in the bowel: a 'whirlpool' effect.

F. What are the methods for treatment and prevention of this infection? (2 marks)

Treatment

1. **Mebendazole.**
   - 100 mg/kg, 3 days
   - Blocks the uptake of glucose by the worm.
2. **Pyrantel pamoate**
   - Contraindicated in intestinal obstruction
3. **Piperazine citrate.**
   - Effective in intestinal obstruction secondary to ascariasis.

Prevention of Infection

1. **By prevention of soil pollution:**
   - By treating the infected persons—deworming of the school children
   - Use of sanitary latrines
2. **By prevention of ingestion of eggs:**
   - Improved personal hygiene—washing hands before eating
   - Avoiding eating uncooked vegetables, fruits

---

3. A 27-year-old patient presented to the OPD with h/o profuse watery diarrhoea. After a day, he is pale and weak due to dehydration by loose motions and vomiting. Macroscopic examination of the stool revealed rice watery stool. Stool was collected for culture.

A. What is the probable diagnosis and the etiological agent? (1 mark)

Probable Diagnosis

- Cholera.

Aetiological Agent

- *Vibrio cholerae.*

B. Discuss the pathogenesis and clinical features of this infection. (3+3 marks)

Pathogenesis

Source of Infection

- Patients and carriers

Mode of Transmission

- Faeco–oral route

Incubation Period

- <24 hours to about 5 days.

Host Factors

1. Gastric pH—Achlorhydria predisposes to cholera.
2. *Blood group:* Blood group 'O' people are more prone to cholera than people with other blood group.
3. Malnutrition.

Risk Factors

1. Poor sanitation
2. Overcrowding
3. Inadequate medical service

Virulence Factors

1. Cholera toxin
2. Toxin co-regulated pilus (TCP)
3. Mucinase
4. Motility
5. Lipopolysaccharide (LPS O antigen, endotoxin).
6. β-haemolysin

Sequence of Events

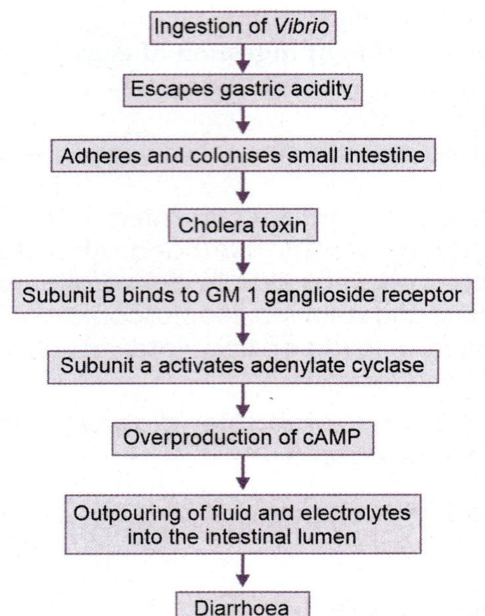

Clinical Features

- Begins with sudden onset of nausea, diarrhoea accompanied by abdominal cramps that starts 24–48 hours after ingestion.
- Faeces are like clouded water, with mucous flakes and inoffensive smell (rice water stool).
- Electrolyte imbalance leads to acidosis and vomiting.
- Hypokalaemia accounts for the leg cramps in aged patients.
- Signs and symptoms of dehydration (fluid loss >5% of body weight).
  - Dry mouth
  - Absence of tears
  - Increasing thirst
  - Loss of skin turgor (Washerwoman's hand)
- *In severe form:* Copious effortless vomiting and profuse painless watery diarrhoea may lead to hypovolaemic shock and death.

C. Discuss the laboratory diagnosis of this condition. (4 marks)

Specimen Collection

1. **Stool**
   - Collected before antibiotic administration
   - *Rectal swab:* Moistened with transport medium before sampling
2. **Food samples**
3. **Water**
   - Enrichment method and filtration method.

Transportation

- Transport media used are:

1. *Venkatraman—Ramakrishnan (VR) medium:* About 1–3 ml stool is to be added to 10–15 ml of the medium.
2. *Cary–Blair medium:* Suitable for *Salmonella*, *Shigella* as well as *Vibrio*.
3. Alkaline peptone water (pH 8.2).
4. Monsur's taurocholate tellurite peptone water (pH 9.2).
5. Autoclaved sea water.

Direct Examination

1. **Macroscopy**
   - Rice water stool
   - Non-bloody effluent
   - Fluid, mucus, and few epithelial cells.
2. **Microscopy**
   i. *Motility*
      - Darting *"shooting star"* motility is observed under wet mount.
      - Actively motile vibrios suggest *"swarm of gnats"*.

ii. *Immobilisation test*
- Motility ceases on mixing with polyvalent anti-cholera diagnostic serum (e.g. 01 antiserum)

iii. *Stained smears*
- Arranged in parallel rows *"fish in stream"* appearance.
- Dilute carbol fuchsin stain: Comma-shaped bacilli (Fig. 3.1.5)

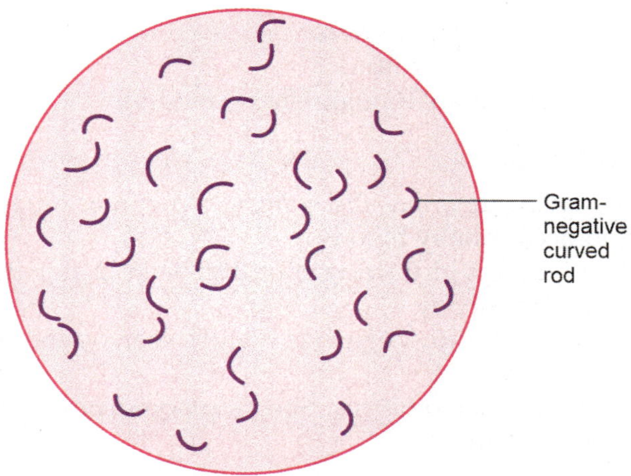

Fig. 3.1.5: Comma-shaped bacilli—*Vibrio cholerae*

Culture Methods

- Specimen sent in transport/holding media should be inoculated into enrichment media.
- Incubated for 6–8 hours (including transit time).
- Streak on selective and non-selective media.
- Incubated at 37°C for 24 hours (overnight >18 hours).
- Media used—Liquid and solid.

I. Liquid (Enrichment) Media

1. Alkaline peptone water
2. Monsur's taurocholate tellurite peptone water.

II. Solid Media

1. *Non-selective media.*
   i. Nutrient agar.
   ii. Blood agar.
2. *Selective media.*
   a. Low selective and differential media.
      i. MacConkey agar.
   b. High selective media.
      i. Thiosulphate citrate bile salt sucrose (TCBS).
      ii. Alkaline bile salt agar (BSA, pH 8.2).
      iii. Monsur's gelatin taurocholate trypticase tellurite agar (GTTA).

Biochemical Identification

- Oxidase positive and other tests.

Special Tests

1. **Cholera-red reaction.**
   - *Reagent used:* Concentrated H_2SO_4
   - *Positive reaction:* a reddish pink colour
2. **String test.**
   - *Reagent used:* 0.5% sodium deoxycholate
   - *Positive reaction:* Forms a string when loop is lifted slowly

Confirmation of the Identification

- *Confirmed by agglutination test:* Polyvalent 01 or non-01 antiserum
- *0139 strains:* 0139 antiserum
- Strains which do not agglutinate both may be non-01, non-0139 strains of *V. cholerae* or other closely related vibrios.
- 01 positive strains are serotyped using Ogawa and Inaba sera to identify serotypes: Ogawa, Inaba, Hikojima

D. Differentiation between Classical and El Tor Biotypes of Vibrio cholerae O1

Test	*Classical biotype*	*ElTor biotype*
Haemolysis	–	+
Vogues-Proskauer	–	+
Chick erythrocyte agglutination	–	+
Polymyxin B sensitivity	Sensitive	Resistant
Group IV phage susceptibility	Susceptible	Resistant
El Tor phage 5 susceptibility	Resistant	Susceptible

E. Discuss the Treatment. (4 marks)

- Prompt fluid and electrolyte replacement.
- Intravenous polyelectrolyte fluids such as Ringer's lactate.
- Oral rehydration solution (ORS) can be used to replace loss in patients who are able to take orally.
- Antibiotics in severely dehydrated patients.

Age Group	*First Line Drug Choice*	*Alternate Drug Choice*
Children <12 years old	Doxycycline 2–4 mg/kg p.o single dose	Azithromycin 20 mg/kg (max 1 g) p.o. single dose, or ciprofloxacin 20 mg/kg (max 1 g) p.o. single dose
Children ≥12 years old and adults, including pregnant women	Doxycycline 300 mg p.o. single dose	Azithromycin 1g p.o. single dose, or ciprofloxacin 1g p.o. single dose

4. An outbreak of 4 cases which developed loose watery severe diarrhoea after consumption of crab salad.

A. What is the most probable diagnosis and the aetiological agent? (1 mark)

Most Probable Diagnosis

- Diarrhoea.

Aetiological Agent

- *Vibrio parahaemolyticus*.

B. Pathogenesis and clinical features of this condition. (3 marks)

Pathogenesis

- *Incubation period: Vibrio parahaemolyticus*: 12–24 hours
- *Mode of infection:* Ingestion of raw or uncooked sea food, e.g., oyster
- *Virulence Factors*
  1. *Adhesion:* to the host cells.
  2. *Toxins: tdh* and TDH-related haemolysin (*trh*): responsible for haemolysis and cytotoxicity in the host cell.
  3. *Type III secretion systems:* needle-like bacterial machine to inject bacterial protein effectors directly into the host cells.

Clinical Features

- Acute dysentery
- Abdominal pain
- Accompanied by nausea, vomiting, fever, chills.

C. Work up for diagnosis of this outbreak. (2 marks)

Epidemiologic Data

- Geographic distribution, time period and outbreaks in the past.
- Foods or other exposures occurring more often in sick people than expected.
- Clusters of cases who ate at the same restaurant .

Traceback Data

- A common point of contamination in the distribution chain, identified by reviewing records collected from restaurants where sick people ate.
- Findings of environmental assessments in food production facilities, farms, and restaurants identifying food safety risks.

Food and Environmental Testing Data

- Recovery of bacteria from food item collected from a sick person's home or outside eatery.
- Similar DNA fingerprint pattern linking bacteria found in food item to bacteria recovered from the cases.

D. Discuss the laboratory diagnosis in this case. (4 marks)

Specimen Collection

1. *Stool:* In case of gastroenteritis.
2. *Food sample and water sample:* In suspected case of *Vibrio* contamination.

Transport Media

1. Alkaline peptone water.
2. Cary–Blair medium.
3. Venkatraman–Ramakrishnan medium.

Macroscopy

- *Stool:* Characteristically watery, sometimes mucoid, and occasionally bloody
- *Motility:* Rapid darting motility, seen under dark field microscopy
- *Staining:* Gram-negative bacilli seen, generally comma-shaped
- *Vibrio parahaemolyticus:* Shows pleomorphism and bipolar staining

Culture

I. **Liquid Media**
  1. Alkaline peptone water
  2. Nutrient broth.

II. **Solid Media**
  1. *Nonselective media.*
     i. Nutrient agar (with added NaCl)
     ii. Blood agar
  2. *Selective media.*
     i. Thiosulphate citrate bile salt sucrose agar (TCBS).
     ii. Taurocholate tellurite gelatin agar (TTGA or Monsur's agar).
  3. *Differential media.*
     i. MacConkey agar.

Vibrio parahaemolyticus: Cultural and Biochemical Characteristics

- *MacConkey agar:* Non-lactose fermenting flat colonies
- *TCBS agar:* Green with opaque raised center (sucrose non fermenting)
- Kanagawa phenomenon-β haemolysis on Wagatsuma agar
- Swarming on blood agar
- Urease test is positive in few strains
- Salt tolerance test-resist maximum of 8% NaCl.

5. *Entamoeba histolytica* is the primary cause for amoebiasis affecting both intestinal and extra intestinal system. Supporting the given statement, describe in detail about the parasite concerned under the following headings.

A. Morphology and life cycle of the trophozoite and cyst. (2+3 marks)

Trophozoites

Morphology

- 12–60 μm.
- Invasive form of the parasite
- Found in the lumen, mucosa, submucosa of LI.
- Nucleus is spherical with fine peripheral chromatin and central karyosome
- Cytoplasm
  - Clear ectoplasm and granular endoplasm
  - Numerous food vacuoles and RBCs are found in the endoplasm
  - Ingested erythrocytes are a feature of *E. histolytica* not *E. dispar*
- Motile by pseudopodia

Cyst

Morphology (Figs 3.1.6 and 3.1.7)

- Infective stage
- 10–16 μm
- Mature cyst is quadrinucleate.
- Nucleus is same as trophozoite, with chromatoid bars and glycogen vacuole in the cytoplasm.

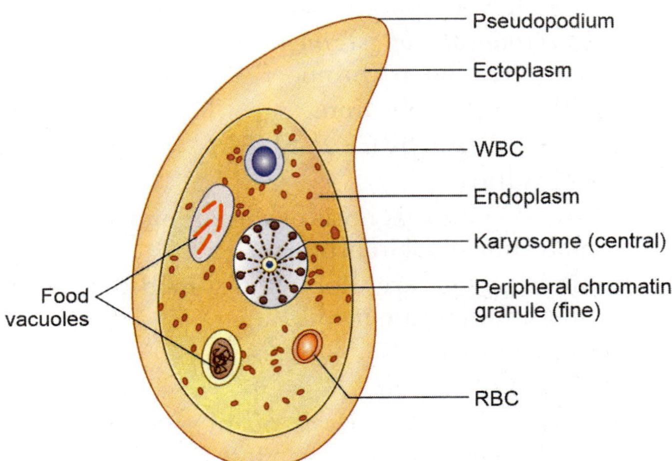

Fig. 3.1.6: Trophozoite of *Entamoeba histolytica*

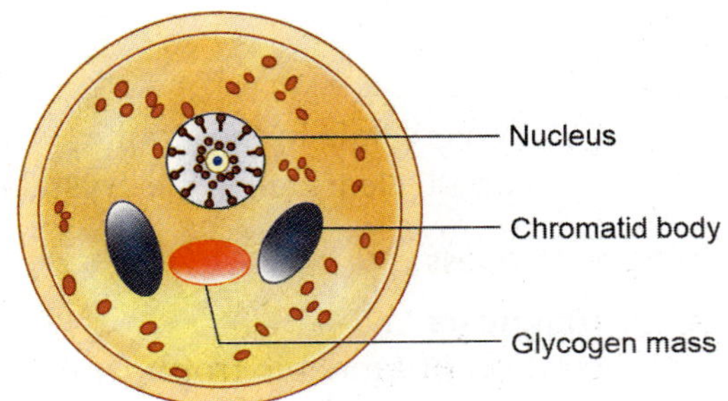

Fig. 3.1.7: Uninucleate cyst of *Entamoeba histolytica*

- Surrounded by a thin chitinous wall, which confers resistance.
- As the cyst matures, the glycogen mass and chromatoid bodies disappear.

Life Cycle (Fig. 3.1.8)

- *Host:* single host: Man
- *Infective form:* Mature quadrinucleate cyst
- *Mode of transmission.*
  - Faeco-oral route (most common).
  - Sexual (oral, anal).

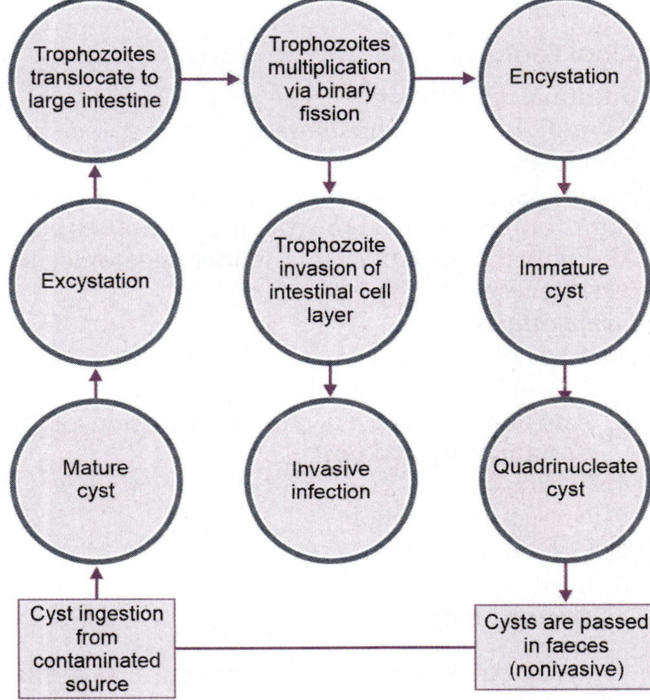

Fig. 3.1.8: Life cycle of *Entamoeba histolytica*

B. Discuss the pathogenesis and clinical presentation of intestinal amoebiasis. (4 marks)

Pathogenesis

- *Source of infection:* Food, water contaminated by human faeces that contain cysts
- *Transmission of infection*
  - Faeco–oral route
  - Ingestion of food, water contaminated by faeces containing the quadrinucleate cysts.
  - Man can also acquire infection by anogenital or orogenital sexual contact.
- *Virulence factors.*
  1. *Amoebic lectin:* Adherence to intestinal mucosa.
  2. *Ionophore like protein:* Leakage of ions from the target cells.
  3. *Hydrolytic enzymes:* Phosphatase, proteinase, RNAse.
  4. *Toxins and enzymes.*

Sequence of Events

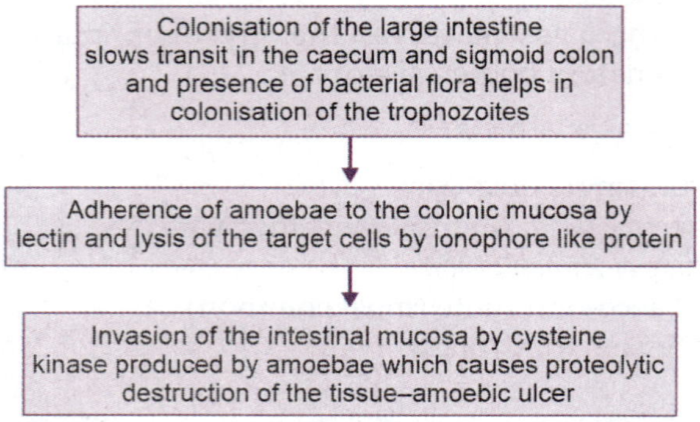

Colonisation of the large intestine slows transit in the caecum and sigmoid colon and presence of bacterial flora helps in colonisation of the trophozoites

↓

Adherence of amoebae to the colonic mucosa by lectin and lysis of the target cells by ionophore like protein

↓

Invasion of the intestinal mucosa by cysteine kinase produced by amoebae which causes proteolytic destruction of the tissue–amoebic ulcer

Clinical Features

- Intestinal amoebiasis.
- Asymptomatic intestinal infection (cyst passers).
- Nondysenteric colitis.
- *Acute amoebic dysentery:* Common form of symptomatic invasive intestinal amoebiasis. Abdominal pain, tenderness, tender hepatomegaly, rectal tenesmus
- *Complications.*
  1. Toxic megacolon
  2. Fulminant amoebic colitis
  3. Ameboma (localised chronic infection of the caecum or the rectum)
  4. Peritonitis
  5. Urogenital infection
  6. Colonic stricture
  7. Intussusceptions
  8. Haemorrhage

C. Write about Amoebic liver abscess. (4 marks)

- *Extraintestinal invasion of the tissue and serum:* From the intestine it is carried by portal circulation to the liver and then to lungs, spleen, heart, brain and stomach
- Evade the complement mediated lysis by cysteine proteinase.

Amoebic Liver Abscess

- Seen in 10–50% cases of extraintestinal amoebiasis
- Single or multiple
- occurs in any part of the liver
- Common in right lobe, confined to the postero-superior surface.
- Abscess is reddish brown with semifluid consistency.
- Microscopically—3 zones:
  1. *Inner central zone* is necrotic and has lysed hepatocytes with no amoebae.
  2. *Intermediate zone* has degenerated liver cells, connective tissue cells, red cells, few leucocytes and occasional trophozoites.
  3. *Outer zone* is a layer of normal liver tissue invaded by amoebic trophozoites.
- Pus—thick chocolate brown, anchovy sauce pus.
- It has liquified and necrotic liver cells.

Clinical Manifestations

- Most common form, in 10–50% of invasive amoebiasis
- Sudden onset of fever, right upper abdominal pain and tenderness radiating to right scapula, right shoulder
- H/o intestinal amoebiasis is present in 30% cases.

Complications

1. Rupture of the liver abscess into abdomen and right pleural space
2. Secondary bacterial infection
3. Infections of retroperitoneal space, stomach, oesophagus
4. Amoebic pericarditis, pneumopericardium

D. Laboratory diagnosis of amoebiasis. (2 marks)

Intestinal Amoebiasis

1. **Stool Microscopy**
   - Iodine mount or saline mount
   - Demonstration of mature quadrinucleate cyst or haematophagous trophozoites.
   - Examination of at least 3 consecutive stool specimens will identify 90% cases.
   - *Examination of stool after concentration:* Formalin ether for the concentration of the cysts
   - *Examination of stained stool smears:* Iron haematoxylin, trichrome, PAS
2. **Stool antigen detection.**
   - Coproantigen by CIEP, ELISA.
3. **Stool culture**
   - Useful in the diagnosis of chronic and asymptomatic intestinal infections
   - Media used are Robinson's medium, NIH polyxenic culture media.
4. **Serodiagnosis**
   - IHA, IFA
   - Useful in the diagnosis of invasive intestinal amoebiasis but positive in less than 50% cases
5. **Molecular diagnosis**
   - DNA Probe
   - PCR
6. **Others**
   - Charcot leyden crystals in the stool
   - Diamond-shaped, clear, refractile crystals

Amoebic Liver Abscess

1. **Parasitic diagnosis**
   - Demonstration of amoebic trophozoites in the aspirated liver pus, in the last part of the pus (in 15% cases).

2. **Serodiagnosis**
   - Detection of amoebic antibodies
     - IHA
     - IFA
     - ELISA
   - Detection of antigens
     - ELISA, CIEP
     - Present in serum only in active infections
3. **Molecular diagnosis**
   - PCR
4. **Imaging methods**
   - X-ray
   - USG
   - CT scan
5. **Others**
   - Leucocytosis
   - Mild anaemia
   - ESR
   - LFT
   - Serum cholesterol and albumin decreased
   - Proteinuria present

---

6. 40-year-old man presented to the Medicine OPD with abdominal discomfort. He has past history of abdominal pain, nausea, passing proglottids of worms in the stool for 2 years. He consumes beef regularly. Stool examination revealed bile-stained eggs with radial striations and hexacanth embryo.

A. What is the probable diagnosis? (1 mark)

- Intestinal taeniasis caused by *Taenia* spp.

B. Explain the life cycle of this parasite. (3 marks)

Life Cycle

- *See* Figure 3.1.9.

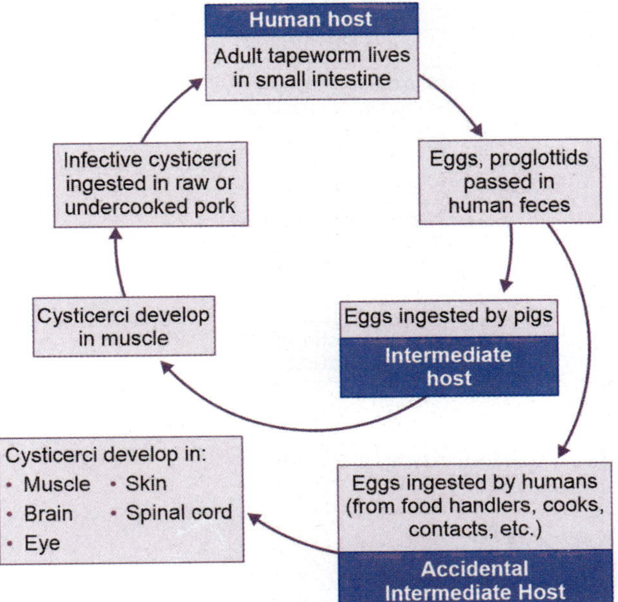

Fig. 3.1.9: Life cycle of *Taenia* spp.

C. Discuss the pathogenesis and clinical manifestations of this condition. (2+2 marks)

Pathogenesis

- Taeniasis is an intestinal infection with the adult form of the beef tapeworm, *Taenia saginata*, or the pork tapeworm, *T. solium*.
- *Mode of infection:* Ingestion of the larva (cysticerci) in undercooked and infected pork, beef
- Adult worm is nonpathogenic. Rarely cause any damage to the intestinal mucosa.

Clinical Manifestations

- Intestinal taeniasis
  - Mostly asymptomatic
  - In symptomatic cases: nausea, abdominal discomfort, weight loss, chronic indigestion
- Complications
  1. Intestinal obstruction
  2. Appendicitis
  3. Pancreatitis

D. Discuss the laboratory diagnosis of this condition. (2 marks)

Specimen

- Stool

Methods of Examination

1. **Stool Microscopy**
   - Demonstration of eggs in the faeces and less frequently of scolex and proglottids (Fig. 3.1.10).
   - Eggs are demonstrated by thick faecal smear examination.
   - Essential to collect 2–3 stool samples because eggs are shed irregularly in the stool
   - Perianal swabs are also used in case of demonstration of eggs
   - *Advantage:* will detect eggs in 85–90% of cases
   - *Disadvantages:* Identification of species cannot be made as eggs of both the species are similar

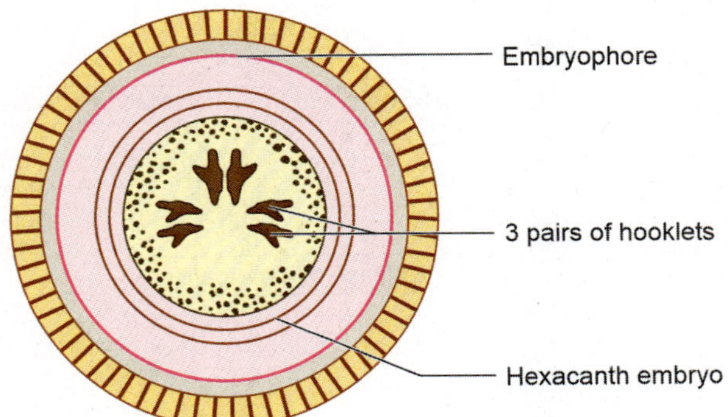

Fig. 3.1.10: Egg of *Taenia* spp

- Species diagnosis is done by identifying the features of gravid proglottids in the faeces and also the presence of Scolex.
- The gravid segments are washed in clean water and placed between two slides.
- Two slides are held together by adhesive tape at each end examined by hand lens.
- Demonstration of 10–20 lateral branches on each side of uterine stem in the uterus-helps in the identification of *T. saginata* (in case of *T. solium* 7–12 lateral branches are present).

2. **Detection of *Taenia* antigen in faeces**
   - Antigen capture ELISA in faeces
   - *Advantages*
     1. Most sensitive method
     2. Useful for screening of intestinal taeniasis.
   - *Disadvantage:* Does not differentiate between *T. saginata* and *T. solium*
3. **Serodiagnosis**
   - Indirect haemagglutination (IHA)
   - Indirect fluorescent antibody (IFA)
   - Enzyme-linked immunosorbent assay (ELISA).
   - Useful for demonstration of specific antibodies in the serum, tests are of limited vale in diagnosis of intestinal taeniasis.
4. **Molecular diagnosis.**
   - PCR.
     - To detect genome of the egg in stool.
     - Advantage: It is reported that the procedure can detect even a single egg in stool and differentiate between two species.
   - DNA probes.
     - Detects and differentiates between the eggs of *T. saginata and T. solium* in stool specimen.
     - Distinguishes between the proglottids of *T. saginata* and *T. solium.*

7. A 50-year-old man with HIV presented to casualty with severe diarrhoea of 6–7 episodes for 6 days duration. The stool specimen showed oocysts with four sporozoites on modified acid staining.

A. Identify the causative agent in this case. (1 mark)

- *Cryptosporidium parvum.*

B. List the other coccidian parasites causing diarrhoea in HIV positive individuals. (1 mark)

1. *Cryptosporidium* sp.
2. *Isospora belli.*
3. *Cyclospora* sp.
4. *Microsporidium* sp.

C. Write briefly about the life cycle of this agent (2 marks)

Life Cycle

- *See* Figure 3.1.11.

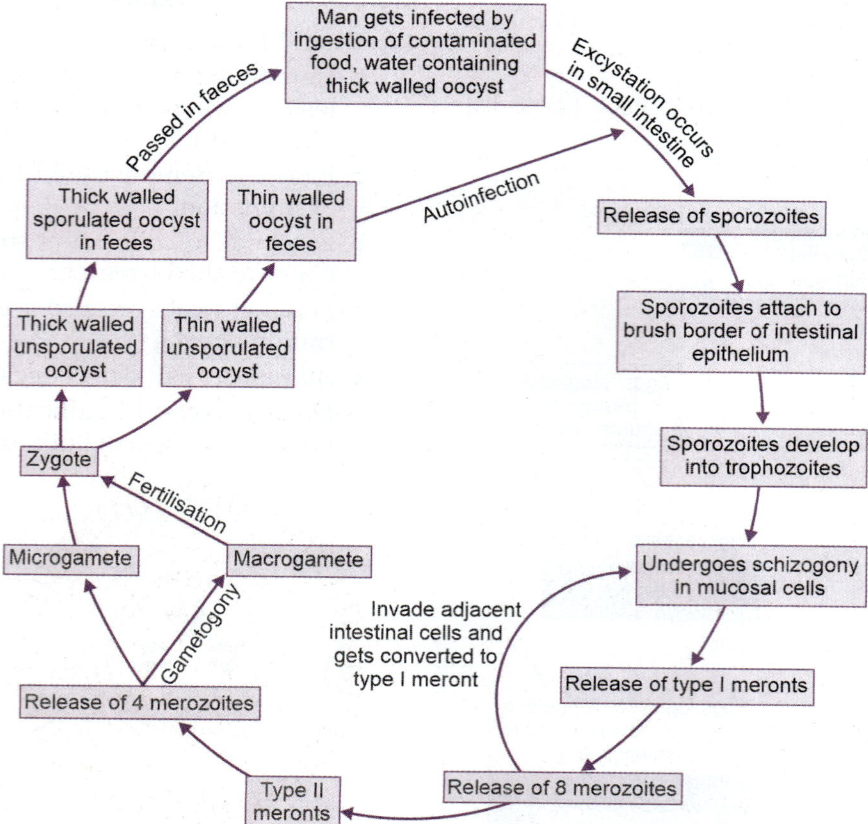

Fig. 3.1.11: Life cycle of *Cryptosporidium parvum*

D. Discuss the pathogenesis and clinical presentation of this condition. (2 marks)

Pathogenesis

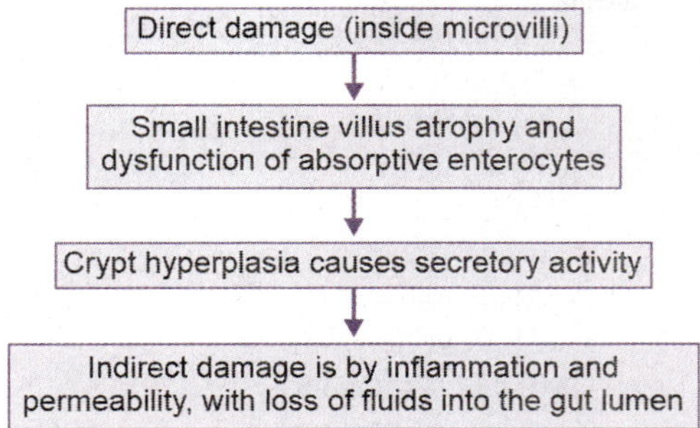

Clinical Features

- *In immunocompromised patients:* Watery, non-bloody diarrhoea causing large fluid loss
- Symptoms persist for long periods in immunocompromised patients, whereas they are self-limited in immunocompetent patients.

E. What are the various diagnostic modalities? (3 marks)

1. **Stool microscopy**
   - Direct wet mount
   - Wet mount after concentration—Sheather's sugar flotation technique is preferred.
   - Modified acid-fast staining and calcofluor white staining.
   - Direct fluorescent antibody staining
   - *Observation:* Round 4–6 µm size oocyst containing four sporozoites
2. **Antigen detection** from stool by ELISA, ICT
3. Antibody detection from serum by ELISA
4. Molecular diagnosis by PCR
5. Histopathology of intestinal biopsy specimen to demonstrate the oocysts

F. How will you treat this patient? (1 mark)

- Fluid resuscitation
- Nitazoxanide has been FDA approved for treatment of diarrhoea caused by *Cryptosporidium* in people with healthy immune systems
- Paromomycin and macrolide antibiotics (alternative).

---

8. A 40-year-old HIV positive patient comes to the Medicine OPD with symptoms of weight loss, cough and diarrhoea. Routine stool examination is ordered as a part of evaluation. Stool wet mount reveals rhabditiform larvae of the parasite. Eosinophil count is normal.

A. Which is the probable agent in this case? (1 mark)

- The nematode associated with diarrhoea in this case is *Strongyloides stercoralis*.

B. Discuss the pathogenesis and life cycle of this nematode. (3+3 marks)

Pathogenesis

- *Infective stage:* Filariform larvae (L3)
- *Mode of infection:* Penetration of the skin by filariform larvae in the soil and internal autoinfection
- Effect due to migrating larva.
  - Asymptomatic infection
  - Macules, papule at the site of invasion
  - Cutaneous larva migrans
  - Pulmonary symptoms: Bronchopneumonia or pneumonitis
- Effect Due to adult worm
  - Mild-to-moderate worm load: Epigastric pain, nausea, diarrhoea, and blood loss
  - Heavy larva load: Hyperinfection syndrome and disseminated strongyloidiasis

Life Cycle

- *See* Figure 3.1.12.

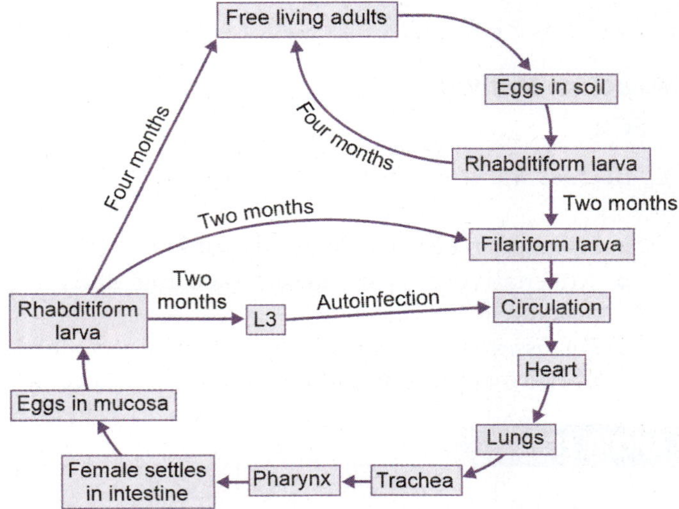

Fig. 3.1.12: Life cycle of *Strongyloides stercoralis*

C. Discuss the complications of this infection. (3 marks)

Hyperinfection Syndrome and Disseminated Strongyloidiasis

- Repeated autoinfection resulting in massive larval invasion of lungs and CNS.
- Risk factors
  - Immunosuppressive therapy
  - Organ transplantation
  - Haematological malignancy
  - AIDS, HTLV 1 infection
  - End-stage renal disease

- Clinical features
  - Pulmonary infiltrate, gram-negative septicaemia, meningitis, brain abscess, severe diarrhoea, paralytic ileus.

D. What are the laboratory methods for diagnosis of this infection? (3 marks)

Specimen Collection

- Stool, duodenal aspirate (Entero test), sputum.

Microscopy

- Demonstration of rhabditiform larva.

Culture

- Stool is cultured to demonstrate the formation of filariform larvae in 2 days.
- Harada Mori filter paper method
- Baermann funnel method
- Agar plate method (sensitive method)

Serodiagnosis

- Antibody by ELISA

Molecular Method

- PCR

E. Discuss the treatment of this infection. (2 marks)

- Ivermectin (200 mg/kg daily for 2 days)
- Alternatively, albendazole (400 mg daily for 3 days)
- *For disseminated strongyloidiasis:* Prolonged course of Ivermectin until the parasites are eradicated.

SHORT ESSAYS

1. Compare and contrast between amoebic dysentery and bacillary dysentery. (4 marks)

Feature	Amoebic dysentery	Bacillary dysentery
Caused by	• *Entamoeba histolytica*	• *Shigella sp.*
Occurrence	• Sporadic	• Outbreak
Onset	• Gradual	• Acute
Signs and symptoms	• 6–8 episodes of loose motions per day	• More than 10 episodes of bloody diarrhoea
Stool characteristics	• Relatively copious • Dark in colour • Offensive odour	• Scant • Colour of fresh blood • Odourless
Microscopic examination	• RBCs—clumped together with a reddish yellow colour • Numerous eosinophils • Few pus cells and macrophages • Also seen—Charcot–Leyden (C-L) crystals and pyknotic bodies	• RBCs—discrete amounts, Rouleaux formation • Fewer eosinophils • Numerous pus cells and macrophages • Have ghost cells

Contd.

2. Enumerate various types of diarrhoeagenic *Escherichia coli*. Write in detail about the diarrhoeagenic *Escherichia coli* causing traveller's diarrhoea and infantile diarrhoea. (1+2+2 marks)

Diarrhoeagenic *Escherichia Coli*

1. Enteropathogenic *E. coli (EPEC)*
2. Enterotoxigenic *E. coli (ETEC)*
3. Enteroinvasive *E. coli (EIEC)*
4. Enterohaemorrhagic *E. coli (EHEC)*
5. Enteroaggregative *E. coli (EAEC)*
6. Diffusely adherent *E. coli (DAEC)*

Traveler's Diarrhoea and Infantile Diarrhoea

- Caused by *enterotoxigenic Escherichia coli.*
- Endemic in developing countries in all age groups
- Spectrum ranges from mild watery diarrhoea to fatal disease, similar to cholera
- *Traveler's diarrhoea (25–75%):* In persons visiting endemic areas
- *Weaning diarrhoea:* 10–30% of infants in endemic areas during the time of weaning (4–6 months)

Pathogenesis

- Adherence to intestinal mucosa mediated by colonisation factor antigens (CFA I, II, III and IV).
- Production of enterotoxin (plasmid mediated): Labile and stable toxin LT bind to specific ganglioside receptors (GM1) on the epithelial cells of small intestine and facilitate the entry of A subunit where it activates adenylate cyclase. Stimulation of adenylate cyclase causes an increased production of cAMP, which leads to hypersecretion of water and electrolytes into the lumen.
- Infective dose 10^6 bacilli.

Diagnosis

- *Specimen collection:* Faeces—within 4 days of onset of illness

- *Transport media:* Cary Blair, Stuarts, buffered glycerol saline
- *Macroscopic appearance*
  - Watery stool.
- *Microscopic appearance.*
  - *Saline wet mount:* To observe pus cells and RBCs.
  - *In secretory diarrhoea:* Leukocytes are absent or scanty.
- *Direct methods—Antigen detection.*
  - Immunoassays for ST (ETEC), Shiga toxin (EHEC) and LPS (O157).
  - Nucleic acid detection—Specific probes for genes encoding the toxins.

3. Describe the pathogenesis, clinical features of diarrhoea due to campylobacter jejuni. (2+2 marks)

Diarrhoea due to *Campylobacter jejuni*

- Associated with acute diarrhoea worldwide.
- Inhabits the intestinal tracts of animals, especially poultry; contamination from these sources can lead to foodborne disease.

Pathogenesis (Fig. 3.1.13)

- *Source:* Zoonotic
- *Mode of infection:* Water-borne outbreaks, poultry, raw milk and direct contact with animals or animal products
- *Virulence factors.*
  1. Motility
  2. Adhesion
  3. Produce a heat-labile, cholera like enterotoxin: watery diarrhoea.
  4. *Cytotoxin production:* Bloody diarrhoea. The infection is rarely associated with haemolytic-uremic syndrome and thrombotic thrombocytopenic purpura.

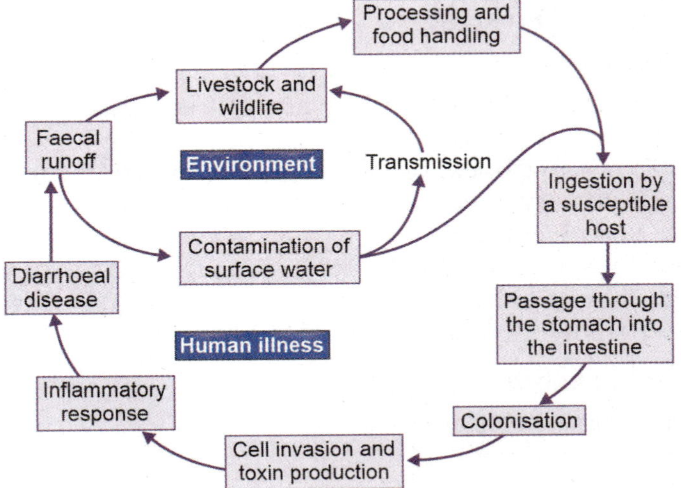

Fig. 3.1.13: Pathogenesis of *Campylobacter jejuni*

- *Effects*
  1. The bacteria cause diffuse, bloody, edematous, and exudative enteritis.
  2. The inflammatory infiltrate comprises of neutrophils, mononuclear cells, and eosinophils.
  3. Crypt abscesses develop in the epithelial glands, and ulceration of the mucosal epithelium occurs.

Clinical Features

- Seen in young children, elderly patients, AIDS.
- *Incubation period:* 2–5 days
- Clinical symptoms are:
  - Diarrhoea (frequently bloody)
  - Abdominal pain
  - Fever
  - Headache
  - Nausea and/or vomiting
  - Symptoms typically last 3–6 days.
- Death is rare.
- Complications
  1. Bacteraemia
  2. Hepatitis
  3. Pancreatitis
- Post-infection complications
  1. Reactive arthritis
  2. Neurological disorders—Guillain-Barré syndrome, severe neurological dysfunction.

4. Write in brief about non-typhoidal *Salmonellae* under the following headings.

A. Species of *Salmonella* included under Non Typhoidal Salmonella. (1 mark)

- Includes the Salmonella strains other than *S. typhi* and *S. paratyphi.*
- They are:
  1. *S. typhimurium*
  2. *S. enteritidis*
  3. *Others: S. newport, S. javiana, S. Heidelberg, S. choleraesuis* and *S. dublin.*

B. Mode of transmission, prevalence, Seasonality (1 mark)

- Zoonotic.

Mode of Transmission

- Food contaminated with animal products-seafood, eggs, poultry, meat, dairy, vegetables, salads.

Prevalence

- Prevalent in developed as well as developing nations.

Seasonality

- Rainy season in tropical region and warmer months in temperate region.
- Outbreaks are common in hospitals.

C. Discuss gastroenteritis due to non-typhoidal *Salmonella*. (3 marks)

Source of Infection

- Usually animal products (zoonosis)
- Poultry—chicken, eggs and egg products, meat, milk and milk products
- Salads/uncooked vegetables contaminated by manure.
- Food contaminated by droppings of rats/lizards.

Route of Transmission

- Faecal–oral route.

Infective Dose

- 10^5–10^6 bacilli.

Incubation Period

- 12–36 hours.

Pathogenesis

- The bacteria penetrate the epithelial cells lining small intestine.
- Bacterial multiplication in the lamina propria → neutrophils → inflammation.
- LPS causes fever. Prostaglandins are released from epithelial cells, which causes outpouring of fluid and electrolytes into the lumen of the intestine.

Symptoms

- Fever, abdominal pain, vomiting, diarrhoea—self-limiting, subside in 2–4 days.
- Rarely—typhoidal/septicemic type of fever in immunosuppressed.

Diagnosis

- Isolation from faeces and food item.

Treatment

- Symptomatic, antibiotics—prolong faecal shedding.
- For serious invasive illness—antibiotics given.

---

5. Discuss in brief the major epidemiological aspects of cholera. Add a note on O139 Strain. (3+2 marks)

Epidemiological Aspects of Cholera

- Cholera has been endemic in the Ganges Delta since time immemorial.
- Annual epidemics reported in West Bengal and Bangladesh.
- Worldwide spread resulting in six pandemics from 1817 to 1926.
- The seventh pandemic started in 1961 from Indonesia has spread to South Asia, Middle East, Africa, Southern Europe and Western Pacific regions.
- 7th Pandemic—differed from previous pandemics.
  - Only pandemic that originated outside India i.e., from Indonesia.
  - Caused by El Tor biotype.
  - Milder cholera with more carrier rate
  - Rapid spread of El Tor, involving the entire globe including some unusual parts
  - Isolated first from Chennai in 1992.

O139 Strain

- O139 strain—Not agglutinated by any of the antisera available at that time (O1 to O138).
- Organism did not belong to any of the O serogroups previously described for *V. cholerae* but to a new serogroup, which was given the designation O139 Bengal after the area where the strains were first isolated.
- *Vibrio cholerae* O139 is identified non-O1V. cholerae strain responsible for outbreaks of epidemic cholera in India, Bangladesh, and Thailand.
- Bengal strain—spread rapidly along the coastal region of bay of Bengal.
- Derivative of O1 El Tor—differs in having a distinct LPS and capsulated.
- Invasive → bacteraemia and extraintestinal manifestations.
- No cross protection between O1 and O139.
- By 1994, O1 El Tor replaced with O139.

---

6. Enumerate the viruses causing diarrhoea. Discuss in brief the pathogenesis, clinical features of diarrhoea in children due to rotavirus. (1+4 marks)

Viruses Causing Diarrhoea

1. Rotavirus
2. Adenovirus
   - Types 40 and 41
3. Norovirus
4. Astrovirus

Rotavirus

- Member of the Reovirus family (reo; respiratory enteric orphan).
- Non-enveloped, dsRNA viruses with icosahedral symmetry
- 11 segments RNA
- RNA-dependent RNA polymerase
- The capsid has double shell
- 6 serotypes (A-F).

Pathogenesis

- *Transmission:* Faecal–oral route.
- *Season:* winter.
- Majority of children by 6 years of age have antibodies to at least one serotype.

- Rotavirus replicates in the mucosal cells of the small intestine, damaging the transport mechanisms with consequent loss of fluids and electrolytes.
- No inflammation occurs and the diarrhoea is non-bloody.
- Babies under 2 years are the main victims.

Clinical Features

- Nausea, vomiting and watery, non-bloody diarrhoea.
- Dehydration is the main complication.

7. Prolonged antimicrobial use especially of cephalosporins can disturb the flora of large intestine and lead to diarrhoea. Which is the organism responsible for this condition and describe its pathogenesis and diagnosis. (1+2+1 marks)

Organism Responsible for this Condition

- *Clostridium difficile.*

Toxins

- Two large protein exotoxins: toxin A, a 308-kd enterotoxin, and toxin B, a 250-to-270-kd cytotoxin

Pathogenesis

- Disruption of flora and colonisation of *C. difficile* followed by toxin release, which causes mucosal damage by altering the actin cytoskeleton and causes inflammation.

Diagnosis

- By culture
- Detection of toxin by EIA, ICT, latex agglutination, molecular methods.

8. What is a mycotoxin? Discuss in brief about important mycotoxins and their significance. (1+2+2 marks)

Mycotoxins

- Secondary metabolites produced by microfungi that can cause disease and death in humans.
- For example, aflatoxin, citrinin, ergot alkaloids, fumonisins, ochratoxin A, patulin, trichothecenes, and zearalenone

Mycotoxicosis

- Disease produced following consumption of food contaminated by toxins liberated by certain fungi.

Aflatoxin

- *Produced by Aspergillus species: A. flavus* and *A. parasiticus*
- *Four types:* B_1, B_2, G_1, and G_2
- Aflatoxin B_1, the most toxic, is a potent carcinogen and has been directly correlated to adverse health effects, such as liver cancer in many animal species.
- associated with commodities produced in the tropics and subtropics, such as cotton, peanut, spices, and maize.
- *Associated conditions:* Hepatoma, hepatitis, Indian childhood cirrhosis, Reye's syndrome

Ochratoxin

- Produced by *Penicillium* and *Aspergillus* species.
- *Aspergillus ochraceus* is found as a contaminant of a wide range of commodities including beverages such as beer and wine.
- *Associated conditions:* Nephropathies (Balkan endemic nephropathy)

Fumonisins

- Produced by *Fusarium moniliforme*
- Associated with maize.
- Associated conditions
  - Equine leukoencephalomalacia
  - Porcine pulmonary oedema
  - Carcinoma oesophagus

Trichothecenes

- Produced by *Fusarium graminearum.*
- Associated with.
  - Alimentary toxic aleukia.
  - Biological warfare (yellow rain).

9. Define halophilic *Vibrios* with examples. Discuss the pathogenesis and clinical manifestations of Halophilic *Vibrios*. (1+1+3 marks)

Halophilic Vibrios

Definition

- *Vibrios* that require a high concentration of sodium chloride for growth known as halophilic *Vibrios*.
- Halophilic *Vibrios* are a part of normal marine microbial flora.

Examples

1. *Vibrio parahaemolyticus.*
2. *Vibrio vulnificus.*
3. *Vibrio alginolyticus.*

Vibrio parahaemolyticus

Pathogenesis

- *Source:* Crabs, prawns, oysters having *Vibrio parahaemolyticus* as their normal microflora
- *Mode of transmission:* Consumption of raw or undercooked sea food

- *Virulence factors.*
  1. Thermostable direct haemolysin (vp-TDH)
  2. Thermostable related haemolysin (vp_TRH)
  3. Urease
  4. Pili—which help in the colonisation

Clinical Manifestations

- *Incubation period:* 4–96 hours
- Onset of the illness is within 24 hours of ingestion of contaminated sea food
- Enteric illness ranging from mild watery diarrhoea to frank dysentery like syndrome.

Vibrio vulnificus

Pathogenesis

- *Source:* Oysters and crabs
- *Mode of transmission:* Consumption of raw oysters and crabs
- Sometimes exposed wounds coming in direct contact with contaminated sea water leads to the skin and soft tissue infection.

Clinical Manifestations

- *Incubation period:* About 7 days
- *Predisposing conditions:* Liver disorders, immunosupression, iron overload
- Soft tissue infection or septicaemia or both.
- Erythematous lesions evolving to bullae or vesicles and necrotic ulcer.

10. A 3-month-old infant is brought to the casualty by her mother. The child has not been eating well, seems lethargic, and has lax muscle tone. The mother notes that she seemed "floppy" when lifted. The infant does not have a fever. Her mother indicates that she had recently started the child on solid foods including cereal with honey.

A. What is the most likely infection and its aetiology? (1 mark)

Infection

- Infant botulism.

Aetiology

- *Clostridium botulinum.*

B. Mechanism of action of this toxin and its clinical manifestations. (2 marks)

Mechanism of Action of Toxin

- Neurotoxin 'botulinum toxin' (BT).
- *Serotype:* Eight serotypes—A, B, C1, C2, D, E, F and G
- Entry (ingested, inhaled, from wound) → via blood to peripheral cholinergic nerve terminals (neuromuscular junctions, postganglionic parasympathetic nerve endings, and peripheral ganglia) → bind to Ach receptors at neuromuscular junction → blockage of release of Ach → Flaccid paralysis.

Clinical Manifestations

- Diplopia, dysphasia, dysarthria
- Descending symmetric flaccid paralysis of voluntary muscles
- Decreased deep tendon reflexes
- Constipation
- Respiratory muscle paralysis may lead to death.
- No sensory or cognitive deficits.

SHORT ANSWERS

1. Describe in brief about the immunoprophylaxis of cholera (4 marks)

See Table 3.1.1

2. Discuss briefly about enteroinvasive *Escherichia coli.* (2 marks)

- Have the capacity to invade the interstitial epithelial cells *in vivo* (plasmid mediated).

Table 3.1.1 Immunoprophylaxis of cholera

Vaccine	*Type*	*Route*	*No. of doses*	*Efficacy*	*Duration*	*Advantages*	*Disadvantages*
Whole cell/B subunit (Dukarol)	• Killed organisms *V. cholerae* O1 and B subunit of toxin	Oral	• 2/3 • (10–24 days apart)	50–60%	2/3 years	• More potent stimulator of intestinal immune response • Safe • Easy to administer	• Unsuitable in children and O blood group patients • Less protection against El Tor biotype

Contd.

Table 3.1.1 Immunoprophylaxis of cholera

Vaccine	Type	Route	No. of doses	Efficacy	Duration	Advantages	Disadvantages
CVD 103-HgR	• Live attenuated organism (classical, O1, Inaba)	Oral	• 1	59%	At least 6 months	• Safe for adult and children • Immune response within 7days • Increased intestinal immune response • Better immune response in O blood group • 80% protection against El Tor	• Can't prevent cholera transmission
Cholera vaccine	• Extract or killed	IM	• 2 • (7–24 days apart)	50%	3–6 months		• Short lived immunity • Doesn't reduce severity

- Mediated by a plasmid-coded antigen called virulence marker antigen (VMA)
- Serogroups—028a, 0112ac, 0124, 0136, 0143, 0114, 0152, 0154.
- Clinically resembles shigellosis.
- *Manifestations:* Ulceration of bowel, dysentery
- *Diagnosis:* Detection of VMA by ELISA, HeLa cell invasion assay, Sereny test

3. What is Shiga-like toxin? Enumerate the complications of Shiga-like toxin. (1+2 marks)

Shiga-like Toxins (Stx)

- Shiga-like toxins (Stx) represent a group of bacterial toxins involved in human and animal diseases.
- Stx is produced by enterohaemorrhagic *Escherichia coli, Shigella dysenteriae type 1, Citrobacter freundii,* and *Aeromonas spp.*

Complications

1. Bloody diarrhoea.
2. Hemolytic-uremic syndrome (HUS).

4. Mention the parasite causing fatty diarrhoea? Discuss in brief about the pathogenesis and diagnosis of this condition. (1+2+2 marks)

Parasite Causing Fatty Diarrhoea (Giardiasis)

- *Giardia lamblia*

Pathogenesis of Fatty Diarrhoea

- *Transmission:* Ingestion of cysts in fecally contaminated food and water.
- *Risk group:* Male homosexuals, children in day care centers and patients in mental hospitals
- *Sequence of events.*
  - Excystation in the duodenum
  - Attachment of the trophozoite attaches to the intestinal mucosa (no invasion)
  - Inflammation of the duodenal mucosa, leading to protein and fat malabsorption
  - 50% of the infected are asymptomatic carriers who excrete the cysts for years

Diagnosis

- *Stool wet mount:* Trophozoite (falling leaf motility) and cysts (Figs 3.1.14 and 3.1.15)
- *Entero test:* Duodenal aspirate for the presence of cysts and trophozoites
- Antigen detection in stool.
- *Molecular methods:* PCR, probes

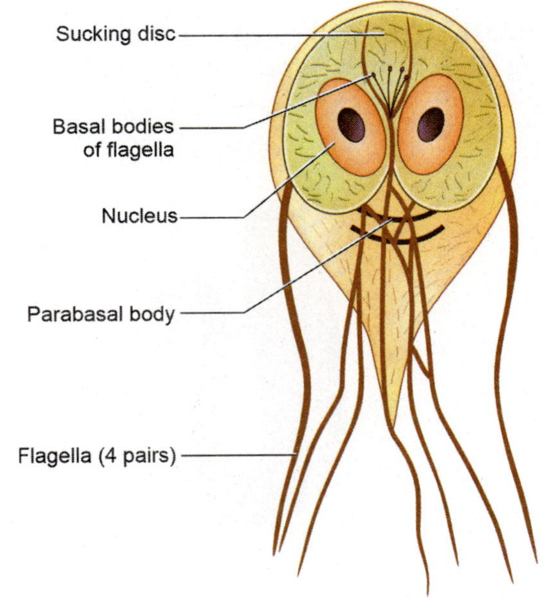

Fig. 3.1.14: Trophozoite of *Giardia lamblia*

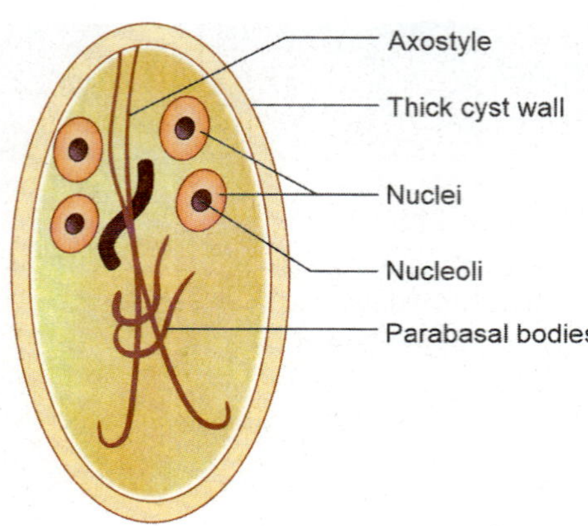

Fig. 3.1.15: Cyst of *Giardia lamblia*

5. A toddler accompanied by his mother visits a paediatrician with c/o of itching around the anal region especially at night. Doctor examines the child and confirms by presence of short white worms around the anus. What is the disease and its etiological agent? What is the mode for transmission and diagnostic tool used for the diagnosis? Draw a neat, labelled diagram of the egg seen under microscopy in this case. (1+2+1 marks)

Disease

- Pinworm infection (Enterobiasis).

Aetiological Agent

- *Enterobius vermicularis.*

Mode of Transmission

- Faecal–oral route.
- Or via contact with contaminated clothes, bedding, personal care products, and furniture.

Diagnostic Tool Used

- Demonstration of the eggs in perianal skin by using the Scotch tape technique, NIH swab (Fig. 3.1.16).

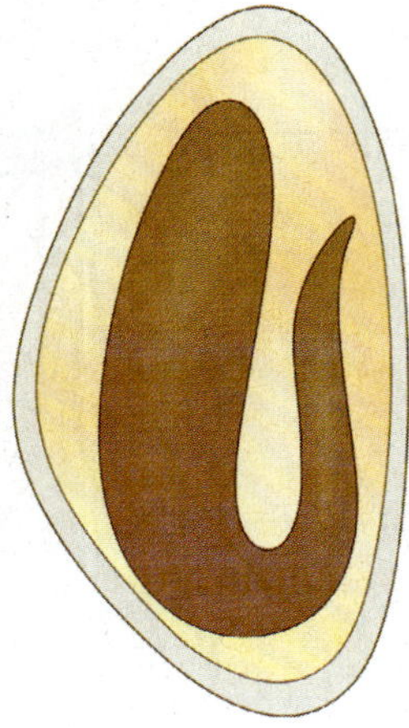

Fig. 3.1.16: Egg of *Enterobius vermicularis* with tadpole-shaped embryo

6. Discuss the pathogenesis, clinical features, and diagnosis of diarrhoea due to *Bacillus cereus*. (2+1+1 marks)

Pathogenesis

- *Transmission:* Spores on rice grains survives steaming and frying. The spores germinate when rice is kept warm for many hours (e.g. reheated fried rice). The portal of entry is the GI tract
- *Virulence factors.*
  - 2 enterotoxins.
    - The mode of action of one of the enterotoxins is the same as that of cholera. Heat labile. Long incubation period. Associated with meat or vegetable-containing foods after cooking
    - The mode of action of the other enterotoxin is the same as the staphylococcal enterotoxin (superantigen). Heat stable. Short incubation period. Associated with fried rice

Clinical Features

- Two syndromes:
  1. *Emetic type:* Short incubation period (4 hours), nausea and vomiting, similar to staphylococcal food poisoning.
  2. *Diarrhoeal type:* As a long incubation period (18 hours), watery, non-bloody diarrhoea, resembling clostridial gastroenteritis.

Laboratory Diagnosis

- *Sample collection:* Food, faeces, vomitus
- *Culture isolation.*
  - *MYPA (mannitol, egg yolk, polymyxin, phenol red and agar):* Colonies are rough with a violet-red background, surrounded by white precipitated egg yolk.
  - *PEMBA (polymyxin B, egg yolk, mannitol, bromo-thymol blue, agar):* Peacock blue colour colonies after 48 hrs.
  - Motile, non-capsulated and not susceptible to gamma phage.

7. Mention the cause of food poisoning due to *Clostridium botulinum*. Enumerate the virulence factor and clinical manifestations of botulinum food poisoning. (2+2 marks)

Cause of Food Poisoning Due to *Clostridium botulinum*

- Food-borne botulism occurs when *C. botulinum* grows and produces toxins in food prior to consumption. The spores of *C. botulinum* exists in soil, river and sea water, in lightly preserved foods and in inadequately processed, home-canned or home-bottled foods.
- *Food:* Low-acid preserved vegetables, such as green beans, spinach, mushrooms, and beets; fish, including canned tuna, fermented, salted and smoked fish; and meat products, such as ham and sausage

- Pathogenesis.
  1. Toxin (A, B, C1, D, E, F, and G).
  2. Toxin binds to presynaptic receptors in peripheral NMJ
  3. Blocks the release of Ach
  4. Flaccid paralysis

Clinical Manifestations of Botulinum Food Poisoning

- Diplopia, dysphasia, dysarthria
- Descending symmetric flaccid paralysis of voluntary muscles
- Decreased deep tendon reflexes
- Constipation
- Respiratory muscle paralysis, may lead to death
- No sensory or cognitive deficits.

8. Name the ciliated protozoa causing dysentery in man. Discuss its pathogenesis, diagnosis in brief. (1+2+2 marks)

Ciliated Protozoa Causing Dysentery in Man

- *Balantidium coli.*

Pathogenesis

- *Reservoir:* Domestic animals, especially pigs
- *Mode of infection:* Ingesting the cysts in food or water contaminated with animal or human faeces.
- Excystation happens in the small intestine, the trophozoites reach the colon, burrow into the wall and cause an ulcer similar to that of *Entamoeba histolytica.*
- No extraintestinal lesions.

Diagnosis

- Demonstration of large ciliated trophozoites or large cysts with a characteristic V-shaped nucleus in the stool (Figs 3.1.17 and 3.1.18).
- There are no serologic tests available.

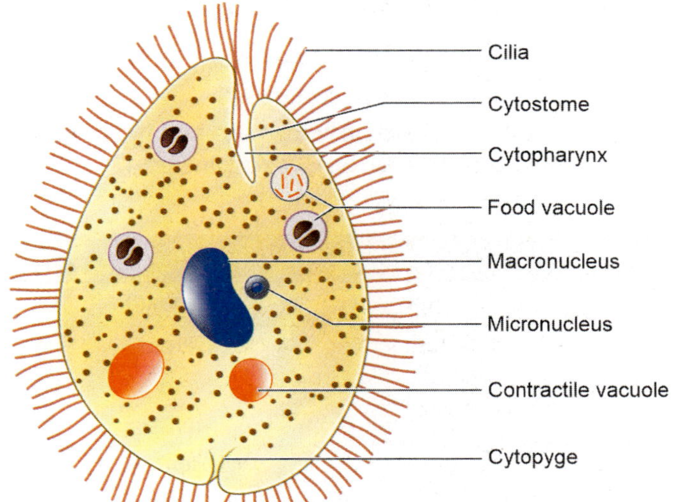

Fig. 3.1.17: Trophozoite of *Balantidium coli*

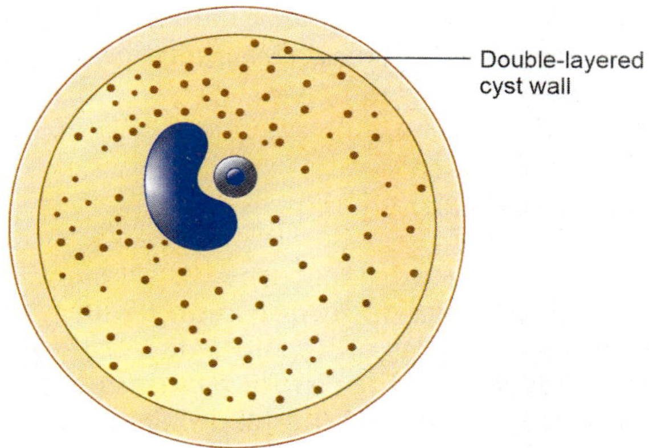

Fig. 3.1.18: Cyst of *Balantidium coli*

9. A 5-year-old school going child visited the paediatrician for c/o of itching in the perianal region especially during night times. The sample was sent for investigation to the microbiology laboratory. The stool microscopy revealed the following parasite.

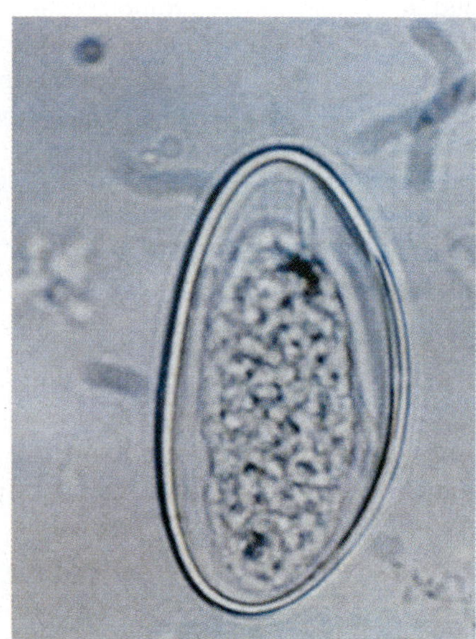

A. What is your diagnosis? (1 mark)

- Pinworm infection (Enterobiasis) caused by *Enterobius vermicularis.*

B. What is the appropriate sample to be collected? (1 mark)

- Specimen can be collected by using NIH (National Institute of Health, USA) or Scotch tape method.

C. Write the identifying features of the egg? (1 mark)

- *Shape:* Planoconvex
- Non-bile stained.
- Embryonated ovum with larva inside.

D. Name the other non-bile-stained eggs. (1 mark)

- Hookworm (Eggs of *Ancylostoma duodenale* or *Nectar americanus*).
  - *Shape:* Oval
  - Non bile stained
  - Segmented egg

10. A 6-year-old toddler came to a clinic with c/o severe pain abdomen along with nausea vomiting. On examination the child was malnourished. The stool examination on microscopy revealed the following picture.

- *See* Figure 3.1.1.

A. Identify the causative agent? (1 mark)

- Ascariasis caused by *Ascaris lumbricoides.*

B. Draw a neat, labelled diagram describing the morphology of the egg. (1 mark)

Bile-stained Eggs

Fertilised egg	*Unfertilised egg*
• Albuminated thick coat • Shape: Round to oval • Crescentic space at the poles • Floats in saturated salt solution • Unembryonated large ovum	• Albinous coat is thin • Shape: Elongated • No crescentic space • Sinks in saturated salt solution • Ovum is atrophied with refractile granules

C. Name the other bile-stained eggs. (1 mark)

1. *Trichuris trichiura* egg
2. *Taenia* egg.

11. Compare diarrhoea and dysentery with the aetiological agents. (4 marks)

Feature	*Diarrhoea*	*Dysentery*
Symptoms	• Loose, watery, and possibly more-frequent bowel movements	• Stomach cramps and diarrhoea with blood or mucus in the faeces
Associated with	• Nausea, vomiting, abdominal pain or weight loss	• Fever, abdominal pain, tenesmus
Aetiological agents	• *E. coli, Vibrio cholerae, Clostridium perfringens, Bacillus cereus, Clostridium difficile, Aeromonas hydrophilia* • Viruses: Rotavirus, Norwalk virus, adenovirus 40, 41, astrovirus • Parasites: *Giardia lamblia, Cryptosporidium, isospora*	• Bacteria: *Shigella spp. Campylobacter jejuni, Vibrio parahaemolyticus, Yersinia enterocolitica,* non-typhoidal *Salmonella* • Parasites: *Entamoeba histolytica, Balantidium coli, Schistosoma haematobium*

12. Write about the clinical significance of Yersinia enterocolitica. (3 marks)

Clinical Significance

- Enterocolitis that is clinically indistinguishable from that caused by *Salmonella* or *Shigella*.
- Mesenteric adenitis that clinically resembles acute appendicitis.
- Bacteraemia, liver or splenic abscess , mainly in persons with underlying disease.
- *Associated with two autoimmune diseases:* reactive arthritis and Reiter's syndrome.

MI 3.2 IDENTIFY THE COMMON AETIOLOGIC AGENTS OF DIARRHOEA AND DYSENTERY

SHORT ESSAY

1. After a party, approximately 36 hours after the meal, the children of a family developed abdominal cramps, fever, and watery diarrhoea. The parents had developed similar symptoms 6 and 8 hours earlier.

A. What is your clinical diagnosis and probable aetiology?

Clinical Diagnosis

- Dysentery.

Probable Aetiology

- *Shigella* spp. or *Entamoeba histolytica.*

B. Which sample needs to be collected?

- Stool sample in a sterile container.

C. How to differentiate between the two types of this infection on microscopic examination?

- Through microscopy.

Feature	*Amoebic dysentery*	*Bacillary dysentery*
Cellular exudate	Scanty	Abundant
Red blood cells	Clumped	Discrete
Macrophages	Few	Severe
Cells	Eosinophils	PMNLs
Charcot–Leyden crystals	Present	Absent
Motile bacteria	Present	Absent (non-motile)
Amoeba	Motile trophozoites	Absent

MI 3.3 DESCRIBE THE ENTERIC FEVER PATHOGENS. DESCRIBE THE EVOLUTION OF THE CLINICAL COURSE AND LABORATORY DIAGNOSIS OF THE DISEASES CAUSED BY THEM

LONG ESSAYS

1. A 40-year-old male businessman presented with history of coated tongue, pyrexia, weakness, anorexia and vomiting for the last 4 days. He gives history of eating food outside. Physician advised for complete blood profile, blood for culture and sensitivity. On general physical examination, patient complaint of mild tenderness at right lower hypochondrium of the abdomen. Blood culture grew typical non-lactose fermenting colonies on MacConkey agar. Answer the following questions related to the case discussed.

A. What could be the most probable diagnosis of the above case. Enumerate the causative agent and modes of transmission. (3 marks)

Most Probable Diagnosis

- Enteric/Typhoid fever.

Causative Agent

- Typhoid fever caused by *Salmonella enterica* serovar typhi strains (*S. typhi*).
- Paratyphoid fevers caused by *S. paratyphi A*, *S. paratyphi B* and *S. paratyphi C*.

B. Pathogenesis, clinical features of this condition. (4 marks)

Pathogenesis

- *Source of infection:* Patients and carriers
- *Mode of infection:* Ingestion; contaminated food and water
- *Infective dose:* 10^5–10^8 bacilli
- *Incubation period:* 7–14 days
- *Host factors.*
  1. Gastric acidity
  2. Normal flora
  3. Gastric disorders—Inflammatory bowel disease.
- *Virulence factors.*
  1. Type I fimbriae
  2. Intracellular survival
  3. Endotoxin.
  4. Vi antigen—inhibits phagocytosis.
- Sequence of events.

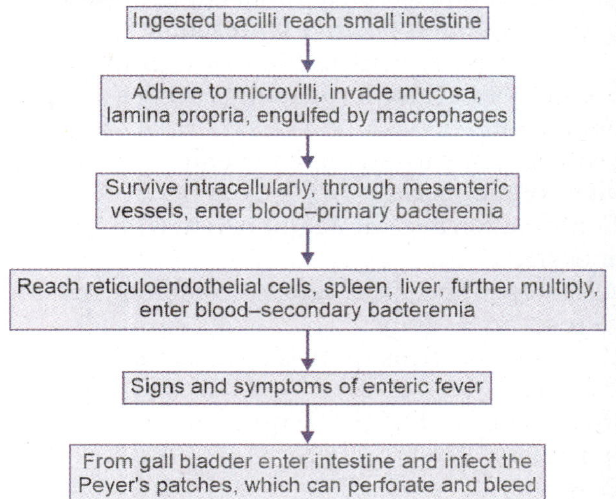

Clinical Features

- Fever (step ladder pyrexia).
- Headache.
- Hepatosplenomegaly.
- Alternate diarrhoea and constipation.
- Fine rose-pink rash—rose spots.
- Complications.
  1. Perforation.
  2. Peritonitis.
  3. Hemorrhage.

C. Describe the specimen collection and laboratory diagnosis of the above case. (3 marks)

Specimen Collection

- Specimen collection depends on stage of disease.
  - 1st week: Blood culture, Bone marrow aspirate, Duodenal aspirate.
  - 2nd week: Serology, Blood culture, Stool culture, Urine culture.
  - 3rd week: Serology, Stool culture, Urine culture, Blood culture.
- *Other specimens:* bile, biopsy of rose spots

Laboratory Diagnosis

Blood Culture

- 1st and 2nd week of enteric fever.
- 10–20 ml of blood collected aseptically by venipuncture.
- Blood is inoculated into 50–100 ml of liquid culture medium.
- Incubate at 37°C for 7 days.

- In conventional method, subcultures are done on MacConkey and blood agar at 24 hours, 96 hours, and 7 days.
- In semi-automated system, subculture is done if the bottle flags off as positive by machine.
- Growth on subculture shows gram-negative bacilli, non-lactose fermenting colonies and motile organism.
- Oxidase test (negative), biochemical tests done to identify the species.
- Confirmation by slide agglutination with 'O' and 'H' antisera.
- *Advantages:* Specific diagnosis, antibiotic sensitivity testing can be done
- *Disadvantages:* Sensitivity is low, useful only in early infection
- Ideal method for diagnosis in 1st week (positivity=90%).
- Positivity decreases 75% in 2nd week, 60% in 3rd week, 25% till fever subsides.

Clot Culture

- Variation of blood culture
- 5 ml of blood collected and allowed to clot
- Clot transferred to bile broth with streptokinase
- Clot lysed and bacilli released to grow
- The serum obtained is used for serology
- *Advantages:* Yield is more, more sensitive
- *Disadvantages:* Chances of contamination are more, expensive

Stool Culture

- Usually positive from 2nd week, highest rate of isolation in 3rd week.
- Stool is cultured.
- Directly on to Mac Conkey agar, DCA, XLD, Wilson Blairs agar.
- Enrichment broth like selenite F broth, tetrathionate broth.
- Growth is identified by biochemical reactions and agglutination.
- *Advantages:* To detect carriers, useful in later stages
- *Disadvantage:* In endemic area cannot differentiate between patients and carriers

Serology

Detection of Antigen

- *In serum:* ELISA
- *In urine:* Co-agglutination
- Vi antigen detection in case of carriers.
- *Advantage:* partially treated cases, acute infections

Detection of Antibody

- *Tube agglutination:* Widal test
  - Second week onwards
  - Detects antibodies to O and H Ag in patient's serum.
- ELISA.

---

2. A 15-year-old 11th grade student admitted in the hospital with history of fever since 3 weeks. Dengue NS1 Ag test is negative and peripheral blood smear examination is negative for malarial parasites.

A. Most probable diagnosis of the above case. List the infectious causes of it. Discuss the work up to be done for this case. (5 marks)

Most Probable Diagnosis

- Pyrexia of unknown origin (PUO)

Infectious Causes of PUO

1. Pneumonia
2. Urinary tract infection
3. Cellulitis (or line infection)
4. Abdominal/pelvic abscess
5. Endocarditis
6. Meningitis
7. Brucellosis
8. Leptospirosis
9. TB—Pulmonary or extrapulmonary.
10. Viral.
    i. Gastroenteritis
    ii. Hepatitis
    iii. HIV
    iv. EBV
    v. CMV
    vi. Recent vaccination
11. Parasitic.
    i. Malaria

Workup in a Case of PUO

History	*Examination*	*Investigation*
• Drenching night sweats • Weight loss • Headache • Haemoptysis • Altered bowel habits • Occupation • Travel • Recreational activities • Injecting drug use • Medications	• Measurement of fever • Lymphadenopathy • Scalp tenderness • Hepatosplenomegaly • Cardiac murmurs • Respiratory auscultation • Rashes	• Full blood count • Liver function tests • ESR, CRP • HBV, HCV, HIV • Urine cultures • Blood cultures • ANA, RF • EPG • Chest X-ray • Abdominal CT • Echocardiography

B. What is the best clinical sample for the diagnosis of enteric fever in the 1st week of illness? (1 marks)

- Blood culture.

C. Method of detection of typhoid carriers (2 marks)

- 2–5% of typhoid patients fail to fully clear the infection within one year of recovery, instead progressing to a state of carriage.

Site of Carriage

- Biliary tract and gallbladder.
- Faecal carriers or Urinary carriers.

Duration of Shedding

- Convalescent carriers 3 weeks to 3 months
- Temporary carriers 3 months to 1 year
- Chronic carriers for more than 1 year

Detection of Carriers

Limitations

1. Intermittent shedding of bacilli
2. Low numbers

Specimen

- Stool
- Urine
- Cultures of duodenal specimens by aspiration or string device have slightly better sensitivity but limited public health utility.
- Bile, gallbladder stones, or tissue of afebrile individuals undergoing elective cholecystectomy is considered a gold standard of diagnosis.

Serology

- Detection of Vi antibody in the serum.
- *Drawback:* This antibody is found in the serum of healthy individuals in endemic arars.
- However, may remain useful in outbreak investigations in non-endemic areas.
- *Titre of* 1:10 is also considered as significant.

Isolation of Salmonellae from Sewage

- Sewer–swab technique and filtration.

Polymerase Chain Reaction (PCR) Amplification

- For *S. typhi* specific genes (e.g. fimbrial gene *staA* or *fliC*) have performed well in detecting organisms in bile or gallbladder specimen.

SHORT ESSAYS

1. Discuss the importance of blood cultures and serological tests in the diagnosis of Typhoid fever. (2+2 marks)

Blood Culture

- The standard diagnostic method for enteric fever.
- Multiple blood cultures with larger sample volumes always yield better results.
- 1st and 2nd week of enteric fever.
- Ideal method for diagnosis in 1st week (positivity—90%). Positivity decreases to 75% in 2nd week, 60% in 3rd week, 25% till fever subsides.
- *Advantages.*
  1. Specific diagnosis.
  2. Antibiotic sensitivity testing can be done.
- *Disadvantages.*
  1. Sensitivity is low.
  2. Useful only in early infection.

Serology

Widal Test

- For presumptive diagnosis of enteric fever.
- Single high titre or 4-fold rise in O and H agglutinins in patients serum is diagnostic of enteric fever.
- *Advantages.*
  1. Used in developing nations where enteric fever is endemic.
  2. Affordable testing alternative.
- *Disadvantages.*
  1. *False positive results:* repeated exposures to *S. typhi* in endemic regions, cross-reactivity with other non-Salmonella organisms.
  2. *Requires demonstration* of a rising titre of antibodies in paired samples 10–14 days apart.

2. Discuss in brief about the immunoprophylaxis of Typhoid fever. Compare and contrast the available vaccines for typhoid fever. (3+2 marks)

Immunoprophylaxis of Typhoid Fever

- The vaccines available against typhoid fever provide short-term protection.
- *Recommendations.*
  - Travelers to endemic area
  - People in close contact with a typhoid carrier
  - Laboratory workers working with *Salmonella typhi.*

Comparison of Enteric Fever Vaccines

Feature	*Inactivated typhoid vaccine: Parenteral Vi vaccine*	*Live typhoid vaccine: Typhoral (oral live attenuated S. Typhi Ty2 1a vaccine)*
Route of administration	• IM or subcutaneous single dose	• Administered orally
Age	• 2 years and older	• 6 years and older

Contd.

Feature	Inactivated typhoid vaccine: Parenteral Vi vaccine	Live typhoid vaccine: Typhoral (oral live attenuated S. Typhi Ty2 1a vaccine)
Dose	• One dose taken at least 2 weeks before travel	• One capsule is taken on alternate days (3 capsules). The last dose should be taken at least 1 week before travel
Booster	• Every 2 years for people who remain at risk	• Every 5 years for people who remain at risk
Duration of immunity	• 2 years	• 4 years

3. Define PUO. Compare and contrast the types of PUO/FUO according to "Durack and Street Classification" (1 + 3 marks)

Pyrexia of Unknown Origin Definition

- Pyrexia of unknown origin (PUO) is a state of febrile illness for more than three weeks, with a body temperature greater than 38.3°C on several occasions' minimum diagnostic evaluation of three outpatient visits or three days of in-hospital investigation.

Types of PUO/FUO

1. Classical FUO
2. Nosocomial FUO
3. Immune deficient/neutropenic FUO
4. HIV-associated FUO

Category of FUO	Definition	Common aetiologies
Classic	• Temperature >38.3°C (100.9°F) • Duration of >3 weeks • Evaluation of at least 3 outpatient visits or 3 days in hospital	• Infection • Malignancy • Collagen vascular disease
Nosocomial	• Temperature >38.3°C • Patient hospitalised ≥24 hours but no fever or incubating on admission • Evaluation of at least 3 days	• *Clostridium difficile* • Enterocolitis • Drug-induced • Pulmonary embolism • Septic thrombophlebitis • Sinusitis
Immune deficient (Neutropenic)	• Temperature >38.3°C • Neutrophil count ≤500 per mm³ • Evaluation of at least 3 days	• Opportunistic bacterial infections • Aspergillosis • Candidiasis • Herpes virus
• HIV-associated	• Temperature >38.3°C • Duration of >4 weeks for outpatients, >3 days for inpatients • HIV infection confirmed	• Cytomegalovirus • *Mycobacterium avium-intracellulare* complex • *Pneumocystis carinii* pneumonia • Drug-induced • Kaposi's sarcoma • Lymphoma

Contd.

4. Discuss the principle, procedure, significance and limitations of Widal test. (5 marks)

Widal Test

- Detect antibodies against enteric fever group of organisms (*S. typhi 'O', S. typhi 'H,' S. paratyphi A 'H', S. paratyphi B 'H)'* in patient's serum.

Principle

- Tube agglutination test.
  - Patients serum contains specific antibodies which agglutinate antigens of enteric fever group of organisms at 37°C in 18 hours.

Procedure

- Antigens used.
  - Four antigens are used.

1. antigens of *S. typhi (TO)*
2. H antigens of *S. typhi (TH)*
3. H antigens of *S. paratyphi A (AH)*
4. H antigens of *S. paratyphi B (BH)*

- Patient 's serum (serially diluted 1 in 20 to 1 in 640) is mixed with antigen suspensions.
- If the patients serum contains antibodies, there will be agglutination, when incubated at 37°C for 18 hours.
- Observation.
  - *O agglutination:* Compact and granular deposit with top clearing if positive.
  - *H agglutination:* Loose and floccular deposit with top clearing if positive.
- **O antibody:** Appears and disappears early—recent infection
- **H antibody:** Appears and disappears late (convalescent stage)

Significance

- Interpretation of the titre depends on the endemic or baseline titre.
- Four-fold rise in the titre is significant.
- **Significant titre:** O antibody >1 in 100, H antibody >1 in 200

Limitations

False Positives

1. Immunisation
2. Previously infected
3. Anamnestic response

False Negatives

1. Negative in upto 30% of culture proven cases of typhoid fever due to prior antibiotic therapy
2. Early stage (1st week).
3. Late stage (2nd week).
4. Relapses of typhoid fever
5. Carriers
6. Prozone

SHORT ANSWERS

1. Define (3 marks)

A. Clot culture and advantages
B. Anamnestic response
C. Baseline titre and its significance

A. Clot Culture

- Modification of a blood culture, where the blood is allowed to clot, and the clot is added to the blood culture broth with streptokinase (for lysis of the clot).

Advantages

1. Higher rate of isolation of the pathogen compared to blood culture (no bactericidal effect from serum).
2. Serum can also be collected and investigated for serological tests.

B. Anamnestic Response

- Transient rise of H antibody titre to *Salmonella Typhi, Salmonella Paratyphi* due to unrelated infections (malaria, dengue) in persons who have had prior enteric fever.
- Differentiated from true infection by lack of any rise in titre on repetition of test after a week.

C. Baseline Titre

- The antibody titre of O and H agglutinins to Salmonella group in the healthy population in endemic area.
- The titre is attributed to past exposure, TAB vaccination and cross-reacting antigens.
- Varies widely from place to place.
- Interpretation of Widal test depends on the baseline titre of that area.

2. Discuss in brief about MDR Salmonella (3 marks)

Multidrug-Resistant Typhoid Fever (MDRTF)

Definition

- Defined as typhoid fever caused by *Salmonella enterica* serovar typhi strains (*S. typhi*), which are resistant to the first-line recommended drugs for treatment such as chloramphenicol, ampicillin and Trimethoprim-sulfamethoxazole.

Mechanisms of Antibiotic Resistance in S. typhi

- Inactivation of drug, alteration of the target site, and active efflux.
- Chromosomal or plasmid mediated.

Treatment

- Ciprofloxacin, Azithromycin and ceftriaxone are the drugs most commonly used for treatment of MDRTF.

MI 3.4 IDENTIFY THE DIFFERENT MODALITIES OF DIAGNOSIS OF ENTERIC FEVER. CHOOSE THE APPROPRIATE TEST RELATED TO DURATION OF ILLNESS

LONG ESSAY

1. A 58-year-old male admitted with history of fever for 10 days. Blood sample is negative for malarial parasite. Widal test is ordered to diagnose enteric fever.

A. What is the significance of the test? (1 mark)

- **Diagnosis of Enteric fever:** High titre of O and H agglutinins or 4-fold rise in the antibody titre is diagnostic of enteric fever

B. What is the appropriate duration for performing this test? (1 mark)

- Second and third week of fever.

C. Describe in brief about the procedure of the test. (3 marks)

Requirements

1. Test tubes
2. Antigen suspensions
   - *S. typhi* 'O' antigen suspension.
   - *S. typhi* 'H' antigen suspension.

- *S. paratyphi* A 'AH' antigen suspension.
- S. paratyphi B "BH" Antigen suspension.
- H antigen is type specific; O antigen is group specific.

Method

- 1st row with patient's diluted serum *S. typhi* 'O' antigen is incubated.
- 2nd row with patient's diluted serum *S. typhi* 'H' antigen is incubated.
- 3rd row with patient's diluted serum *S. paratyphi* A 'AH' antigen is incubated.
- Tubes incubated at 37°C for 18 hours in water bath.
- *Patient's serum double diluted:* 1 in 20–1 in 320.

Observation

- O agglutination—compact and granular deposit with top clearing if positive.
- H agglutination—loose and floccular deposit with top clearing if positive.
- Titre is highest dilution which produces agglutination.

D. Write about the interpretation of the test. (4 marks)

STO	STH	SPAH	SPBH	Interpretation
+	—	—	—	Enteric fever
+	+	—	—	Typhoid fever
—	+	—	—	Typhoid fever
+	—	+	—	Paratyphoid (A) fever
—	—	+	—	Paratyphoid (A) fever
—	+	+	—	TA vaccination
+	+	+	—	Recent TA vaccination
—	—	—	+	*Salmonella* group B infection
—	+	+	+	Anamnestic reaction

Titre	Comment
+80 for any one antigen only	Could be due to enteric fever (typhoid or paratyphoid)
+80 for both STO and any one H	Suggestive of enteric fever (typhoid or paratyphoid)
+160 for any one antigen only	Suggestive of enteric fever (typhoid or paratyphoid)
+160 for both STO and any one H	Diagnostic of enteric fever (typhoid or paratyphoid)
+320 for any one antigen only	Diagnostic of enteric fever (typhoid or paratyphoid)

E. Define "Anamnestic Response". (1 mark)

- Transient rise of titre due to unrelated infections (malaria, dengue) in persons who have had prior enteric fever.

SHORT ESSAY

1. A young adult female doctor admitted in the hospital with severe headache, abdominal pain, vomiting for the last 5 days. She consumed food from a nearby restaurant the previous week. Fever is of remittent type and rises gradually. On examination, she had a temperature of 101°F and mild splenomegaly. Blood culture is positive with the growth of non-lactose fermenting bacilli, which are motile. Answer the following questions related to the case discussed above.

A. What is the most probable diagnosis? (1 mark)

- Enteric fever.

B. Differential diagnosis for the above condition. (2 marks)

1. Dengue fever
2. Malaria
3. Amebiasis
4. Leptospirosis
5. Giardiasis
6. Bacterial gastroenteritis
7. Rickettsial infection
8. Toxoplasmosis
9. Tuberculosis
10. Brucellosis

C. Specimen collection for the above condition. (2 marks)

- *Specimen sources:* Blood for culture and serology, stool, urine
- Specimen collection depends on stage of disease:
  - *1st week:* Blood culture, bone marrow aspirate, duodenal aspirate
  - *2nd week:* Serology, blood culture, stool culture, urine culture
  - *3rd week:* Serology, stool culture, urine culture, blood culture.
- *Other specimens:* Bile, biopsy of rose spots.

D. Mention the appropriate test in the first 5 days of illness. (1 mark)

- Culture of blood, bone marrow aspirate, duodenal aspirate.

MI 3.5 ENUMERATE THE CAUSATIVE AGENTS OF FOOD POISONING AND DISCUSS THE PATHOGENESIS, CLINICAL COURSE AND LABORATORY DIAGNOSIS

LONG ESSAY

1. A 30-year-old bachelor attended a night party with his friends. 18 hours later he had severe diarrhoea, nausea and vomiting. Patient was taken to a nearby hospital and treatment initiated. Patient revealed that he consumed some poultry food and egg salads in the party.

A. What could be the most probable diagnosis of the above case and enumerate the causative agents of the above case and mention the incubation period. (3 marks)

Most Probable Diagnosis

- Food poisoning due to non-typhoidal *Salmonella*.

Causative Agents

- Nontyphoidal *Salmonella: S. enterica* subspecies *enterica* serotypes—*S. enteritidis, S. typhimurium, S. newport, S. Heidelberg, and S. javiana*

Incubation Period

- 12–36 hours.

B. Discuss in detail about the effects of key virulence factors in the pathogenesis. (4 marks)

- *Transmission:* Food contaminated with animal products—seafood, eggs, poultry, meat, dairy, vegetables, salads
- *Prevalence:* Developed as well as developing nations
- *Outbreaks:* Common in hospitals.

Pathogenesis

- **Interaction of *Salmonellae* with enteric host defense.**
  - Ability to adapt to low pH
  - Compete with the normal intestinal microbial flora.
  - Must withstand bile salts, pancreatic enzymes, Paneth cell antimicrobial peptides and secretory IgA
- **Mechanisms of adherence and invasion**
  - *Adherence:* Fimbriae, biofilms
  - Invasion of the M cells, columnar epithelium. Non-phagocytic cells such as enterocytes internalize *Salmonella* by bacterial-mediated endocytosis
  - Bacteria remain within a modified phagosome: *Salmonella*-containing vacuole (SCV), within which they survive and replicate.
- **Pathogenicity islands:** SPI-1 and 2,.
  - Type III secretion systems creates a hypodermic needle-like apparatus and injects proteins into the cells, facilitating uptake of the bacteria into those cells.
  - SPI-1 encodes genes needed for nonphagocytic cell invasion
  - SPI-2 contains genes needed for survival and replication within macrophages
- **Inflammatory response mechanisms:** *Salmonella* induces migration of subepithelial neutrophils across polarised epithelial cells: *Salmonella typhimurium*-induced colitis in humans
- **Survival within phagocytes:** Contributes to the dissemination of the microorganism from the submucosa to the circulation and the reticulo-endothelial system.

C. Enumerate the bacteria causing food poisoning and the food sources. (3 marks)

Causes of food poisoning	*Food sources*
Staphylococcus aureus	• Potato/egg salad, poultry,mayonnaise, ham, cream pastries
Bacillus cereus	• Fried rice
Clostridium perfringens	• Beef, poultry, legumes, gravies
Clostridium botulinum	• Canned or bottled meat, vegetables, and fish
Vibrio parahaemolyticus	• Uncooked or undercooked crabs, prawns, shrimps and other seafoods
Non-typhoidal Salmonella	• Beef, poultry, eggs, dairy products, raw milk

SHORT ESSAYS

1. Enumerate the causative agents of watery diarrhoea, bloody diarrhoea (5 marks)

- *See* Table 3.5.1.

2. A 28-year-old with c/o double vision, paralysis of upper limbs came to the ED. The patient attenders gave a h/o consumption of sausage burger the previous day.

A. What is the most probable diagnosis and the causative agent? (1 mark)

Most Probable Diagnosis

- Food botulism.

Table 3.5.1 Mechanism and causative agents of diarrhoea

Mechanism	*Location*	*Illness*	*Stool M/E*	*Examples*
Non-inflammatory (enterotoxin)	Proximal small intestine	Watery diarrhoea	No faeco-leukocytes	• *Vibrio cholerae* • ETEC • EAggEC • *Clostridium perfringens* • *Bacillus cereus* • *Staphylococcus aureus* • Rotavirus • Norovirus • Enteric adenoviruses • *Giardia lamblia* • *Cryptosporidium* spp. • *Cyclospora* spp. • *Microsporidia* spp.
Inflammatory (invasion/cytotoxin)	Colon/distal small intestine	Dysentery/ inflammatory diarrhoea	PMN faecal leukocytes	• *Shigella* spp. • *Salmonella* spp. • *C. jejuni* • EHEC • *Yersinia enterocolitica* • *Vibrio parahaemolyticus* • *Clostridium difficile* • *Entamoeba histolytica*
Penetrating	Distal small intestine	Enteric fever	Mono-nuclear faecal leukocytes	• *Salmonella typhi* • *Y. enterocolitica* • *Campylobacter fetus*

Causative Agent

- *Clostridium botulinum* serotypes A, B, E.

B. Mechanism of action of the virulent toxin responsible and the clinical presentation of this condition. (2 marks)

Mechanism of Action of the Virulent Toxin

- Ingestion of preformed neurotoxin.
- *Source:* Improperly home-canned vegetables or fermented fish
- Prevents the release of the neurotransmitter acetylcholine from axon endings at the neuromuscular junction by binding to the Ach receptors, thus causing flaccid paralysis.

Clinical Features

- Gastrointestinal signs (i.e. nausea, vomiting, diarrhoea), followed acutely by neurological signs, such as bilateral cranial nerve deficits
- Diplopia, dysphasia, dysarthria
- Descending symmetric flaccid paralysis of voluntary muscles.
- Decreased deep tendon reflexes.
- Respiratory muscle paralysis, may lead to death.

C. Write a brief note on laboratory methods for diagnosis. (2 marks)

- Food is inoculated in Robertson cooked meat medium and blood agar or egg-yolk agar.
- The toxin can be demonstrated by injecting intraperitoneally the extract of food or culture into mice or guinea pig.

---

3. A 25-year-old software engineer after her hectic duty consumed fried rice from a nearby Chinese restaurant. After 10 hours she started suffering with abdominal pain, vomiting. Her friends take her to a nearby clinic. Answer the following questions.

A. What could be the probable causative agent for this condition? (1 mark)

- Food poisoning by *Bacillus cereus*.

B. What are the selective media used for the isolation of the causative agent. (1 mark)

1. MYPA (mannitol, egg yolk, polymyxin, phenol red and agar).
2. PEMBA (polymyxin B, egg yolk, mannitol, bromothymol blue, agar).

C. Clinical manifestations of food poisoning due to the above organism. (2 marks)

- Two types of gastrointestinal illness.

1. Emetic Syndrome

- Food contaminated with the emetic toxin.
- Associated with starchy food such as pasta or rice dishes.
- Clinical features:
  - Vomiting, nausea sometimes diarrhoea
  - *IP* : 0.5–5 hours after ingestion of contaminated food
  - Symptoms disappear in 6–24 hours

2. Diarrhoeal Syndrome

- Bacilli produce enterotoxin in the small intestine.
- Meat products, stews, soups, sauces, vegetables and milk products.
- Clinical features.
  - Diarrhoea, sometimes with blood and/or mucus
  - Nausea
  - Abdominal pain
  - Symptoms usually start 8–16 hours after ingestion of contaminated food
  - Symptoms disappear in 12–24 hours

D. Available antibiotics with activity against *Bacillus cereus* (1 mark)

- Clindamycin, vancomycin, gentamicin, chloramphenicol, and erythromycin.

---

4. A 30-year-old young businessman hailing from Delhi went to Mexico on a company trip. During a company gathering at Mexico, he consumed some sea food which included raw oysters, edible fish. After 12 hours he suffered from nausea, abdominal cramps, and mild fever. He passed stool with blood and mucus. Answer the following questions related to the case.

A. Define Gastroenteritis. (1 mark)

- Acute infectious syndrome of the stomach lining and the intestine
- Characterised by diarrhoea, vomiting, and abdominal cramps
- Other symptoms can include nausea, fever, and chills

B. Which strain of *Vibrio* causes food poisoning due to oyster consumption. (1 mark)

- *Vibrio parahaemolyticus.*

C. Clinical manifestations of food poisoning in the above case. (2 marks)

- Infections by eating raw or undercooked shellfish, particularly oysters
- Symptoms start within 24 hours
- Watery diarrhoea
- Abdominal cramps
- Nausea
- Vomiting
- Fever
- Headache

D. Available drug therapy for the above condition. (1 mark)

- Prompt rehydration
- Antibiotics such as tetracycline, ampicillin or ciprofloxacin can be used in severe cases.

---

5. Classify food poisoning based on the incubation period, symptoms, and pathogenesis. (5 marks)

A. Based on Symptoms and Duration of Onset

• Nausea and vomiting within six hours	• *Staphylococcus aureus* • *Bacillus cereus*
• Abdominal cramps and diarrhoea within 8–16 hours	• *Clostridium perfringens* • *Bacillus cereus*
• Fever, abdominal cramps, and diarrhoea within 16–48 hours	• *Salmonella* spp. • *Shigella* spp. • *Vibrio parahaemolyticus* • *Enteroinvasive E. coli* • *Campylobacter jejuni*
• Fever and abdominal cramps within 16–48 hours	• *Yersinia enterocolitica*
• Bloody diarrhoea without fever within 72–120 hours	• *Enterohaemorrhagic E.coli O157:H7*
• Nausea, vomiting, diarrhoea and paralysis within 18–36 hours	• *Clostridium botulinum*

B. Based on Pathogenesis

Ingestion of preformed bacterial toxins	• *Staphylococcus aureus* • *Bacillus cereus* • *Clostridium botulinum* • *Clostridium perfringens*
Non-invasive bacteria that secrete toxins while adhering to the intestinal wall	• *Enterotoxigenic E. coli* • *Vibrio cholerae* • *Campylobacter jejuni*
Intracellular invasion of the intestinal epithelial cells	• *Shigella spp.* • *Salmonella spp.*
Diseases caused by bacteria that enter the bloodstream via the intestinal tract	• *Salmonella typhi* • *Listeria monocytogenes*

SHORT ANSWERS

1. Enumerate bacteria causing food poisoning due to:

A. Canned food

B. Poultry, raw eggs

C. Molluscs, crustaceans (1+1+1 marks)

A. **Canned food:** *Clostridium botulinum*

B. **Poultry, raw eggs:** *Non-typhoidal Salmonella, Staphylococcus aureus*

C. **Molluscs, crustaceans:** *Vibrio parahaemolyticus.*

2. Mention.

A. The sources for food poisoning due to Enterotoxin of *S. aureus*. (1 mark)

- Ham, poultry, potato/egg salad, mayonnaise, cream pastries, milk products.

B. Incubation period. (1 mark)

- 1–6 hours.

C. Pathogenesis of Staphylococcal food poisoning. (2 marks)

- **Enterotoxin :** Superantigen → massive release of IL-2 and TNF-alpha, which induces diarrhoea. The toxin acts on the receptors in the gut and sensory stimulus is carried to the vomiting center in the brain by vagus and sympathetic nerves.

D. Two major clinical manifestations. (1 mark)

1. Sudden onset of nausea, vomiting, stomach cramps, diarrhoea.
2. Develop within 30 minutes to 8 hours after eating or drinking an item containing toxin, and last no longer than 1 day. Severe illness is rare.

3. Compare and contrast non-inflammatory and inflammatory diarrhoea due to food poisoning. (3 marks)

- *See* Table 3.5.2.

4. Mention the food sources for diarrhoea and dysentery due to:

A. ETEC. (1 mark)

- Raw fruits and vegetables (e.g., salads), raw seafood or undercooked meat or poultry, unpasteurised dairy products, food from street vendors, and untreated water.

B. *Shigella* species. (1 mark)

- Salads (potato, tuna, shrimp, macaroni, and chicken), raw vegetables, milk and dairy products, and poultry.

C. *Clostridium perfringens*. (1 mark)

- Meat, poultry, gravies, and other foods cooked in large batches and held at an unsafe temperature.

Table 3.5.2 Differentiating features of non-inflammatory and inflammatory diarrhoea due to food poisoning.

Mechanism	*Location*	*Illness*	*Stool M/E*	*Examples*
Non-inflammatory (enterotoxin)	• Proximal small intestine	• Watery diarrhoea	• No faecal leukocytes	• *Vibrio cholerae* • ETEC • EAggEC • *Clostridium perfringens* • *Bacillus cereus* • *Staphylococcus aureus* • Rotavirus • Norovirus • Enteric adenoviruses • *Giardia lamblia* • Cryptosporidium spp. • Cyclospora spp. • Microsporidia spp.
Inflammatory (invasion/ cytotoxin)	• Colon/distal small intestine	• Dysentery/ inflammatory diarrhoea	• PMN faecal leukocytes	• *Shigella* spp. • *Salmonella* spp. • *Campylobacter jejuni* • EHEC • *Yersinia enterocolitica* • *Vibrio parahaemolyticus* • *Clostridium difficile* • *Entamoeba histolytica*

MI 3.6 DESCRIBE THE AETIOPATHOGENESIS OF ACID PEPTIC DISEASE AND THE CLINICAL COURSE. DISCUSS THE DIAGNOSIS AND MANAGEMENT OF THE CAUSATIVE AGENT OF APD

LONG ESSAY

1. Discuss in detail about acid peptic disease (APD) under the following headings.

A. Morphology and virulence factors of the causative agent. (3 marks)

Causative Agent

- *Helicobacter pylori.*

Morphology

- Gram-negative, S-shaped or curved rod, six polar flagella.
- Actively motile in hanging drop preparations.
- spherical, V or U shaped (ox-bow) and straightened forms in culture or in vivo.

Virulence Factors

1. **Colonisation**
   - Adhesins, flagella.
2. **Immune escape**
   - LPS (molecular mimicry, anti-inflammatory).
   - CagA Type 4 secretion system, Vac A (anti-phagocytic blocks T cell response).
3. **Disease induction**
   - CagA Type 4 secretion system, Vac A (gastric carcinoma, peptic ulcer disease).

B. Risk factors associated and pathogenesis of APD. (1+3 marks)

Risk Factors

1. ***H. pylori* infection.**
2. **Medicines**
   i. Nonsteroidal anti-inflammatory medications (NSAIDs)
   ii. Oral corticosteroids
   iii. Potassium chloride
   iv. Chemotherapy drugs used to treat cancer
3. **Health problems**
   i. Cytomegalovirus infection
   ii. Crohn disease
4. **Other factors**
   i. Smoking
   ii. Drinking alcohol
   iii. Type O blood.
   iv. Having other family members with peptic ulcer disease.

Pathogenesis (Fig. 3.6.1)

- Acid peptic disease includes gastric ulcers, duodenal ulcers, and gastroesophageal reflux disease The pathogenesis of these disorders involves an imbalance between acid secretion and gastric mucosal defences.

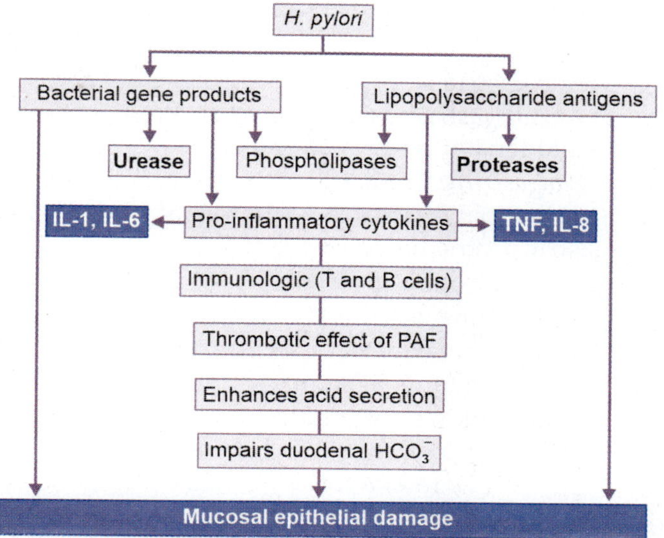

Fig. 3.6.1: Pathogenesis of acid peptic disease

C. Different types of diagnostic tests available in the diagnosis of APD. (3 marks)

Diagnostic Tests Available

I. **Non-invasive tests**
   1. Urea breath tests
   2. Stool monoclonal antigen tests: ELISA, ICT
   3. Antibody testing

II. **Invasive tests**
   1. Endoscopy with biopsy
   2. Rapid urease test

Culture

- *Specimen collection:* Gastric biopsy, duodenal biopsy
- Microscopy reveals curved gram-negative rods resembling *Helicobacter* in 60–100% of the culture-positive biopsies.
- Culture media.
  - Skirrow's media (selective media)
  - Chocolate agar
  - Incubated at 37°C under microaerophilic condition (5% O_2, 10% CO_2 and 85% nitrogen).

Importance of Serological Tests

Stool Antigen (Coproantigen) Assay

- Used to monitor treatment response
- Useful for screening of children

Antibody (IgG) Detection by ELISA

- Screening before endoscopy, sero epidemiological study.

SHORT ESSAY

1. Discuss in brief about the clinical manifestations of acid peptic disease caused by *H. pylori*. (4 marks)

1. Acute gastritis
   - *Antral gastritis (most common):* Predisposes to duodenal ulcers
   - *Pangastritis:* Predisposes to adenocarcinoma
2. *Peptic ulcer disease:* 80% duodenal and 60% of gastric ulcers due to *H. pylori*.
3. Chronic atrophic gastritis
4. Autoimmune gastritis
5. Pernicious anaemia
6. Adenocarcinoma of stomach
7. Non-Hodgkin's gastric lymphoma (Fig. 3.6.2).

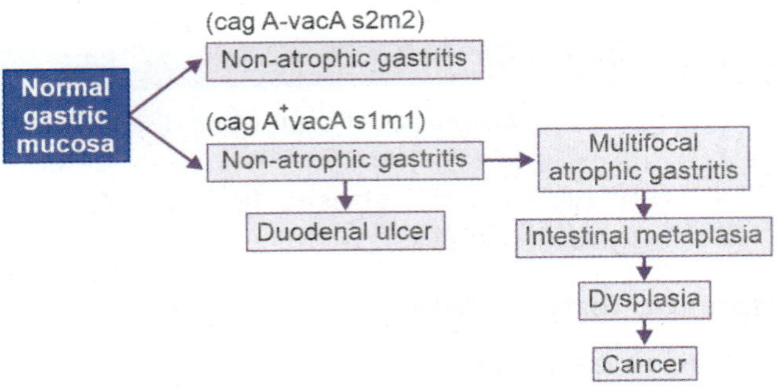

Fig. 3.6.2: Clinical manifestations of *H. pylori*

SHORT ANSWER

1. Discuss in brief about the recommended treatment guidelines for *H. pylori* infection. (3 marks)

Recommended Treatment Guidelines for *H. pylori* Infection

First Line: Triple Therapy

Clarithromycin triple	• PPI (Omeprazole) (standard or double dose) with Clarithromycin (500 mg) and • Amoxicillin (1 g) or Metronidazole (500 mg TID)	BID	14 days

- Urea breath test is done after one month of therapy and if the first line fails → second line quadruple therapy.

Second Line: Quadruple Therapy

Bismuth quadruple	• PPI (standard dose) • Bismuth subcitrate (120–300 mg) or subsalicylate (300 mg) • Tetracycline (500 mg) • Metronidazole (250–500 mg)	• BID • QID • QID • QID (250) • TID to QID (500)	• 10–14 days

MI 3.7 DESCRIBE THE EPIDEMIOLOGY, AETIOPATHOGENESIS AND DISCUSS THE VIRAL MARKERS IN THE EVOLUTION OF VIRAL HEPATITIS. DISCUSS THE MODALITIES IN THE DIAGNOSIS AND PREVENTION OF VIRAL HEPATITIS

LONG ESSAYS

1. A 30-year-old male presented with history of anorexia, weakness, icterus for the last 6 weeks. He consulted a Gastroenterologist and on examination mild liver enlargement with tenderness in the right hypochondrium is elicited. On complete evaluation, patient gave the history of sharing of needles, drug injection during his postgraduate period in the college. Serological reports revealed that he is reactive for HBsAg. Treatment initiated and patient is under observation.

A. List the viruses causing hepatitis. (2 marks)

Common Viruses

1. Hepatitis A virus
2. Hepatitis B virus
3. Hepatitis C virus
4. Hepatitis D virus
5. Hepatitis E virus

Infrequent Viruses

1. Epstein–Barr virus
2. Herpes simplex
3. Cytomegalovirus
4. Yellow fever

B. Modes of transmission, pathogenesis, clinical manifestations of HBV infection. (3 marks)

Modes of Transmission

1. *Parenteral:* Needle stick injury, transfusion.
2. Sexual
3. *Perinatal:* Mother to child
   i. During delivery
   ii. Transplacental: Rare
   iii. No evidence that transmission occurs during breastfeeding.

Pathogenesis

- *Reservoir:* Humans only
- *Source of infection:* Infected persons, carriers, infected blood and blood products/other body fluids

- *High risk group:* IV Drug abusers, healthcare personnel, repeated blood transfusion patients, homosexuals, newborns of HBV infected mothers
- *Incubation period:* 45–90 days
- *Sequence of events.*

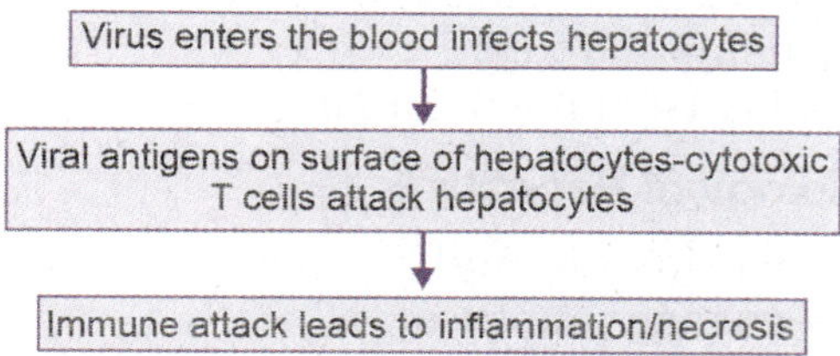

Clinical Features

Acute Infection

- *Incubation period:* 10–12 weeks
- Prodromal or preicteric phase.
  - Insidious
  - 1–2 weeks
  - Malaise, low grade fever, fatigue, myalgia, anorexia, nausea, vomiting
  - Appearance of dark urine, pale faeces, elevated transaminases, jaundice
  - Lasts for 1 month
  - Usually subsides
  - Some may develop extrahepatic manifestations like serum sickness, acute necrotising vasculitis, membranous glomerulonephritis.

Fulminant Hepatitis

- Rare.
- Seen in 0.1–0.5%.
- Rapidly progressive acute hepatitis within 28 days with liver failure (coagulopathy, enteropathy)
- *HBsAg:* Negative because of early clearance, but shows IgM anti HBc, + HBV DNA
- Due to massive immune response.

Chronic Hepatitis

- At least 6 months of persistent HBV
- 90% of infected neonates, 5% of infected adults.

C. Serological and molecular assays for the diagnosis of HBV infection. (5 marks)

Serological Assays

1. **HBsAg:** Hepatitis B surface antigen.
   - Represents the surface component of the Dane particle and also the spherical and filamentous forms.
   - *Appears:* 1 month after exposure
   - 1st serological marker to appear.
   - Detectable in the incubation period, prodrome and acute phase.
   - *Disappears:* In uncomplicated cases: Within 3–6 months-in convalescence
   - In chronic carriers, persists beyond 6 months.
   - *Significance:* Acute infection/Chronic Carrier state
2. **AntiHBs:** Antibody against HBsAg
   - Only neutralising antibody.
   - Produced in response to infection and vaccination
   - *Appears:* By about 6 months after exposure i.e. After the disappearance of HBsAg
   - *Disappears:* Once present, persists for years providing lifelong immunity
   - *Significance:* Indicates recovery from infection/vaccination
3. **AntiHBc:** Antibody against HBcAg
   - Not a neutralising antibody
   - IgM AntiHBc
     - *Appears:* At the onset of Acute illness—2–3 months after exposure
     - Detectable in prodrome and acute phase.
     - *Disappears:* At 6 months.
   - IgG AntiHBc.
     - *Appears* after IgM AntiHBc disappears—6 months.
     - Detectable in early convalescence and chronic carrier state.
     - *Persists* for years
   - *Significance*
     - Only marker present and detected during Core window/window phase (When HBsAg has disappeared and antiHBs has not yet appeared)
     - IgM AntiHBc indicates acute infection
     - IgG AntiHBc indicates chronic infection/past infection
4. **HBeAg**
   - Soluble form of the core antigen.
   - Detectable during incubation period, prodrome and acute illness.
   - *Disappearance.*
     - In uncomplicated cases: Within 6 months
     - In chronic carriers: May persist longer
   - *Significance:* Indicates high likelihood of transmissibility, marker for infectivity
5. **AntiHBe:** Antibody formed against HbeAg
   - Not a neutralising antibody.
   - *Appears:* After HBeAg disappears—Persists for years
   - *Significance:* Indicates low infectivity

Assay Results			Interpretation
HBsAg	Anti HBs	Anti HBc	
+ +	–	–	• Incubation period or very early infection
+ +	–	+ +	• Acute Infection or chronic infection (IgM or IgG) • Recommend HBeAg or HBV DNA to check infectivity
–	+ +	+ +	• Past infection, recovery
–	–	+ +	• Core window
–	–	–	• Never infected with HBV • Rule out other causes
–	+ +	—	• Vaccinated

Molecular Assays

- *Detection of HBV DNA:* PCR
- HBV-DNA is an indicator of active replication of virus.
- More accurate than HBeAg in cases of escape mutants.
- Used for monitoring response to therapy.

2. Write in detail about hepatitis panel of viruses causing jaundice in humans transmitted faeco-orally under the following headings.

A. Morphology of the viruses transmitted faeco-orally as mentioned in the question given above. (2 marks)

Morphology

Hepatitis A virus	• *Family:* Picorna viridae • *Genus:* Hepatovirus • Naked ssRNA virus • Icosahedral • One serotype • Replicates in cytoplasm
Hepatitis E virus	• *Family:* Hepeviridae • *Genus:* Hepevirus • Small non-enveloped • Single-stranded RNA • Icosahedral • Capsid consists of one single protein

B. Epidemiology, pathogenesis, clinical features. (5 marks)

Epidemiology of Hepatitis A

- *Reservoirs:* Humans: Infected food handlers
- *Risk of infection:* Close contacts, infected food handlers
- *Greatest period of communicability:* 2 weeks before onset of jaundice to 2 weeks after the appearance of jaundice
- Virus is stable in environment for months.
- *Age:*
  - Children and adolescents (5–14 years of age) are most affected, subclinical infection.
  - Adults icteric (75–90%).
- Outbreaks are common in summer camps, day care centers, families and institutions, neonatal ICUs, and among military troops.
- Seasonality late rainfall and in early winter.

Epidemiology of Hepatitis E

- Found worldwide and is common in low- and middle-income countries.
- Occurs as outbreaks and as sporadic cases.
- Outbreaks usually follow periods of faecal contamination of drinking water supplies and may affect several people especially in camps.
- Sporadic cases are reported in areas with better sanitation and water supply. Sporadic cases are caused by genotype 3 virus, originating in animals. Mode is through ingestion of undercooked animal meat (including animal liver, particularly pork).

Pathogenesis

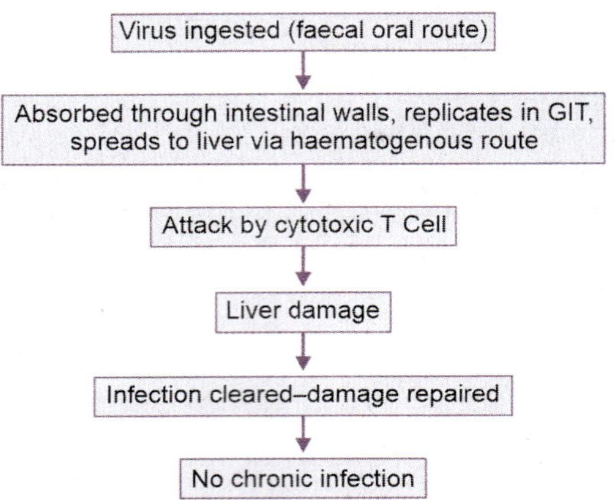

Clinical Features of Hepatitis A

- *Incubation period:* 3–4 weeks
- Mild fever, anorexia, nausea, vomiting, jaundice
- Dark coloured urine, pale faeces
- Resolve in 10–12 weeks
- <1% fulminant hepatitis
- No chronic infection.

Clinical Features of Hepatitis E

- Incubation period is about 14–60 days (average 40 days).
- Most of the patients present as self-limiting acute hepatitis lasting for several weeks followed by complete recovery.
- Fulminant hepatitis may occur rarely in 1–2% of cases.
- *Pregnant women* who are particularly at higher risk (20%) of developing fulminant hepatitis.
- There is no chronic infection or carrier state.

C. Laboratory diagnosis and prophylaxis. (3 marks)

Laboratory Diagnosis

- The methods include:
  - *Detection of antibody IgM (acute infection) and IgG (past infection):* By ELISA: Most important.
  - *Demonstration of virus in faeces:* Immunoelectron microscopy—Rarely done.
  - *Molecular diagnosis:* RT PCR of faeces.

Prophylaxis

General Measures

- Proper handwashing
- Sanitary disposal of infected feces by disinfection with 0.5% hypochlorite
- Purification of drinking water by effective filtration and chlorination
- Use of boiled water.

Immunoprophylaxis

Hepatitis A

- *Active immunisation:* Inactivated HAV
  - 2 doses: 6–12 months apart
  - To children >1 year age.
  - Protection begins 4 weeks after injection; lasts 10–20 years.
  - Recommended for travelers to endemic countries, children 2–18 years.
- Live attenuated vaccine is given as single dose, subcutaneously.

Hepatitis E

- First HEV vaccine using recombinant proteins.

3. A 30-year-old man presented with complaints of pain in the right hypochondrium. Ultrasound abdomen revealed a cystic lesion with daughter cysts in right lobe of liver. The biopsy was sent for histopathology evaluation which revealed brood capsules attached to the cyst wall.

A. Identify the disease and the causative agent. (1 mark)

Disease is:

- Hydatid disease.

Causative Agent

- *Echinococcus granulosus.*

B. Life cycle of the aetiological agent and mode of transmission. (3 marks)

Life Cycle (Fig. 3.7.1)

- *Definitive host:* Dogs and other canine animals
- *Intermediate host:* Sheep and other herbivores
- Man acts as an accidental intermediate host (dead end).

Mode of Transmission

- Humans get infected by ingestion of food contaminated with dog faeces or while handling dogs or by contaminated water.

C. Discuss the clinical features of this condition. (4 marks)

- Hydatid cysts in liver (1st filter) in 60–70% of human infections, as hexacanth embryos after hatching out penetrates intestinal wall and enter radical of portal vein.
- Can occur in lungs (2nd filter) the embryo passes through hepatic capillaries and enter the pulmonary circulation.
- Few embryos may pass through pulmonary circulation too and enter various organs.
- Thus rarely, the cysts may be found in the brain. eye, kidney, muscles, bones, spleen, genital organs.

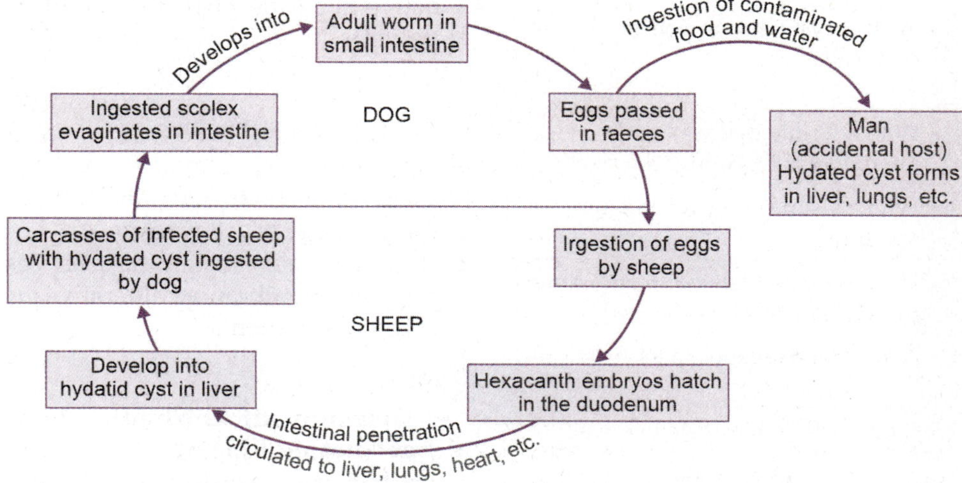

Fig. 3.7.1: Life cycle of *Echinococcus granulosus*

Clinical Features

- Mostly asymptomatic, discovered accidentally.
- Hepatic echinococcosis: abdominal pain or palpable mass in the right upper quadrant.
- Compression of a bile duct or leakage of cyst fluid into the biliary tree may mimic recurrent cholelithiasis, and biliary obstruction can result in jaundice.
- Pulmonary hydatid cysts may rupture into the bronchial tree or peritoneal cavity and produce cough, dyspnoea, chest pain, or haemoptysis.
- Rupture during surgery or episodic leakage from a hydatid cyst may produce fever, pruritus, urticaria, eosinophilia, or anaphylaxis or may lead to multifocal dissemination of protoscolices, which can form additional cysts.

D. Describe the various diagnostic modalities and therapy for this disease. (2+2 marks)

Diagnostic Modalities

1. Radiodiagnosis to study the cysts in lung, liver—X-ray, USG (water lily sign), CT scan, MRI.
2. Examination of aspirated fluid for protoscolices or hooklets—usually not recommended because of the risk of fluid leakage.
3. Antibody detection.
   i. Can be useful, although a negative test does not exclude the diagnosis of echinococcosis.
   ii. Sensitivity in hepatic cysts: 85–98%.
   iii. Can be carried out by ELISA, indirect IF, IHA (indirect haemagglutination).
4. *Antigen detection:* Double diffusion, CIEP, sera/CSF.
5. Others.
   i. *Blood:* Eosinophilia.
   ii. *Molecular diagnosis:* DNA probes, PCR.

Therapy

- Ultrasound staging

Active cysts include types of CL	• With a cystic lesion and no visible cyst wall
CE1	• With a visible cyst wall and internal echoes (Snowflake sign)
CE2	• With a visible cyst wall and internal septation
Transitional cysts (CE3)	• Have detached laminar membranes or may be partially collapsed
Inactive cysts include types CE4	• A nonhomogeneous mass
CE5	• A cyst with a thick calcified wall

- Small C1, CE1, and CE3 lesions may respond to chemotherapy with **albendazole**
- For CE1 lesions and uncomplicated CE3 lesions, PAIR (*puncture, a*spiration, *i*nfusion of scolicidal agents, and reaspiration) is now recommended instead of surgery.

SHORT ESSAYS

1. Mention various modes of transmission of NANB Serum hepatitis virus. Briefly discuss its pathogenesis, clinical features, diagnosis. (1+4 marks)

NANB Serum Hepatitis Virus

- Hepatitis C virus is a member of flavivirus family (NON-A NON-B).

Modes of Transmission

- Humans are reservoirs.
- Transmitted primarily by blood.
- Parenteral:
  i. Recipients of contaminated blood transfusions, blood products or organ transplantations.
  ii. Contaminated needles and sharps pricks.
  iii. Injection drug users.
- Sexual and vertical transmission is rare.

Pathogenesis

- Infects hepatocytes primarily. Death of the hepatocytes is due to immune attack by cytotoxic T cells.
- HCV infection strongly predisposes to hepatocellular carcinoma. Cancer is caused by prolonged liver damage, consequent rapid growth of hepatocytes as cells attempt to regenerate rather than the direct oncogenic effect of HCV.
- Antibodies against HCV are formed, but 75% are chronically infected and produce virus for at least 1 year.
- Rate of chronic carriage is high (75–80%), chronic active hepatitis, cirrhosis occurs in 10–20% of these patients.

Clinical Features

- Milder than HBV.
- Fever, anorexia, nausea, vomiting, jaundice, dark urine, pale faeces, elevated transaminases.
- *Incubation period:* 8 weeks
- *Also leads to autoimmune reactions:* Vasculitis, arthralgia, purpura, membranoproliferative glomerulonephritis, cryoglobulinaemia

Diagnosis

1. **Detection of antibodies to HCV Ag by 3rd generation ELISA.**
   - Increased sensitivity and specificity (>99%).
   - Can detect Abs within 6–8 weeks of exposure.

- Does not distinguish between IgM, IgG.
- False positive result—seen in with autoimmune diseases, mononucleosis, and pregnancy.
- False-negative result—seen in with immunosuppression such as HIV infection, transplant recipients, etc.

2. **HCV core antigen (HCV Ag) detection ELISA or CLIA based.**
   - *Advantages:* can be used as an alternative to HCV RNA testing for diagnosis of active infection and prognostic purpose
   - *Disadvantage:* Less sensitive than RT-PCR
3. **HCV RNA testing in plasma, serum by RTPCR.**
   - Detectable 2–14 days of exposure
   - Used to screen for infection in HCV EIA negative cases (HIV, dialysis)
   - Used to monitor treatment.

2. HBV and HDV are associated with co-infection. Distinguish between the co-infection and superinfection with respect to HBV and HDV. (5 marks)

Hepatitis Delta Virus (HDV)

- Transmitted sexually, by blood, perinatally.
- May be acquired as co-infection with HBV (infection with both the viruses simultaneously), or superinfection of HBV infection.
- Exacerbates HBV induced disease.

Consequences of Hepatitis Delta Virus Infection

- Delta virus (δ) requires the presence of hepatitis B virus (HBV) infection.
- Superinfection of a person already infected with HBV (carrier) causes more rapid, severe progression than coinfection.

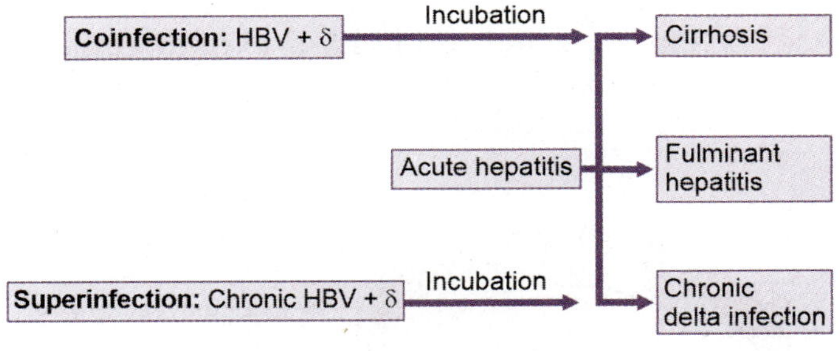

3. Discuss in brief the genomic diversity of HCV. Add a note on treatment module of HCV. (3+2 marks)

Genomic Diversity of HCV

- HCV has at least six genotypes and multiple subgenotypes based on differences in the genes that encode one of its two envelope glycoproteins.
- This genetic variation results in a "hypervariable" region in the envelope glycoprotein.
- The genetic variability is due to the high mutation rate in the envelope gene coupled with the absence of a proofreading function in the virion-encoded RNA polymerase.
- As a result, multiple subspecies (quasi species) often occur in the blood of an infected individual at the same time.

Treatment

- Treatment of acute hepatitis C with peg interferon alfa significantly decreases the carrier rate.
- *Chronic hepatitis C:* Combination of drugs from three classes
  1. RNA polymerase inhibitors.
  2. NS5A inhibitors.
  3. Protease inhibitors.
- Administered orally, which is an improvement over the drugs in previous regimens.
- *Preexposure prevention:* Blood found to have HCV Abs is discarded
- *Post-exposure prevention:* An individual with documented exposure should be screened for HCV Abs and ALT to exclude prior infection, repeated every 6 months later.

4. A 33-year-old man is admitted to the hospital because of jaundice. He is found to be reactive to HCV Antibodies. Briefly discuss the laboratory work-up of Hepatitis C. (4 marks)

Laboratory Work-up

1. **Serology:** Detection of antibody.
   - Enzyme immunoassays for detection of Hepatitis C Antibody.
   - Used for initial screening for hepatitis C.
   - Third generation EIAs have a sensitivity/specificity of approximately 99%.
   - The presence of HCV Ab does not indicate whether the infection is acute, chronic, or resolved. A positive antibody test result should be followed up with an HCV RNA test to confirm that viraemia is present.
   - *False-negative results:* window period, immunocompromised
   - *False-positive:* cross-reactivity with other viral antigens or the presence of immunologic disorders, such as lupus or rheumatoid arthritis
2. **HCV RNA Testing**
   - HCV RNA tests can detect virus within 1–2 weeks following exposure by real-time PCR.
   - Indications of HCV RNA testing.
     - To confirm a positive HCV Ab result and make the diagnosis of current HCV infection.
     - To measure a patient's baseline viral load prior to starting HCV therapy.
     - To monitor a patient's response to therapy.

5. Enumerate the medically important flukes affecting the liver. Discuss the life cycle, clinical features, and diagnosis of any 2 of them. (1+4 marks)

Medically Important Flukes Affecting the Liver

1. Liver flukes
2. Fasciola hepatica
3. Clonorchis sinensis

Feature	*Fasciola hepatica*	*Clonorchis sinensis*
Life cycle	• Humans are infected by eating watercress (or other aquatic plants) contaminated by larvae (metacercariae) that excyst in the duodenum, penetrate the gut wall, and reach the liver, where they mature into adults • Hermaphroditic adults in the bile ducts produce eggs, which are excreted in the faeces	• Humans are infected by eating raw or undercooked fish containing the encysted larvae (metacercariae) • After excystation in the duodenum, immature flukes enter the biliary ducts and differentiate into adults • The hermaphroditic adults produce eggs, which are excreted in the faeces
	• The eggs hatch in fresh water, and miracidia enter the snails	• Upon reaching fresh water, the eggs are ingested by snails, which are the first intermediate hosts
	• Miracidia develop into cercariae, which then encyst on aquatic vegetation • Sheep and humans eat the plants, thus completing the life cycle	• The eggs hatch within the gut and differentiate first into larvae (rediae) and then into many free-swimming cercariae • Cercariae encyst under the scales of certain freshwater fish (second intermediate hosts), which are then eaten by humans
Clinical Features	• Symptoms are due primarily to the presence of the adult worm in the biliary tract • In early infection, right-upper quadrant pain, fever, and hepatomegaly can occur, but most infections are asymptomatic • Months or years later, obstructive jaundice can occur	• Most infections are asymptomatic • In patients with a heavy worm burden, upper abdominal pain, anorexia, hepatomegaly, and eosinophilia can occur
Diagnosis	• Identification of eggs in the faeces	• Diagnosis is made by finding the typical small, brownish, operculated eggs in the stool

6. Describe the larval stage of *Echinococcus granulosus* with a neat, labelled diagram. (4 marks)

Hydatid Cyst (Fig 3.7.2)

- Represents the larval form of parasite, found in liver, viscera of man, herbivores.
- Measures from few mm—30 cm.
- It has 3 layers.
  1. **Endocyst.**
     - Inner or germinal layer.
     - Gives rise to brood capsule and scolices on inside and ectocyst on outside.
  2. **Ectocyst.**
     - Acellular chitinous, tough, laminated, hyaline membrane.
     - Elastic, when ruptured or excised curls on itself exposing inner layer containing brood capsules, scolices and daughter cyst.

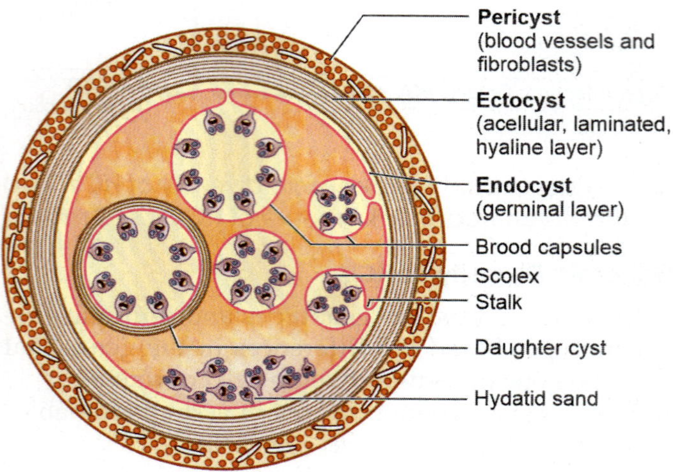

Fig. 3.7.2: Hydatid cyst

3. **Pericyst.**
   - Outer host inflammatory response, fibroblastic proliferation, mononuclear cells, eosinophils, giant cells developing into fibrous capsule which may calcify.
   - Ectocyst and endocyst are secreted by embryo.

- **Hydatid sand:** When embryo break free from the membrane and float in the fluid within the cyst, called hydatid sand.
- **Hydatid fluid.**
  - Clear, colourless, or pale yellow.
  - Acidic.
  - Contains sodium chloride, sodium phosphate, sodium, and calcium salts of succinic acid.
  - Antigenic so used for Casoni test.
  - Toxic, anaphylactic.

SHORT ANSWERS

1. Define.

A. Super Carriers. (1 mark)

B. Simple Carriers with respect to HBV. (1 mark)

A. Simple Carriers

- Low infectivity.
- Low level of HBsAg and no HBeAg.

B. Super Carriers

- Highly infectious and transmit the virus efficiently.
- Higher levels of HBsAg, HBeAg, DNA polymerase, and HBV DNA.

2. Discuss in brief the available immunoprophylaxis module for HBV. (3 marks)

Active Immunisation

- Recombinant vaccines.
  1. Engerix B (20 μg of HBsAg/ml).
  2. Recombivax HB (10 μg of HBsAg/ml).
- *Indication:* Persons exposed frequently to blood and body fluids (students, surgeons, lab workers), patients receiving multiple transfusions or dialysis, patients with STD or IV drug users
- *Dosages.*
  - *Adults:* 0, 1–2, 6–12 months, IM deltoid.
  - *Infants:* at 6, 10, 14 weeks (along with DPT vaccine) on anterolateral aspect of thigh.
- Booster dose for high risk every 5 years.
- Protective level AntiHBs >10 IU/ml.

Passive Immunisation

- HBIg 0.05–0.07 ml/kg
- 2 doses one month apart
- *Indications.*
  - Exposure to HBsAg positive blood, e.g., surgeons, nurses, laboratory workers.
  - Sexual contact of patient.
  - Neonates borne to hepatitis B carrier mothers.
  - HBIG should be started immediately (ideally within 6 hr, but not later than 48 hours).

Combined Immunisation

- With HB Ig, vaccine for all non-immune who have had percutaneous, sexual contact, mucous membrane exposure to blood.
- First dose 0.06 ml/kg HB Ig given within 72 hours along with first dose of vaccine at different site followed by remainder of series.
- After Needle stick injury from HBsAg positive person.
- Infants born to HBsAg positive mothers should have HB Ig within 12 hours of delivery with vaccine at different site.

3. Draw a neat, labelled diagram of structure of HBV and highlight the major serological markers playing a vital role in the diagnosis of HBV. (2 marks)

Structure of HBV (Fig. 3.7.3)

- *Dane particle:* An outer shell (envelope, HBsAg) and an inner body (core: HBcAg, HBeAg, HBV-DNA and DNA polymerase)

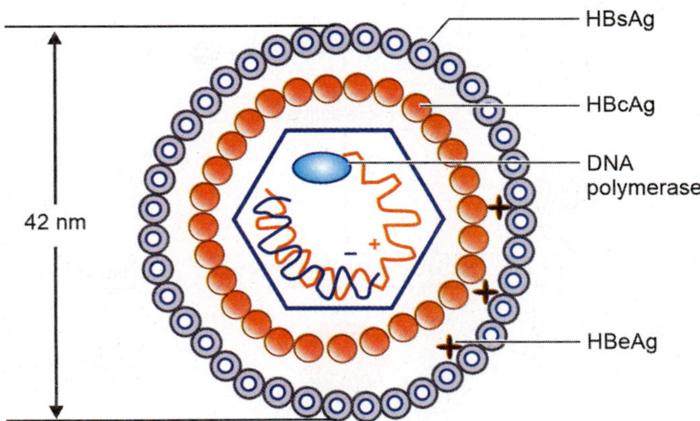

Fig. 3.7.3: Complete Dane particle: Hepatitis B virus

MI 3.8 CHOOSE THE APPROPRIATE LABORATORY TEST IN THE DIAGNOSIS OF VIRAL HEPATITIS WITH EMPHASIS ON VIRAL MARKERS

SHORT ESSAYS

1. Discuss in brief the role of molecular assays in the diagnosis of HBV (4 marks)

Types of Assays

1. Quantitative viral load tests
2. Genotyping assays
3. Drug resistance mutation tests
4. Core promoter/precore mutation assays.

Role of Molecular Assays in the Diagnosis of Hepatitis B

- Quantitative HBV DNA assay by real-time PCR.
- Detection of as few as 10 copies/ml of HBV DNA in serum.
- Initial evaluation of chronic hepatitis B and during management, particularly in the decision to initiate treatment and in therapeutic monitoring.
- Diagnosis of HBeAg⁻ CHB and occult HBV (definition, detectable HBV DNA in peripheral blood or liver in the absence of HBsAg, where viral loads can be quite low.
- Measurement of viral load at 3–6-month intervals during treatment.
- Posttreatment monitoring intervals vary from every 1–3 months for 12 months and then every 6–12 months to monthly for 3 months then once again at 6 months, with continued monitoring only for non-responders to identify delayed therapeutic responses or the need to reinitiate treatment.

2. Briefly discuss the diagnostic algorithm of HCV infection. (4 marks)

- See Figure 3.8.1

3. Interpret the significance of HBsAg, anti-HBs and HBeAg in the diagnosis of Hepatitis B. (4 marks)

Assay results			*Interpretation*
HBsAg	*Anti HBs*	*Anti HBc IgM/ IgG*	
++	–	–	• Incubation period or very early infection
++	–	++	• Acute infection or chronic infection (IgM or IgG) • Recommend HBeAg or HBV DNA to check infectivity
–	++	++	• Past-infection, recovery
–	–	++	• Core window
–	–	–	• Never infected with HBV • Rule out other causes
–	++	–	• Vaccinated

SHORT ANSWER

1. Enumerate various major serological markers in the diagnosis of NANB enteric hepatitis. (2 marks)

- Antibody detection by ELISA.
  1. IgM anti-HEV appears in serum at the same time with the appearance of liver enzymes and indicates acute infection.
  2. IgG anti-HEV replaces IgM in 2–4 weeks (once the symptoms resolve) and persists for years; indicates recovery or past infection.

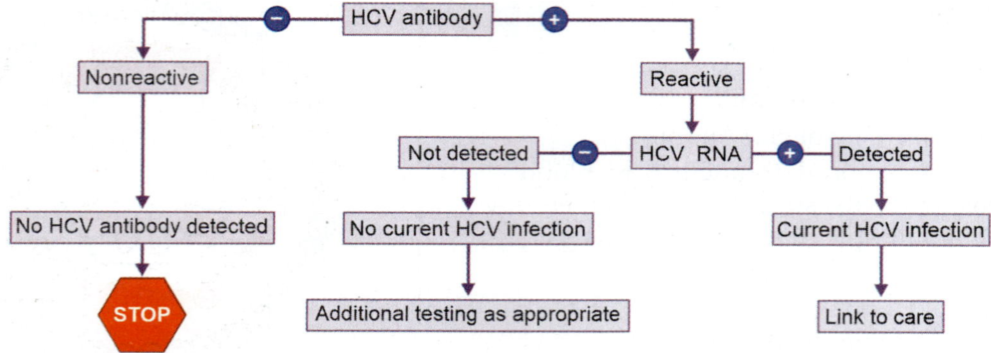

Fig. 3.8.1: Complete Dane particle: Hepatitis B virus

CHAPTER 4

Musculoskeletal System, Skin and Soft Tissue Infections

MI 4.1 ENUMERATE THE MICROBIAL AGENTS CAUSING ANAEROBIC INFECTIONS. DESCRIBE THE AETIOPATHOGENESIS, CLINICAL COURSE AND DESCRIBE THE LABORATORY DIAGNOSIS OF ANAEROBIC INFECTIONS

LONG ESSAYS

1. A 30-year-old male person working in a sugar cane industry exposed to a crush injury in a machine. He was admitted to a nearby hospital 4 days after the exposure. On examination, the site of crush injury was tied with a bandage improperly, contaminated with soil, dust particles and local muscles were crushed. Crepitus was felt on palpation Patient complaint of pain and swelling at the site. Crushed muscle fragments were sent for anaerobic culture to microbiology laboratory and treatment initiated immediately.

A. What is your diagnosis? List the aetiological agents causing this condition. (1+2 marks)

Diagnosis

- Gas gangrene (Flesh eating disease).

Aetiological Agents

- Established agents.
  1. *C. perfringens*—Most common
  2. *C. novyi*
  3. *C. septicum*
- Probable agents.
  1. *C. histolyticum*
  2. *C. sporogenes*
  3. *C. bifermentans*
  4. *C. sordellii*
  5. *C. tertium*

B. Pathogenesis of this disease and its complications. (3+1 marks)

Pathogenesis

Source of Infection

- Exogenous and endogenous.

Mode of Transmission

- Although spores may contaminate the wounds, they will germinate only if certain predisposing factors prevail such as deep puncture wounds, foreign body, etc.

Toxins

- Four major toxins.
  1. Alpha (α)
     - Lethal
     - Dermonecrotic
     - Hemolytic
     - Lysis of hot-cold variety
     - Damages the cell membrane.
     - Causes haemolytic anaemia and haemoglobinuria.
  2. Beta (β).
  3. Epsilon (ε)
  4. Iota (ι).

  (2–4: Lethal and necrotising activity)

Complications

1. Shock
2. Organ failure
3. Mortality rate (50%).

Sequence of Events

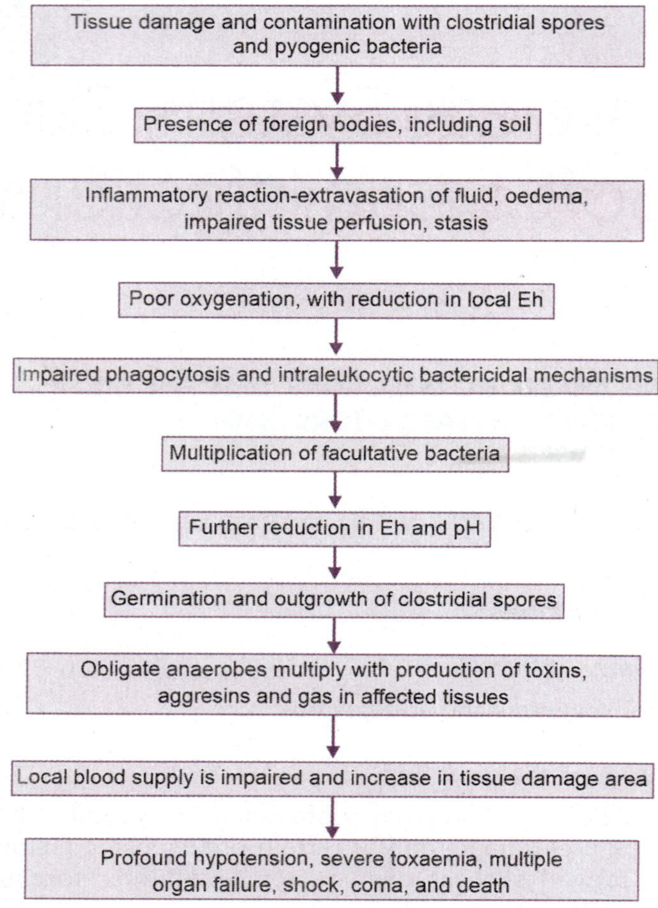

C. Mention the appropriate specimen to be collected. Mention the laboratory workup for this condition. Outline the treatment with respect to the case discussed above. (3 marks)

Specimen to be Collected

- Necrotic tissue, muscle tissue, exudate from deep part of wound.

Laboratory Workup

1. **Direct microscopy.**
   - Thick, stubby, boxcar-shaped gram-positive bacilli without spore suggestive of *Clostridium perfringens* with scanty or absence of pus cells.
2. **Culture media.**
   - Robertson's cooked meat broth, egg yolk agar incubated anaerobically in gas pak or anoxomat.
3. **For confirmation of clinical diagnosis and species identification**
   i. *Target haemolysis on blood agar:* Double zone haemolysis.
   ii. *Nagler's reaction:* Opalescence which surrounds the streaked line on egg yolk agar due to lecithinase activity of α toxin.
   iii. *Reverse CAMP test with S agalactiae:* Presence of arrow-shaped haemolysis pointing towards *Cl. perfringens.*
   iv. *Heat tolerance test in RCM broth:* Positive.
   v. *Litmus milk test:* Stormy clot reaction due to acid and gas production.

Treatment

1. Debridement of wound.
2. Antibiotics—Penicillin and clindamycin for 10–14 days.
3. Hyperbaric oxygen.
4. Passive immunisation with anti α toxin.

---

2. A farmer sustained an injury when a stick pierced his leg. A few days later he noticed spasm in the leg muscles, progressed to become generalised involving jaws. In the hospital ED, when the door slammed, he developed arching of the back.

A. What is the most probable diagnosis and the responsible aetiological agent? (1 mark)

Most Probable Diagnosis

- Tetanus.

Aetiological Agent

- *Clostridium tetani.*

B. Mechanism of action of toxin and various modes of transmission responsible for this disease. (3 marks)

Mechanism of Action of Toxin (Fig. 4.1.1)

Modes of Transmission

1. Trivial pin prick
2. Puncture wounds
3. Unsterile surgery
4. Intra- uterine death
5. Unsterile division-umbilical cord
6. Otitis media
7. Chronic skin ulcers
8. Gangrenous limbs
9. Burns.

C. Clinical manifestations, complications seen with this disease. (4 marks)

Clinical Manifestations

- *Incubation period:* 4–5 days to as many weeks
- *Generalised tetanus.*
  - Affects skeletal muscles—most common.
  - Trismus or lockjaw—most common presentation.
  - Irritability, muscle cramps, sore muscles, weakness, or difficulty swallowing, descending spastic paralysis.

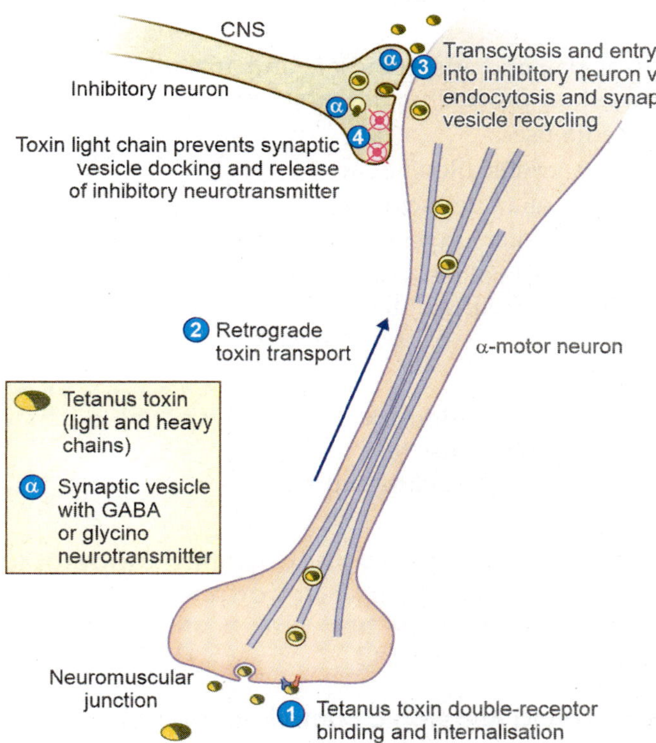

Fig. 4.1.1: Mechanism of action of toxin

- *Local tetanus:* Muscle spasms at or near the wound
- *Cephalic tetanus:* Trismus (lockjaw)
- *Neonatal tetanus:* Neck stiffness, irritable, poor sucking ability, difficulty swallowing and opisthotonos
- *Autonomic disturbances:* High BP, tachycardia, sweating, increased tracheal secretions

Complications

1. Risus sardonicus—spasm of facial muscles.
2. Opisthotonus—generalised spasm of extensor muscles leading to abnormal position of the body.
3. Airway obstruction
4. 50% mortality depending on severity and treatment.

D. Add a note on immunoprophylaxis available for its prevention. (2 marks)

Immunoprophylaxis

Active Immunisation

- Most effective method.
- Stimulates the production of the protective antibodies.
- Two preparations.
  1. *Combined vaccines.*
     i. DPT (Diphtheria toxoid, pertussis whole cell killed, tetanus toxoid).
     ii. TD (Tetanus toxoid and adult diphtheria toxoid).
     iii. Pentavalent (DPT, hepatitis B, Hib).
     iv. DTaP (Diphtheria toxoid, tetanus toxoid, acellular pertussis).
  2. *Monovalent Vaccines.*
     i. TT (Alum absorbed tetanus toxoid).
     ii. Tetanus vaccine, adsorbed (PTAP, APT).
- *3 doses of DPT:* 4–8 weeks apart; starting at 6 ,10, 14 weeks of birth
- *Second booster (only DT):* 5–6 years
- *Third booster (only TT):* After 10 and 16 years
- *Site:* Deep intramuscular deltoid in adults and anterolateral aspect of thigh in children.

Passive Immunisation

- Emergency procedure, used once.
- Provided by human tetanus hyperimmunoglobulin (TIG) or antitetanus serum (ATS).
- Human TIG dose for all ages—250–500 IU, Intramuscular.
- *Advantage:* Does not cause any anaphylaxis as associated with ATS (equine origin).

SHORT ESSAYS

1. A lady presented with double vision and difficulty in talking to ED. Last night she had tasted canned olives before cooking it for dinner. On examination there was paralysis of cranial nerves, hands and trunk. No others from her family had such symptoms. What is the condition the patient suffering from? Describe the clinical manifestations of this condition and the mechanism of action virulence factor responsible for paralysis. (1+2+2 marks)

The Condition the Patient Suffering from is

- Botulism.

Clinical Manifestations

- Nausea, vomiting, abdominal cramps, or diarrhoea.
- After the onset of neurologic symptoms—constipation.
- *Neurologic symptoms:* Dry mouth, blurred vision, and diplopia followed by dysphonia, dysarthria, dysphagia, and peripheral muscle weakness
- *Symmetric descending paralysis.*
  - Characteristic of botulism.
  - Paralysis begins with the cranial nerves, then affects the upper extremities, the respiratory muscles, and, finally, the lower extremities.
  - In severe cases, extensive respiratory muscle paralysis leads to respiratory failure and death.

Mechanism of Action Virulence Factor

- Preformed toxin.

- The most frequent source is home-canned foods, the spores survive an inadequate cooking and canning process germinates and produce toxin.

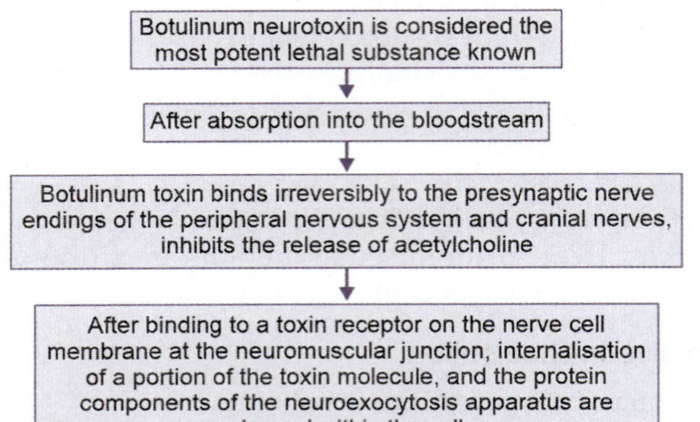

2. Enumerate the virulence factors of *Bacteroides fragilis*. Write the clinical infections caused and laboratory diagnosis of *Bacteroides fragilis*. (1+2+2 marks)

Virulence Factors of *Bacteroides Fragilis*

1. *Capsular polysaccharide:* Acts as antiphagocytic and chemo tactic.
2. *Adherence factors:* Pili and fimbriae.
3. Endotoxin.
4. *Succinic acid:* Helps to inhibit phagocytosis.
5. *Enzymes:* Hyaluronidase, collagenase, neuraminidase, heparinase and fibrinolysins.

Clinical Infections

1. Peritonitis
2. Intra-abdominal abscess
3. Brain abscess
4. Acute bacterial pharyngitis, tonsillitis, chronic suppurative otitis media
5. Pelvic inflammatory disease
6. Endocarditis
7. Bacteraemia.

Laboratory Diagnosis

Specimen Collection and Transport

- Aspirated abscess, fluids, tissue, blood.
- Specimen is collected and transported in pre-reduced anaerobically sterilised plated media (PRAS).
- Pus or fluids can be collected in airtight containers.
- Swabs are not recommended, but if required accu-CulShure collection instrument is used.

Microscopy

- Kopeloff`s modified Gram's stain—gram-negative bacilli.

Culture

- Gas pak and anaerobic jars and anaerobic chamber used for processing the samples.
- Media used.
  - Anaerobic blood agar.
  - Brucella bile esculin agar.
  - Laked kanamycin, vancomycin blood agar.
  - Thioglycolate and Robertson`s cooked meat broth- facilitate the growth of anaerobes.

Others

- Biochemical identification and special potency antimicrobial disc test.
- Gas-liquid chromatography.

3. Give examples for non-sporing anaerobic bacteria of dental importance. Describe the pathogenesis and give a brief outline on laboratory diagnosis. (1+2+2 marks)

Non-sporing Anaerobic Bacteria of Dental Importance

1. **Root canal infections**
   i. *Porphyromonas gingivalis*
   ii. *Porphyromonas endodontalis*
   iii. *Prevotella intermedia*
2. **Dental abscess**
   i. *P. melaninogenica*
   ii. *Fusobacterium* spp
3. **Periodontitis.**
   i. *P. gingivalis*
   ii. *P. intermedia*
   iii. *Eubacterium*

Pathogenesis

- Anaerobic bacteria are present on skin, mouth, nasopharynx, upper respiratory tract.
- Precipitating factors such as trauma, necrosis, impaired circulation, haematoma, malnutrition, diabetes.

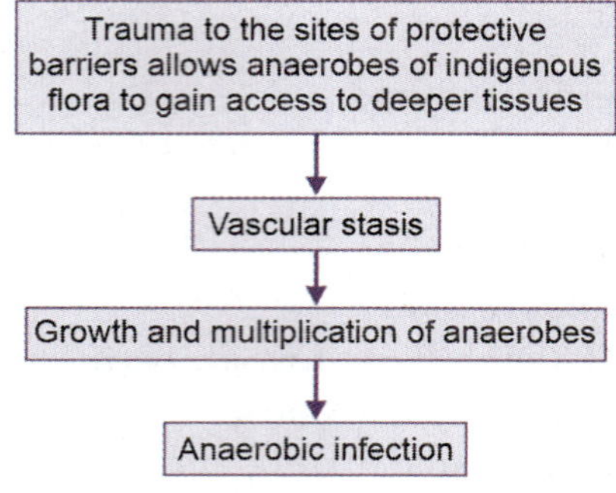

Laboratory Diagnosis

Specimen Collection

- Aspirated abscess, fluids, tissue, blood.
- Specimen is collected and transported in pre-reduced anaerobically sterilised plated media (PRAS).
- Pus or fluids can be collected in airtight containers.
- Swabs not recommended—But if required, Accu-culshure collection instrument is used.
- Gas pak and anaerobic jars and anaerobic chamber used for processing the samples.
  - A gas mixture of 5%carbon dioxide + 10% hydrogen + 85% nitrogen and a pallidum catalyst maintain the anaerobic environment inside the chamber.
- Thioglycolate and Robertson's cooked meat broth—facilitate the growth of anaerobes.

Microscopy

- Kopeloff's modified Gram's stain—gram-negative bacilli.

Culture

- Media used.
  - Anaerobic blood agar.
  - Brucella bile esculin agar.
  - Laked kanamycin, vancomycin blood agar.

Biochemical identification and Special potency antimicrobial disk test

Species Identification by PCR

Gas Liquid Chromatography

SHORT ANSWERS

1. List out six important clinical clues in anaerobic infections. (3 marks)

1. Foul smelling discharge
2. Crepitus
3. Black discolouration
4. Cold clammy shiny skin
5. Infection near mucosal surfaces
6. Tendency to form closed space infections either as discrete abscess (lung, brain, pleura).

2. Enumerate six important non-sporing anaerobes and the infections produced by them. (3 marks)

1. *B. fragilis:* Brain abscess
2. *Fusobacterium:* Periodontal disease
3. *P. gingivalis:* Periodontal disease
4. *Mobiluncus:* Bacterial vaginosis
5. *Prevotella* spp.: Pelvic inflammatory diseases
6. *Peptostreptococcus* spp.: Brain abscess.

MI 4.2 DESCRIBE THE ETIOPATHOGENESIS, CLINICAL COURSE AND DISCUSS THE LABORATORY DIAGNOSIS OF BONE AND JOINT INFECTIONS

LONG ESSAYS

1. Staphylococci cause localised pyogenic infections of varying severity. Supporting this statement, describe in detail about *S. aureus* under the following headings.

A. Virulence factors of *Staphylococcus aureus*. (4 marks)

Virulence Factors

Cell-associated polymers	• *Cell wall:* Polysaccharide peptidoglycan • *Teichoic acid:* Adhesion, prevents complement mediated opsonisation • *Capsular polysaccharide:* In some strains only/ prevent opsonisation
Cell-surface proteins	• *Protein A:* Chemotactic, anti-phagocytic, anti-complementary • *Clumping factor:* Bound coagulase is a surface protein. Demonstrated by slide coagulase test • *Protein receptors:* Help to bind to host cells and tissues
Extracellular enzymes	• *Coagulase:* Enzyme which clots human or rabbit plasma. It acts with coagulase reacting factor in plasma, binds with prothrombin and convert fibrinogen to fibrin. Demonstrated by tube coagulase test • *Lipid hydrolases:* Break down phospholipids and lipids • *Hyaluronidase:* Break down connective tissue • *Nuclease:* DNase specific for *S. aureus*
Toxins	• *Cytolytic toxins:* Four haemolysins and a leucocidin; Alpha, Beta, Gamma, Delta, and Leucocidin (Panton Valentine toxin)—Lethal, dermonecrotic, leucocidal • *Enterotoxin:* Preformed, food poisoning with 6 hours • *Toxic shock syndrome toxin:* Toxic shock syndrome; Superantigen • *Exfoliative (epidermolytic) toxin:* Staphylococcal-scalded skin syndrome

Contd.

B. Musculo-skeletal Infections caused by *S. aureus.* (2 marks)

1. Septic arthritis
2. Osteomyelitis
3. Pyomyositis
4. *Abscess:* psoas abscess, epidural abscess
5. Lung abscess

C. Laboratory work-up for bone and joint infections caused by *S. aureus.* (4 marks)

Specimen Collection

- Pus, blood, synovial fluid, or tissue.

Microscopy

- *Gram stain:* Pus cells with gram-positive cocci in pairs and clusters

Culture

- Blood agar—Beta haemolytic colonies
- Nutrient agar—Golden yellow colonies
- Selective medium—Ludlam's medium, salt milk agar, mannitol salt agar
- Identification of the culture growth
  - Catalase test: 3% H_2O_2 + growth = effervescence means *Staphylococcus*.

Biochemical Identification

1. **Coagulase test**
   i. *Slide coagulase test.*
      - Colony in drop of saline + plasma = clumps.
      - Clumps—*S. aureus*; bound coagulase detected.
      - No clumps—Possible cons; rule out by tube coagulase test.

   ii. *Tube coagulase test.*
      - Colony emulsified in diluted plasma and incubated at 37°c for 4 hours.
      - The free coagulase cause clotting of plasma.
2. **DNase test.**
   - Positive for *S. aureus*.
3. **Phosphatase test**
   - Positive for *S. aureus*.

Typing of *S. aureus* for Epidemiological Studies

1. Bacteriophage typing.
2. *Molecular methods:* PCR—RFLP, PFGE.

---

2. A 50-year-old male carpenter exposed to a hard surface while working on the hand. After 3 days he noticed a swelling, redness, pain which progressed slowly. Purulent discharge was noticed from the affected site after 2 days. He is a known diabetic, but on irregular treatment. Pus sample collected and sent for Gram's staining, culture and sensitivity. Gram's stain report revealed the presence of many pus cells, with gram-positive cocci in clusters. Answer the following questions related to the case.

A. Enumerate the culture media required to isolate the organism. (3 marks)

Culture Media Required

1. *Nutrient agar:* Golden yellow pigment colonies.
2. *Blood agar:* Colonies with β haemolysis.
3. *Selective media:* Mannitol salt agar, Ludlam`s media, salt milk agar.

B. What could be the organism discussed above and enumerate its species and their special characters. (3 marks)

Organism Discussed Above

- *Staphylococcus* spp.

Organism Species

1. *S. aureus*
2. *S. epidermidis*
3. *S. lugdunensis*

Special Characters of the Organism

1. ***S. aureus.***
   - More virulent than coagulase-negative *Staphylococcus*.
   - Slide and tube coagulase test—Positive, phosphatase test—positive.
   - Several enzymes and toxins such as clumping factor, haemolysins, panton valentine leucocidin, enterotoxin, *Staphylococcus* toxic shock syndrome toxin.
   - It causes infections such as.
     - Abscess, boil, carbuncle, folliculitis, furuncle, impetigo, septic arthritis, osteomyelitis.
     - Toxin-mediated diseases such *Staphylococcus* toxic shock syndrome, food poisoning, scalding skin syndrome.
     - Ventilator associated pneumonia, lung abscess.
     - Endocarditis.
     - Sepsis.
2. ***S. epidermidis, S. lugdunensis.***
   - Less virulent, can produce biofilms.
   - Slide coagulase test—negative, phosphatase test—positive.
   - Colonisation.
   - Cause prosthetic valve device infections—endocarditis, ventricular shunt infections.
3. ***S. lugdunensis.***
   - Express virulence factor, such as clumping factor, lipase.

- Slide coagulase test: Positive
- Tube coagulase test: Negative
- Causes native valve endocarditis.

C. Enumerate the deep-seated infections produced by the isolate. (2 marks)

1. Septic arthritis.
2. Osteomyelitis.
3. Pyomyositis.
4. Abscess—Psoas abscess, epidural abscess.
5. Lung abscess.

D. Significance of MRSA. (2 marks)

- MRSA (Methicillin resistant *S. aureus*) is a type of *S. aureus* that is resistant to currently available beta-lactam antibiotics, anti-staphylococcal penicillins (e.g. methicillin, oxacillin, nafcillin) and cephalosporins.

Mechanism

1. Presence of an altered penicillin binding protein, PBP2a.
2. Modification of normal penicillin binding proteins (PBP 1,2,4).
3. Hyperproduction of beta-lactamases.

Types of MRSA

Feature	CA-MRSA	HA-MRSA
Age group	Young	Old
Predisposing factors	Absent	Present
History of hospitalisation	No	Yes
PVL gene association	Present	Absent
mecA gene	Mobile	Non mobile
Size of SCCmec	Small	Large
Types of SCCmec	4, 5	1, 2, 3
Antibiotic resistance	Resistant to few antibiotics	Many antibiotics
Infections	SSTI, necrotising pneumonia, severe sepsis	Pneumonia, bacteraemia, invasive infections

Detection of MRSA

- *Antimicrobial susceptibility test:* Cefoxitin disc or oxacillin (MIC-based method), the antibiotics are surrogate markers for identification of MRSA.
- *Oxacillin screen agar:* Adding oxacillin 6 μg/ml and NaCl (2–4%) to the medium
- PCR for mec A gene.
- Latex agglutination for detection of PBP2a.

SHORT ESSAYS

1. Give 4 examples for the bacteria causing bone and joint infections. Briefly discuss the clinical manifestations of bone and joint infections. (2+3 marks)

Examples for the Bacteria Causing Bone and Joint Infections

1. *Staphylococcus aureus*
2. Streptococci (Group A and B)
3. *Haemophilus influenza*
4. *Neisseria gonorrhoeae*

Clinical Manifestations of Bone and Joint Infections

- Localised tenderness and bone pain at the site of infection.
- Constitutional symptoms such as fever, night sweats, and fatigue.
- Limited range of motion of an affected extremity is seen.

2. Discuss in brief with examples regarding bone and joint infections caused by non-sporing anaerobes. (5 marks)

- Non-sporing anaerobes causing bone and joint infections such as osteomyelitis are *peptostreptococci*, *Bacteroides* spp., *Fusobacterium* spp.

Clinical Features

- Bone pain and localised tenderness at the site of infection.
- Constitutional symptoms, such as fever, sweating, and fatigue.
- Limited range of motion of an affected extremity is seen.

Laboratory Diagnosis

Specimen Collection and Transport

- Aspirated abscess, fluids, tissue, blood.
- Specimen is collected and transported in pre-reduced anaerobically sterilised plated media (PRAS).
- Pus or fluids can be collected in airtight containers.
- Swabs are not recommended, but if required Accu-CulShure collection instrument is used.

Microscopy

- Kopeloff's modified Gram's stain—gram-negative bacilli or gram-positive cocci in chains.

Culture

- Gas pak and anaerobic jars and anaerobic chamber used for processing the samples.
- Media used.

- Anaerobic blood agar.
- Brucella bile esculin agar.
- Laked kanamycin, vancomycin, blood agar.
- Thioglycolate and Robertson`s cooked meat broth—facilitate the growth of anaerobes.

Others

- Biochemical identification and special potency antimicrobial disc test.
- Gas liquid chromatography.

3. A 30-year-old patient develops swelling, pain, and difficulty in movement of the joint after post knee surgery. What is the probable diagnosis? List the causative agents, mode of acquiring this condition, investigations to be performed and management of the case. (1 + 1 + 1 + 1 + 1 marks)

Probable Diagnosis

- The signs and symptoms along with the history of knee surgery indicates it to be a probable case of osteomyelitis.

Aetiological Agents

1. *S aureus*
2. *Streptococci* spp.
3. Gram negative bacilli—*E coli, Pseudomonas*

Mode of Acquiring the Infection

- Direct invasion secondary to trauma, surgery, prosthesis, foreign bodies, etc.
- Haematogenous spread.

Investigations

1. *Sample to be collected:* Bone fragment, blood, bone biopsy.
2. *Culture:* Blood culture for haematogenous spread, enriched media like blood agar is used.
3. *Radiology:* X-ray-periosteal thickening, CT, MRI.

Management

- Early detection of the pathogen and antibiotic therapy.
- Surgery—debridement of necrotic tissue.
- Drainage of abscess if present.

4. A researcher concluded that some pink-coloured long bacilli isolated from water bodies of Central South America can cause cutaneous lesions, bone infections. He found that the bacteria are having a narrow temperature range of 31–33°C. Answer the following questions related to the discussion.

A. Mention the examples for non-photochromogens. (2 marks)

1. *M. avium-intracellulare complex (MAC)*
2. *M. ulcerans*
3. *M. xenopi*
4. *M. paratuberculosis*
5. *M. malmoense.*

B. What is Buruli ulcer and its aetiological agent? (2 marks)

Buruli Ulcer

- A chronic debilitating disease that affects mainly affects the skin and sometimes bone.

Aetiological Agent

- *Mycobacterium ulcerans.*
- A waterborne skin pathogen, found mainly in the tropics of Africa, America, and Southeast Asia.

C. Name of the toxin produced by the causative agent of Buruli ulcer. (1 marks)

- Mycolactone—an exotoxin.

SHORT ANSWERS

1. Mention the bony deformities seen in a person with severe Hansen's disease. (3 marks)

Face

1. Leonine facies
2. Sagging face
3. Loss of eyebrow/eye lashes
4. Corneal ulcers.

Hands

1. Claw hand
2. Wrist drop

Feet

1. Foot drop
2. Clawing of toes
3. Inversion of foot
4. Plantar ulcers.

2. Gram's stain of a pus sample is interpreted as follows.

Gram-positive cocci in pairs with angular arrangement along with plenty of polymorphs
Age of the patient: 25 years
Gender: Male
Occupation: Dock worker
Answer the following questions related to the short case:

A. Most probable bacteria with above said description. (1 mark)

- *Enterococcus* species.

B. Morphology/growth pattern on MacConkey agar. (1 mark)

- Magenta pink coloured small sized colonies on Mac Coney's agar.

C. Any one special test of identification. (1 mark)

- Bile esculin agar test—Positive.

3. Synovial fluid is collected from a 22-year-old football player with history of pain in the medial aspect of knee, History of severe arthralgia is elicited. Swollen patella is observed. Collected sample is sent for culture and sensitivity. Answer the following questions related to the case.

A. Method of collection of synovial fluid. (1 mark)

- Blood cultures are positive in about 50% of cases with acute bone and joint infections.
- Aspirated joint fluid can be cultured.
- Imaging-directed aspiration of fluid collections, pus, or biopsies of bone, periosteum or synovium can be performed in difficult cases.
- Direct aspiration of material from infected bone is possible in infants and small children.

B. Examples for bacteria causing synovial joint infections. (2 marks)

1. *Staphylococcus aureus* (70% in adults, 50% in children).
2. *Streptococcus pyogenes* (16% in children, 7% in adults).
3. Gram-negative rods—*E coli*, *Pseudomonas* spp (15% in adults).
4. *Streptococcus pneumoniae*.
5. *Neisseria gonorrhoeae* (3%).
6. *Borrelia burgdorferi* (Lyme arthritis).

4. Enumerate the pathogens causing osteomyelitis along with their predisposing factors. (3 marks)

Pathogens causing osteomyelitis	Predisposing factors
• *Streptococcus agalactiae* (group B *Streptococcus*)	• Neonates
• *Staphylococcus aureus*	• Children and adults
• *Staphylococcus epidermidis*	• Prosthetic joints
• *S. aureus* • *Mycobacterium tuberculosis*	• Adults with vertebral osteomyelitis
• *S. aureus* • *Pseudomonas aeruginosa* • *Serratia marcescens* • *Candida albicans*	• Intravenous drug users
• *S. aureus* • Anaerobes	• Skin infection in diabetic patient
• *P. aeruginosa*	• Puncture wounds of foot
• *Pasteurella multocida*	• Cat bite
• *Salmonella* species	• Sickle cell anaemia
• *Coccidioides immitis*, *Histoplasma capsulatum*	• Exposure in endemic area

Contd.

5. In case of osteomyelitis, during debridement, samples were sent for cultures which grew *S. aureus*. What are the different modes of acquiring such infection? (3 marks)

1. Haematogenous spread from distant site of infection.
2. Direct inoculation during surgery or fracture.
3. From contiguous infected site.

6. Reactive polyarthritis is caused by *S. aureus*. The statement is true or false. Justify your answer.

Statement is

- False.

Justification

- Reactive arthritis is seen in:
  - Nongonococcal urethritis
  - *Yersinia enterocolitica*
  - *Sh. flexneri*
  - *C. jejuni*
  - *Salmonella* spp.
- It may be associated with other infections, such as conjunctivitis, urethritis, uveitis.

MI 4.3 DESCRIBE THE AETIOPATHOGENESIS, CLINICAL COURSE AND DISCUSS THE LABORATORY DIAGNOSIS OF SKIN AND SOFT TISSUE INFECTIONS

LONG ESSAYS

1. A 45-year-old farmer is admitted to a nearby hospital with chief complaints of fever, severe pain in the lateral aspect of the left leg and pus discharge from the left ankle region. On physical examination, the infected area was red, tender, and warm. Pus sample was collected and sent for Gram's stain, culture, and antibiotic sensitivity. The Gram's stain picture shows gram-positive cocci in clusters which was resistance to methicillin. Answer the following questions related to the case.

A. Skin and soft tissue infections caused by the organism. (4 marks)

Skin and Soft Tissue Infections

1. **Superficial infections**
   - Folliculitis
   - Furuncle (boil)
   - Carbuncle
   - Impetigo
   - Paronychia
2. **Deep infections**
   - Abscess (breast abscess, psoas abscess and epidural abscess)
   - Wound infection
   - Cellulitis
   - Botryomycosis (mycetoma-like condition)
   - Surgical site wound infection
   - Hidradenitis suppurativa
   - Postoperative parotitis
3. **Musculoskeletal**
   - Osteomyelitis
   - Arthritis
   - Bursitis
   - Pyomyositis
   - *Pyomyositis (skeletal muscle infection):* In tropics and HIV infected people.

B. Role of epidermolytic toxin in the pathogenesis in this case. (3 marks)

Epidermolytic Toxin

- The generalised desquamation by dissolving the mucopolysaccharide matrix of the epidermis.
- The toxins are superantigens.

Role of Epidermolytic Toxin (Exfoliative Toxin)

- Mainly belong to phage group II.
- Scalded skin syndrome (Nikolsky's sign—epidermal layer separated).
- *Severe:* Ritter disease (newborn), toxic epidermal necrolysis (TEN) (adult).
- *Milder form:* Pemphigus neonatorum, bullous impetigo.

C. Clinical significance of MRSA. (3 marks)

- MRSA (Methicillin resistant *S. aureus*) is a type of *S. aureus* that is resistant to currently available beta-lactam antibiotics, anti-staphylococcal penicillins (e.g. methicillin, oxacillin, nafcillin) and cephalosporins

Mechanism

1. Presence of an altered penicillin binding protein, PBP2a.
2. Modification of normal penicillin binding proteins (PBP 1,2,4).
3. Hyper production of beta-lactamases.

Types of MRSA

Feature	*CA-MRSA*	*HA-MRSA*
Age group	• Young	• Old
Predisposing factors	• Absent	• Present
History of hospitalisation	• No	• Yes
PVL gene association	• Present	• Absent
mecA gene	• Mobile	• Non mobile
Size of SCCmec	• Small	• Large
Types of SCCmec	• 4, 5	• 1, 2, 3
Antibiotic resistance	• Resistant to few antibiotics	• Many antibiotics
Infections	• SSTI, necrotising pneumonia, severe sepsis	• Pneumonia, bacteremia, invasive infections

Detection of MRSA

- Antimicrobial susceptibility test—Cefoxitin disc or oxacillin (MIC-based method), the antibiotics are surrogate markers for identification of MRSA.
- *Oxacillin screen agar:* Adding oxacillin 6 µg/ml and NaCl (2–4%) to the medium
- PCR for mec A gene.
- Latex agglutination for detection of PBP2a.

---

2. Discuss in detail about group-A streptococci under the following headings.

A. Superficial skin and soft tissue infections caused by group-A streptococci. (3 marks)

Superficial Skin and Soft Tissue Infections

1. **Impetigo (Pyoderma)**
   - Seen in children, poor hygiene, warm climate.
   - Characterised by pustular lesions that become honeycomb like crusts, no fever, painless.
   - Associated with higher M types, and nephritogenic strains.
2. **Cellulitis and Erysipelas.**
   - Tender, bright red, swollen and indurated peau d'orange texture of skin (due to involvement of the superficial lymphatics) along with fever and chills.
   - *Most common site:* Malar area of the face, seen in older people

B. Deep soft tissue infections caused by group-A streptococci. (4 marks)

Deep Soft Tissue Infections

1. Necrotising fasciitis or streptococcal haemolytic gangrene—*S. pyogenes* is MC cause (60%), it is rapidly spreading, hence *S. pyogenes* is also called flesh eating bacteria.

2. Toxic shock syndrome (staphylococcal TSS is MC, but bacteremia is MC in streptococcal TSS).
3. Streptococcal myositis (*S. aureus* is the most common cause of myositis).

C. Laboratory diagnosis of Group-A Streptococci in relation to skin and soft tissue Infections. (3 marks)

Laboratory Diagnosis

Specimen Collection

- Pus, exudate, tissue, swab from deep wounds.

Transport Medium

- Pike's medium.

Direct Smear Microscopy

- Pus cells with gram-positive cocci in short chains.

Culture

- *Blood agar:* Pinpoint colony with a wide zone of β-haemolysis
- *Selective media:* Crystal violet blood agar and PNF (polymyxin B, neomycin, fusidic acid) media
- *Liquid media:* Granular turbidity with powdery deposit

Biochemical Identification

- Catalase negative.
- Bacitracin sensitive.
- Pyrrolidonyl arylamidase (PYR) test is positive.

Typing

- *Lancefield grouping:* Shows group A *Streptococcus*
- *Typing of group A Streptococcus:* Griffith typing and emm typing

Serological Tests

- Anti-DNase-B Ab—Titer > 300–350 units/ml is diagnostic of pyoderma.
- Other antibodies elevated are antihyaluronidase and antistreptokinase antibodies.

---

3. 50-year-old man, who is an avid gardener, suffers a puncture wound on his right hand while clearing brush and debris. Within a few days of the injury, he suffers from myalgia and spasms in the wound but no fever. He visits a clinic where the physician orders a wound culture. Bacteria with swarming growth on anaerobic blood agar plates was observed. The physician prescribes antibiotics, antitoxin, and vaccination.

A. What is the most likely aetiology and infection? (2 marks)

Aetiology

- *Clostridium tetani.*

Infection

- Tetanus.

B. What is the mechanism of action of this toxin? (2 marks)

- *Refer to Page 160, Q. No. 2 of Long Essays.*

C. Describe the clinical presentation and sample collection and lab methods in the diagnosis of this condition (4 marks)

Clinical Presentation

- *Refer to Page 160, Q. No. 2 of Long Essays.*

Sample Collection

- *Specimen:* Bits of excised tissue from the necrotic depths of wounds

Lab Methods

Gram Staining

- Reveal gram-positive bacilli with terminal and round spores (drumstick appearance).
- However, unreliable to distinguish *C. tetani* from morphologically similar clostridia like *C. tetanomorphum* and *C. sphenoides* by microscopy.

Culture

- Culture is more reliable than microscopy.
- *In RCM broth:* *C. tetani*, being proteolytic turns the meat black and produces foul odour
- *Blood agar:* *C. tetani* produces characteristic swarming growth

Toxigenicity Test

- For demonstration of toxin production.
  - *In vitro* haemolysis inhibition test detects tetanolysin.
  - *In vivo* mouse inoculation test detects tetanospasmin.

D. What is the immediate treatment for this condition? (2 marks)

Passive Immunisation (Tetanus Immunoglobulin)

- It is the treatment of choice
- Two preparations are available:
  1. HTIG (Human tetanus immunoglobulin): 250 IU (protects for 30 days).
  2. ATS (antitetanus serum, equine derived): 1500 IU (protects for 7–10 days).
- HTIG is preferred as ATS is associated with side effects, such as serum sickness and anaphylactoid reactions.

Combined Immunisation (Both Active and Passive Immunisation)

- Indicated in non-vaccinated person.

- Tetanus toxoid.
  - Four doses of TT are given I.M.
  - 2 doses of TT at 1 month interval followed by 2 booster doses at 1 year and 6 years.

Antibiotics

- Antibiotics has minor role as they cannot neutralise the toxin once released.
- They are useful.
  - In early infection before expression of the toxin (before 6 hours).
  - To prevent further release of toxin.
- Metronidazole is the drug of choice. Penicillin can be given alternatively.

4. Write the differential diagnosis of hypo-pigmented patch. Classify leprosy based on skin lesions and nerve involvement. How is this disease transmitted? Explain the specimen collection and lab methods useful in the diagnosis of Leprosy. (2+3+5 marks)

Differential Diagnosis of Hypopigmented Patch

1. Tinea versicolour
2. Vitiligo
3. Leprosy
4. Pityriasis alba

Leprosy Classification Based on Skin Lesions and Nerve Involvement

Ridley Jopling classification	*Madrid classification*	*Indian classification*
Lepromatous leprosy (LL)	Lepromatous type	Lepromatous type
Borderline lepro-matous leprosy (BL)	Borderline	Borderline
Borderline Leprosy (BB)	Indeterminate Type	Indeterminate type
Borderline tuberculoid leprosy (BT)	Tuberculoid type	Pure neurotic type
Tuberculoid leprosy (TT)	—	Tuberculoid type

Disease Transmission

Source of Infection

- Patients.
- Non-human source—Armadillos, Mangabey monkeys, Chimpanzees.

Mode of Transmission

- Person to person through aerosols from asymptomatic lesion in upper respiratory tract.
- Prolonged and intimate contact with infected person.
- Ulcerated or broken skin lesion.

Specimen Collection

- Slit-skin scrapings—Ideally 6 sites sampled: Skin lesions, earlobes, fingers, elbow, knees, nasal mucosa
- Nasal discharge
- Nasal scrapings
- Skin/nerve biopsies

Laboratory Diagnosis

1. **Microscopy.**
   - Ziehl–Neelsen stain using 5% H_2SO_4.
   - Stained smear shows:
     - Solid and uniformly stained—viable bacilli
     - Fragmented and granular—dead bacilli
   - Grading of smears is done using bacteriological and morphological indices.

	Lepromatous leprosy	*Borderline (BB, BL) leprosy*	*Tuberculoid leprosy*
Skin Lesions	• Many • Symmetrical • Margin is irregular • Lesions appear as multiple nodules (lepromata), plaques and xanthoma like papules • Leonine facies and eyebrow alopecia	• Few or many ill-defined plaques	• One or few, asymmetrical • Margin is sharp • Lesions appear as hypo- pigmented, annular macules with elevated borders • Tendency towards central clearing
Nerve lesions	• Appear late • Hypoaesthesia is a late sign	• Hypoaesthetic • Nerve trunk palsies	• Early anaesthetic skin lesion • Enlarged thickened nerves (MC nerves involved are ulnar nerve followed by post-auricular nerve) • Nerve abscess seen (common in BT)

2. **Serological tests.**
   - *ELISA:* detects antibodies against phenolic glycolipid 1 (PGL 1) antigen
   - *ML flow test (serum Lateral flow test):* Detect IgM antibodies against PGL-1, suggestive of current MB infection
3. **Molecular method.**
   - To detect *M. leprae* DNA.
   - *PCR:* Real time PCR, conventional PCR
4. **Mouse foot pad cultivation.**
   - *M. leprae* is not cultivable either in artificial culture media or in tissue culture.
   - *M. leprae* is cultivated by inoculating the specimens into:
     - Nine banded armadillos.
     - Foot pad of mice.

5. Compare and contrast between the skin lesions seen in tuberculoid leprosy and lepromatous Leprosy (Hansen's Disease). Add a note on Lepromin test. (7+3 marks)

Skin Lesions Seen in Tuberculoid Leprosy and Lepromatous Leprosy (Hansen's Disease)

See Table 4.3.1.

Lepromin Test

- The test demonstrates the delayed hypersensitivity reaction and an intact CMI against the lepra antigen.

Procedure

- 0.1 ml of lepromin antigen is given intradermally to forearm and reading is taken twice; at 48 hours and 21 days.

Early Reading or Fernandez Reaction at 48 Hours

- Induration and erythema (red area) of >10 mm diameter indicates delayed hypersensitivity reaction and hence past exposure to lepra bacilli. However, it does not indicate active infection.

Late Reading or Mitsuda Reaction at 21 Days

- Nodule of >5 mm size formed at the site of inoculation which ulcerates later. It indicates that the patient's CMI is intact.

Uses of Lepromin Test

- The late reaction measures the CMI, hence can be used for.
  1. *Classifying lesions of leprosy:* In TT patients with intact CMI, the test is strongly positive. In LL patients, the test is negative indicating a low CMI.
  2. *Assessing prognosis:* Intact CMI (as in TT patients) indicates good prognosis.
  3. *Assessing resistance to leprosy in individuals:* Lepromin negative persons are at higher risk of developing multibacillary leprosy than lepromin positive persons.

6. A high school boy developed multiple painful papulovesicular lesions over lips and buccal cavity. Another child also complained of similar lesions. Scrapings taken from the lesion demonstrated multinucleated giant cells.

A. What is the probable diagnosis? (1 marks)

- Chickenpox or varicella caused by varicella zoster virus.

Table 4.3.1 Features of Tuberculoid, borderline and lepromatous

Feature	Tuberculoid (TT, BT) leprosy	Borderline (BB, BL) leprosy	Lepromatous (LL) leprosy
Skin lesions	• One or a few asymmetric hypopigmented skin lesions—macules, papules, plaques, erythematous • Dry and scaly • Central clearing	• Few or many ill-defined plaques	• Symmetric • Poorly marginated • Multiple infiltrated nodules • Leonine facies • Plaques and xanthoma-like papules • Loss of eyebrow
Nerve lesions	• Asymmetric enlargement of one/few peripheral nerves	• Hypoesthetic nerve trunk palsies	• Symmetric nerve enlargement and anaesthesia
Acid-fast bacilli (BI)	0–1+	3–5+	4–6+
Lepromin skin test	+++	—	—
Prognosis (CMI)	Good	Variable	Poor
CD4+/CD8+ T cell ratio in lesions	1.2	BB (Not tested) BL: 0.48	2:1
Antibodies to PGL-1	60%	85%	95%
Acid-fast bacilli (BI)	0–1+	3–5+	4–6+
Lepromin skin test	+++	—	—
Prognosis (CMI)	Good	Variable	Poor

B. Pathogenesis, clinical manifestations, and complications of this disease. (4 marks)

Pathogenesis

- *Source:* Patient or carrier
- *Mode of transmission:* respiratory droplets or contact with infected patients
- *Incubation period:* 14–21 days
- *Sequence of events.*

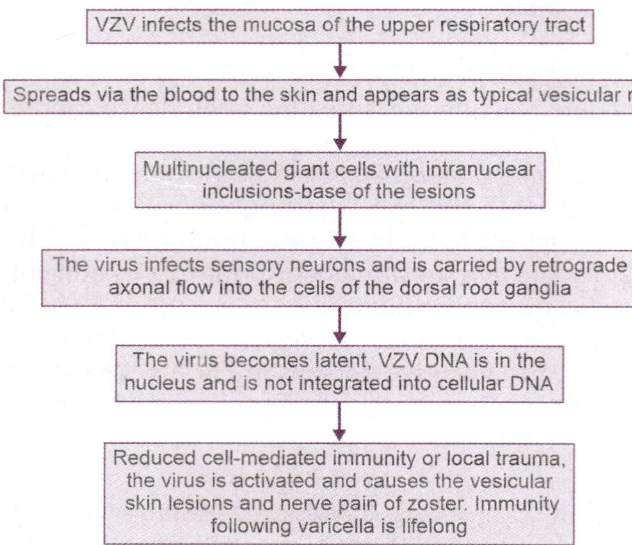

Clinical Manifestations

- Brief prodromal symptoms—fever and malaise.
- A papulovesicular rash appears in crops on the trunk and spreads to the head and extremities.
- The rash evolves from papules to vesicles, pustules, and, finally, crusts.
- Itching (pruritus) is a prominent symptom.
- In children mild infection and more severe in adults.

Complications

1. Varicella pneumonia
2. Encephalitis
3. Reye's syndrome, characterised by encephalopathy and liver degeneration, is associated with VZV and influenza B virus infection, especially in children given aspirin.

C. Laboratory investigations in the diagnosis of this disease. (3 marks)

Specimen Collection

- Vesicular fluid from the base of the lesion.

Cytopathology

- Tzanck smear using Wright's or Giemsa stain.
- Detects inclusion bodies (Lipschutz body) and formation of multinucleated giant cells, ballooning of infected cells.

Virus Isolation

- Remains the most definitive tool.
- *Conventional cell lines:* Detects diffuse rounding and ballooning of cell lines

Viral Antigen Detection

- In specimen by direct IF. It is sensitive.

HSV DNA detection by PCR

- The most sensitive test and can differentiate HSV-1 and HSV-2.

Antibody detection by ELISA or other formats

- Most available tests usually detect IgG or total antibodies.

D. Preventive Prophylaxis Available for This Infection. (2 marks)

Active Immunisation

- Live attenuated vaccine using *Oka strain* of VZV is available.
- *Age:* It is given to children after 1 year of age
- *Dose:* 2 doses, first dose is given at 12–15 months and second dose at 4–6 years

Passive Immunisation

- PEP given <96 hours of exposure
- Varicella zoster immunoglobulin
  - Immunodeficient exposed to virus.
  - Neonates born to mothers suffering from chickenpox if the mother had the infection between <5 days before delivery till 48 hours after delivery.

---

7. Enumerate the various cutaneous presentations seen in herpes virus type 1. Explain the pathogenesis of these lesions. Describe specimen collection and lab methods utilised in the diagnosis of this disease. (2+3+5 marks)

Cutaneous Presentations Seen in Herpes Virus Type 1

1. *Gingivostomatitis:* Fever and vesicular lesions in the mouth.
2. *Orolabial herpes:* Vesicles, near lips or nose.
3. *Keratoconjunctivitis:* Corneal ulcers and lesions of the conjunctival epithelium, may lead to scarring and blindness.
4. *Encephalitis necrotic lesion:* Necrotic lesion in one temporal lobe. Fever, headache, vomiting, seizures, and altered mental status.
5. *Herpetic whitlow:* Pustular lesion of the skin of hand.
6. *Herpes gladiatorum:* Lesions in head, neck and trunk.

7. Eczema herpeticum (Kaposi's varicelliform eruption)—atopic dermatitis. Seen in children.
8. *Disseminated infections:* Pneumonia and esophagitis in immunocompromised individuals.
9. Erythema multiforme.

Pathogenesis

- *Source:* Patient or carrier
- *Mode of transmission:* Horizontal/vertical **contact**—Saliva
- *Incubation period:* 1–2 days
- *Sequence of events.*

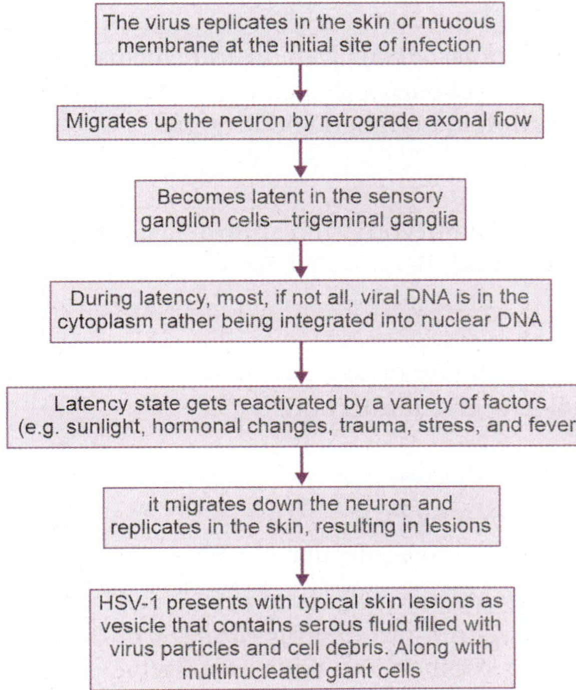

Specimen Collection

- Vesicular fluid from skin lesions, cells from base of the vesicle.

Lab Diagnosis

1. **Cytopathology.**
   - Tzanck smear using Wright's or Giemsa stain.
   - Detects inclusion bodies (Lipschutz body) and formation of multinucleated giant cells, ballooning of infected cells.
   - It cannot differentiate between HSV-1, HSV-2, and VZV.
   - Sensitivity of staining is low (<30% for mucosal swabs).
2. **Virus isolation.**
   - Remains the most definitive tool for HSV diagnosis.
   - *Conventional cell lines:* Detects diffuse rounding and ballooning of cell lines
3. **Viral antigen detection**
   - In specimen by direct IF
   - It is sensitive, specific and can differentiate HSV-1 from HSV-2
4. **HSV DNA detection by PCR**
   - The most sensitive test and can differentiate HSV-1 and HSV-2.
5. **Antibody detection by ELISA or other formats**
   - Most available tests usually detect IgM and IgG or total antibodies
   - Serologic assays based on the type-specific antigens can differentiate between HSV-1

SHORT ESSAYS

1. A woman visits a dermatologist with c/o cluster of vesicular rashes in a single area. The physician suspects that the woman is experiencing a reactivation of a latent form of the virus. What is the most likely infection and its aetiology? Discuss in brief the pathogenesis and lab diagnosis of this disease. (1+3+2 marks)

Most Likely Infection

- Herpes zoster.

Aetiological Agent

- Varicella zoster virus.

Pathogenesis

- *Source:* Reactivation—the dorsal root ganglia
- *Predisposing factors:* Local trauma, old age, reduced cell mediated immunity
- *Sites:* Ophthalmic nerve, T3—L2
- *Sequence of events.*

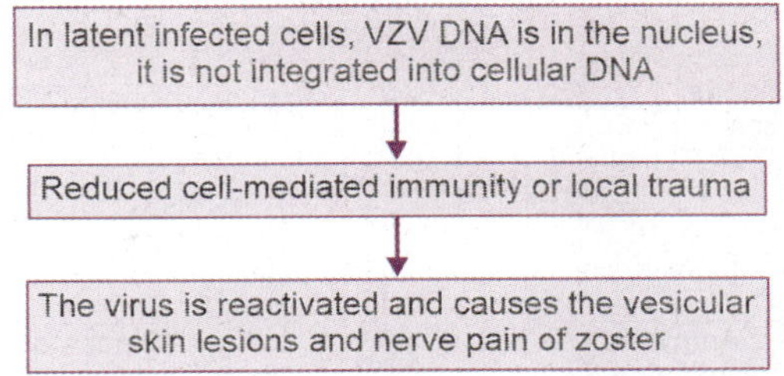

- Initially starts with severe pain and unilateral in skin or mucosa supplied by one or more groups of sensory nerves and ganglia. Crops of vesicles are common in neck head and trunk region.

Lab Diagnosis

Specimen Collection

- Material from base of the vesicle (scrapings), blood, CSF.

Microscopy

- *Tzanck smear:* Multinucleated giant cells
- *Direct fluorescent antigen assay:* Intracellular viral antigens can be demonstrated
- Electron microscopy.

Culture

- Tissue—Human diploid fibroblast cells, rabbit kidney cell lines, HeLa cells.
- Growth detected by ballooning of cells (CPE) and virus in the fluid.

Serology

- *By ELISA:* Detection of IgM antibody.

Molecular Methods

- Viral DNA by PCR.

2. A paediatrician notices rash over the trunk and distended abdomen of a newborn after birth. O/E hepatosplenomegaly is present. The doctor notifies the parents that the child may be severely impaired with mental retardation, deafness, and blindness. What is the probable infection and its aetiological agent? How is it transmitted and lab diagnosis in this case? (1+2+2 marks)

Probable Infection

- Cytomegalic inclusion disease.

Aetiological Agent

- Cytomegalo virus (CMV).

Transmission of the Disease (Fig. 4.3.1)

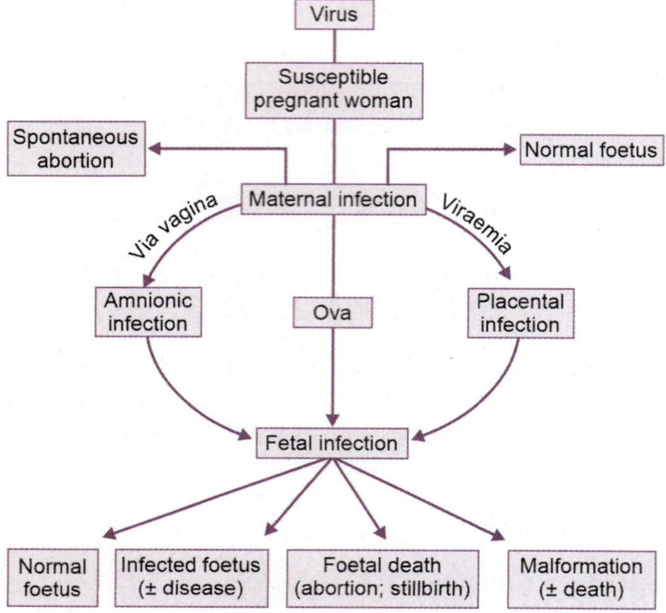

Fig. 4.3.1: Transmission of the disease

- *Source:* Patient/asymptomatic carrier
- *Intrauterine:* Congenital
- *Other modes:*
  - *Perinatal:* Breast milk, saliva.
  - *Post-natal:* Saliva, sexual contact, parenteral (blood transfusion or organ transplantation)

Lab Diagnosis

Specimen Collection

- Saliva, urine, throat washings, blood, biopsy samples.

Microscopy

- *Histological staining:* Demonstrate inclusion bodies
- *Immunohistochemical staining:* CMV pp65 antigen detection in peripheral neutrophils

Culture

- Human embryonic lung fibroblasts—CPE (cytopathogenic effect)—Owl eye.

Serology

- IgM—primary or seroconversion.
- IgG—recurrent infection.

Molecular Methods

- CMV DNA by PCR.
- To detect active infection—mRNA detection.

3. A 14-month-old child is brought to emergency by his mother. The child is suffering from fever, cough, runny nose, and conjunctivitis. O/E, a macular rash covers most of the child's body and blanches when pressed. White spots with bright red edges are obvious in the child's mouth. The mother has not vaccinated the child due to the fear of complications. What is the most likely infection and its aetiology? Describe the pathogenesis, lesions seen, complications and lab diagnosis for this case. (1+2+1+2 marks)

Most Likely Infection

- Measles rash.

Aetiological Agent

- Measles virus.

Pathogenesis

- *Mode of transmission:* Inhalation via droplets
- *Incubation period:* 4–10 days

- *Sequence of events.*

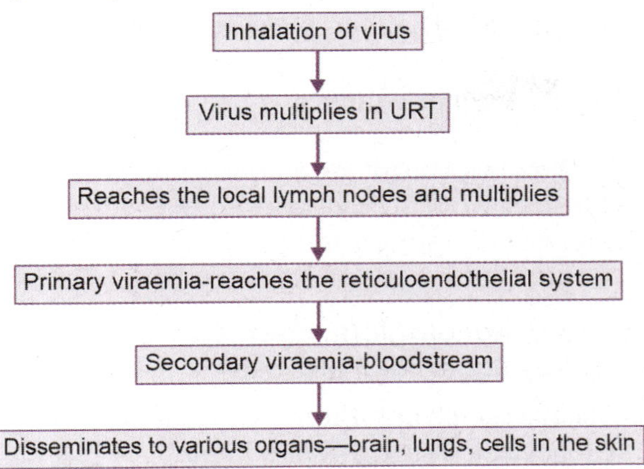

  - CMI is suppressed transiently as the virus binds to CD46 receptors in humans and IL-12 production is suppressed.

Clinical Features

- Multinucleated giant cells—characteristic of these lesions.
- Life ling immunity once infected with the virus.
- Prodrome with coryza, conjunctivitis, brassy cough.
- Kolpik spots—lesions are bright red with a white, central dot that are located on the buccal mucosa.
- Rash begins in hair line, forehead, moves down and covers entire body. Becomes confluent before it fades by desquamation.
- Rash is maculopapular, light pink, discrete to confluent.

Complications

1. Secondary infection of lungs and ears due to damage to respiratory epithelium: Pneumonia.
2. *Encephalitis:* Post measles encephalomyelitis.
3. Otitis media.
4. Subacute sclerosing pan-encephalitis.

Lab Diagnosis

- Clinically diagnosed

Specimen Collection

- Nasopharyngeal secretions

Immunofluorescence

- Direct IF for measles Ag
- *Cell culture:* Monkey/human kidney cells—Multinucleate giant cells with intranuclear and cytoplasmic inclusions
- Demonstrate IgM or IgG—4-fold rise.

Molecular Method

- RT PCR.

---

4. Discuss in brief about the role of the enzymes produced by group-A streptococci. (5 marks)

Role of the Enzymes produced by Group-A Streptococci

See Table 4.3.2

---

5. A 60-year-old woman had a fall resulting in a fracture femur and the prosthesis had to be replaced. Three weeks later, fluid was noticed from the wound site. The patient was afebrile. Two days later, because of increasing drainage, the wound was debrided, and exudate was sent for Gram's stain evaluation, which was negative, but an acid-fast stain revealed pink bacilli. What is your diagnosis and probable etiological agent? What is the other skin and soft tissue infections caused by this pathogen? Laboratory work-up required for diagnosis of this case. (1+2+3 marks)

Diagnosis

- Prosthetic joint infection.

Table 4.3.2 Role of enzyme produced by group A streptococci

Enzymes	*Role*	*Uses*
Streptokinase	Fibrinolysin (activates plasminogen) Rapid spread: By preventing the formation of fibrin barrier.	1. In treatment of coronary thrombosis 2. To liquefy the thick exudates in empyema cases. Facilitates removal of pus and necrotic tissue
DNase (4 types: A, B, C, D)	Liquefy the thick exudates	1. To liquefy the thick exudates in empyema cases. Facilitates removal of pus and necrotic tissue 2. Anti-DNase B >300–350 U is useful for the retrospective diagnosis of skin infections (pyoderma) and acute glomerulonephritis where ASO titer is low
Hyaluronidase	It breaks down the hyaluronic acid of the tissues, thus helps in the spread of infection along the intercellular space	---

Probable Aetiological Agent

- Nontuberculous *Mycobacterium* (NTM) such as *Mycobacterium fortuitum*.

Skin and Soft Tissue Infections by NTM

1. Post injection (post-traumatic abscess): *M. fortuitum—chelonae complex.*
2. Swimming pool granuloma: *M. marinum.*
3. Buruli ulcer or Bairnsdale ulcer: *M. ulcerans.*
4. Infection of tendon sheath, bone and joint: *Mycobacterium avium* intracellulare complex *(MAC).*
5. Catheter related infection: *M. fortuitum chelonae complex.*

Laboratory Work-up

Specimen Collection

- Cutaneous lesions—pus, exudate, skin biopsy material.

Specimen Processing

- Commonly used decontamination and concentration methods are N–acetyl–L–cysteine (NALC)—NaOH method or Petroff's method.

Microscopy

- *Acid fast staining:* Gabbet's stain or ZN stain: Acid fast bacilli
- *Flurochrome stain:* Auromine O: NTM fluoresce bright yellow to orange

Culture

- *Solid media:* Nonselective media—Lowenstein—Jensen medium (L J), Middle brooks 7H10
- *Liquid media:* Middle brook 7H9, BACTEC
- *Colony morphology.*

M. kansasii	*Smooth, non-pigmented in dark, lemon yellow in light*
MAC	• Smooth, dome shaped, buff coloured
M. fortuitum	• Soft, butyrous, multilobate and appear green

- *NTM differentiated from MTB complex by.*
  - Resistance to para nitrobenzoic acid (PNB), but sensitive to thiophen-2-carboxylic acid hydrazide (TCH).
  - Aryl sulfatase test positive
  - Strong catalase positive
  - Resistant to antitubercular drugs
- Further identification of NTM is based on growth rate, pigment production and biochemical tests.

Chromatographic Analysis

- Differentiation is based on pattern of long chain fatty acid.

Molecular Methods

- Gene probe (*M. avium, M. kansasii)*
- PCR
- 16S rRNA gene sequence.

---

6. List the important aetiological agents and the diseases caused by superficial mycoses. Add a brief note on specimen collection and laboratory diagnosis for superficial mycoses. (2+3 marks)

Important Aetiological Agents and the Diseases Caused by Superficial Mycoses

1. *Malassezia furfur*—Pityriasis versicolour.
2. *Exophiala werneckii—Tinea nigra.*
3. *Piedraia hortae*—Black piedra
4. *Trichosporon* species—White piedra

Specimen Collection

- Skin scrapings
- Hair
- The affected skin area is thoroughly cleaned with 70% alcohol to remove surface contaminants. After drying active edges of lesions are scrapped by using sterile blade.
- Another method, particularly in children is by applying piece of scotch tape with its adhesive side down, followed by pressing tape firmly to recover scales.
- Infected hair is removed by plucking with forceps.

Laboratory Diagnosis

Direct Examination

- Wood's lamp examination for *Malassezia* infection: Scaly lesions usually show golden yellow fluore-scence
- KOH mount (10–20%).
- In case of *Malassezia* infections the skin scrapings are examined in KOH with DMSO, methylene blue or Albert stain.

Fungal infection	*Observation in KOH mount*
Malassezia	• Short, curved hyphal elements along with round yeast cells • The characteristic spaghetti and meatball' forms are seen in *M. furfur* infections
Tinea nigra	• Brownish to olivaceous, multiple branched septate hyphae 5–6 µm and budding yeast cells (2–8 mm) are seen
Black piedra	• Oval asci, containing 2–8 aseptate ascorpores • Ascospores are spindle shaped and have a filament at each pole
White piedra	• Intertwined hyphae and oval or rectangular arthroconidea and budding cells are present

Culture

See Table 4.3.3

7. Discuss the pathogenesis, clinical presentation, and lab diagnosis of cutaneous mycoses. (1 + 1 + 3 marks)

Pathogenesis

- *Source of infection:* Infected person or fomites
- *Mode of transmission:* Direct contact or indirectly through fomites
- *Predisposing factors.*
  1. Hydration of stratum corneum
  2. Environmental conditions like warm, moist and CO_2 content
  3. Atopic dermatitis
  4. Collagen vascular disease, Cushing's syndrome, diabetes mellitus, haematological malignancy, and old age.
- *Sequence of events.*

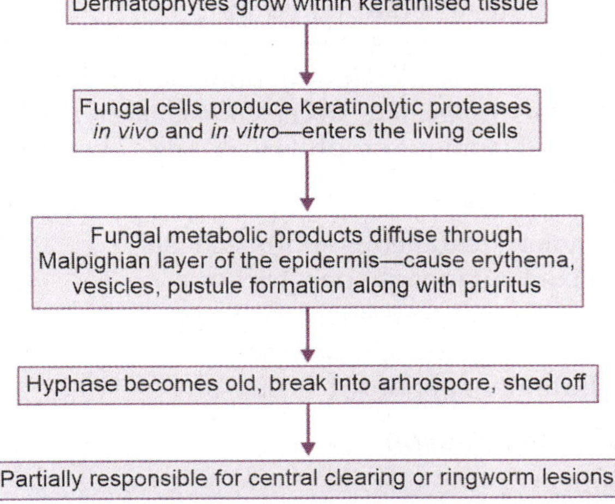

Clinical Presentation

- Dermatophytosis—Tinea or ringworm.
  1. Tinea capitis.
     i. Favus (Tinea favosa)
     ii. Kerion
  2. Tinea barbae (face)
  3. Tinea corporis (face, arms, legs)
  4. Tinea imbricata (face, trunk, arms, legs)
  5. Tinea cruris (inguinal region)
  6. Tinea unguium (nail)
  7. Tinea manuum (hand)
  8. Tinea pedis (foot)
  9. Tinea gladiatorum (arm, trunk, head, neck)

Lab Diagnosis

Specimen Collection

1. Skin scrapping
2. Skin stripping
3. Nail
4. Hair

Specimen Transport

- Specimen should be wrapped by paper and send to laboratory.

Methods

- *Wood's lamp:* Certain dermatophytes fluoresce such as *Microsporum* species and *Trichophyton schoenleinii* when the infected lesions are viewed under Woods lamp.

Microscopy

- *KOH mount:* For skin and hair—10% and for nails—20%
- *Calcofluor white:* Colourless fluorochrome dye

Table 4.3.3 Laboratory investigationn of gungal agents causing superficial mycoses

Fungi	*Malassezia species*	*Exophiala werneckii*	*Piedra hortae*	*Trichosporon species*
Culture media	• Sabourad's dextrose agar (SDA)with chloramphenicol, actidione, Tween 80 and a film of sterile olive oil • Dixon agar	• SDA with actidione lacking cycloheximide	• SDA with chloramphenicol without actidione	• SDA with chloramphenicol without actidione
Temperature and time	• 32–35°C for 5–7 days	• 25–30°C for 3 weeks	• 25°C for 2–3 weeks	• 25°C for 2–3 weeks
Macroscopic appearance on SDA	• Fried egg colony • Urease test positive	• Colonies are pasty, black, yeast like in appearance	• Slow growing appears brown to black with reddish brown diffusible pigment and produce aerial mycelium	• Culture is white and has pasty to yellowish with a creamy texture
Tease mount	• Yeast cells and short hyphae are seen.	• Yeast cells showing transverse septa are seen	• Dark coloured hyphae are seen	• Hyphae, blastospores and arthrospores are seen

Culture

- Sabourad's dextrose agar with antibiotics (gentamicin 0.04 mg/L or chloramphenicol 0.05 mg/L) and antifungal agent cycloheximide 0.5 mg.
- *Dermatophyte test medium:* Colour change is from yellow to red.
- *Dermatophyte identification medium:* Colour change from greenish blue to purple.
- Potato dextrose agar or potato flake agar.
- Cornmeal agar with 1% dextrose.

Species	Colony (Macroscopy)	Microscopy
T. rubrum	• Velvety, red pigment on reverse	• Few, long, pencil-shaped macroconidia
T. mentagrophytes	• White, cottony, or powdery pigment variable	• Clusters of microconidia • Cigar shaped macroconidia with terminal rat-tail filaments
M. gypseum	• Powdery, buff coloured	• Abundant, thin-walled macroconidia with 4–6 septa
E. floccosum	• Yellowish green, powdery	• Club-shaped macroconidia in clusters

8. A 45-year farmer has sustained blunt trauma to the right forearm while at work. He presented to the hospital after 1 month with a developed nodular lesion at the site of trauma. The surgeon sent the biopsy specimen for microbiological investigation after resecting the lesion. On KOH mount, "copper penny bodies" were seen.

A. What is the probable diagnosis and list the causative agents of this condition? (2 marks)

Probable Diagnosis

- Chromoblastomycosis.

Aetiological Agents

1. *Phialophora verrucosa.*
2. *Rhinocladiella aquaspersa.*
3. *Fonsecaea pedrosoi.*
4. *Fonsecaea compacta.*
5. *Cladophialophora carrionii.*

B. Laboratory workup required for diagnosis of this case. (3 marks)

Specimen Collection

- Tissue, biopsy.

Microscopy

- *10% KOH mount:* Small, round thick-walled septate bodies *(Sclerotic bodies)*
- *H&E, Fontana Masson stain:* Sclerotic bodies in the tissue
- *Culture:* Sabourad's dextrose agar with or without antimicrobial agents
  - Colonies are compact, deep brown to black, and develop a velvety, often wrinkled surface and black reverse.
  - *Microscopy morphology:* Brown septate branching hyphae with phialides, chains of blastoconidia or sympodial type of conidiation.

9. Write about the clinical presentation, laboratory work-up for a suspected case of sporotrichosis. (2+3 marks)

Sporotrichosis/Rose Gardener's Disease

- It is caused by *Sporothrix schenckii.*

Clinical Presentation

- A chronic pyogranulomatous fungal infection characterised by nodular lesions of the cutaneous or subcutaneous tissues and adjacent lymphatics that suppurate, ulcerate, and drain.
- The asteroid bodies of sporotrichosis consist of central yeast of *S. schenckii*, surrounded by eosinophilic spicules *(Splendore Hoeppli Phenomenon)* probably derived from neutrophils of abscess at center.

Clinical Types

1. Lymphocutaneous sporotrichosis
2. Fixed cutaneous sporotrichosis
3. Mucocutaneous sporotrichosis
4. Disseminated sporotrichosis
5. Pulmonary sporotrichosis

Source of Infection

- Soil
- Decaying vegetation

Mode of Transmission

- Infection acquired through thorn prick or minor injuries

Lab Diagnosis

Specimen Collection

- Pus, aspirate from nodules, biopsy materials.

Microscopy

- Direct examination in sporotrichosis
- *10% KOH mount:* Small, elongated yeast cells
- Haematoxylin and eosin staining (H–E staining), Periodic acid—Schiff stain (PAS), Gomori's methenamine silver stain (GMS): Round, oval or cigar-shaped yeast cells and asteroid body in abscess.
- Culture
  - Sabourad's dextrose agar with or without antimicrobial agents

- Cream white mold colonies which change to brown-black colour with wrinkled surface
- On LPCB (Lactophenol cotton blue)—hyphae with conidia and conidiophores.

10. Describe the lesions seen in a suspected case of rhinosporidiosis and the methods used in its diagnosis and treatment. (2+2+1 marks)

Lesions seen in Rhinosporidiosis

- Rhinosporidiosis is a chronic granulomatous disease.
- Characterised by large friable polyps in the nose, conjunctiva and occasionally in ears, larynx, bronchus, and genitalia.

Methods Used in Diagnosis

Specimen Collection

- Tissue, biopsy from lesion.

Microscopy

- *10% KOH:* Mature sporangia and spores
- Histopathology of tissue—spherules (large sporangia containing numerous endospores).
- *Mucicarmine stain/GMS:* Mature sporangia and spores

Culture

- Cannot been cultivated yet.

Treatment

- *Radical surgery:* Excision/electrocautery

11. A gardener sustained an injury over his left foot while at work. Few weeks later his foot was swollen and developed a discharging sinus with granules. The pus along with granules was sent for microscopy and culture.

A. What is the probable diagnosis and list the causative agents of this condition? (2 marks)

Probable Diagnosis

- Mycetoma.
- Also known as Madura foot or *Madura mycosis* presents with a triad of swelling, sinus, granules.

Causative Agents

Eumycetoma agent	*Grain colour*
• Madurella mycetomatis	• Black to dark red
• Pseudallescheria boydii	• White
• Exophiala jeanselmei	• Black
• Curvularia geniculate	• Black
• Madurella grisea	• Black
• Aspergillus nidulans	• White
• Fusarium spp	• White

Actinomycetoma agent	*Grain colour*
• Nocardia spp	• White to yellow
• *Actinomadura madurae*	• White to yellow or pink

B. Laboratory workup required for diagnosis of this case. (3 marks)

Specimen Collection

- Pus, exudates, or biopsy material from the patient may be examined for the presence of grains and gauze bandage over the lesion.

Direct Examination

A. Macroscopic

- Grains looked for morphology, texture, shape, colour.
- The granules are washed in sterile saline, crushed between two slides, and examined.

B. Microscopic

1. **KOH Mount.**
   - Grains are mounted in 5–10% potassium hydroxide.
   - Staining method.
     i. *Gram's stain:* Actinomycetoma shows gram-positive branching filamentous bacteria.
     ii. *Modified acid—fast staining (Kinyoun's method): Nocardia.*
     iii. *Tissue section stained with H and E* shows a suppurative granuloma, Splendore-Hoeppli phenomenon.
     iv. *Periodic acid-Schiff:* For eumycetoma.
2. **Culture methods:** Blood agar
   i. Brain—heart infusion agar and thioglycolate broth.
   ii. *Lowenstein–Jensen media (LJ media):* Orange colour colonies-seen in *Nocardia.*
   iii. *Sabouraud dextrose agar without antibiotics:* White to black velvety to leathery colonies.
3. **Serology**
   i. Counter-immuno-electrophoresis (CIE)
   ii. Immunodiffusion (ID)
   iii. Enzyme-linked immunosorbent assay (ELISA).

12. Describe the clinical features and laboratory diagnosis of cutaneous leishmaniasis. (3+3 marks)

Cutaneous Leishmaniasis (CL)

Clinical Features

- *Infective form:* Promastigote
- *Mode of transmission:* By bite of female sandfly
- Single or several ulcers or nodules on the skin.

- Ulcers heal spontaneously within a period of 6 months in immunocompetent, causing disfiguring scars.

Diffuse Cutaneous Leishmaniasis (DCL)

- Caused by *L. aethiopica.*
- It is an anergic form of CL, in which neither humoral nor cell-mediated immune response are functional.
- Prevalent in Venezuela, Brazil, and Mexico.
- Large swollen papules, nodules appear on the skin resembling lepromatous leprosy.

Muco-cutaneous Leishmaniasis (MCL)/Espundia

- Caused by *L. braziliensis.*
- It is confined to central and South America.
- It occurs as intracellular parasite in macrophages and mucous membrane of nose and buccal cavity.
- It shows progressively destructive ulceration of mucosa.
- It extends from nose and mouth to pharynx and larynx.
- Not self-healing seen for months or years after CL.
- The lesions are chronic and progressive, may lead to death due to secondary infections.

Lab Diagnosis

Specimen Collection

- In CL and MCL
- Biopsy material from the cutaneous lesions.

Microscopy

- Smears are stained by Leishman, Giemsa, or Wright stains.
- Amastigotes are present inside the monocytes.
- Cytoplasm appears as blue, purple stained kinetoplast and a red nucleus.

Culture

1. *In vitro.*
   - Novy-McNeal-Nicolle (NNN) medium—Examined for promastigotes.
2. *In vivo.*
   - Animal inoculation.
   - Hamster is used; Specimen is inoculated intra-peritoneally or intradermally.

Demonstration of Antibodies or Antigens

1. **Specific leishmanial antigens**
   - Complement fixation test—Using tubercle bacilli antigen like WKK antigen.
   - Counter-immunoelectrophoresis (CIE)
   - Indirect fluorescent antibody test (IFAT)
   - ELISA
   - rk39-based ICT—antibody detection
   - Direct agglutination test (DAT)—antigen detection
   - *Hypergammaglobulinemia:* Detected by Napier's aldehyde and Chopra's antimony test
2. **Leishmanin (Montenegro) skin test**
   - Indicates delayed hypersensitivity reaction.
   - It is positive in people with good cell mediated immunity.
   - Observed in patients with CL, leishmaniasis recidivans, recovered from visceral leishmaniasis.

13. Distinguish between cutaneous larva migrans and visceral larva migrans (5 marks)

Feature	*Cutaneous larva migrans*	*Visceral larva migrans*
Aetiology	• Causes ground itch • Caused by: ✦ *A. brasiliensis* ✦ *A. caninum* ✦ *Ancylostoma duodenale* ✦ Strongyloides stercoralis: *Larva currens*	• *Main cause: Toxocara* • *Other agents:* ✦ Angiostrongylus cantonensis: Causes ✦ Eosinophilic meningoencephalitis ✦ *Gnathostoma spinigerum*
Lesions	• Creeping eruption • Larva migration occurs in skin and subcutaneous tissue	• Larva migration takes place in viscera • Eosinophilic granulomas
Mode of infection	• Penetration of skin by larvae	• Through ingestion of eggs

14. Discuss the pathogenesis, clinical presentation, and laboratory evaluation of trichinellosis. (5 marks)

Trichinellosis/Trichinosis

Pathogenesis

- Caused by *Trichinella spiralis.*
- Humans are infected by eating raw or undercooked meat containing larvae encysted in the muscle.
- *Reservoirs:* Pigs, the larvae excyst and mature into adults within the mucosa of the small intestine
- Eggs hatch within the adult females, and larvae are released and distributed via the bloodstream to many organs; They develop only in striated muscle cells.

Clinical Presentation

- Diarrhoea followed 1–2 weeks later by fever, muscle pain, periorbital edema, and eosinophilia
- Subconjunctival haemorrhages are an important diagnostic criterion.
- Larvae migrate to these tissues—resulting in cardiac and central nervous system disease.
- Death, which is rare, is usually due to congestive heart failure or respiratory paralysis.

Laboratory Evaluation

Specimen Collection

- Tissue biopsy, serum.

Microscopy

- *H and E:* Muscle biopsy reveals larvae within striated muscle

Serology

- The bentonite flocculation test—becomes positive 3 weeks after infection.

15. Briefly explain the characteristic clinical features of exanthematous fevers. (5 marks)

Exanthematous Fevers

- Fever due to systemic effects of a microorganism infects the skin leading to cutaneous lesions.

Exanthematous fever	*Characteristic clinical features*
Measles (First disease) *ssRNA* *Paramyxoviridae* *Morbillivirus*	• Inhalation of respiratory droplets • Incubation period: 8–15 days • Prodromal period with 2–4 days fever, cough, coryza, conjunctivitis, Koplik's spots (Enanthem) • Maculopapular extensive rash
Rubella (German measles, third disease) *ssRNA* *Togaviridae* *Rubivirus*	• Inhalation of respiratory droplets • Incubation period: 14–21 days • Prodromal period with 2–5 days low grade fever, sore throat, red eye • Rash on face, neck → trunk and extremities
Erythema infectiosum (Fifth disease) *Parvoviridae* *Erythrovirus* *Parvovirus B19*	• Inhalation of respiratory droplets, blood transfusion, trans placental transmission • Incubation period: 4–28 days • Prodromal period with 7–10 days low grade fever, headache, chills, myalgia, recticulocytopenia • Erythematous facial and lace like rash with a classic *"slapped cheek appearance"*
Roseola infantum (Sixth disease, Exanthem subitum) *Herpesviridae* *Roseolavirus* *Herpes virus 6 and 7*	• Oral secretions, trans placental transmission • Incubation period: 4–7 days • Abrupt onset of high fever • Faint pink or rose coloured non-pruritic • 2–3 mm morbilliform rash → trunk → face → extremities

Contd.

Exanthematous fever	*Characteristic clinical features*
Chickenpox *dS DNA* *Herpesviridae* *Varicello* *Herpes zoster virus*	• Respiratory droplets and direct contact • Incubation period: 14–16 days • Prodromal period 2–3 days fever, malaise, anorexia, headache occurs 24–48 hours before rash • Lesion appears first on scalp, face, trunk then extremities
Hand foot mouth disease ss RNA Picorna viridae Enterovirus Coxsackie virus	• Faeco-oral route, infected hands and fomites, Inhalation of infectious aerosols • Incubation period: 2–9 days • Mild fever, oral and pharyngeal ulceration • Vesicular rash of palms and soles

16. A 5-year-old girl has a rash on her face that appeared 1 day before. The rash is erythematous and located over the malar eminences bilaterally. The rash is macular; A h/o runny nose and anorexia was present. What is the diagnosis and the causative agent? How is it transmitted? Enumerate the other manifestations seen in this infection. Laboratory work-up available for this condition. (1+1+2+1 marks)

Diagnosis is

- Erythema infectiosum (Slapped cheek syndrome or fifth disease).

Causative Agent

- Parvovirus B19.

Transmission

- Respiratory route or trans placental.

Other Manifestations

- Aplastic anaemia because it preferentially infects and kills erythroblasts-seen in children with chronic anaemia.
- It also infects the foetus, resulting in hydrops foetalis.
- immune complex–mediated arthritis, especially in adult women.
- Chronic B19 infection-in immunodeficiency or HIV infected.

Laboratory Work-up

- *Specimen collection:* Blood, amniotic fluid in fetal infection
- Serology
- IgM antibodies to parvovirus B19
- *Molecular method:* PCR analysis

SHORT ANSWERS

1. Distinguish between suppurative and non-suppurative manifestations of *Streptococcus pyogenes* (4 marks)

- See Table 4.3.4.

2. Discuss in brief about.
A. Toxic shock syndrome due to *Streptococcus pyogenes* (2 marks)
B. Scarlet fever. (2 marks)

A. Toxic Shock Syndrome due to *Streptococcus pyogenes*

- Streptococcal pyrogenic exotoxin (Erythrogenic toxin).
  - Three antigenically distinct types: SPE A, B and C.
  - Have super antigen activity.
  - SPE A and C are associated with streptococcal toxic shock syndrome and scarlet fever.
  - Mechanism.

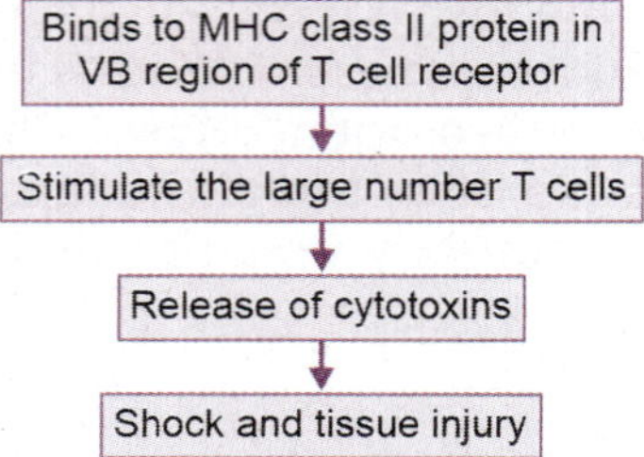

- Streptokinase (fibrinolysin).
  - Spreading factor.
  - Converts plasminogen into plasmin and hinders buildup of fibrin barriers.
- Streptodornase (deoxyribonucleases).
  - Hydrolyses nucleic acid and liquefies viscous exudates.
  - Facilitates removal of pus and necrotic tissue.
- Hyaluronidase.
  - Splits hyaluronic acid of connective tissue and helps in spread of infections.
- Clinical manifestations.
  - Mediated by TSST—superantigen.
  - Pyogenic inflammation and blood cultures are often positive, whereas staphylococcal toxic shock syndrome typically has both negative.

B. Scarlet Fever

- Characterised by.
  - Pharyngitis and sandpaper rashes, strawberry tongue.
  - Pastia's lines—prominent rashes in skin fold.
- Pathogenesis is due to SPE toxin (Dick test is positive).

3. Give examples of non-sporing anaerobic bacteria causing skin and soft tissue to infections and outline their major clinical features. (3 marks)

Table 4.3.4 Differentiating features of suppurative and non-suppururative manifestations of *Streptococcus pyogenes*

Feature	*Suppurative manifestations*	*Non-suppurative manifestations*
Types of infections	• Respiratory infections ✦ Pharyngitis/sore throat (Most common cause, 20–40% of all cases) ✦ Pneumonia and empyema ✦ Scarlet fever • Skin and soft tissue infections ✦ Impetigo (pyoderma) ✦ Cellulitis and erysipelas • Deep soft tissue infections ✦ Necrotising fasciitis or streptococcal haemolytic gangrene ✦ Toxic shock syndrome	• Acute rheumatic fever • Poststreptococcal glomerulonephritis (PSGN) • Reactive arthritis • Pediatric autoimmune neuropsychiatric disorders associated with *Streptococcus pyogenes* (PANDAS)
Mechanism	• *Streptokinase:* Fibrinolysin (activates plasminogen) • *Rapid spread:* By preventing the formation of fibrin barrier • *DNase:* liquefies exudate • *Hyaluronidase:* It breaks down the hyaluronic acid of the tissues	• Streptococcal antigens show molecular mimicry with human antigens. Due to antigenic cross reactivity, antibodies produced against previous streptococcal infections cross react with human tissues to produce lesions
Investigations	• *Microscopy:* Gram-positive cocci in chains • *Culture:* Beta haemolytic colonies on blood agar • Bacitracin sensitive • PYR test positive	• Serological assay 1. ASO antibodies titer is elevated >200 Todd unit/ml in most streptococcal infections except in pyoderma and PSGN. 2. Anti-DNase-B Ab—Titer >300–350 units/ml is diagnostic of PSGN and pyoderma

Non-Sporing anaerobic bacteria	*Major clinical features*
Peptostreptococcus	• Wounds infections: breast abscess • In postpartum endometritis • After rupture of an abdominal viscus • Brain abscess • In chronic suppuration of the lung
Bacteriodes fragilis	• Intra-abdominal infections, usually following perforations related to surgery or trauma • Acute appendicitis, and diverticulitis-polymicrobial • Pelvic inflammatory disease and ovarian abscesses
Fusobacterium necrophorum	• Severe infections of the head and neck • Lemierre's disease—It is characterised by acute jugular vein septic thrombophlebitis that progresses to sepsis with metastatic abscesses of the lungs, mediastinum, pleural space, and liver

4. Classify different types of bacterial skin and soft tissue infections based on the anatomic site along with one example for each. (3 marks)

Site	*Lesion*	*Organism*
Superficial (Hair follicle)	Folliculitis	*Staphylococcus aureus*
	Furuncle	*Staphylococcus aureus*
	Carbuncle	*Staphylococcus aureus*
Epidermidis	Impetigo	*Streptococcus pyogenes*
Dermis	Erysipelas	*Streptococcus pyogenes*
Sweat gland	Hidradenitis	*Staphylococcus aureus*
	Sebaceous cyst	*Staphylococcus aureus*
Subcutaneous	Cellulitis	*Streptococcus pyogenes*
Fascia	Necrotising fasciitis	Anaerobes and mixed infections
Muscle	Myonecrosis gangrene	*Clostridium*

5. Enumerate the organisms causing necrotising fasciitis. (3 marks)

1. *Facultative gram-negative bacilli: Vibrio* species.
2. *Anaerobes:* Clostridia spp.
3. *Gram-positive cocci:* Group A streptococci.

6. Enumerate the fungi causing subcutaneous infections. (4 marks)

I. Sporotrichosis

1. *Sporothrix schenckii*

II. Mycetoma

A. **Eumycetoma**
   1. *Madurella mycetomatis*
   2. *Madurella grisea*
   3. *Pseudallescheria boydii*
   4. *Exophiala jeanselmei*

B. **Actinomycetoma**
   1. *Actinomyces*
   2. *Actinomadura madurai*
   3. *Actinomadura pelletiere*
   4. *Nocardia asteroides*
   5. *Nocardia brasiliensis*
   6. *Streptomyces somaliensis*

III. Chromomycosis/Chromoblastomycosis

1. *Fonsecaea pedrosoi*
2. *Fonsecaea compacta*
3. *Phialophora verrucosa*
4. *Cladosporium carrionii*

IV. Rhinosporidiosis

1. *Rhinosporidium seeberi*

V. Lobomycosis

1. *Loboa loboi*

VI. Subcutaneous Phycomycosis

1. *Conidiobolus* spp.
2. *Basidiobolus* spp.

7. List the SSTI caused by non-tuberculous *Mycobacterium* and the aetiological agents. (3 marks)

1. *M. marinum:* Swimming pool granuloma or fish tank granuloma.
2. *M. ulcerans:* Buruli ulcer.
3. *M. fortuitum and M. chelonae:* Post-trauma injection abscess.
4. *Mycobacterium avium complex (MAC):* Causes opportunistic infection in HIV.

8. A 25-year-old woman is seen in the emergency department suffering from fever, nausea, vomiting, diarrhoea, hypotension, and a diffuse rash. She is currently menstruating and has been using tampons for 7 days. A culture from the genital tract grew the bacteria. What is the most likely infection and aetiology? Which is the key virulence factor responsible for this condition and its activity? (1 + 1 + 1 marks)

Most Likely Infection

- The patient most likely has toxic shock syndrome.

Aetiology

- *Staphylococcus aureus.*

Virulence Factor Responsible

- Toxic shock syndrome toxin (TSST).
- TSST is a superantigen that activates massive numbers of T cells resulting in release of cytokines (including IFN- γ and TNF- α), which causes skin desquamation during convalescence.

9. 40 days after undergoing knee replacement surgery, a 60-year-old woman develops fever and malaise. The area of the replaced joint and incision is tender and erythematous. Blood cultures are positive for the bacteria which is catalase-positive, coagulase negative, and novobiocin sensitive. What is the most likely infection and aetiology? Which is the most important virulence factor in this case? (1+1+1 marks)

Most Likely Infection

- The patient most likely has bacteraemia and artificial joint infection.

Aetiology

- *Staphylococcus epidermidis.*

Virulence Factor Responsible

- Extracellular polysaccharide material (slime), which enables the bacterium to produce biofilms on prosthetic surfaces, is its most important virulence factor.

10. Compare and contrast actinomycetoma and eumycetoma. (3 marks)

Clinical Features	*Actinomycetoma*	*Eumycetoma*
Causative organisms	• Aerobic, Actinomycetes	• Hyaline and Phaeoid hyphomycetes
Tumor mass	• Multiple, diffuse with ill—defined margins	• Usually single, with well—defined margins
Sinuses	• Appear early and more in number	• Appear late and relatively less in number
Opening of sinuses	• Raised, inflamed, and flared up	• Flat opening and not flared up
Flap of opening	• Easily removed	• Not easily removed
Discharge	• Usually, purulent	• Serous or sero-sanguineous
Grains	• White except *A. pelletieri* which is red	• Black or white
Extent of involvement	• More extensive and obliterative with hypertrophic, punched out osteolytic lesions	• Less extensive, only osteosclerotic lesions of bone

11. Enumerate 6 viral exanthematous fever. (3 marks)

1. *Measles:* Measles virus
2. *Dengue fever:* Dengue virus
3. *Chicken pox:* Varicella zoster virus
4. *Hand foot Mouth disease:* Enterovirus, coxsackie virus.
5. *Roseola subitem:* Herpes viridae
6. *Erythema infectiosum:* Parvovirus

12. Actinomycetes are aerobes and cause actinomycetoma and pulmonary infections. Statement is true or false. Justify your answer. (3 marks)

Statement is

- False.

Justification

- *Actinomycetes* is anaerobic and produce clinical condition called actinomycosis.
- Clinical manifestations
  1. Oral cervicofacial actinomycosis (lumpy jaw)
  2. Thoracic actinomycosis- cavitary lung lesions
  3. *Pelvic actinomycosis:* due to IUCD
  4. *Disseminated actinomycosis:* Lungs, liver
  5. Dental caries and periodontal diseases.

13. Pearly white umblicated lesions are characteristic of what type of infection? How is it acquired and characteristic cytopathic effects seen? (3 marks).

Characteristic of:

- Molluscum contagiosum by *Molluscum contagiosum* virus.

Method of Transmission

- Spread by direct and indirect contact in children or rarely sexual transmission in adults.

Characteristic Cytopathic Effects

- *On H and E:* Molluscum bodies—intracytoplasmic eosinophilic inclusions seen in skin scrapings.

CHAPTER 5

Central Nervous System Infections

MI 5.1 DESCRIBE THE AETIOPATHOGENESIS, CLINICAL COURSE AND DISCUSS THE LABORATORY DIAGNOSIS OF MENINGITIS

LONG ESSAYS

1. A 58-year-old male presented to clinician with complaints of fever, headache, pain in cervical joint movement and nausea. Clinician examined and suggested the person for complete CSF analysis for further confirmation. Assuming it as a confirmed case of pyogenic meningitis, discuss this infection under the given below headings.

A. Bacterial aetiology of pyogenic meningitis. (2 marks)

Age group	Organisms
Neonates/infants up to 3 months	• Group B *Streptococcus* • Coliforms: *E. coli*, *Klebsiella* spp. • *Listeria monocytogenes*
6 months–5 years	• *Haemophilus influenzae* • *Streptococcus pneumoniae* • *Neisseria meningitidis*
Older children and adults	• *S. pneumoniae* • *N. meningitidis*
Elderly	• *S. pneumoniae* • *N. meningitidis* • *Listeria monocytogenes*

B. Viruses causing meningitis and type of meningitis caused by them. (2 marks)

Viral Meningitis

A. **Primarily neurotropic**
   1. Poliovirus
   2. Arbovirus
   3. Lymphocytic choriomeningitis virus

B. **Not primarily neurotropic**
   1. *Enteroviruses:* Echo virus, coxsackie virus
   2. *Paramyxoviruses:* Mumps, measles viruses
   3. HSV, VZV, EBV
   4. Adenovirus

C. Pathogenesis, clinical features of pyogenic meningitis. (5 marks)

Pathogenesis

Source of Infection

- *Endogenous:* Nasopharyngeal colonisation
- Exogenous
  - Trauma
  - Surgery
  - Indwelling devices example: shunts.

Predisposing Factors

1. **Age**
   - Neonates—highly susceptible to meningitis because:
     - Immature immune system.
     - Acquiring organisms from mother's genital tract (*Listeria*, GBS).
     - ↑ permeability of blood–brain barrier
2. **Vaccination**
   - Widespread vaccination reduces the incidence of meningitis by that particular agent, e.g. *H. influenzae* meningitis incidence is less after introduction of Hib vaccine
3. Alcoholism, diabetes, malignancy, immunosuppression, splenectomy
4. Presence of CSF shunt
5. Breach in blood–brain barrier

Routes of Infection

1. *Hematogenous route:* Most common, through choroid plexus/ other blood vessels of the brain/ infected WBCs
2. *Direct spread:* From an infected site close to the brain—otitis media, sinusitis, mastoiditis
3. *Anatomical defect in the CNS:* Trauma, surgery, congenital defects- allow easy entry
4. *Invasion along the nerves:* Least common, e.g. rabies, HSV

Microbial Virulence Factors

- Some of them play an important role
- Examples
  - Capsule—adhesion, invasion, and intracellular survival
  - IgA protease—invasion and intracellular survival.
  - Pili—adhesion
  - Endotoxin—Invasion and intracellular survival.
  - Outer membrane proteins

Sequence of Events

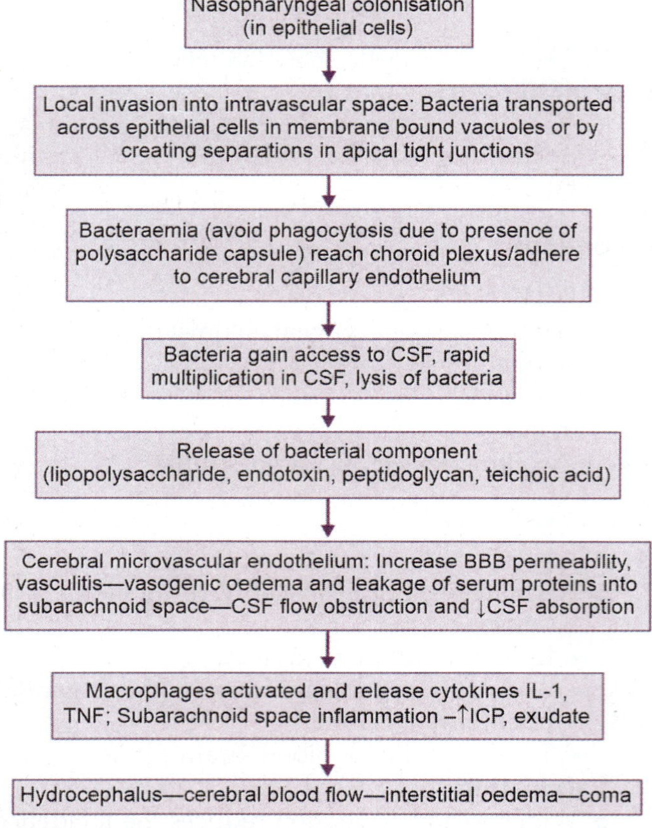

Clinical Features

Symptoms

- High-grade fever, vomiting
- Intense headache
- Photophobia
- Drowsiness, convulsions, altered mental status, coma
- *In neonates:* Poor feeding, lethargy, drowsiness

Signs

1. Neck rigidity
2. Kernig's sign—inability to extend leg when knees are flexed to 90°
3. Brudzinski's sign—flexion of knee and hip when neck is flexed
4. In meningococcal meningitis: non-blanching purpuric rash may be seen

D. Laboratory diagnosis of pyogenic meningitis. (6 marks)

- Serves 2 purposes:
  1. To differentiate acute pyogenic, chronic, and aseptic meningitis (treatment is different for each)
  2. To differentiate infective and non-infective causes

Specimen Collection

1. *CSF:* Gram's stain, culture, antigen detection.
2. *Blood:* For culture.
3. *Serum:* Antigen or antibody detection.
4. *Urine:* Antigen detection.
5. *Nasopharyngeal swab:* For detection meningococcal carriers.

CSF Sample Collection and Transport

- By lumbar puncture under strict aseptic precautions.
- Collected in 3 sterile containers—for cell count, biochemical analysis and for bacteriological examination.
- Transport immediately to lab.
- No transport media to be used.
- Never refrigerate CSF sample for culture. If delay is expected, keep in incubator at 37°C (cold sensitive pathogens like *H. influenzae and N. meningitidis* will die if refrigerated).

Methods for Evaluation

1. Macroscopic Appearance

- *Normal CSF:* Clear, bright, colourless
- *Turbid:* Indicates bacterial meningitis—acute, purulent
- *Cobweb formation on standing:* Tubercular meningitis
- *No turbidity/clear:* In aseptic meningitis, early infection, treated bacterial meningitis
- *Blood in CSF:* trauma, haemorrhage

2. Biochemical analysis and Cell count of CSF

- Provide a preliminary clue about type of meningitis:
- *See* Table 5.1.1

3. Microscopy

i. Gram's staining of centrifuged deposit of CSF.
   - Inflammatory cells: PMNLs/lymphocytes
   - Causative organism may be seen (gram-positive cocci, gram-negative coccobacilli, gram-negative diplococci—in pyogenic meningitis).
   - *Advantages.*
     1. Gives preliminary clue of aetiological agent.
     2. Differentiates purulent and chronic meningitis.
     3. Aids in selection of culture media.

Table 5.1.1 Biochemical analysis of CSF

Diagnosis	Cell Count (per μl); Cell Type	Glucose (mg/dL)	Pressure	Protein (mg/dL)
Normal	0–5; lymphocytes	45–85	70–180 mm H_2O	• 15–45
Purulent (bacterial)	200–20,000; PMNLS	Low (<45)	+ + + +	High (>250) (Marked increase)
Granulomatous (mycobacterial, fungal)	100–1000; Mostly lymphocytes	Low (<45)	+ + +	High (100–500) (Moderate to marked rise)
Aseptic (viral)	100–1000; lymphocytes	Normal	Normal to +	Normal to moderate rise (20–80)

- Morphological clues.

Morphology of bacteria	Suggestive of
Gram-positive cocci in pairs, lanceolate shaped	*Streptococcus pneumoniae*
Gram-positive cocci in short chains (in neonates)	*Streptococcus agalactiae* (Group B *Streptococcus*)
Gram-negative cocci in pairs, intracellular	*Neisseria meningitidis*
Gram-negative pleomorphic coccobacilli	*Haemophilus influenzae*
Gram-negative bacilli	*Escherichia coli, Klebsiella* spp., other GNB

ii. *Methylene Blue Stain.*
   - Better appreciation of cellular morphology.

4. Antigen Detection Tests: Rapid Diagnosis

- Can be done on CSF, urine
- CSF
  - Supernatant of centrifuged CSF is used for antigen detection
  - Method: Latex agglutination
  - Available for:
    - *Streptococcus pneumoniae*
    - *Streptococcus agalactiae* (Group B *streptococcus*)
    - *N. meningitidis*
    - *H. influenzae*
- Urine.
  - Ag detection can be done for *Streptococcus pneumoniae* (by immunochromatography).

5. Culture (Bacteriological)

- Media ideally should be inoculated within ½ hour.
- Centrifuged deposit of CSF is cultured.
- Media used.
  1. *Blood agar and Chocolate agar:* for *S. pneumoniae, N. meningitidis, H. influenzae.*
  2. *Mac Conkey's agar:* To differentiate lactose fermenter and non-lactose fermenters (coliforms).
- Incubate at 37°C for 18–48 hours.
- Growth identified by colony morphology, biochemical tests.
- *Blood culture:* Mandatory, as most cases of meningitis also have septicemia, BacTalert
- *Nasopharyngeal culture:* for detection of meningococcal and *H. influenzae* carriers (Thayer–Martin medium, chocolate agar)

6. Molecular Methods

- *In pyogenic meningitis:* Multiplex PCR using multiple primers to detect common aetiological agents like *S. pneumoniae, N. meningitidis, H. influenzae*

---

2. Classify and describe the aetiological agents of meningitis under the following headings.

A. Classify the aetiological agents of pyogenic meningitis based on age group infected. (4 marks)

Neonates/infants up to 3 months	• Group B *Streptococcus* • Coliforms: *E. coli, Klebsiella* spp. • *Listeria monocytogenes*
6 months—5 years	• *Haemophilus influenzae* • *Streptococcus pneumoniae* • *Neisseria meningitidis*
Older children and adults	• *S. pneumoniae* • *N. meningitidis*
Elderly	• *S. pneumoniae* • *N. meningitidis* • *Listeria monocytogenes*

B. Distinguish between pyogenic meningitis and tubercular meningitis. (4 marks)

Diagnosis	Bacterial meningitis	Tubercular meningitis
Presentation	• Acute	• Chronic
Cell count (per μl); Cell type	200–20,000; PMNLS	100–1000; Mostly lymphocytes

Contd.

Diagnosis	*Bacterial meningitis*	*Tubercular meningitis*
Glucose (mg/dl)	Low (<45)	Low (<45)
Pressure	+ + + +	+ + +
	High (>250) (Marked increase)	High (100–500) (Moderate to marked rise)
Gram stain	Bacteria with Pus cells	Bacteria with lymphocytes
Ziehl–Neelsen stain	Negative	Acid fast bacilli
Culture	Blood agar, Chocolate agar, Bac Talert	Lowenstein–Jensen`s media, MGIT
Treatment	Antibacterial agents—Third generation cephalosporins	Anti-tubercular therapy

C. Immunoprophylaxis of Hi-b. (2 marks)

- The phospho ribosyl protein (PRP) capsular antigen of *H. influenzae* type b is used as vaccine.
- As capsular antigens by itself are poorly immunogenic to children, they are conjugated with adjuvants such as diphtheria toxoid, tetanus toxoid.
- It reduces the rates of pharyngeal colonisation with Hib.
- Conjugate vaccines have contributed to reducing the incidence of Hib disease.

3. A 37-year-old woman who had an episode of seizure. A CT scan shows a ring-enhancing lesion in her brain. History reveals that she is an intravenous drug user and is HIV antibody positive with a CD4 count of 40. Serologic tests confirm that the patient is infected with *Toxoplasma gondii*. How is the disease transmitted? Explain the pathogenesis and laboratory diagnosis of this disease. (2+4+4 marks)

Modes of Transmission

1. Congenital.
2. Acquired.
   - Ingestion of either sporulated oocysts from contaminated soil, water, food or bradyzoites from undercooked meat.
   - Via seropositive blood or organ donors.
   - Inhalation/abraded skin or mucous membrane coming in contact cats' faeces.

Pathogenesis

- *Definitive host:* Cat
- *Intermediate host:* Humans and other animals
- *Sequence of events.*

See Figure 5.1.1

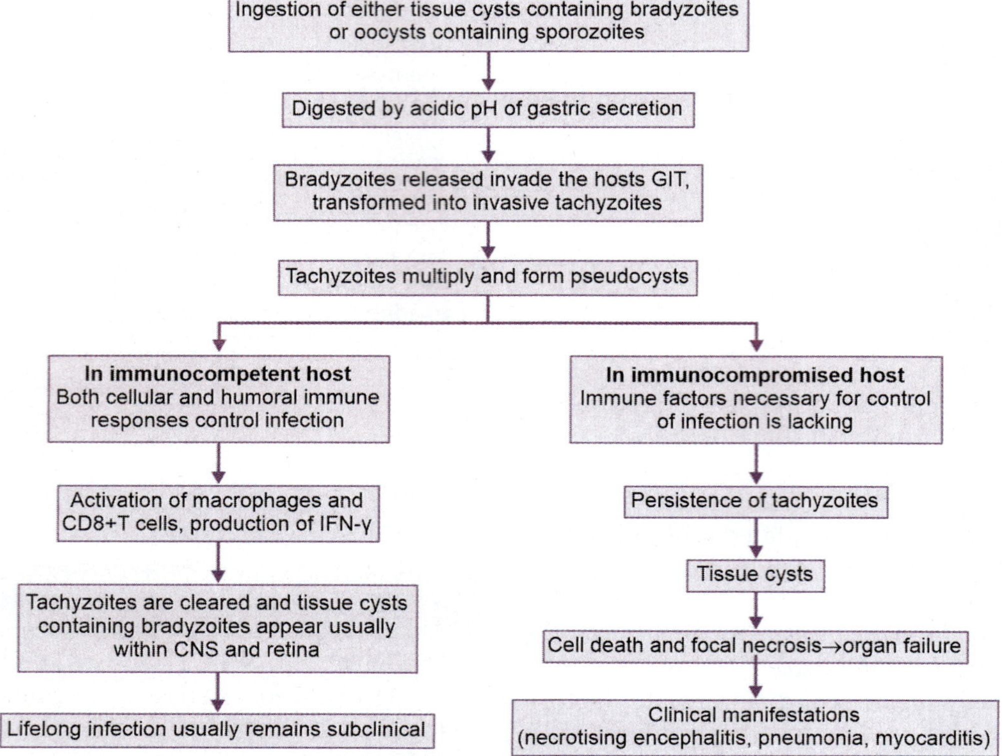

Fig. 5.1.1: Pathogenesis of *Toxoplasmosis gondii*

1. **Toxoplasmosis in Immunocompetent Host**
   - The most common manifestation is cervical lymphadenopathy
     - Headache, malaise, fatigue, fever
     - Myalgia, sore throat, meningo-encephalitis, confusion
     - Pneumonia, myocarditis, pericarditis, polymyositis
2. **Toxoplasmosis in AIDS Patients**
   - It is due to recrudescent infection
   - Patients develop toxoplasmosis when CD4+T cell count <200/µl.
   - Clinical findings:
     - Encephalopathy, meningoencephalitis, and mass lesion
     - Altered mental status, seizures, and focal neurologic deficits
     - Pneumonitis

Laboratory Diagnosis

Microscopy

- *Blood smear:* Comma-shaped tachyzoites (indicates active lesion)
- *Smear from biopsy from organs:* Tissue cyst with bradyzoites (indicates chronic or past infection)

Serology (Antibody Detection (IgG))

- Sabin Feldman test.
  - Gold standard method, highly sensitive and specific but cannot differentiate recent and past infection.
  - Patient's serum + live tachyzoites + complement + methylene blue—Incubated.
  - Antibody in patient's serum binds to tachyzoites along with complement that leads to tachyzoites becomes distorted and colourless. The dye test titre is that dilution of antiserum capable of preventing the cytoplasm of 50% of the *Toxoplasma* from being stained with methylene blue.
- ELISA—double-sandwich IgM-ELISA.
- Indirect fluorescent antibody test—IgM detection in acute infections.

Molecular Method

- PCR.

Animal Inoculation

- Mice.

Radiological Method

- MRI Image shows ring enhancing lesion in patients with toxoplasmic encephalitis.

Diagnosis of Toxoplasmosis

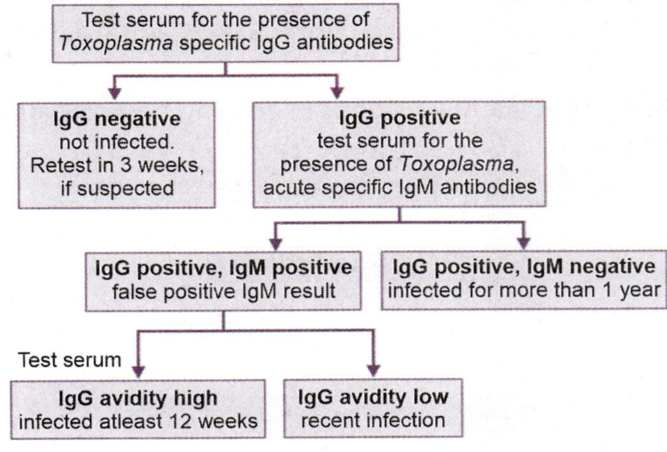

SHORT ESSAYS

1. What are the features seen in aseptic meningitis and enumerate the viral aetiological agents? (2+2 marks)

Features Seen in Aseptic Meningitis

1. Predominantly mononuclear pleocytosis
2. No apparent cause initially
3. Predominantly viral aetiology
4. Non-bacterial granulomatous meningitis

Aetiological Agents

1. Infectious causes
2. Viral:
   i. Enteroviruses
   ii. Enteroviruses (echoviruses, polioviruses, coxsackieviruses)
   iii. Mumps (including post-immunisation)
   iv. Herpes (herpes simplex and varicella-zoster)
   v. Arboviruses

2. Infection with *Toxoplasma gondii* can be seen in women with bad obstetric history. Justify the statement with relevant explanation and role of the infective stages in causing neurological lesions. (2+2 marks)

Statement Justification

- Infection can be contracted during pregnancy by.
  - Ingestion of either sporulated oocysts from contaminated soil, water, food or bradyzoites from undercooked meat
  - Via seropositive blood or organ donors
  - Inhalation/ abraded skin or mucous membrane coming in contact cats' faeces
- Toxoplasmosis in pregnancy
  - Asymptomatic

- Regional lymphadenopathy
- Abortion or stillbirths
- Full term or premature babies with severe manifestations

Role of the infective stages in causing neurological lesions

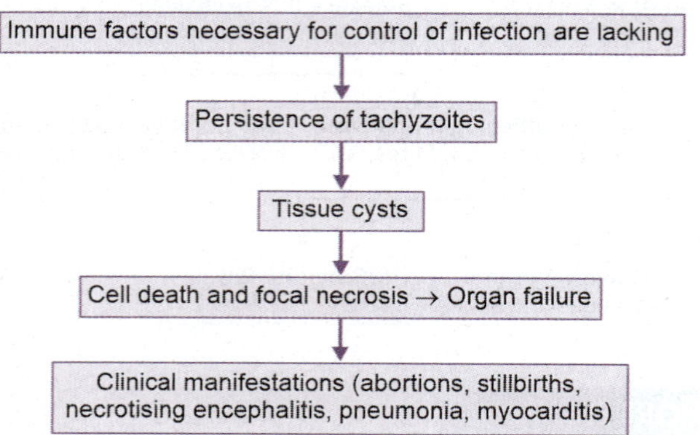

3. A 1-week-old neonate presents to the paediatric emergency room with fever, irritability, poor feeding, and a bulging anterior fontanelle. Lumbar puncture is performed, and the cerebrospinal fluid (CSF) grows group B *Streptococcus* (GBS). Describe the clinical manifestations and lab workup in this disease. What are the preventive measures that can be taken for this case. (2+2+1 marks)

Clinical Manifestations

- Sources of infections
  - Asymptomatic carriers
  - Present as colonizer in genitourinary, lower gastrointestinal tract
  - Transient vaginal carriage
- Neonatal infections
  - Early onset infection.
    - Occurs during the first 7 days of birth—vertical transmission
    - Systemic infections—meningitis, septicemia, pneumonia
  - Late onset infection
    - 7 days–3 months
    - Meningitis, bacteraemia, osteomyelitis
    - Sources: nosocomial, during handling by colonised mother, hospital staff

Lab Work-up

Specimen Collection

- Blood for culture, CSF, pus/exudate, vaginal swab.

Direct Microscopy

- GPC in chains.

Culture

- Blood agar—beta haemolysis.

Biochemical Identification

- *Catalase:* Negative
- *Bacitracin, sulfamethoxazole trimethoprim susceptibility:* Group B is resistant to both
- *Hippurate hydrolysis:* Positive
- *CAMP test:* Single streak of *Streptococcus* to be tested and a *Staphylococcus aureus* are made perpendicular to each other. Arrowhead-shaped zone of complete haemolysis is seen in GBS.

Preventive Measures

- GBS can be reduced by intrapartum administration of penicillin. An aminoglycoside such as gentamicin may be added due to the relative reduced susceptibility of some strains.
- *Early onset:* Screening pregnant females early in pregnancy
- *Late onset:* Hand hygiene and hospital environmental cleaning

SHORT ANSWERS

1. Describe in brief the morphology of *Cladophialophora* with a neat, labelled diagram. Mention the neurological effects caused by it. (2+2 marks)

Morphology of *Cladophialophora* (Fig. 5.1.2)

- Variably brown- or olivaceous-pigmented hyphae (2–6 mm wide) occur singly or in small aggregate.

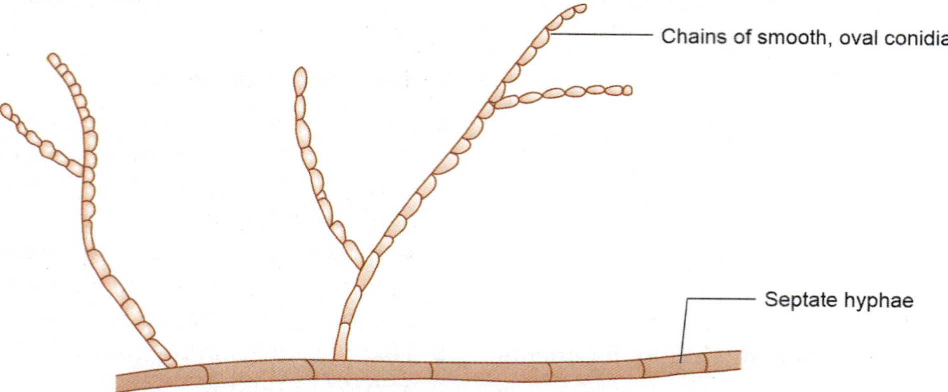

Fig. 5.1.2: Morphology of *Cladophialophora*

- Brown, septate hyphae with conidiophores that are similar to the vegetative hyphae; long, sparsely branched, wavy chains of smooth, oval conidia.

Neurological Effects

Cladophialophora bantiana

- It is neurotrophic dematiaceous fungi.
- Produces brain abscess, affects frontal lobe.
- In cerebral infections, the characteristic inflammatory response is suppurative and granulomatous with abscess formation—Cerebral phaeohyphomycosis.
- The infection may present initially as a brain tumor.
- Cerebral lesions that are solitary and encapsulated carry a more favourable prognosis, while lesions with satellite abscesses, or ones that are poorly encapsulated, carry a worse prognosis.
- Optimal outcome has been best achieved with combined medical and surgical interventions.

2. Enumerate the bacterial causes for aseptic meningitis. (3 marks)

1. *Treponema pallidum*
2. *Leptospira*
3. *Borrelia burgdorferi*
4. *Mycoplasma pneumoniae*
5. *Chlamydia*

3. Enumerate aetiological agents causing neonatal meningitis along with the important virulence factors responsible for meningitis. Mention important signs of meningism. (3+1 marks)

Etiological Agents of Neonatal Meningitis with the Virulence Factors Responsible

Organism causing neonatal meningitis	*Virulence factors*
Group B *Streptococcus*	• Polysaccharide rich sialic acid
Coliforms: *E. coli, Klebsiella* spp	• K1 polysaccharide rich sialic acid
Listeria monocytogenes	• Listeriolysin O

Important Signs of Meningism

- Meningism is characterised by the signs and symptoms of nuchal rigidity (neck stiffness), photophobia, headache.
- In Kernig's sign, the patient is supine with the knee bent at right angles. Subsequent knee extension is painful.
- In Brudzinski's sign, when the neck is flexed, it causes flexion of the hips and knees.

4. A 50-year-old female presents with headache, neck stiffness. India ink staining of CSF reveals spherical budding yeast cells with a clear halo.

A. What is the most likely aetiological agent in this case. (1 mark)

- Cryptococcal meningitis caused by *Cryptococcus neoformans.*

B. Mention other staining methods to demonstrate the structure of the organism discussed in this case. (1 mark)

1. Gram stain—Gram-positive round budding yeast cells.
2. Mucicarmine stain—Stains the cell wall of *C neoformans.*
3. Masson Fontana stain—It demonstrates the production of melanin.
4. Alcian blue stain—Demonstrates the capsule.

C. What is the structure mentioned and its significance in the case. (1 mark)

Structure Mentioned

- Capsule made up of capsular polysaccharide.

Its Significance

- It has antiphagocytic activity and enhances fungal migration.

5. Mention the parasites affecting CNS. Discuss the role of imaging techniques in identifying space-occupying lesions in brain due to the infective stage of pork tape worm. (2+2 marks)

Parasites Causing Meningitis

1. *Acanthamoeba species.*
2. *Naegleria* species.
3. Leptomeningitis caused by *T. brucei, T. cruzi.*
4. *T. gondii.*
5. *Angiostrongylus cantonensis.*

Imaging Techniques in Neurocysticercosis

- Detection of the cyst by CT/MRI
- CT scan is superior to detect calcified nodular cysts—appears as hyperdense dots
- MRI is superior to CT scan to detect the extra-parenchymal cysts in ventricle and cisterns, inflammatory changes, vesicular, necrotic lesions, and non-cystic lesions
- Del Brutto criteria—neurocysticercosis
- A ringlike pattern of enhancement is often evident in postcontrast MRI.

MI 5.2 DESCRIBE THE AETIOPATHOGENESIS, CLINICAL COURSE AND DESCRIBE THE LABORATORY DIAGNOSIS OF ENCEPHALITIS

LONG ESSAY

1. A 66-year-old man with acute onset of fever, nausea, vomiting and headache. In the emergency department, he was delirious. He had a h/o dementia due to Alzheimer's. No h/o use of antibiotics in the recent past. Diagnosed to have viral encephalitis.

A. Differential diagnosis for organisms causing encephalitis. (3 marks)

1. Herpes simplex virus—most common
2. Japanese encephalitis
3. Mumps
4. Coxsackie virus
5. Enterovirus 71
6. HIV
7. Rabies

B. Pathogenesis, clinical features of viral encephalitis. (5 marks)

Pathogenesis

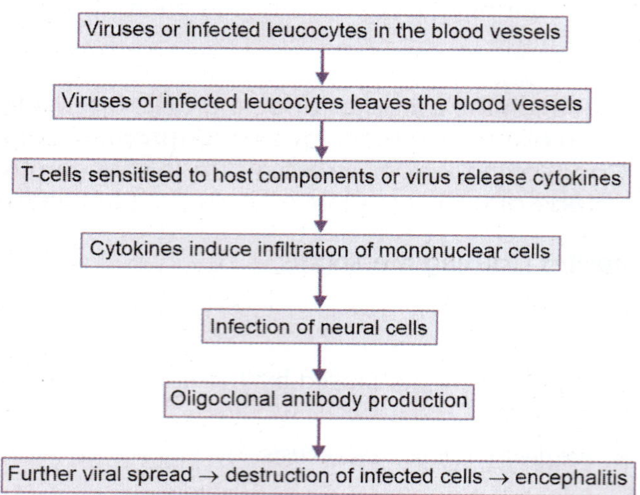

Clinical Features

- Signs of cerebral dysfunction
- Lining of the brain is inflamed
- Abnormal behaviour, confusion, seizures and altered consciousness, often with nausea, vomiting and fever.
- Irritability, drowsiness, ataxia, excessively brisk tendon reflexes, up-going plantar responses.
- Signs of cerebral or brainstem failure (sluggish or absent pupil reflexes, intermittent breathing patterns).
- Signs of brain swelling (focal neurological signs, papilloedema.
- Emerging viruses that can cause encephalitis—Nipah virus, bat lyssaviruses, and avian influenza A H5N1 virus infections.

C. Diagnostic work-up for viral encephalitis. (2 marks)

CSF Analysis

- Mild elevation of lymphocytes, increased protein, and normal glucose.

Serology

- ELISA for detecting pathogen specific antibodies.

Radiological Methods

- CT scan or MRI—to note oedematous change in brain.

Molecular Methods

- RT PCR assay for specific aetiology.

SHORT ESSAYS

1. Compare and contrast in terms of pathogenesis, clinical presentation, and laboratory diagnosis of amoebic meningoencephalitis. (5 marks)

Feature	*Naegleria fowleri*	*Acanthamoeba castellanii*
Age group	• Children and young adults	• Debilitated chronically ill low immunity
Lesion	• Diffuse meningoencephalitis	• Focal, granulomatous, space-occupying lesion
Disease course	• Runs rapidly fatal course (death within 3–6 days)	• Runs sub-acute or chronic course (lasts for weeks, months or years)
Disease	• Primary amoebic meningoencephalitis	• Granulomatous amoebic encephalitis • Ulcerative keratitis • Cutaneous acanthamoebiasis
Risk factor	• History of swimming in natural water or swimming pools	• Immunodeficiency
Infective form and diagnostic form	• Trophozoites	• Trophozoites and cysts

Contd.

Feature	Naegleria fowleri	Acanthamoeba castellanii
Pathogenesis	• Infection occurs through: • The nasal route → cribriform plate → olfactory nerve → brain	• Cyst and trophozoites can enter humans • Nasal mucosa, eyes or ulcerated or broken skin • Infection occurs in: • Lower respiratory tract, ulcerated skin or mucosa → blood stream → CNS
Trophozoite form	• Two forms, amoeboid and flagellated • Form blunt pseudopodium (lobopodia) • 8–15 μm size	• One form, no flagellated form • Thorn like pseudopodium • (acanthopodia) • 15–25 μm size
Cyst form	• Not present in tissue or CSF • Small (7–15 μm), thick smooth double wall	• Can be found in tissue or CSF • Larger (12–20 μm), thin wrinkled • double wall
CSF cells	• Neutrophils	• Lymphocytes
Culture	• Require bacterial supplement	• Does not require bacterial supplement

2. A 55-year-old man came with complains of poor memory and vision that was progressing rapidly and myoclonic jerks. Cerebrospinal fluid examination at a reference laboratory revealed the presence of 14–3-3 protein. Over the next 6 months his cognitive deterioration became severe, and he died 3 months later. At an autopsy, spongiform encephalopathy was noted. Which of the following is the most appropriate diagnosis for this man? Add a note on the types of this condition. (1+4 marks)

Most Appropriate Diagnosis

Rapidly progressive dementia and myoclonus associated with presence of 14–3-3 protein is strongly suggestive of ***Creutzfeldt–Jakob Disease (CJD)***, which was confirmed by the presence of spongiform encephalopathy at autopsy.

Types of CJD

1. **Sporadic CJD.**
   - It has a median age of onset of 62 years (60–74).
   - Results from spontaneous conversion of normal PrPC to PrPSC or spontaneous mutation of the PRNP gene leading to production of PrPSC, the abnormal form.
   - Myoclonus is an important component of symptoms; death usually occurs within 8 months after onset of symptoms.
2. **Familial CJD.**
   - Associated with an autosomal dominant inheritance of mutations in the PRNP gene.
   - Onsets between 45 and 49 years of age.
   - Progression is slower and death occurs in about 2 years.
3. **Variant CJD.**
   - It is acquired through eating meat from cattle with bovine spongiform encephalopathy.
   - Age of onset varies, but median is 28 years of age.
   - Psychiatric abnormalities and sensory symptoms are predominant; death occurs in approximately 14 months.
4. **Iatrogenic CJD.**
   - It has transmitted following corneal transplants, dura grafts, administration of human pituitary-derived gonadotropins, and use of contaminated surgical instruments and EEG electrodes, from blood transfusion.

3. A 27-year-old is brought to the emergency department with altered sensorium in Dakshina Kannada, Karnataka. A history of fever and headache two days back and on conducting laboratory investigations revealed low platelet count, increased ferritin levels, QBC was negative for malaria and NS1 antigen was positive by immunochromatographic test. MRI showed oedematous lesions in the brain. What is your likely diagnosis? Explain the pathogenesis, clinical presentation and laboratory work-up for this case. (1+4+2 marks)

Likely Diagnosis

- Dengue encephalitis.
- Caused by dengue virus.

Pathogenesis

- *Vector: Aedes aegypti, A. albopictus*
- *Reservoir:* Man, mosquito
- *Primary dengue infection:* First time with any 1 serotype
- *Secondary dengue infection:* Months—years later, more severe form, due to infection with another second serotype
- Type 2 and serotype 1 followed by serotype 2 which is more dangerous.
- Antibody response in dengue.
  - Neutralising antibodies.
    - Protective
    - Against infective serotype (lifelong) and against other serotypes (lasts for some time)

- Non-neutralising antibodies.
  - Lasts lifelong
  - Heterotypic (produced against other serotypes, not against infective serotype)
  - In secondary infection, instead of neutralising the second serotype, these Abs protect the virus from immune system by inhibiting the bystander B cell activation (**Antibody dependent enhancement)**
- In individuals with passively acquired maternal antibody or preexisting non-neutralising heterotypic Ab due to previous infection with different serotype of the virus.
- Immune complexes activate complement, causing Increased vascular permeability, thrombocytopenia.
- Ab increase the entry of virus into monocytes, macrophages with liberation of large number of cytokines leading to DIC, shock in both.

Clinical Presentation

1. **Classic dengue**
   - *Incubation period:* 4–7 days
   - Fever (saddle back/biphasic/break bone), malaise chills, headache
   - Maculopapular rash on chest, upper limbs
   - Severe frontal headache
   - Muscle, joint pain
   - Lymphadenopathy
   - Retro orbital pain
   - Loss of appetite, nausea, vomiting
2. **Dengue haemorrhagic fever**
   - High grade continuous fever
   - Hepatomegaly
   - Thrombocytopenia
   - Raised haematocrit by 20%
   - Positive tourniquet test/spontaneous bleeding from skin, nose, mouth, gums
3. **Dengue shock syndrome**
   - DHF+ features of shock
   - Rapid and weak pulse
   - Hypotension
   - Cold clammy skin
   - Restlessness

Laboratory Work-up

1. **Specimen collection**
   - Blood
   - Serum or plasma
   - CSF
2. **NS 1Ag detection**
   - ELISA, ICT
   - 1–18 days
   - Highly specific
3. **Antibody detection**
   - Primary infection: IgM (5–90 days), IgG in 14–21 days, the titre then increases
   - Secondary infection: IgG titres rise rapidly. Cross reaction with many flaviviruses, IgM: low or undetectable
4. **Virus detection (1–5 days)**
   - Virus isolation in mosquito cell line
   - RT PCR

4. Describe the pathogenesis, clinical features, lab investigations and preventive measures for Japanese encephalitis. (3+2+1 marks)

Japanese Encephalitis

Pathogenesis (Fig. 5.2.1)

- Flavivirus
- Japan, Korea, India, Malaysia
- Epidemics in summer, autumn in temperate regions
- *Reservoir:* Ardeid birds (herons, egrets)
- *Amplifier hosts:* Pigs
- *Vector: Culex tritaeniorhynchus*
- Humans act as dead-end host.

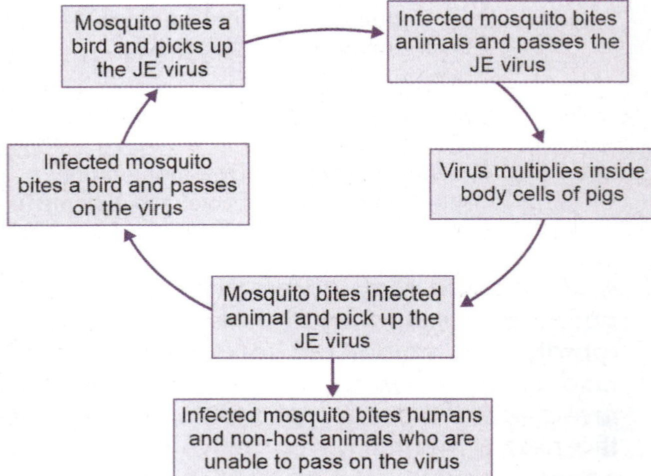

Fig. 5.2.1: Life cycle of Japanese encephalitis

Clinical Features

- Large majority of infections are asymptomatic.
- Abrupt onset of fever, headache, vomiting.
- *After incubation period of 1–6 days:* Nuchal rigidity, convulsions, altered sensorium, coma
- Mortality 50% in epidemics
- Residual neurological changes in 50% survivors (seizures, paresis, movement disorders, or mental retardation)
- *In utero* infection can also occur in humans, resulting in abortion of the fetus
- *Postmortem lesion:* Pan-encephalitis
  - Infected neurons throughout CNS
  - Occasional microscopic necrotic foci
  - Thalamus generally severely affected

Lab Investigations

Sample Collection

- CSF, blood, or serum

Tentative Diagnosis

- *Antibody titre:* Haemagglutination inhibition, indirect fluorescent antibody test, CF, ELISA
- JE-specific IgM in serum or CSF.

Definitive Diagnosis

- *Virus isolation:* CSF, brain
- Mosquito cell lines
- Wide range of mammalian cell lines
- Suckling mouse brain
- *Molecular methods:* Reverse transcriptase PCR

Preventive Measures

1. Mosquito control, locating piggeries away from human dwellings, mass slaughter of pigs during epidemics.
2. Formalin inactivated mouse brain vaccine—Nakayama strain.
   - 2 doses at 2-week intervals, booster 6–12 months later.
   - *Immunity:* Short lived (human use)
   - Used for endemic or epidemic areas especially among travelers, military, laboratory workers.
3. Live attenuated JE- SA14–14-2.
   - Produced in baby hamster kidney cells, passed through weaning mice
   - 2 doses, 1 year apart
   - Successful for reducing incidence

SHORT ANSWERS

1. Give examples for the parasites causing encephalitis. Mention the clinical features of amoebic meningo encephalitis. (1+2 marks)

Parasites Causing Encephalitis

1. *Naegleria fowleri.*
2. *Acanthamoeba* spp.
3. *Toxoplasma gondii.*

Primary Amoebic Meningoencephalitis (PAM)

- Acute, necrotising, rapidly fatal, fulminating, haemorrhagic meningoencephalitis.
- Occurs in previously healthy children and young adults.
- *Source:* Contaminated domestic water used for bathing, recent exposure to warm fresh water and contaminated swimming pools
- Fever, headache, stiffness of neck, nausea, vomiting, convulsions.
- Photophobia, diplopia, loss of sense of smell, cranial nerve palsies
- Coma and death within 5–10 days from infection.
- Increased intracranial pressure with brain herniation, leading to cardiopulmonary arrest and pulmonary oedema
- Rapidly fatal disease

Granulomatous Amoebic Meningoencephalitis

- Granulomatous amoebic encephalitis (GAE)—seen in immunocompromised individuals
- Cutaneous acanthamoebiasis—seen in HIV patients—hard erythematous nontender nodules, papules, or ulcers
- Acanthamoeba keratitis (AK)—seen in contact lens wearers

2. Enumerate the Arboviral infections in India. (3 marks)

1. Genus *alphavirus* includes chikungunya, sindbis fever.
2. Genus *flavivirus* includes dengue, japanese encephalitis, West Nile fever, Kyasanur Forest disease.
3. Genus *Nairo* virus includes nairobi sheep disease, Bhanja fever.

MI 5.3 IDENTIFY THE MICROBIAL AGENTS CAUSING MENINGITIS

LONG ESSAY

1. A 3-year-old girl was seen in the hospital with progressive leg weakness. She has not been given any vaccination since birth. 9 months ago, she had an illness causing weakness of both legs. Over the course of the illness, she has had progressive left leg weakness suggestive of acute flaccid paralysis. What is the most probable diagnosis? Name the organism causing it and explain its pathogenesis and clinical features of the disease? What are the methods of laboratory diagnosis? (1+1+4+4 marks)

Most Probable Diagnosis

- Poliomyelitis.

Organism Causing It

- Poliovirus.

Pathogenesis

Source

- Patients who shed virus in the GIT and respiratory secretions

Incubation Period

- 4 days to 4 weeks (average 10 days)

Infective Period

- 7–8 days before and after infection

Modes of Transmission

1. Ingestion of contaminated water and food.
2. Droplet infection.

Sequence of Events

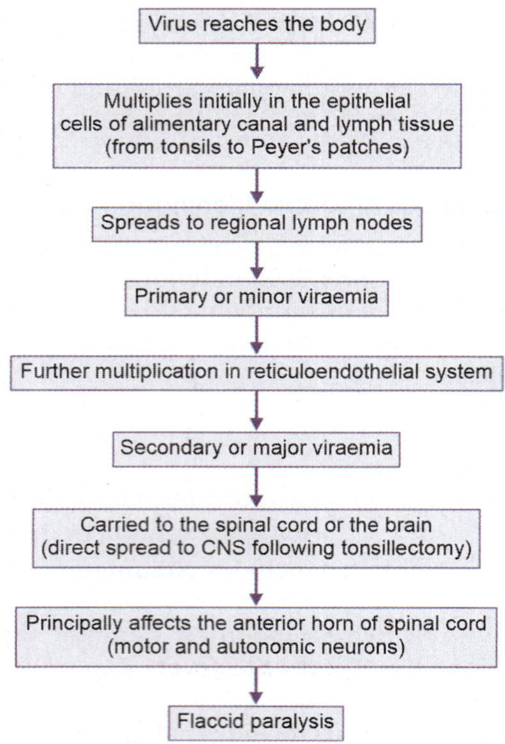

- Degeneration of the Nissl bodies is the earliest change.
- Anterior horn of the spinal cord, motor nuclei of pons and medulla are mostly affected.

Clinical Features

- Inapparent infections.
  1. **Abortive Poliomyelitis/Minor Illness**
     - Most common form
     - Characterised by fever, malaise, drowsiness, headache, nausea, vomiting, constipation, and sore throat
     - Recovery occurs in a few days
  2. **Non-paralytic Poliomyelitis (Aseptic meningitis)**
     - Begins 3–4 days after minor illness
     - Neck stiffness, pain in the back and neck, biphasic fever
     - Recovery is rapid and complete, a small percentage of cases advances to paralysis
  3. **Paralytic Poliomyelitis**
     - Predominant feature is the flaccid paralysis due to the damage to the anterior horn of the spinal cord
     - Spinal paralytic poliomyelitis—quadriplegia, asymmetric pattern
     - Bulbar paralytic poliomyelitis—dysphagia, dysphonia, dyspnoea
  4. **Progressive Post Poliomyelitis Muscle atrophy.**
     - Muscle atrophy leading to weakness.

Laboratory Diagnosis

Specimen Collection

- Throat swab (early stage)
- Blood (early stage)
- CSF
- Feces

Virus Isolation

- Primary monkey kidney cells or human diploid cells—CPE—refractile and pyknotic cells
- Identification done by neutralisation with specific antisera.

Serodiagnosis

- Antibody detection in paired sera by complement fixation test or neutralisation test.

Stool Culture

- Recommended for AFP surveillance and laboratory confirmation.

Molecular Methods

- Reverse transcriptase PCR assays.

SHORT ESSAYS

1. An 18-year-old woman complains of the sudden onset of fever 104°F and severe headache. Physical examination reveals nuchal rigidity. Suspecting it to be meningitis, a spinal tap was done. Gram's stain of the spinal fluid reveals many neutrophils and many gram-negative diplococci. What is the probable agent? Describe in brief its virulence factors, clinical presentation and laboratory work-up for this case.

(1+1+1.5+1.5 marks)

Probable Agent

- *Neisseria meningitides.*

Virulence Factors (Fig. 5.3.1)

1. Capsule-antiphagocytic
2. Porin
3. Pili-adherence to host epithelium and mucosa
4. Opa, Opc: Promotes pilus-mediated adherence and invasion into mucosal surfaces

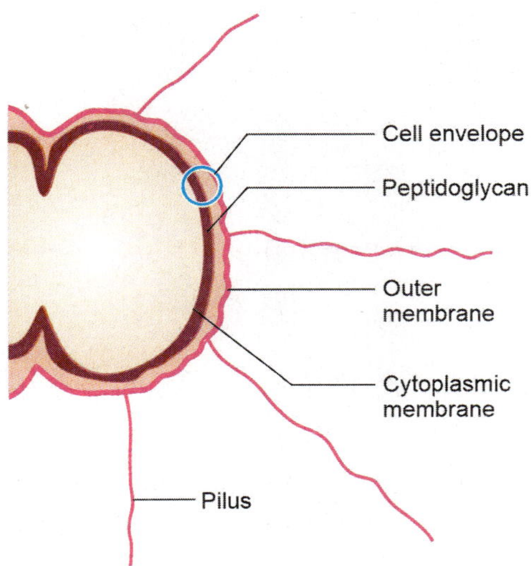

Fig. 5.3.1: Virulence factors of *Neisseria meningitides*

Clinical Presentation

- *Source:* Human nasopharyngeal carriers (mainly children)
- *Mode of transmission:* Droplet inhalation
- *Spread of infection:* From nasopharynx, meningococci reach the meninges either by:
  - Haematogenous route (most common)
  - By direct olfactory nerve spread through cribriform plate
  - Rarely through conjunctiva
- Colonisation of nasopharynx results in subclinical infection (mild upper respiratory tract infection).
- Invasion of the bloodstream—meningococcaemia or meningitis or sepsis.
- Symptoms: Fever, shaking chills, muscle pain, petechial rash in the extremities
- In fulminant form, *Waterhouse–Friderichsen syndrome*—DIC, multisystem failure. Haemorrhage in skin and adrenal glands.
- *Chronic meningococcemia* characterised by recurrent attacks of fever, headache, petechial rash.
- *Post-meningococcal reactive disease*
  - Immune complex mediated
  - Develops after 4–10 days
  - Manifestations seen are arthritis, rash, iritis, pericarditis, polyserositis and fever.

Laboratory Work-up

Specimen Collection

- *For cases:* Blood and CSF
- *For carriers:* Nasopharyngeal swab

CSF Examination

- First portion is centrifuged and used for:
  - Capsular antigen detection—Latex agglutination
  - CSF analysis: ↑ CSF pressure, ↑ protein and ↓ glucose in CSF
  - *Microscopy:* Gram's staining—Pus cells with gram-negative diplococci, kidney bean-shaped
- *Second portion:* For culture on blood agar, chocolate agar
- *Third portion* is enriched in BHI broth and incubated for 7 days.

Nasopharyngeal Swab Culture

- *On Thayer–Martin medium:* Pinkish-brown and translucent colonies

Biochemical Tests

- Oxidase and catalase positive
- Sugar fermentation test—glucose and maltose
- Matrix-assisted laser desorption/ionisation time of flight mass spectrometry (MALDI-ToF) for identification from culture isolate

Serogrouping

- By latex agglutination test.

Molecular Diagnosis

- By multiplex PCR.

---

2. A two-day-old male baby was admitted in a paediatric department of a tertiary-care hospital with fever, listlessness, skin rash, and refusal to feed. There is history of premature rupture of membranes. The baby was meconium stained and did not cry immediately after birth. After 16 hours, he developed fever, irritability, excessive cry, refusal to feed and skin rash. The umbilicus was healthy and there was no focal neurological deficit. The CSF of the baby and the high vaginal swab from the mother were sent to the microbiology laboratory which revealed gram-positive coccobacilli. What is the likely diagnosis? Describe the clinical presentation and lab diagnosis. (1+4 marks)

Likely Diagnosis

- Meningitis caused by *Listeria monocytogenes.*

Clinical Presentation

- Mode of transmission
  - Contaminated food (raw milk, most common)
  - Vertical transmission (mother to foetus)
- Commonly seen in neonates or elderly, immunocompromised individuals
- *Infection in pregnancy:* Before 20 weeks is rare, may lead to abortion, still birth
- *Neonatal disease:* Two types
  1. Early onset
  2. Late onset

- Adult
  - Associated with steroid therapy, HIV, DM, malignancy
  - Bacteraemia > meningitis
  - Most common cause of meningitis in kidney transplanted patient after 1 month
  - Gastroenteritis: Following contaminated milk, meat, and salad

Feature	*Early onset disease*	*Late onset disease*
Onset after delivery	• <5 days	• >5 days
Source of infection	• Intrauterine infection acquired haemato-genously from mother	• Hospital acquired from early onset case, post-natal environmental or maternally acquired during delivery
Site of isolation	• Blood, superficial sites and amniotic fluid	• CSF, rarely blood
Mortality rate	• 30–60%	• 10–12%
• Presentation	• Neonatal sepsis • Granulomatosis infantiseptica occurs rarely	• Neonatal meningitis • Not seen

Lab Diagnosis

Specimen Collection

- CSF, blood in case of meningitis or sepsis, high vaginal swab.
- *For gastroenteritis:* Suspected food, vomitus, stool

Microscopy

- *Gram's stain:* Gram-positive coccobacilli with pus cells
- *Biochemical Identification:* Catalase-positive
- *Motility test:*
  - Shows tumbling type of motility.
  - Motile at 25°C but non-motile at 37°C (Differential motility).
- *Culture.*
  - Growth improves if cultured in thioglycolate broth at 4°C (cold enrichment).
  - *Media:* Blood agar, chocolate agar, PALCAM agar (selective medium): Beta haemolysis seen.
- *Animal inoculation:* Anton test
  - Instillation to rabbit eye results in conjunctivitis.

3. A 4-year-old girl was brought to the emergency room by her parents because of fever and loss of appetite for the past 24 hours and difficulty in arousing her for the past 2 hours. She attended a day care center and had a history of several episodes of presumed viral infections similar to those of other children at the centre. Her childhood immunisations were complete. The CSF Gram's stain picture shows the following. (Fig. 5.3.2).

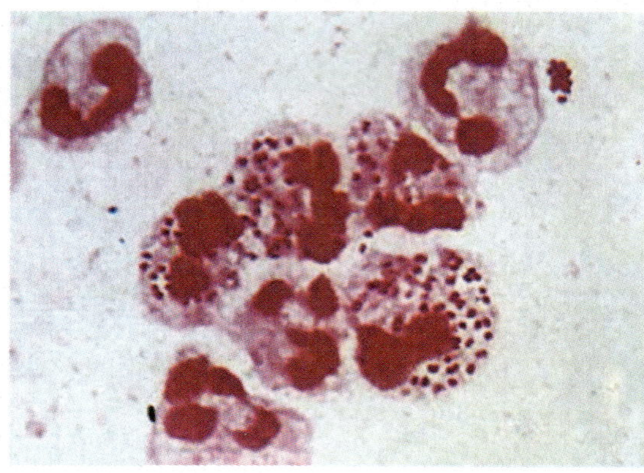

Fig. 5.3.2: CSF Gram's stain

A. What is the clinical diagnosis? (1 mark)

- Meningitis caused by *Neisseria meningitidis.*

B. What is the method for collection of samples? (2 marks)

- CSF is collected by a lumbar puncture using aseptic precautions about 2–3 ml volume and collected in a sterile bottle and transported immediately at room temperature.

C. What are the methods used in the diagnosis? (2 marks)

1. Gram's stain
2. Culture and sensitivity on chocolate agar.
3. Blood and CSF biochemical analysis for protein which is raised; cells predominantly neutrophils and glucose is low.

4. A 40-year-old man who is human immunodeficiency virus (HIV) antibody positive has had a persistent headache and a low-grade fever (temperature, 100°F) for the past 2 weeks. CSF showed the following picture. (Fig. 5.3.3).

A. What is your clinical diagnosis? (1 mark)

- Meningitis caused by *Cryptococcus neoformans.*

B. Which are the staining methods used in the diagnosis? (2 marks)

1. India ink.
2. Periodic acid-Schiff.
3. Mucicarmine stain.

C. Which are the other methods used for diagnosis? (1 mark)

1. SDA culture.
2. Latex agglutination which detects capsular polysaccharide.

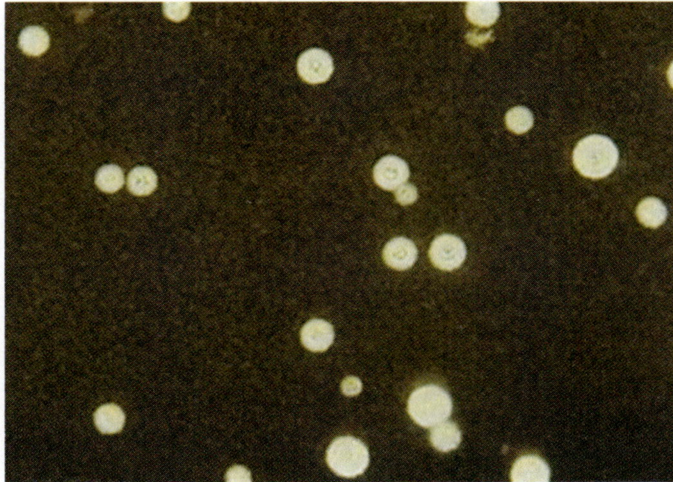

Fig. 5.3.3: CSF

D. Which is the other clinical diagnosis to be kept in mind in this patient? (1 mark)

- Tubercular meningitis.

SHORT ANSWERS

1. Describe in detail about the prophylaxis of meningococcal meningitis. (3 marks)

Vaccine Prophylaxis

- *N meningitides* Polyvalent vaccine contain four groups A, C, Y, W135 or bivalent (serogroups A and C).
- As group B capsule is made up sialic acid residue, which is encephalitogenic and poorly immunogenic, it has not been included in the vaccine.
- *Dose:* Single dose, immunity starts in 10 days, lasts for 3 years.
- Indicated in travelers visiting Hajj, during outbreaks.
- *Contraindications:* Pregnancy and below 3 years (capsule being T independent, is poorly immunogenic <3 years)
- *Chemoprophylaxis among close contacts:* Rifampicin

2. In a case of acute flaccid paralysis due to poliovirus, what are the measures available for prevention of this disease? (1+2 marks)

Methods of Prevention

General Prophylaxis

1. Hand washing
2. Clean food habits
3. Sterilisation of drinking water
4. Environmental sanitation
5. Proper sewage disposal

Specific Prophylaxis

1. **Inactivated killed polio vaccine (Salk)**
   - Contains all 3 types of polio virus inactivated by formalin
   - 4 doses, Intramuscular
   - *Advantages*
     1. Safe in immunocompromised patients
     2. Safe in pregnancy
   - *Disadvantage*
     1. Induces humoural immunity but no local immunity
2. **Oral live polio vaccine**
   - Contains type 1, 2, 3 live attenuated virus grown in primary monkey kidney/human diploid cell culture
   - Given at birth→6 weeks→10 weeks→14 weeks→15–18 months→5 years
   - Dose: 2 drops orally
   - Advantages
     1. Easy to administer
     2. Induces both humoural and intestinal immunity
     3. Herd immunity is produced
     4. Relatively inexpensive
   - Disadvantages
     1. Viral interference by other enteroviruses.
     2. Rare cases of vaccine associated paralytic polio (VAPP)
     3. Frequent diarrhoeal diseases will prevent colonisation

3. Compare and contrast between infections seen in coxsackie A and coxsackie B virus. (3 marks)

Group A coxsackie virus	*Group B coxsackie virus*
• Suckling mouse inoculation • Flaccid paralysis • Generalised myositis	• Suckling mouse inoculation • Spastic paralysis • Focal myositis and necrosis
Manifestations seen (localised)	*Systemic involvement*
• Aseptic meningitis • Herpangina • Hand foot and mouth disease • Acute haemorrhagic conjunctivitis (Coxsackievirus A 24)	• Aseptic meningitis • Pleurodynia • Myocarditis • Hepatitis • Pancreatitis (Coxsackie-virus B4) • Pneumonia • Generalised disease of infants

CHAPTER 6

Respiratory Tract Infections

MI 6.1 DESCRIBE THE AETIOPATHOGENESIS, CLINICAL FEATURES, LABORATORY DIAGNOSIS OF INFECTIONS OF UPPER AND LOWER RESPIRATORY TRACT

LONG ESSAYS

1. An 8-year-old child brought to ENT OPD by her father with history of fever, throat pain for the last 2 days. On examination, the child is running with a fever of 101°F. Throat examination revealed some pustules over the tonsils. Two throat swabs were collected under strict aseptic conditions and were sent to microbiology laboratory. Smear microscopy showed pus cells with gram-positive cocci and short chains.

A. Most probable diagnosis of the above case and bacteria causing the condition. (2 marks)

Most Probable Diagnosis

- Bacterial pharyngitis.

Bacteria Causing the Condition

- *Streptococcus pyogenes* (GAS).

B. Enumerate the infections of URT and LRT with aetiology. (4 marks)

Infections of URT

Type of infection	*Viral aetiology*	*Bacterial aetiology*
Pharyngitis	• Echovirus • Coxsackie A • Adenovirus • Epstein–Barr virus	• *Streptococcus pyogenes* • *C diphtheria* • *Neisseria meningitidis*
Common cold (Coryza)	• Rhinovirus • Coronavirus	–
Acute epiglottitis	• *H. influenzae* type b	• *Streptococcus pyogenes*
Ludwig's angina	–	• *Streptococcus pyogenes* • *Staphylococcus aureus* • *Prevotella melaninogenicus* • *Fusobacterium* spp
Vincent's angina	–	• *Leptotrichia buccalis* • *Borrelia vincentii*
Laryngitis	• Influenza • Parainfluenza virus	–
Acute laryngo-tracheo-bronchitis (croup)	• Parainfluenza virus	–

Contd.

Infections of LRT

Type of infection	*Viral aetiology*	*Bacterial aetiology*
Bronchitis	• Rhinoviruses and corona-viruses	• *H. influenzae* • *Mycoplasma pneumonia* • *S. pneumoniae*
Bronchiolitis	• Respiratory syncytial virus	• *Mycoplasma pneumonia*
Pneumonia	• Influenza • Coronavirus	• *S. pneumoniae,* • *K. pneumoniae* • *Legionella* spp. • *Chlamydophila pneumoniae*

C. Symptoms of URTIs and laboratory diagnosis with respect to bacterial aetiology. (4 marks)

Symptoms of URTI

- Common cold, fever, runny nose, redness of eyes.
- Pharyngitis, sore throat, swollen lymphnodes, difficulty in swallowing.
- Respiratory tract obstruction, difficulty in breathing.

Laboratory Diagnosis

Specimen Collection

- Throat swabs are taken from each of tonsils and the posterior pharyngeal wall without touching the tongue or the buccal mucosa, nasopharyngeal or nasal washings.

Microscopy

1. **Gram stain**
   - *Group A Streptococcus (GAS):* Gram-positive cocci in short chains
   - *Vincent's angina: Leptotrichia buccalis, Borrelia vincentii*-long fusiform and spiral bacilli
2. **Alberts's stain**
   - *Corynebacterium diphtheriae:* Green bacilli with metachromatic granules arranged in Chinese letter pattern

Culture

- *Blood agar:* Haemolytic colonies of GAS
- *Potassium tellurite agar:* Black metallic sheen colonies of CD
- *Vincent's angina:* Anaerobic culture methods

For GAS

- Positive rapid streptococcal antigen test.

Virulence testing for Corynebacterium diphtheriae

- *In vivo*—in animals.
- *In vitro*—ELEK`s gel precipitation.

---

2. An 8-year-old child brought to ED with history of fever, throat pain. O/E, the child had fever, was toxic and revealed white membrane over the tonsils which bleed on touch. The child was covered with only at birth vaccine schedule.

A. What is the clinical diagnosis? Name the aetiological agent causing this condition. (2 marks)

Clinical Diagnosis

- Diphtheria.

Aetiological Agent

- *Corynebacterium diphtheriae.*

B. What is the key virulence factor, its role, and clinical features of this condition? (1+3 marks)

Key Virulence Factor and its Role

- Exotoxin production depends on the presence of a lysogenic β phage, which carries the gene encoding for toxin (tox+).
- The toxin consists of 2 fragments:
  1. *Binding unit:* Receptor domain triggers the entry of toxin into cell through receptor mediated endocytosis.
  2. *Active unit:* ADP ribosylation- transfer of ADP—ribose from NAD to the eukaryotic elongation factor—2 (EF -2).
- The EF—2 is required for the translocation of polypeptidyl—transfer RNA from the acceptor to the donor site of eukaryotic ribosome.

Clinical Features

Source of Infection

- Infected patients or asymptomatic normal carrier.

Mode of Transmission

- Inhalation of aerosolised droplets.
- By direct contact with either respiratory secretions or exudates from infected skin lesion.

Pharyngeal and Tonsillar Diphtheria

- Exudate spreads within 2–3 days and may form adherent membrane
- Membrane may cause respiratory obstruction
- Fever usually not high but patient appears toxic.

Malignant or Hypertoxic

- Severe toxaemia with adenitis (bullneck)
- Death is due to circulatory failure
- Paralytic sequelae are common.

Septic

- Ulceration
- Cellulitis
- Gangrene around the pseudomembrane.

Haemorrhagic

- Bleeding from the edge of the membrane
- Epistaxis
- Conjunctival haemorrhage
- Purpura.

Complications

- Mostly attributes to the toxin
- Extent of local disease is related to severity
- Most common complications are myocarditis and neuritis
- Death occurs in 5–10% for respiratory disease.

C. Discuss the lab diagnosis and management of this condition. (2+2 marks)

Lab Diagnosis

Specimen Collection

- Throat swab
- Nasopharyngeal swab
- Wound swab

Transportation

- The swab should be transported in semisolid transport media such as Amies.

Microscopy

1. *Gram stain*
   - Pleomorphic gram-positive bacillus which is club shaped.
2. *Methylene blue*: Blue pus cells with blue bacilli.
3. *Albert's stain*
   - Green bacilli typically contain granules of polymerised polymetaphosphate called *Volutin granules/Metachromatic granules/Babes Ernst granules/Polar bodies.*

Culture

1. ***Sheep blood agar:*** Grey, white colonies with narrow zone of beta haemolysis.
2. ***Tellurite blood agar:*** Colonies appear black.
3. ***Loeffler's serum slope:*** Metachromatic granules are well developed.

Virulence Test

In Vivo

- Subcutaneously culture emulsions injected into two guinea pigs—one with antidiphtheric toxin and another without → the unprotected animals die.
- Intracutaneously injected the culture emulsions into two guinea pigs.
  - One with anti-toxin given on previous day acts as control
  - Second guinea pig—4 hours after the intracutaneous injection develops reaction at the site of injection only.

In Vitro

- Elek's gel precipitation test.
  - Demonstrates toxin production.
  - The organism is streaked on a plate containing low iron.
  - A filter strip containing antitoxin antibody is placed perpendicular to the streak of the organism.
  - Diffusion of the antibody and secretion of the toxin into the medium occur.
  - At the zone of equivalence, a precipitate will form.

Management

- Protection of the threatened airway by emergency tracheostomy or endotracheal intubation.
- Immediate administration of antitoxin given IM or IV (10,000 to 1,00,000 units).
- *Antibiotics:* Penicillin or erythromycin

---

3. A 60-year-old male with history of alcoholism admitted in a tertiary care hospital with history of non-productive cough, chest pain, and shortness of breath for the last 4 days. Clinical examination revealed dullness over left 6th intercostal space on percussion, abnormal breath sounds in the form of crepitations over left 6th intercostal space on auscultation. CXR depicted clear homology with ground-glass opacity in the left lower lobe. Clinician suspected it to be a case of atypical pneumonia.

A. Enumerate the causative agents of atypical pneumonia. (2 marks)

Bacterial Aetiology

1. *Mycoplasma pneumoniae*
2. *Chlamydophila pneumoniae*
3. *Legionella pneumophila*
4. *Chlamydophila psittaci*
5. *Coxiella burnetii*
6. *Francisella tularensis*

Viral Aetiology

1. Influenza A and B
2. Parainfluenza (types 1–3)
3. Respiratory syncytial virus (RSV)
4. Adenovirus (types 3, 4 and 7)
5. Measles
6. Cytomegalovirus
7. Varicella-zoster virus

Fungal Aetiology

1. *Pneumocystis jirovecii*
2. *Coccidioides immitis*
3. *Histoplasma capsulatum*

B. Distinguish between typical and atypical pneumonia. (2 marks)

Feature	*Typical pneumonia*	*Atypical pneumonia*
Age	• Patients usually present in extremes of ages • Less common in the young	• More common in young
Clinical settings	• Wards/ inpatients/ICU	• Ambulatory patients (OPD)

Contd.

Feature	Typical pneumonia	Atypical pneumonia
Presentation	• Pulmonary disease with mucopurulent sputum, pleural effusion • CXR: Lobar, parenchymal	• Mild pulmonary disease with extrapulmonary component • CXR: Nonlobar, patchy, interstitial pneumonia
Identification	• Cause easily identifiable using routine Gram's stain and culture	• Failure to identify causative organism using routine Gram's stain and culture
Treatment	• Respond to conventional antimicrobial agents	• No response to conventional antimicrobials used in bacterial pneumonia

C. Describe in detail the important bacterial pathogens causing atypical pneumonia. (10 marks)

Important Bacterial Pathogens Causing Atypical Pneumonia

1. *Mycoplasma pneumoniae.*
2. *Chlamydophila pneumoniae.*
3. *Legionella pneumophila.*

1. *Mycoplasma pneumoniae.*

Route of Infection

- Droplet infection.

Incubation Period

- 2–4 weeks.

Population

- **Sporadic:** children, adults

Epidemics

- Closed populations.

Virulence Factors

Mediator	Action
• Interactive adhesins • Accessory proteins on organelle	• Attachment (cytoadherence)
• H_2O_2 mediated killing • ADP-ribosylating and vacuolating cytotoxin	• Injury
• Cell membrane lipoproteins	• Inflammation • Host response

Pathogenesis

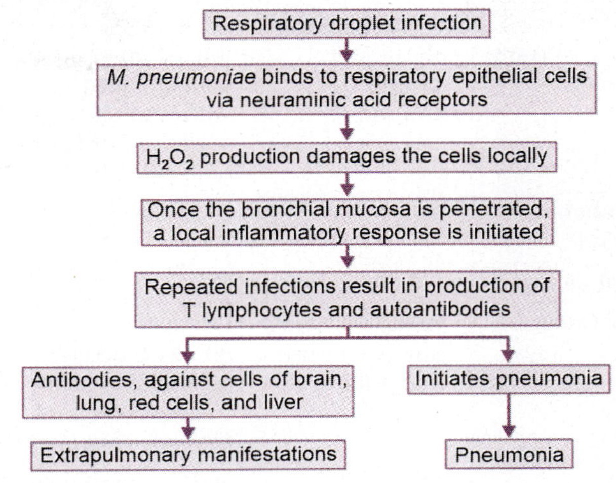

Clinical Manifestations

Constitutional Symptoms

- Headache, malaise, chills, fever.

Pulmonary Symptoms

- Upper respiratory tract symptoms.
  - *Initial:* Sore throat.
  - *Most common:* Cough (non-productive).
  - *High diagnostic value:* Otitis media (± bullous myringitis).

Extrapulmonary Features

Neurological	• Meningoencephalitis • Encephalitis • GBS • Aseptic meningitis
Dermatological	• Erythema multiforme • Erythematous maculopapular/vesicular/petechial/urticarial rash
Cardiac	• Myocarditis • Pericarditis
Rheumatological	• Septic arthritis • Reactive arthritis
Haematological	• Haemolytic anaemia • Aplastic anaemia • Cold agglutinins • DIC • Hypercoagulopathy

2. *Chlamydia*

Feature	*Chlamydia pneumoniae*	*Chlamydia psittaci*
Source of infection	• Human	• Infected psittacine and ornithine birds and their faeces

Contd.

Feature	*Chlamydia pneumoniae*	*Chlamydia psittaci*
Mode of transmission	• Respiratory droplets • (Airborne)	• Inhalation of dust contaminated with respiratory secretions or faeces of infected birds
Incubation period	• 1–3 weeks	• 5–15 days
Host factors	• Elderly	• Elderly
Risk factors	• Associated with atherosclerosis and asthma	• Occupational: poultry workers, pigeon farmers, pet shop owners, bird fanciers, veterinarians
Clinical manifestations	• Pharyngitis, sometimes followed by laryngitis, bronchitis, or interstitial bronchitis • Associated with adult-onset asthma	• Sudden onset with constitutional symptoms • Bilateral patchy pulmonary infiltration • Extrapulmonary manifestations- Liver, heart, spleen, and kidney are often enlarged and congested
Disease	• Pneumonia	• Psittacosis

Life Cycle (Fig. 6.1.1)

- Elementary body (EB), reticulate body (RB)

3. *Legionella pneumophila*

Source of Infection

- Water sources (air conditioners, water cooling towers, shower heads).

Mode of Transmission

- Aerosolised particles (inhalation or aspiration).
- Direct inoculation by respiratory therapy equipment.
- No human-to-human transmission.

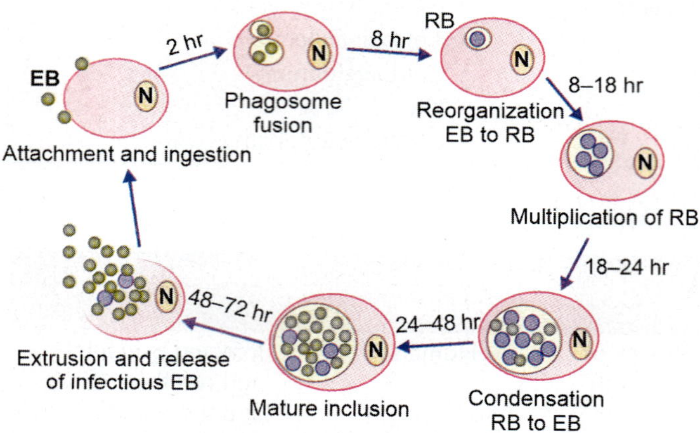

Fig. 6.1.1: Life cycle of *Chlamydia*

Incubation Period

- 2–10 days.

Host Factors

- Ageing > 55 years
- Peaks in 60–70-years age group
- Middle-to-old age—more prone

Risk Factors

- Seen in individuals associated with comorbidities.

Sequence of Events

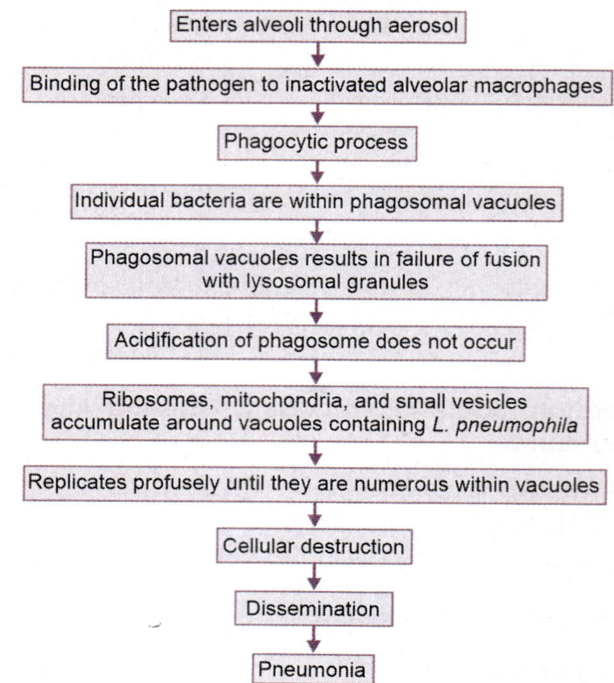

Clinical Features in Legionnaire's Disease

- More severe than other atypical pneumonias.

Constitutional Symptoms

- Malaise, fever (high grade), headache

Pulmonary Symptoms

- Slightly productive cough
- Haemoptysis
- Pleuritic/non-pleuritic chest pain
- Shortness of breath

Extrapulmonary Manifestations

Site	Clinical manifestation
Gastrointestinal	• Watery diarrhoea, abdominal pain, nausea
Neurological	• Confusion, headache • Encephalopathy (rare)
CVS	• Relative bradycardia
Others	• Hyponatraemia, elevated liver enzymes • Haematuria, proteinuria

Lab Diagnosis

Specimen Collection

1. *Sputum: Legionella* infection.
2. *Nasopharyngeal swab: M. pneumoniae* and *C. pneumoniae.*
3. *Bronchoalveolar lavage fluid: Legionella* and *M. pneumoniae* infection
4. *Lung biopsy specimen: Legionella*
5. *Blood: M. pneumoniae, Chlamydiae* and *Legionella.*
6. *Urine: Legionella*

Microscopy

- *Gram's stain* shows plenty of pus cells and no organism or poorly staining gram-negative bacilli.
- Tissue section can be stained by *Silver or Giemsa stain.*
- *Direct fluorescent antibody (DFA)* is used in *Legionella pneumophila* and *Chlamydia.*

Culture

Organisms	*Media*	*Colony Morphology*
M. pneumoniae	• SP4 broth	• Grainy yellowish with thin outer layer, "fried egg appearance"
C. pneumoniae	• HeLa and Hep2 cell lines	• Inclusions detected by fluorescent antibody staining with genus or *C. pneumoniae* specific monoclonal antibody conjugated with fluorescein
L. pneumophila	• Buffered Charcoal Yeast Extract agar (BCYE) with or without antibiotics	• "Cut glass" appearance (grey white to blue green, glistening, convex circular)

Serological Assays

Pathogen	*Test*
Mycoplasma pneumoniae	• Complement fixation test (CFT) • IgM by latex agglutination/ ELISA/Indirect IF
Legionella pneumophila	• Urinary antigen test or rapid microagglutination test
Chlamydophila pneumonia *Chlamydophila psittaci*	• IgM or IgG—Micro immunofluorescence • ELISA using species—specific antigens

Molecular Methods

- DNA probe hybridisation or amplification by PCR are used for rapid identification of specific microorganisms from clinical samples.

Treatment

Causative microbe	*Preferred antimicrobial therapy*
Mycoplasma pneumoniae	• Tetracycline (doxycycline) or macrolide (erythromycin)
Chlamydia	• Doxycycline or azithromycin (adults) • Erythromycin
Legionella	• Erythromycin (IV, high dose) • A macrolide with or without rifampin (severe cases) • Tetracycline

4. A 45-year-old woman presented with 10-day h/o of right-sided facial pain radiating to the right ear, heaviness in her head. She has also recently been diagnosed with diabetes mellitus. On examination, facial swelling and eschar present over right side.

A. What is the most probable diagnosis. (1 mark)

- Mucormycosis.

B. Risk factors, pathogenesis, and clinical presentation seen with this pathogen. (1+1+1 marks)

Risk Factors

1. Diabetes mellitus (ketoacidosis)
2. Leukemias
3. Corticosteroid therapy
4. Intravenous therapy
5. Severe burns

Pathogenesis

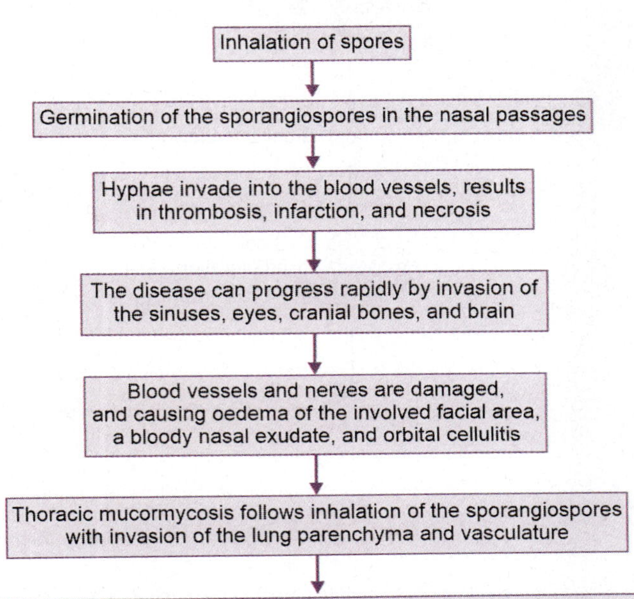

Clinical Presentation

- Rhinocerebral
  - Nose, paranasal sinuses, eye, brain, and meninges are involved
  - Orbital cellulitis
- Thoracic
  - Pulmonary lesions, parenchymal necrosis.
- Local.
  - Post traumatic.
  - Kidney infections.
  - Skin infection following burns or surgery.

C. Laboratory work-up with appropriate sample collection, microscopy and culture characteristics of this pathogen. (5 marks)

Sample Collection

- Sputum, BAL, biopsy of paranasal sinuses.

Microscopy

- *Direct examination on KOH mount:* Non-septate, ribbon-like hyphae which branch at right angles, sporangium
- *Histopathology:* broad, non-septate hyphae, branching angle greater than 90°

Culture

- *Sabouraud dextrose agar (SDA):* cotton candy appearance, fluffy cotton like growth
- *Species:* Mucor, Rhizopus, Absidia

5. Describe the properties, pathogenesis, clinical features (of the URT) of Epstein Barr virus infection and the associated malignancies. (2+3+2+3 marks)

Properties

- ds DNA, enveloped, multiplies in the nucleus of lymphoid cells specially B cells.
- Antigens.
  1. Viral capsid antigens (VCA)—used as diagnostic tool.
  2. Early antigens.
  3. Late antigens.
- EBV infects mainly lymphoid cells, primarily B lymphocytes.

Pathogenesis

- *Source of infection:* Patient active/reactivation
- *Mode of transmission:* contact—saliva
- *Sequence of events* (Fig. 6.1.2).

Clinical Features

See Figure 6.1.3

Associated Malignancies

1. Burkitt's lymphoma—2 types:
   - Epidemic
   - Sporadic
2. EBV associated nasopharyngeal carcinoma
3. Hodgkin's and non-Hodgkin's lymphoma

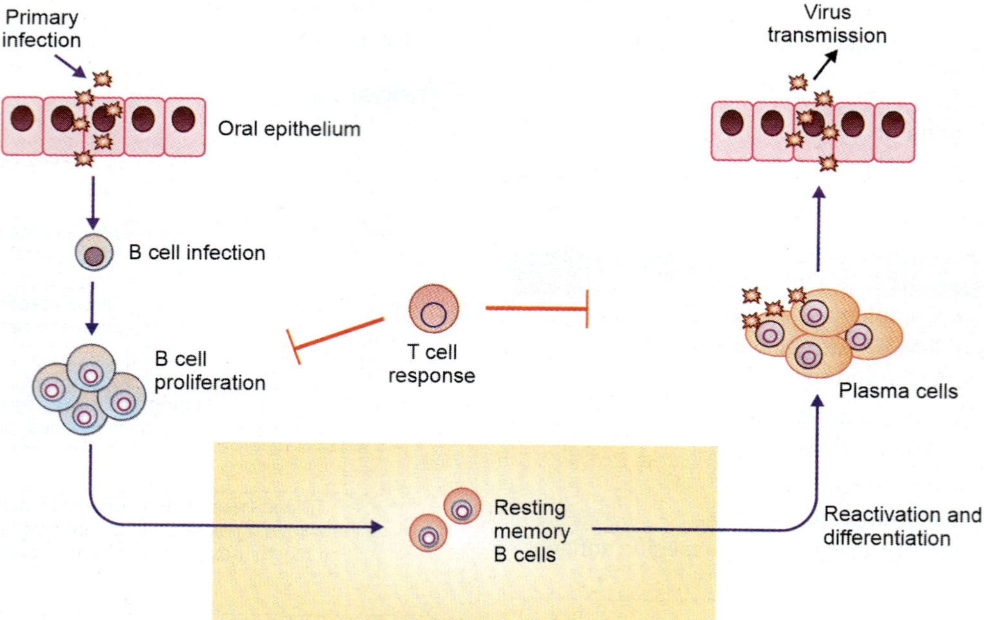

Fig. 6.1.2: Sequence of events in the pathogenesis of Epstein–Barr virus infection

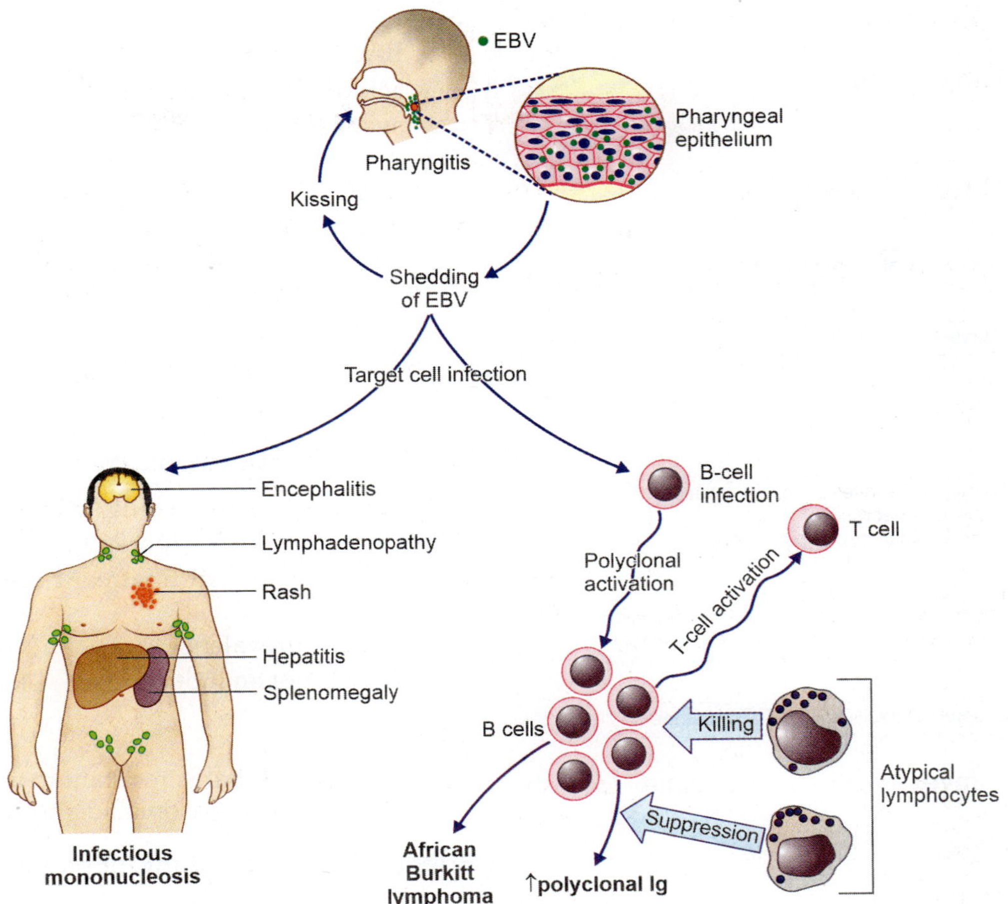

Fig. 6.1.3: Clinical features seen in the Epstein–Barr virus infection

4. Lymphoproliferative changes—immunodeficient
   - Diffuse polyclonal lymphoma
   - Lymphocytic interstitial pneumonia
   - Hairy leukoplakia of tongue

6. Raju, a 35-year-old chronic smoker admitted to the hospital with low grade fever, loss of weight and chronic cough of 2 months duration. Sputum examination revealed acid fast bacilli.

A. What is your provisional diagnosis? (1 mark)

- Pulmonary tuberculosis.

B. Discuss the pathogenesis of this condition. (3 marks)

Pathogenesis

Causative Agents

- *Mycobacterium tuberculosis* complex which includes:
  1. *Mycobacterium tuberculosis*
  2. *Mycobacterium bovis*
  3. *Mycobacterium africanum*
  4. *Mycobacterium microti*

Virulence Factors

1. **Intra-cellular survival.**
   - Mycobacterium produces a protein called "exported repetitive protein" that prevents the phagosome-lysosome fusion.
2. **Cord factor (trehalose-6–6-dimycolate).**
   - Inhibits the migration of leucocytes.
   - Causes chronic granuloma.
3. **Lipids.**
   - Mycolic acids results in granuloma formation.
   - Phospholipids also induce caseous necrosis.
   - Lipoarabinomannan inhibits IFN-γ mediated activation of macrophages and suppression of T-cell proliferation.

Sources of Infection

- Open case of tuberculosis
- Live cultures of the organisms
- Clinical specimens
- Cattles suffering from tuberculosis and their milk.

Modes of Transmission

- Inhalation of respiratory droplet nuclei (1–5 µm) produced during coughing, sneezing, etc.

- Consumption of unpasteurised milk from infected cattle.
- Inoculation into the skin.

Sequence of Events

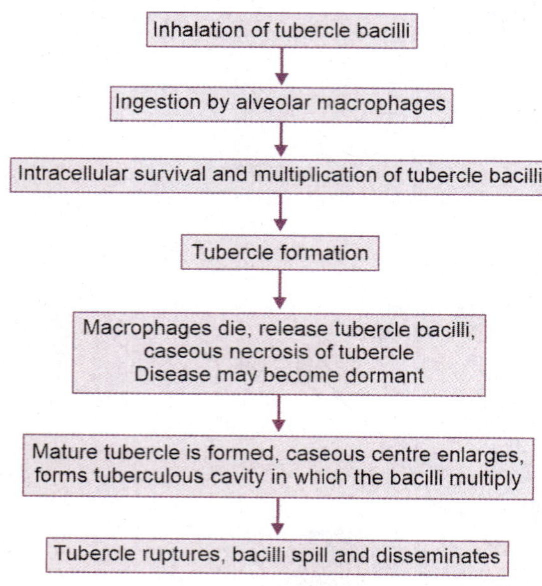

C. Laboratory investigations available for this condition. (4 marks)

Specimen Collection

- For pulmonary tuberculosis:
  - Sputum (2 samples)
  - Difficult to bring out sputum-induced sputum
  - Bronchoalveolar lavage
  - Gastric aspirates
  - Laryngeal swab

Microscopy

- Ziehl–Neelsen (ZN) method (hot method): Acid fast bacilli seen
- Gabbet's method (cold method): Acid fast bacilli seen
- Fluorescent method (Auramine-rhodamine dye): bright fluorescent yellow bacilli

Culture

- Isolation of *Mycobacterium* from the clinical sample remains a gold standard method.
- Contaminated specimens (sputum, urine) require concentration.
- *Modified Petroff's method:* Uses 4% NaOH solution
- N-acetyl L-cysteine method
- Solid media for culture
  - Egg based L-J medium
  - *M. tuberculosis* colony morphology: Rough, tough, and buff colonies
- Agar based
  - Middlebrook 7H10 and7H11
- Liquid media
  - BACTEC 12B medium
  - Middlebrook 7H9 broth
- Newer culture methods
  - Automated continuously monitored systems (BACTEC9000MB, and BACTEC MIGIT): Uses fluorescence quenching system
  - BacT/ALERT uses colourimetric carbon dioxide sensor in each bottle to detect growth: Use broth similar to 7H9 supplemented with

D. Add a note on drug resistance in this aetiological agent. (2 marks)

Risk Factors for Development of MDR-TB

1. Previously unsuccessful TB treatment
2. Interruption of TB therapy
3. Inappropriate TB treatment regimen, dose and duration
4. High TB prevalence
5. HIV+ is not an independent risk factor.

MDR-TB

- MDR-TB is TB that is resistant to at least two of the best anti TB drugs, isoniazid and rifampicin.

Extensively Drug-resistant Tuberculosis (XDRTB)

- TB which is resistant to isoniazid and rifampicin, plus resistant to any fluoroquinolone and at least one of three injectable second line drugs (i.e. amikacin, kanamycin capreomycin).

Methods Used in Detection of Drug Resistance

- Done on solid (LJ, Middlebrook) and liquid media (Bactec 460TB, MGIT).
- Antibiotic proportion method is ideal.
- Detection of drug resistance gene.
- Line probe assays-InnoLipa, Genotype MTBDR, Xpert TB.

---

7. An 80-year-old female presented with severe symptoms of lower respiratory tract infections. There was a history of exposure with her neighbour with similar complaints. Nasopharyngeal swab was collected and sent for evaluation for real-time PCR which was identified as Influenza A/H1N1.

A. Discuss the pathogenesis, clinical manifestations, and lab diagnosis of this aetiological agent. (2+3+2 marks)

Pathogenesis

Incubation Period

- 18–72 hours.

Source of Infection

- Infected persons who shed large number of viruses in their saliva and respiratory secretion.
- Infected bird droppings, faeces of infected animals.

Mode of Transmission

- Mainly by inhalation, by contact.

Sequence of Events

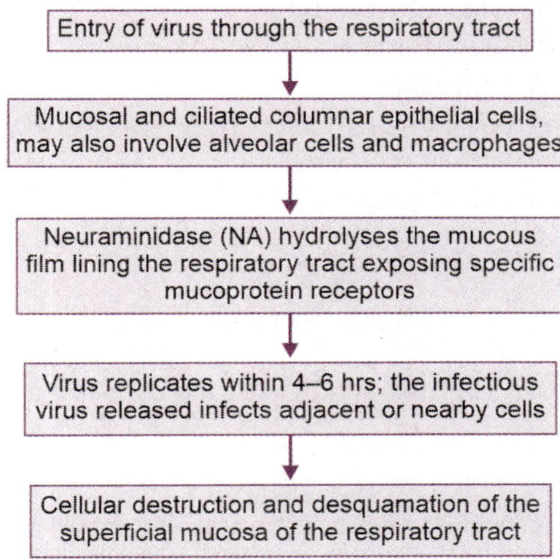

Clinical Manifestations

- *Uncomplicated influenza:* Abrupt onset with chills, headache, dry cough, fever, myalgia, generalised muscular aches and anorexia
- Pulmonary manifestations
  - Croup (acute laryngotracheobronchitis) in young children
  - Symptoms—cough, difficulty in breathing, stridor
  - Primary influenza pneumonia
  - Secondary bacterial pneumonia by *S. aureus*, *S. pneumoniae*, *H. influenzae*

Lab Diagnosis

Specimen Collection

- Throat gargling/ nasal washing/nasopharyngeal swabs
- Serum for serology.

Transport

- Viral transport media (VTM) at 4°C.

Microscopy

- *Direct detection of viral antigen:* By immune electron microscopy and Immunofluorescence.

Culture

- *Isolation and identification by culture:* For primary culture: Primary monkey kidney cells
- *For continuous cell line:* Madin—Darby canine kidney cell line
- *Embryonated chicken egg:* Amniotic cavity
- CPE is characterised by prominent refractile enlarged cells of various shapes, which appears randomly over the monolayer. Debris from disintegrated cells can be found floating in the medium.
- Viruses can be identified by testing the culture fluid for haemagglutination after 5–7 days and by haemadsorption after 3–5 days.

Serology

- *Haemagglutination inhibition, neutralisation, complement fixation and ELISA:* Paired sera and four-fold rise in titre
- Rapid tests:
  1. Flu OIA (Flu optical immunoassay)
  2. Zstat flu

Molecular Method

- By reverse transcriptase PCR.

B. What are the prophylactic measures available and infection control practices in the care of this patient? (3 marks)

General Methods

- Standard infection control measures against influenza like covering the nose and mouth while coughing
- Frequent washing of hands with soap and water or with alcohol-based hand sanitisers
- Avoid touching of eyes, nose, or mouth often
- Social distancing.

Chemoprophylaxis

- Three of the drugs rimantadine, amantadine and oseltamivir can be used in elderly people who have not been immunised or have not been exposed.
- Vaccination
  - A mixture containing two type A viruses and a type B virus of the strains isolated in the previous winter outbreak
  - Indications for vaccination
    1. Individuals at high-risk group (old, debilitated people)
    2. People in closed community
    3. Health care workers.
- Vaccines are either:
  1. Whole virus (WV) vaccine which contains intact, inactivated virus
  2. Surface antigen vaccines contains purified HA and NA glycoproteins
  3. Subvirion (SV) vaccine contains purified virus disrupted with detergents.
- *Inactivated influenza vaccines*
  - Inactivated with formalin or β propiolactone and standardized according to haemagglutinin content

- *Route of administration:* IM
- *Dosage:* one dose containing approximately 15 μg of HA is given, 2nd dose of vaccine given at interval of 3–4 weeks
- *Contraindication:* People who have allergy to eggs or have history of hypersensitivity to previous dose

- *Live attenuated influenza vaccines*
  - A live attenuated, cold-adapted temperature sensitive, trivalent influenza virus vaccine administered by nasal spray.
  - The cold adapted donor virus can grow at 25°C but not at 37°C.
  - Its multiplication stimulates the local production of IgA.
  - *Contraindication:* Pregnant ladies, immuno-suppressed individuals.

8. A 32-year-old man came to the emergency department with c/o fever and pain in his left chest when he coughed along with severe chills and sweating. Five days earlier, he had developed signs of a viral upper respiratory infection with sore throat, runny nose, and increased cough. Further he had a history of drinking moderate to heavy amounts of alcohol and smoking one package of cigarettes daily for about 15 years. On investigation, WBC count was elevated with 80% neutrophils. Gram-stain of sputum revealed lancet shaped gram-positive diplococci. What is your likely diagnosis? Describe the pathogenesis, clinical findings, complications of this condition. What other investigations are required in diagnosis and treatment?

(1+3+1+1+4 marks)

Likely Diagnosis

- Bacterial pneumonia caused by *S pneumoniae.*

Pathogenesis

Predisposing Factors

- Viral and other respiratory tract infections
- Bronchial obstruction and respiratory tract injury
- Alcohol or drug intoxication
- Abnormal circulatory dynamics (pulmonary congestion, heart failure)
- Malnutrition, sickle cell anaemia, hyposplenism, nephrosis and complement deficiency.

Source of Infection

- Patients or carriers.

Mode of Transmission

- Aerosols.

Virulence Factors

1. **Capsular polysaccharide antigen**
   - Major virulence factor, non-capsulated strains are avirulent
   - Antiphagocytic activity.
2. **Pneumolysin**
   - A hemolysin, cytotoxic action, activates complement.
3. **Lipoteichoic acid**
   - Activates complement
   - Induces inflammatory cytokine production.
4. **s-Ig A Protease**
   - Destroys secretory IgA present on the respiratory mucosal surface, thus overcoming local immunity.

Sequence of Events

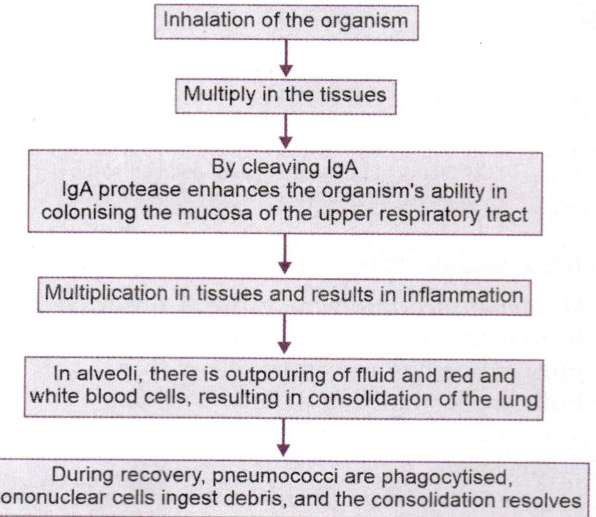

Clinical Findings

- *Most common cause:* Lobar and bronchopneumonia
- They also cause acute tracheobronchitis and empyema.
- Pneumonia is usually sudden with fever, chills, and sharp pleural pain.
- The sputum—bloody or rusty coloured.
- From the respiratory tract it can reach other sites: otitis media, sinusitis, or conjunctivitis —in children
- Meningitis secondary to pneumonia, all ages.
- Bacteraemia from pneumonia has a triad of severe complications—meningitis, endocarditis, and septic arthritis.

Complications

- Suppurative lesions in other parts of the body, usually as complications of pneumonia.
  1. Suppurative arthritis
  2. Conjunctivitis, dacryocystitis
  3. Peritonitis
- Rarely endocarditis, pericarditis.

Other Investigations Required

Specimen Collection

- Depending on site of involvement:
  - Sputum
  - Blood

Microscopy

Gram-stained Smear (Fig. 6.1.4)

- Pneumococci are seen as gram-positive lancet or flame shaped (lanceolate) cocci in pairs surrounded by unstained capsule along with pus cells.

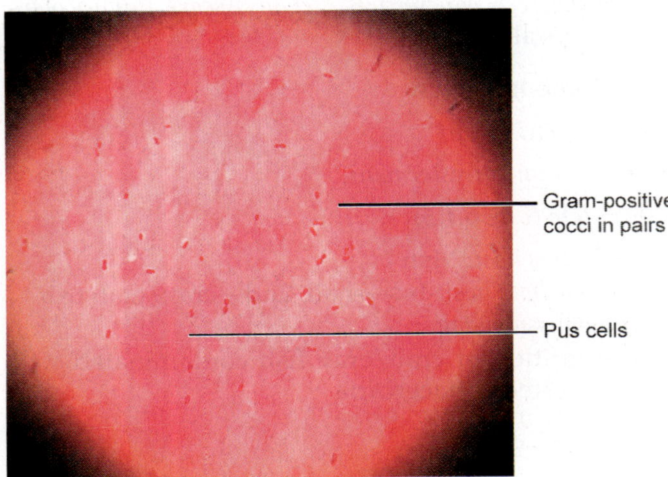

Fig. 6.1.4: Gram-positive cocci in pairs with pus cells

Capsule Demonstration

- By negative staining—India ink or Nigrosin—capsule may be demonstrated as clear halo.
- Quellung reaction (Capsule swelling reaction).

Culture

- *Media used:* Blood agar, chocolate agar—alpha haemolytic colonies dome shaped initially which further has 'Draughtsman' appearance

Bile Solubility Test

- Positive

Optochin Sensitivity Test

- Sensitive

Animal Pathogenicity Test

- Virulent to mouse.

Other Tests

1. C-reactive protein
2. CXR: Lobar pneumonia

SHORT ESSAYS

1. Mention the fungi causing pneumonia. Describe in detail about pulmonary aspergillosis. (2+4 marks)

Fungi Causing Pneumonia

1. *Pneumocystis jirovecii*—pneumonia PCP
2. Zygomycetes—*Mucor*—Zygomycoses
3. *Aspergillus* spp—Aspergillosis
4. *Penicillium* spp—Penicilliosis
5. *Cryptococcus neoformans*—Pulmonary cryptococcosis
6. Systemic mycoses—*Histoplasma* spp, *Coccidioides immitis, Blastomyces dermatitidis, Paracoccidioides brasiliences.*

Pulmonary Aspergillosis

Pathogenesis

Source

- Dust, soil, decomposing organic matter.

Mode of Transmission

- Inhalation of spores.

Sequence of Events

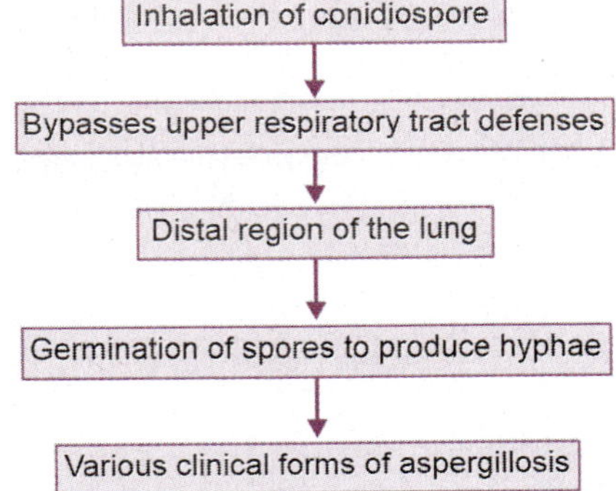

Clinical Presentation

- It is an opportunistic pathogen
- *Invasive aspergillosis:* In immunocompromised patients, invasive disease occurs where the organism invades blood vessels, causing thrombosis and infarction.
- *Aspergilloma:* A person with a lung cavity (e.g. from tuberculosis) may develop a "fungal ball".
- *Otomycosis:* Commonly caused by *Aspergillus niger*
- *Acute bronchopulmonary aspergillosis (ABPA):* An allergic (hypersensitive) person (e.g., one with asthma) is predisposed to this condition mediated by IgE antibody.

Laboratory Work-up

Specimen Collection

- BAL, Sputum, tissue.

Microscopy

- *KOH mount:*
  - Septate hyphae with acute angle branching.
  - Invasion distinguishes disease from colonisation.

Culture Morphology on Sabourad's Agar

Aspergillus species	*Macroscopic features*	*Microscopic features*
A. fumigatus	• Smoky green, velvety to powdery	• Conidia arise only in upper third of conical shaped vesicle • Phialides single row
A. flavus	• Yellow to green velvety	• Conidia arise from upper two third of globular shaped vesicle • Phialides two rows
A. niger	• Black powdery	• Conidia arise from upper two third of globular shaped vesicle • Phialides two rows. Black conidia

Serology

- Antigen detection.
  - *β-d Glucan antigen assay:* Raised in invasive aspergillosis
  - *Galactomannan antigen*: ELISA for early diagnosis.

2. Enumerate the parasites causing pulmonary infections. Describe in detail about the life cycle, clinical features, lab diagnosis and treatment of lung fluke infection. (2+2+1+2+1 marks)

Parasites Causing Pulmonary Infections

1. *Paragonimus westermani:* Pneumonia, lung abscess
2. *Wuchereria bancrofti, B. malayi, Ascaris lumbricoides:* Tropical eosinophilia

Lung Fluke Infection

Aetiological Agent

- *Paragonimus westermani.*

Life Cycle (Fig. 6.1.5)

- *Definitive host:* Man
- *Intermediate host:* 1st—snail, 2nd—cray/crab fish
- *Transmission stage:*
  - Ingestion of crab/cray fish contaminated with encysted metacercaria

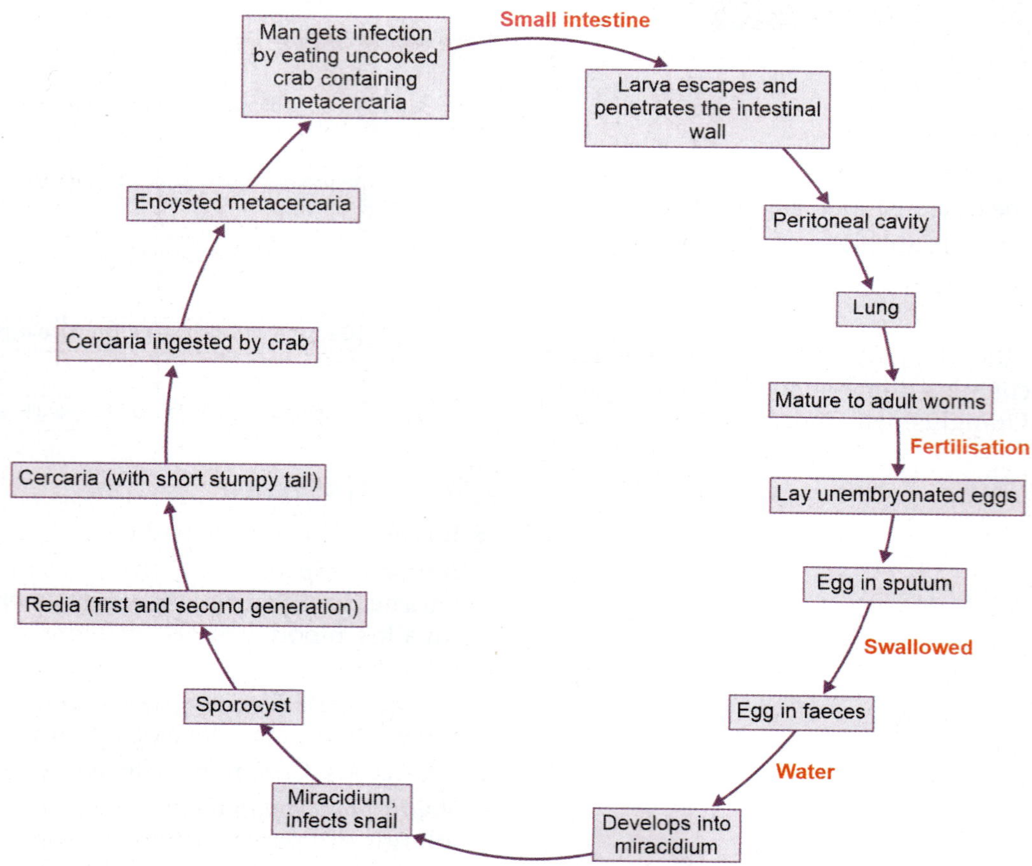

Fig. 6.1.5: Life cycle of *Paragonimus westermani*

- Cyst in right lung (eosinophilic granuloma formation due to egg deposition)
- *Diagnostic stage:* Operculated eggs

Clinical Features

- Productive cough with brownish blood-tinged sputum with offensive fishy odour.
- **In chronic infections:** bronchitis, bronchiectasis, pneumonia, and lung abscess may be seen.
- Cerebral and cutaneous paragonimiasis—seen in severe cases.

Lab Diagnosis

Specimen Collection

- Early morning sputum (multiple specimens required), stool in children

Concentration of Sputum

- Formalin-ether sedimentation.

Microscopy

- *Saline mount:* Operculated eggs, golden brown, unembryonated

Serology

- Antibody detection—ELISA or Western blot
- Antigen detection by ELISA
- Increased eosinophils

Radiology

- MRI or CT to locate cysts
- *Chest X-ray:* Cavity or patchy densities, effusion

Treatment

- Praziquantel—Drug of choice
- Surgical excision for pulmonary/cerebral lesions

3. Discuss the laboratory diagnosis of streptococcal sore throat and the possible complications post infection. (3+2 marks)

Laboratory Diagnosis

Specimen Collection

- Pus, exudate, throat swab from lesion

Transport Medium

- Pike's medium

Direct Smear Microscopy

- Pus cells with gram-positive cocci in short chains.

Culture

- *Blood agar:* Pinpoint colony with a wide zone of β-haemolysis
- *Selective media:* Crystal violet blood agar and PNF (polymyxin B, neomycin, fusidic acid) media
- *Liquid media:* Granular turbidity with powdery deposit

Biochemical Identification

- Catalase negative
- Bacitracin sensitive
- Pyrrolidonyl arylamidase (PYR) test is positive

Typing

- *Lancefield grouping:* shows group A *Streptococcus*
- *Typing of group A Streptococcus:* Griffith typing and emm typing
  - Anti-DNase-B Ab: Titer >300–350 units/ml is diagnostic of pyoderma.
  - Other antibodies elevated are antihyaluronidase and anti-streptokinase antibodies for PSGN.

Acute Rheumatic Fever

- A positive throat culture or positive rapid streptococcal antigen test or a rising anti-streptolysin O antibody titre.

Complications

1. Suppurative
   - Bacteraemia
2. Non suppurative
   - Acute rheumatic fever (ARF)

4. A 25-year-old malnourished male complains of sore throat that has increased in intensity over several days. In addition, the patient also complains of halitosis. O/E, there is submandibular lymphadenopathy. Gram's stain shows gram-negative spiral bacilli and gram-negative fusiform bacilli. What is the probable diagnosis? Causative agent of this disease. Predisposing factors for the condition. How can this clinical condition be diagnosed? (1+1+1+1 marks)

Probable Diagnosis

- Vincent's angina (Trench mouth)

Causative Agents

1. *Treponema vincentii*
2. *Leptotrichia buccalis*

Predisposing Factors

- Malnutrition, viral infection.

Diagnosis

- Pseudomembrane formation which can be peeled off
- Gram's stain of throat swab or exudate reveals spiral and fusiform bacilli

5. Immunoprophylaxis for diphtheria, pertussis and tetanus. (5 marks)

Diphtheria, Pertussis, Tetanus, Toxoid Vaccine

- Contains DT (diphtheria toxoid), pertussis (whole cell) and TT (tetanus toxoid).

Preparation

- *Plain formol toxoid (or fluid toxoid):* Toxoid is prepared by incubating toxin with formalin
- *Adsorbed (alum adsorbed):* Alum acts as adjuvant and increases the immunogenicity of toxoid

Schedule

- At 6, 10, 14 weeks.
- *Booster dose DPT → 1st:* 16–24 months, 2nd: 5–6 years, TT-3rd: 10 years and 16 years

Dose

- 0.5 ml.

Side Effects

- Mild.
  - Fever and local reaction (swelling and indurations) are observed commonly.
- Severe.
  - Whole cell killed *Bordetella pertussis* is encephalitogenic.
  - It is associated with neurological complications. Hence, DPT is not recommended after 6 years of age.

Contraindications

1. Hypersensitivity to previous dose
2. Progressive neurological disorder

- Acelluar pertussis component (aP) is devoid of neurological complication and is safe in older children.

6. Describe the characteristics of hypervirulent Klebsiella. (5 marks)

Characteristics	*Hypervirulent Klebsiella (hvKp)*
Location for the development of infection	• More commonly the community
Host	• All ages; often otherwise healthy
Ethnic background	• Often Asian, Pacific Islander, Hispanic
Hepatic abscess	• Usually occurs in the absence of biliary disease
Number of sites of infection	• Often multiple
Unusual infectious syndromes for *K. pneumoniae*	• Endophthalmitis, meningitis, brain abscess, necrotising fasciitis, splenic abscess, epidural abscess
Drug resistance	• Strains are resistant to antimicrobials due to acquisition of mobile elements carrying resistant determinants

7. Immunoprophylaxis in pneumococcal infection. (5 marks)

- Immunity against pneumococci is type-specific and associated with antibody to capsular polysaccharide (Table 6.1.1).

Table 6.1.1 Vaccines for pneumococcal infection: features, indications and dose

Vaccine	*Features*	*Indications*	*Dose*
23-valent Pneumococcal polysaccharide vaccine (PPSV23)	• A polyvalent vaccine containing capsular polysaccharide of 23 prevalent serotypes is available and administered by single dose injection	1. All adults 65 years or older without certain conditions 2. People 2 through 64 years old with certain medical conditions 3. Adults 19 through 64 years old who smoke cigarettes	• A single dose
13-valent conjugate polysaccharide vaccine (PCV-13)	• Pneumococcal polysaccharide of 13 common childhood serotypes of *Pneumococcus* • The protein conjugate acts as adjuvant and increases the immunogenicity of the polysaccharide antigen—so can be given to children 2 months—24 months of age • This vaccine prevents both bacteraemic infections like meningitis as well as mucosal infections like otitis media	1. All children younger than 2 years old and adults 65 years or older 2. People 2 through 64 years old with certain medical conditions	• 4 doses • One dose at each of these ages → 2 months, 4 months, 6 months, and 12 through 15 months

8. A 3-year-old boy with h/o fever, cough, and dyspnoea for 2 days. Sputum culture grew colonies near streaked line of *S. aureus* on blood agar. What is the etiological agent? Discuss the pathogenesis, clinical manifestations produced by the pathogen. Add a note on preventive prophylaxis available for this condition. (1+1+2+2 marks)

Aetiological Agent

- Pneumonia or laryngotracheobronchitis caused by *Haemophilus influenzae.*

Pathogenesis

- *H. influenzae* infects only humans, there is no animal reservoir.
- *Source of infection:* Endogenous/exogenous
- *Route of Infection:* Inhalation of infective droplets
- *Sequence of Events*
  - Inhalation of *H. influenzae.*
  - Adheres to nasopharyngeal epithelium.
  - Either asymptomatic colonisation or non-invasive disease: Otitis media, sinusitis, pneumonia.
  - Penetrates epithelium → disseminates through blood or direct spread → meninges → meningitis.

Clinical Manifestations

Invasive Infections–Primary Pathogen-type b

- Meningitis
  - >2 years age
  - Subdural effusion
- Laryngoepiglottitis
  - 2–7 years of age
  - Fever, pharyngitis, obstructive laryngitis and difficulty in breathing (life threatening—Tracheostomy)
- Pneumonia in infants
- Cellulitis of neck/head, osteomyelitis, septic arthritis, orbital cellulitis, endophthalmitis, UTI

Noninvasive Infections—Secondary Infections—Non-typable

- Otitis media in children
- Exacerbations of COPD
- Pneumonia in adults
- Sinusitis in adults and children

Preventive Prophylaxis

- *Vaccine:* PRP capsular antigen of *H. influenzae* type b
- As capsular antigens by itself are poorly immunogenic to children, and hence they are conjugated with adjuvants such as diphtheria toxoid, tetanus toxoid.
- It also reduces the rates of pharyngeal colonisation with Hib.
- Conjugate vaccines have dramatically reduced the incidence of Hib disease.

9. A laboratory report of gene Xpert tuberculosis test reads as Isoniazid resistance. What is the clinical significance? Which are the other methods for detection of resistance in this organism? (3+2 marks)

Clinical Significance

- Gene Xpert MTB/RIF test is a promising tool to find new TB and multidrug-resistant (MDR) TB cases earlier, which results in better control of TB transmission
- Also useful in patients with pulmonary TB with sputum negative
- Results are available within 2 hours
- In countries with high TB prevalence, clinicians may suspect TB with low threshold, resulting in overuse of the test

Other Methods Used in Detection of Drug Resistance

- Done on solid (LJ, Middle brook) and liquid media (Bactec 460TB, MGIT)
- Antibiotic proportion method is ideal.
- Detection of drug resistance gene
  - Line probe assays-InnoLipa, Genotype MTBDR.

Test method	*Detection time*
• LJ medium (Middle brook)	• 3–4 weeks
• Liquid media (Bactec 460, MGIT)	• 7–10 days
• Molecular methods (InnoLipa, Genotype MTBDR, Xpert MTB)	• Hours—1 day

10. Describe the medically important nontuberculous mycobacteria causing pulmonary infections and classify them on the growth characteristics. (3+2 marks)

- *Mycobacteria* spp. other than human or bovine tubercle bacilli that may occasionally cause human disease resembling tuberculosis have been called atypical mycobacteria.

Runyon Classification

Group	Group name	Growth characteristics	Examples
I	**Photochromogens**	• Slow growers (≥2 weeks) • Colonies non pigmented in dark but develop pigment when exposed to light	• *M. kansasii* • *M. marinum* • *M. simiae*
II	**Scotochromogens**	• Slow growers(≥2 weeks) • Can produce pigmented colonies both in light and dark	• *M. scrofulaceum* • *M. gordonae (Tap water scotochromogens)*
III	**Non-photochromogens**	• Slow growers (≥2 weeks). • Non pigmented colonies both in dark and light	• *M. avium-intracellulare* complex *(MAC)* • *M. ulcerans* • *M. xenopi*
IV	**Rapid growers**	• Growth in <7 days • Can produce both pigmented and non-pigmented colonies	• *M. fortuitum-chelonae* complex • *M. vaccae* • *M. phlei*

11. Describe the pathogenesis, clinical features, and laboratory diagnosis of measles virus infection. (3+2 marks)

Measles Virus Infection

Pathogenesis

Incubation

- 4–10 days

Mode of Transmission

- Inhalation via droplets

Sequence of Events

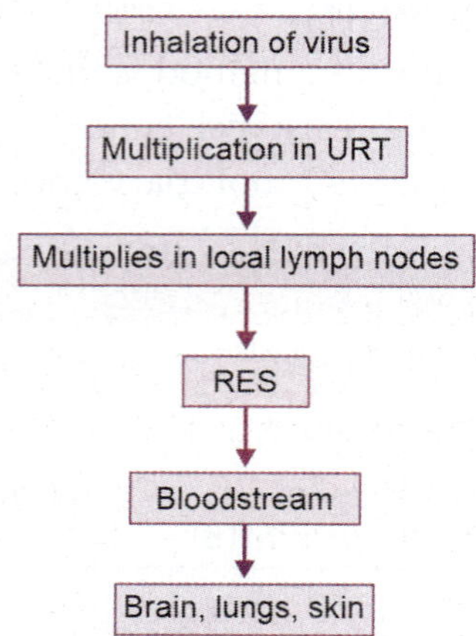

- Cells in the skin infected with virus
- Attacked by T lymphocytes → Skin rash
- CMI is suppressed transiently as the virus binds to CD46 receptors in humans and IL-12 production is suppressed.

Clinical Features

- Multinucleated giant cells-characteristic of these lesions.
- Lifelong immunity once infected with the virus.
- Prodrome with coryza, conjunctivitis, brassy cough
- Kolpik spots—bright red lesions with a white, central dot that are located on the buccal mucosa.
- Rash begins in hairline, forehead, moves down and covers entire body. Becomes confluent before it fades by desquamation.
- Rash is maculopapular, light pink, discrete to confluent.

Laboratory Diagnosis

- Mostly clinically diagnosed

Specimen Collection

- Nasopharyngeal secretions

Antigen Detection

Direct IF for measles Ag

Cell Culture

- Monkey/human kidney cells—Multinucleate giant cells with intranuclear and cytoplasmic inclusions.

Demonstrate IgM or IgG

- 4-fold rise—ELISA

Molecular method

- RT PCR

12. Discuss the pathogenesis, laboratory diagnosis and immunoprophylaxis of pertussis. (3+1+1 marks)

Pertussis

Pathogenesis

Causative Agent

- Gram-negative bacterium *Bordetella pertussis.*

Mode of Transmission

- Spreads from person to person by air-borne droplets.

Virulence Factors

- *B. pertussis* associated with the production of variety of toxins. Such as:
  1. Pertussis toxin
  2. Adenylate cyclase toxin
  3. Tracheal cytotoxin
  4. Endotoxin

Sequence of Events

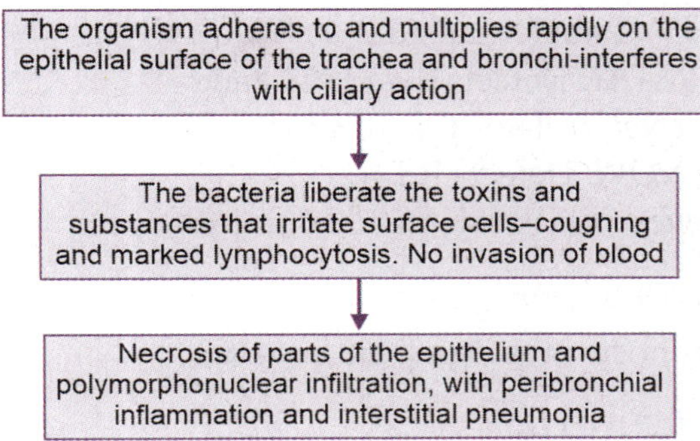

Laboratory Diagnosis

Specimen Collection

- Nasopharyngeal swabs or aspirates using Dacron swab.

Microscopy

- **Gram's stain:** Gram-negative cocco bacilli

Antigen Detection

- Direct fluorescent antibody tests of nasopharyngeal secretions.

Culture

- It is the gold standard method.
- *Media:* Regan and Lowe medium, Bordet-Gengou glycerin-potato-blood agar
- *Colony morphology: Mercury drops or bisected pearls* appearance

Molecular Method

- PCR

Antibody Detection

- Enzyme immunoassays detecting IgA and IgG to pertussis toxin, filamentous haemagglutinin.

Immunoprophylaxis

- A whole cell which is killed preparation of *B. pertussis* as DPT vaccine.
- Now acellular pertussis vaccine is dominant which consists of pertussis toxoid along with other bacterial components.

---

13. Enumerate the causative agents of ventilator associated pneumonia. Briefly discuss the treatment options and drug resistance in VAP associated with *Pseudomonas* spp and *Acinetobacter* spp. (1+2+2 marks)

Causative Agents of Ventilator-associated Pneumonia (VAP)

1. Methicillin-resistant *Staphylococcus aureus* (MRSA)
2. *Pseudomonas aeruginosa*
3. Acinetobacter baumannii.
4. *Enterobacteriaceae* (*Klebsiella pneumoniae, Escherichia coli, Serratia marcescens, Enterobacter* spp.)
5. *Stenotrophomonas maltophilia.*

Treatment for *Pseudomonas* Infections

- *Combination therapy:* Beta lactam piperacillin with aminoglycoside or
- Ceftazidime, cefoperazone, and cefepime or
- Aztreonam or carbapenems such as imipenem or meropenem or.
- Fluoroquinolones, including ciprofloxacin.

Treatment for Acinetobacter Infections

- *Aminoglycosides:* Gentamicin, amikacin, or tobramycin and
- Extended-spectrum penicillins or cephalosporins.
- Antibiotic susceptibility testing must be done because of MDR or PDR.

Drug Resistance in VAP-associated with *Pseudomonas* spp and *Acinetobacter* spp.

- Multidrug resistance has become a major issue in the management of hospital-acquired infections with *P. aeruginosa and Acinetobacter* because
  - Acquisition of chromosomal beta-lactamases, extended-spectrum beta-lactamases
  - Porin channel mutations
  - Efflux pumps

---

14. Describe in detail about viral pneumonia by taking COVID-19 as example under the following headings.

A. Morphology of SARS-CoV. (1 mark)

- Enveloped virus
- Nucleocapsid-helical symmetry
- 4 structural proteins—Nucleocapsid-N, Spike-S, Membrane glycoprotein-M and Envelop protein-E)
- Non-structural proteins—RNA dependent RNA polymerase (RdRp), helicase etc

B. Modes of Transmission. (1 mark)

1. Droplet transmission.
2. Contact transmission.
3. During aerosol generating procedures such as ET intubation.

C. Basic pathology in disease progression. (2 marks)

- *See* Figure 6.1.6.
- ACE-2 receptors are over expressed in the oral mucosa (URT), inducing inflammation which progresses to LRT.
- Leading to reduced surfactant and collapsed alveoli.

D. Clinical presentation in COVID-19. (1 mark)

- Asymptomatic
- ILI-Fever, cough with or without expectoration, fatigue, myalgia, sore throat, runny nose
- Diarrhoea
- Loss of taste and smell
- Shortness of breath
- Complications
  1. ARDS
  2. Sepsis
  3. Septic shock
  4. Thrombotic episodes—Myocardial infarction, deep vein thrombosis, stroke

---

15. Discuss the laboratory diagnosis along with vaccines, their efficacy, side effects and dose for COVID-19. (3+3 marks)

Laboratory Diagnosis

Specimen Collection

- Oropharyngeal swab.
- Nasopharyngeal swab using dacron or polyester flocked swab.

Transport Medium

- Viral transport media (VTM) at –4°C.

Molecular Methods

1. Viral RNA detection by RT-PCR.
   i. Genus specific targets- Spike protein (S).
      - Envelop protein (E)
      - Membrane protein (M)
      - Nucleocapsid protein (N)
   ii. Species specific targets: RNA dependent RNA polymerase (RdRp)
      - Open reading frames (ORF1a/b)
      - N2 nucleocapsid
2. *CBNAAT:* Detects E and N2 gene
3. *TrueNat:* Detects E and RdRp
4. *ID NOW:* Detects RdRp
5. *Sequencing:* For detection of mutations or variants

Antigen Detection

- Immunochromatographic test (ICT).

Antibody Detection

- ELISA, Chemiluminescence and ICT (For sero-surveillance and high-risk population).

Viral Culture

- Not recommended for diagnostics purpose.

Other Tests

1. *Prognostic markers:* C-reactive protein (CRP), increased ferritin, D-dimer, IL-6 levels
2. *CT scan:* Ground-glass appearance and or consolidation.

COVID-19 vaccines

See Table 6.1.2.

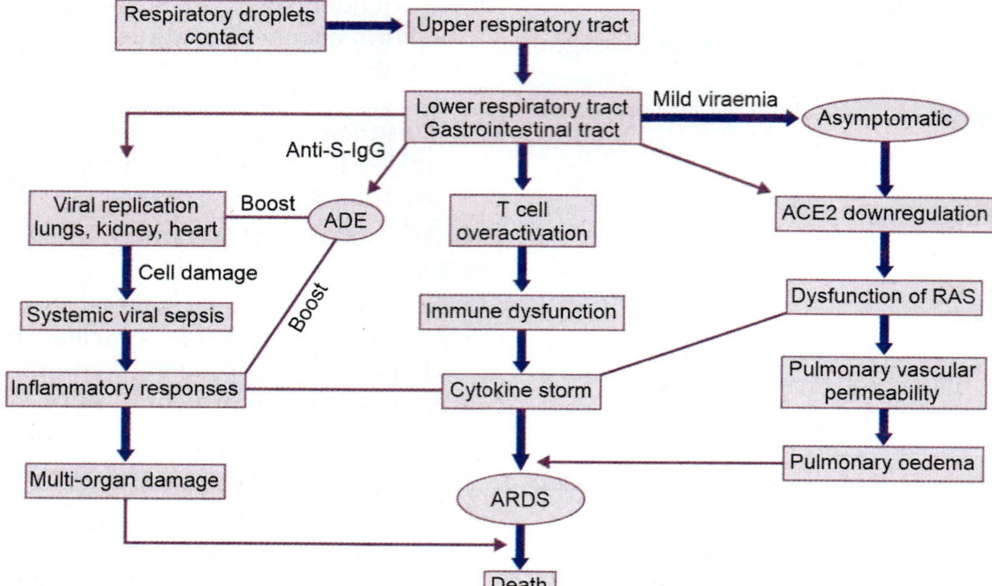

Fig. 6.1.6: Disease progression of COVID-19

Table 6.1.2 COVID-19 vaccines

Type	Vaccine brand	Dose	Schedule	Efficacy	Adverse effects
Viral vector vaccine	• Covishield • (AstraZeneca)	2	12 weeks apart	90%	• Fever, pain at the site of injection, myalgia, thrombosis • Thrombocytopenia
Inactivated virus vaccine	• Covaxin	2	4 weeks apart	82%	• Fever, pain at the site of injection, myalgia
mRNA vaccine	• Moderna	2	4 weeks apart	94.5%	• Anaphylaxis (<0.01)
mRNA vaccine	• Pfizer BioNTech	2	3 weeks apart	95%	• Anaphylaxis (<0.01)
Viral vector vaccine	• Johnson and Johnson	1	—	66%	• Anaphylaxis (<0.01), thrombosis • thrombocytopenia
Inactivated virus vaccine	• Sinopharm-BBIBP	2	3 weeks apart	79%	• Fever, pain at the site of injection, myalgia
Viral vector vaccine	• Sputnik	2	3 weeks apart	90%	• None
Inactivated virus vaccine	• Sinovac	2	2 weeks apart	50%	• None

16. A 70-year-old man with a long history of smoking now has a fever and a cough productive of greenish sputum. The physician suspects pneumonia, which is confirmed by chest X-ray. A sputum sample was plated on chocolate, blood, and MacConkey agars. Colonies only grew on chocolate agar. What is the most likely infection and its aetiology? Briefly explain the pathogenesis, clinical manifestations produced, laboratory work-up plan for this case. (1+2+3 marks)

Most Likely Infection

- Pneumonia

Aetiology

- *Haemophilus influenzae*

Pathogenesis

Source of Infection

- Endogenous/exogenous

Reservoir

- *H. influenzae* infects only humans, there is no animal reservoir

Route of Infection

- Inhalation of infective droplets

Virulence Factors

1. **Capsule**
   - Antiphagocytic.
   - Chemically polyribose-ribitol phosphate (PRP).
   - 6 capsular types: a to f
   - Capsular type b causes most of the severe, invasive diseases like meningitis and sepsis.
   - PRP antigen of Hib induces IgG, IgM, and IgA antibodies which are bactericidal, opsonic, and protective—So Hib PRP is used for immunisation.
2. *s-IgA protease.*
3. *Membrane Lipo-oligosaccharide* (similar to LPS in *E. coli*).
4. *Pili and adhesion proteins.*

Sequence of Events

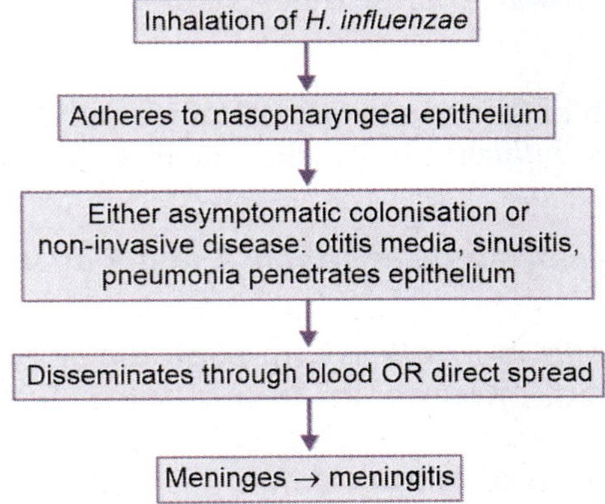

Clinical Manifestations

Invasive Infections—Primary Pathogen Type b

- Meningitis
  - >2 years age
  - Subdural effusion
- Laryngoepiglottitis
  - 2–7 years of age
  - Fever, pharyngitis, obstructive laryngitis, and difficulty in breathing
- Pneumonia in infants
- Cellulitis of neck/head, osteomyelitis, septic arthritis, orbital cellulitis, endophthalmitis, UTI

Noninvasive Infections—Secondary Infections—Non-typable

- Otitis media in children
- Exacerbations of COPD
- Pneumonia in adults
- Sinusitis in adults and children

Laboratory Work-up

Specimen Collection

- Sputum in this case
- CSF, pus and exudates from lesions, blood for culture—for other site infection.

Microscopy

- *Gram's staining:* Pleomorphic gram-negative cocco-bacilli with numerous PMNLs
- *Capsule detection (Quellung reaction):* Using type b antiserum and methylene blue and observing under microscope.

Antigen Detection (Rapid method)

- By Latex agglutination—for CSF and urine.

Culture

- *Chocolate agar:* V factor released from RBCs. *H. influenzae* produces tiny, transparent smooth colonies (dew drop colonies). Requires both X and V factors for growth, fastidious organism.
- *Levinthal medium*
- *Filde's medium* (peptic digest of blood to NA).

Satellitism

- Growth observed near the beta haemolytic *S aureus* when *H influenza* is streaked near it. As it acquires factor V.

Use of commercially available X and V disks

17. *Coxiella burnetii* is an etiological agent for atypical pneumonia. True or false. Justify. How is this disease transmitted and lab work up in the diagnosis of this condition. (2+1+2 marks)

Statement is:

- True

Justification

- *Coxiella burnetii* can cause atypical pneumonia along with extrapulmonary manifestations such as hepatitis, pericarditis, myocarditis, myalgia, headache, arthralgia.

Mode of Transmission

- Inhalation of dust contaminated with infected animal urine or faeces.
- Ingestion of contaminated milk.

Lab Work-up

- *Specimen Collection:* Blood, tissues, serum
- *Microscopy:* Gram's stain—Pleomorphic gram-negative coccobacilli
- *Culture:* Using human embryonic lung fibroblasts cell lines
- *Serology:* Antibody detection
- *Indirect immunofluorescence assay:* Acute infection—rise in phase II antigens
- *Chronic infection:* Rise in phase I antigens
- *Molecular methods:* PCR

18. A 45-year-old woman has a painless ulcer on her tongue. She is HIV antibody positive. Other investigations done were CD4 count of 25 and VDRL test was non-reactive. Biopsy of the lesion revealed yeasts within macrophages. What is the clinical diagnosis and the aetiological agent? Explain the other clinical manifestations caused by this pathogen and plan the laboratory work-up in this case.

(1+2+2 marks)

Clinical Diagnosis

- Disseminated histoplasmosis

Aetiological Agent

- *Histoplasma capsulatum*

Clinical Manifestations

- The infection is acquired through inhalation of spores (microconidia)
- Endemic in United States (central and eastern parts), especially in the Ohio and Mississippi river valleys
- Asymptomatic
- pneumonia and cavitary lung lesions
- Mucocutaneous oral lesions—Ulcer
- Disseminated infection in AIDS patients

Laboratory Work-up

- *Specimen collection:* Sputum, tissue biopsy, bone marrow aspirates
- *Microscopy:* Giemsa stain, periodic acid-Schiff (PAS stain)—oval yeast cells within the macrophages
- *Culture*
  - Sabourad's agar, BHI agar at 37°C—pasty white colonies—yeasts visible within macrophages.
  - At 25°C, mycelial form—tuberculate chlamydo-spores and microconidia.
- *Serology:* Complement fixation (CF) and immuno-diffusion (ID): A rise in antibody titre is noted.
- *Skin test:* A mycelial extract, histoplasmin, is antigen used.

SHORT ANSWERS

1. Define croup. Which age group is commonly infected with croup? Mention the symptoms of croup. Enumerate the causative agents. (1+1+1+1 marks)

Croup

Definition

- An inflammation of the respiratory tract such as larynx, trachea, and large bronchi (laryngo-tracheobronchitis).

Age Group is Commonly Infected with Croup

- Seen in children

Symptoms of Croup

- Hoarseness and a burning retrosternal pain
- Dry cough and inspiratory stridor ('crowing')
- Respiratory tract obstruction
- Nasal irritation and congestion which could acutely progress to stridor over a day

Causative Agents

1. Influenza virus
2. Parainfluenza virus
3. Respiratory syncytial virus

2. Distinguish between community-acquired pneumonia and hospital-acquired pneumonia. (4 marks)

See Table 6.1.3.

3. Mention six examples for the viruses causing Bronchiolitis. (3 marks)

1. Parainfluenza virus—most common
2. Influenza virus
3. Respiratory syncytial virus
4. Adenoviruses.
5. SARS CoV2.
6. Human Metapneumovirus.

4. A 15-year-old student presented to the ENT OPD with history of throat pain of 2 days duration. On examination, inflammation of the tonsils and posterior pharyngeal wall was noted. What is the possible infectious cause for sore throat? (3 marks)

Viral Causes

1. Influenza virus
2. Parainfluenza virus
3. Coxsackievirus A
4. Rhinovirus

Bacterial Causes

1. *Streptococcus pyogenes*—Most common bacterial cause
2. *Corynebacterium diphtheria*
3. *Borrelia vincentii* and *Leptotrichia buccalis*

Fungal Causes

1. *Candida*.

Table 6.1.3 Differentiating features of community-acquired and hospital-acquired pneumonias

Feature	*Community-acquired pneumonia*	*Hospital-acquired pneumonia*
Definition	• Pneumonia in individuals who become ill outside the hospital or within 4–8 hours of admission to hospital	• Pneumonia acquired by an individual within the hospital setting usually at least two days following admission and up till 48 hours after discharge
Aetiology agents	• *S. pneumoniae* • *H. influenzae* • *C. pneumoniae* • *L. pneumophila* • Gram-negative rods	• *Enterobacteriaceae* (*K. pneumoniae, E. coli, S. marcescens, Enterobacter* spp.) • *Pseudomonas* spp. • *Acinetobacter* spp.
Source of infection	• Patients • Carriers • Contaminated fomites	• Contaminated health care devices • Patients • Environment (air, water, fomites)
Risk factors	• Age: young adults • Personal habits: smoking • Risk of aspiration • Comorbidities—pulmonary, extrapulmonary	• Age: >70 years • Malnutrition • Coma • Metabolic acidosis • Severe underlying diseases • Presence of co morbid illness • Ventilatory support

5. A 62-year-old man presents to his physician with fever, cough, and evidence of pneumonia. Sputum and blood cultures are collected for analysis. Alfa haemolytic colonies grew on blood agar. What is the most likely infection and aetiology? What key virulence factor produced by this bacterium is responsible for evading immunity and is part of a protective vaccine? (3 marks)

Most Likely Infection

- Pneumonia

Aetiology

- *Streptococcus pneumoniae*

Key Virulence Factor

- Polysaccharide capsule

6. A 4-year-old girl has a temperature of 102.4°F, nausea, and has sore throat. Upon examination, the doctor notes swollen lymph nodes and a purulent exudate on the nasopharynx. A rapid antigen test is negative, but a second throat swab was plated on blood agar for confirmation. The colony was beta haemolytic and gram-positive cocci in short chains. What is the most likely infection and aetiology? Which is the key virulence factor responsible and its role? (3 marks)

Most Likely Infection

- Streptococcal pharyngitis

Aetiology

- *Streptococcus pyogenes*

Key Virulence Factor

- M protein is the virulence factor that emanates from the cell surface, is antigenically variable between strains, and has antiphagocytic activity.

7. What tests can be used to identify the capsule surrounding the lanceolate-shaped cocci? Since penicillin resistance has emerged within this species of bacteria, what is the current drug of choice for empiric treatment of invasive infections with this pathogen? (3 marks)

To Demonstrate the Capsule

1. By negative staining—India ink or Nigrosin—capsule may be demonstrated as clear halo.
2. Quellung reaction (capsule swelling reaction).

Drug of Choice

- Third generation cephalosporins (e.g. ceftriaxone) and vancomycin

8. At the emergency department, a cystic fibrosis patient suffers from sudden, decreased lung function. Sputum samples were collected and plated on MacConkey agar. The resulting colourless colonies yielded gram-negative, rod-shaped bacteria with fruity odour. What is the most likely infection and aetiology? Briefly explain the important virulence factor responsible for the pathogenesis in this case. (3 marks)

Most Likely Infection

- Lung infection or LRTI

Aetiology

- *Pseudomonas aeruginosa*

Key Virulence Factor

- The capsular material alginate, composed of a repeating polymer of mannuronic and glucuronic acids, provides resistance to phagocytosis and lung clearance.

9. A patient on immunosuppressive drugs, presents at the emergency department with pneumonia. The patient c/o chest pain, coughing, and fever gradual in onset. Sputum samples revealed long filamentous gram-positive bacilli which were also acid fast. What is the most likely infection and aetiology? How is it transmitted and treatment for this condition? (3 marks)

Most Likely Infection

- Nocardiosis

Aetiology

- *Nocardia asteroides*

Mode of Transmission

- Inhalation of contaminated soils

Treatment

- Cotrimoxazole is the drug of choice

10. Enumerate the systemic mycoses? Briefly mention their characteristic features. (3 marks)

Systemic Mycoses

1. Histoplasmosis—*Histoplasma capsulatum*
2. Blastomycosis—*Blastomyces dermatitidis*
3. Coccidioidomycosis—*Coccidioides immitis*
4. Paracoccidioidomycosis—*Paracoccidioides brasiliensis*

Characteristic Features of Systemic Mycoses

- Caused by dimorphic fungi

- Self-limiting and asymptomatic in more than 95% patients
- Infection acquired by inhalation
- Primary infection is in lung
- Disseminate to other parts of the body through hematogenous route
- Seen in immunocompetent individuals
- Exhibit some amount of geographic restriction

11. A 6-year-old develops sore throat, fever, and nasal congestion. The child also has redness of conjunctiva. The child`s mother gives a h/o of similar complaints in 2 or 3 other children in the same class. The doctor says no therapy is required except for rest at home. What is the most probable disease condition and its aetiological agent? What are the other clinical manifestations seen by this pathogen? (3 marks)

Most Likely Infection

- Pharyngoconjunctival fever

Aetiology

- Adenovirus

Other Clinical Manifestations

- Haemorrhagic conjunctivitis
- Infant diarrhoea
- Epidemic keratoconjunctivitis
- Upper respiratory tract infection
- Pneumonia
- ARDS

12. Influenza A, H1N1 develops due to quadruple re-assortment. Statement is true or false? Justify your answer. (3 marks)

Statement is

- True

Justification

- Various species of animals (e.g. chickens, aquatic birds, swine, and horses) have their own influenza A viruses.
- The viruses in these animals are the source of the RNA segments that encode the antigenic shift variants that can lead to epidemics among humans.
- The new virus has 2 genes from flu viruses in pigs from Europe and Asia that acts a mixing vessel, 1 avian and 1 human gene—quadruple re- assortment (Fig. 6.1.7).

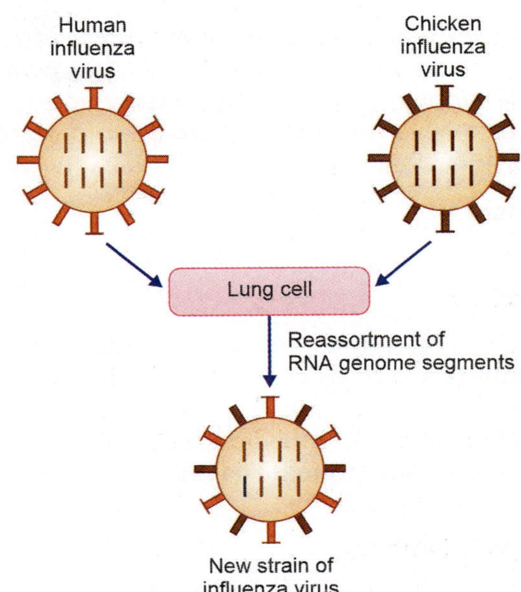

Fig. 6.1.7: New strain of influenza virus contains 1 avian gene and 1 human gene

13. Pulmonary nocardiosis presents with Lobar pneumonia. True or false? Justify your answer. What are the methods used in the diagnosis of this condition? (2+2 marks)

Statement is

- True

Justification

- Pulmonary nocardiosis manifests with subacute onset of cough and purulent sputum.
- It can disseminate to other organs leading to pericarditis, mediastinitis, laryngitis and bronchitis.

Methods Used in the Diagnosis

- *Specimen collection:* Sputum, BAL
- *Microscopy.*
  - *Gram stain:* Pus cells with gram-positive branching and filamentous bacilli.
  - *Modified acid-fast stain:* 1% H_2SO_4—Branching and filamentous acid-fast bacilli.
  - *H and E:* Sun ray appearance.
- *Culture.*
  - Brain heart infusion agar, Sabourad's dextrose agar.
  - *Colony morphology:* Creamy, wrinkled pigmented colonies.
  - *Lowenstein's Jensen media:* Glabrous pigmented colonies.
  - *Paraffin bait technique:* Media with paraffin as a sole source of carbon.
- *Biochemical Identification:* Catalase-positive, use of sugars oxidatively

14. Risk factors are associated with chronic respiratory tract infections caused by *Pseudomonas aeruginosa*. True or False. Justify your answer. Give a brief laboratory work-up in diagnosis of this infection. (2+2 marks)

Statement is

- True

Justification

- Chronic infections occur with underlying co morbidities such as cystic fibrosis, bronchiectasis, or chronic bronchiolitis.
- *Factors responsible:* Mucoid strains of *Pseudomonas* possessing the alginate layer, structural abnormalities of airways.

Laboratory Work-up

- *Specimen collection:* BAL, ET secretions
- *Microscopy:* Gram's stain—slender gram-negative bacilli
- *Culture.*
  - *Peptone water:* Surface pellicle formation with turbidity.
  - *Nutrient agar:* Large irregular colonies with metallic sheen.
  - *Blood agar:* Beta haemolytic colonies.
  - *Mac Conkey's agar:* Non-lactose fermenting colonies.
  - *Selective media:* Cetrimide agar
- *Biochemical identification.*
  - Non-fermenter of sugars, citrate positive.

15. Respiratory viruses are non-enveloped viruses. Statement true or false? Justify the statement. (3 marks)

Statement is

- False

Justification

- Respiratory viruses are enveloped viruses and transmitted through contact or droplet.
- **Enteric viruses** are non-enveloped transmitted via the faecal-oral route and are important causes of a wide range of human infections, both gastrointestinal and extra-intestinal, if enteric viruses were enveloped, the viruses will be destroyed with the gastric acidity.

16. A 28-day old neonate develops cough, wheezing. Nasopharyngeal secretions were sent for culture which revealed syncytial pattern. What is the diagnosis and aetiological agent? How is it transmitted? (3 marks)

Diagnosis

- Bronchiolitis

Etiological Agent

- Respiratory syncytial virus

Mode of Transmission

- Direct contact—transmitted through contaminated fingers or fomites
- Inhalation of large droplets

MI 6.2 IDENTIFY THE COMMON AETIOLOGIC AGENTS OF UPPER RESPIRATORY TRACT INFECTIONS (GRAM'S STAIN)

SHORT ESSAYS

1. A 4-year-old boy presents to the paediatrician with sore throat, high-grade fever and difficulty in swallowing in the past 2 days. On examination there is congestion of the tonsils and posterior pharyngeal wall.

A. What is the probable diagnosis? (1 mark)

- Exudative pharyngitis.

B. What is the specimen to be collected and how is it collected? (1 mark)

Specimen to be collected

- Throat swab.

Method

- It is collected after depressing the tongue with depressor and the tonsillar area and pillars are swabbed.
- Bits of pseudo membrane if present can be collected.
- *2 swabs:* one for microscopy and one for culture

C. Perform appropriate staining and comment. (1 mark)

- Gram's stain shows the presence of polymorphonuclear leucocytes with gram-positive cocci in pairs and chains (Fig. 6.2.1).

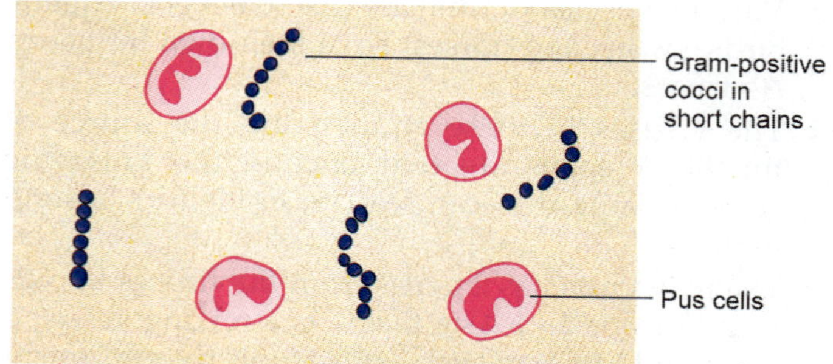

Fig. 6.2.1: Polymorphonuclear leucocytes with gram-positive cocci

D. What investigations are requested to confirm the identity of the pathogen in this case? (1 mark)

- *Culture:* Blood agar—beta haemolytic colonies, Gram positive cocci in chains
- *Biochemical tests:* Catalase negative, Bacitracin sensitive

2. An 8-year-old boy is referred to hospital from PHC with low grade fever and sore throat of 6 days' duration. On examination, his tonsils were inflamed with white patches. The child is not immunised.

A. What is the probable diagnosis? (1 mark)

- Diphtheria.

B. What is the specimen to be collected and how is it collected? (1 mark)

Specimen to be collected

- Throat swab.

Method

- It is collected after depressing the tongue with depressor and the tonsillar area and pillars are swabbed.
- Bits of pseudomembrane if present can be collected.
- *2 swabs:* One for microscopy and one for culture.

C. Choose the appropriate stain and report and draw a neat, labelled diagram. (1 mark)

- Albert stain.
- Green bacilli arranged in Chinese letter pattern with bluish black metachromatic granules seen, morphologically resembling *Corynebacterium diphtheria* (Fig. 6.2.2).

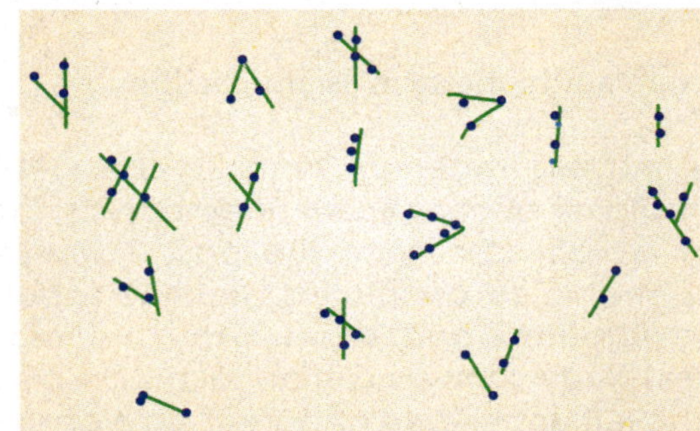

Fig. 6.2.2: Green bacilli arranged in chinese letter pattern with bluish black metachromatic granules resembling C diphtheriae

D. What are the other names given to the granules? (1 mark)

- Volutin granules
- Babes Ernst granules
- Polar bodies

E. What are the granules chemically made up of? (1 mark)

- *Polymetaphosphate:* Energy source to the bacteria

F. What is the investigation required to confirm the identity of the pathogen? (1 mark)

- Culture for *Corynebacterium diphtheria.*

MI 6.3 IDENTIFY THE COMMON AETIOLOGIC AGENTS OF LOWER RESPIRATORY TRACT INFECTIONS (GRAM'S STAIN AND ACID-FAST STAIN)

SHORT ESSAYS

1. A 35-year-old male, presents with fever and cough productive of small amounts of purulent secretions. He noticed bright red blood flecks in his sputum. The patient has no significant history of familial illness, hospitalisations, or trauma. Sputum is sent for ordinary culture and sensitivity. Comment on the Gram's stain. (Fig. 6.3.1).

A. Report on the Gram's stain (1 mark)

- The sputum smear shows the presence of polymorphonuclear leucocytes with gram-positive cocci lanceolate-shaped diplococci morphologically resembling *Streptococcus pneumoniae.*

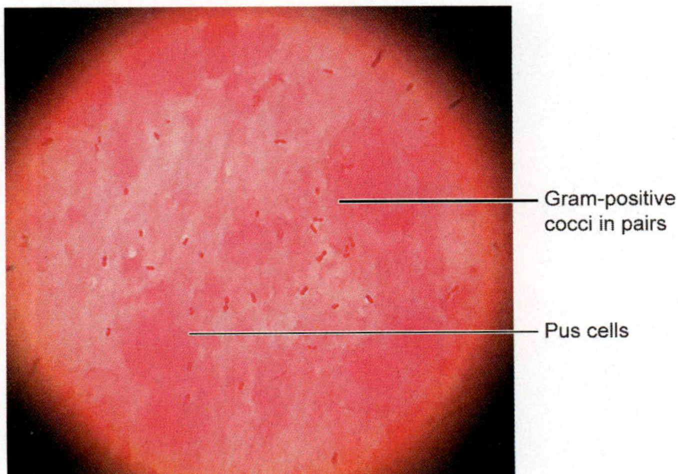

Fig. 6.3.1: Gram-positive cocci in pairs with pus cells

B. What type of pneumonia does the patient have? (1 mark)

- Community acquired pneumonia.
- *Explanation:* No history of familial illness, hospitalisation, or trauma

C. Give one example of an organism that usually causes CAP? (1 mark)

- *Streptococcus pneumoniae* (in 20–60% of cases).

D. What type of antibiotic is suitable in his case? (1 mark)

- β lactam antibiotic such as amoxicillin

2. 36-year-old male presents to the OPD with complaints of cough with haemoptysis, fatigue, and weight loss since the past 2 weeks, not responding to antibiotics. Routine laboratory investigations and chest X-ray are ordered. Chest X-ray showed a triangular consolidation of the left upper lobe and small cavitary lesions. Sputum is sent to the microbiology laboratory. Do the appropriate staining on sputum and report?.

A. Choose the appropriate staining method. (1 mark)

- Ziehl–Neelsen stain/Gabbet's stain.

B. Draw a neat, labelled diagram. (1 mark)

- See Figure 6.3.2.

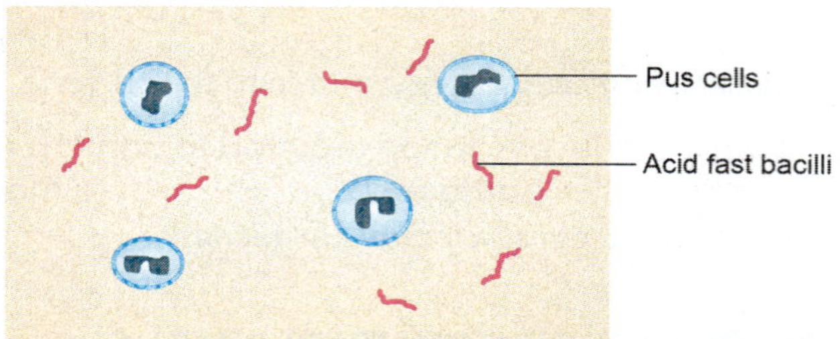

Fig. 6.3.2: Acid fast bacilli with pus cells

C. What are the instructions to be given to the patient on sample collection and how many specimens are recommended in this scenario? (1 mark)

Instructions to be Given to the Patient on Sample Collection

- Sputum specimen is collected following deep cough in a sterile wide mouthed leak proof container in a well-ventilated area.

Specimens Recommended

- **Two sputum specimens are collected:** spot and early morning for suspected case of pulmonary tuberculosis

D. Comment on the smear. (1 mark)

- Acid fast bacilli are seen.

E. Give the reason for acid fastness in *Mycobacterium tuberculosis*. (1 mark)

- Mycolic acid present in the cell wall of *Mycobacterium tuberculosis*.

F. Give other examples of acid-fast organisms and structures, with the degree of acid fastness. (1 mark)

Examples of Acid-fast Organisms

1. *Mycobacterium leprae* (5% H_2SO_4)
2. Nocardia (1% H_2SO_4)

Examples of Structures

1. Oocysts of *Cryptosporidium* spp. *Cyclospora* spp., *Microsporidia* spp. (0.5% H_2SO_4)
2. Bacterial spore (0.25% H_2SO_4).

CHAPTER 7

Genitourinary and Sexually Transmitted Infections

MI 7.1 DESCRIBE THE AETIOPATHOGENESIS AND DESCRIBE THE LABORATORY DIAGNOSIS OF INFECTIONS OF GENITOURINARY SYSTEM

LONG ESSAYS

1. Describe in detail the diseases of genitourinary system under the following headings.

A. Mention the bacteria and the diseases causing genitourinary infections. (2 marks)

Bacteria	*Disease caused*
Treponema pallidum	• Syphilis
Neisseria gonorrhoeae	• Gonorrhoea
Chlamydia trachomatis L1, 2, 3	• Lymphogranuloma venereum
Haemophilus ducreyi	• Chancroid
Klebsiella granulomatis	• Granuloma inguinale
Mycoplasma *Ureaplasma*	• Non-conococcal urethritis

B. Examples of viruses causing STDs. (2 marks)

1. *HIV/AIDS:* HIV 1, 2
2. Hepatitis B, Hepatitis C
3. *Genital Herpes:* Herpes Simplex virus 2
4. *Genital warts:* Human papilloma virus
5. *Molluscum contagiosum:* Poxvirus.

C. Pathogenesis, clinical features of HSV type-2. (4 marks)

Pathogenesis

- *Source:* Patient or carrier
- *Mode of transmission:* contact/vertical
- *Incubation period:* 1–2 days
- *Contact:*
  - Saliva, sexual contact, during birth
  - Spread via nerves by retrograde axonal flow to dorsal root ganglia: latency
  - HSV 2: Sacral ganglia
- *Sequence of events*
  - Disease is initiated by direct contact and depends on infected tissue (e.g., oral, genital, brain)
  - Direct cytopathogenic effects—Lesıons
  - Avoids antibody by cell-to-cell spread (syncytia)
  - Establishes latency in neurons (hides from immune response)
  - Reactivated from latency by stress or immune suppression
  - CMI is *required* for resolution with limited role for antibody
  - Cell-mediated immunopathologic effects contribute to symptoms
  - Lesions:
    - Thin walled umbilicated vesicles, roof of which breaks down to form superficial ulcers
    - Primary infection: though self-limited are severe, widespread associated with systemic manifestations
    - May be inapparent or vesicular (vesicle fluid contains infectious virons)
  - Viral pathology + immunopathology: tissue damage
  - Heals without a scar.

Clinical Features of Genital Herpes

- Painful vesicular lesions of male and female genitals
- Primary disease more severe with fever, inguinal lymphadenopathy
- Many infections are asymptomatic.

Neonatal Herpes

- Either during passage through genital tract or rarely *in utero*.
- Postnatally from family or hospital personel
- Weak immune system
- Ranges from asymptomatic infection, local lesions (skin, mouth, eye) to severe disease (disseminated, encephalitis).

D. Laboratory diagnosis of HSV-2. (2 marks)

Specimen Collection

- Material from base of the vesicle (scrapings).
- Blood
- CSF

Microscopy

- *Tzanck smear (scraping of the base of a lesion):*
  - Presence of multinucleated giant cells with faceted nuclei and ground glass chromatin.
  - Intranuclear type A inclusion bodies: Giemsa.
- *Electron microscopy*
- *Direct IF*

Virus Isolation

- CPE in 1–3 days in HeLa, Hep-2 cells, human diploid fibroblasts and rabbit kidney cells.
- Isolates are identified by antigen detection by IFA or by type specific antibody by ELISA (differentiates HSV-1 and HSV-2).
- *Cytopathic effects:* syncytia, ballooning of cytoplasm, Cowdry A intranuclear inclusions

Molecular Method

- *In situ* hybridisation or PCR in tissue or vesicle fluid.

Serology

- Primary infection, ELISA.

2. A 25-year-old man presents with a history of unprotected sex with multiple partners. He has an ulcerated lesion on his penis that is not painful. Dark-field microscopy of fluid from the lesion reveals the presence of motile spirochetes.

A. What is the probable diagnosis? (1 mark)

- Syphilis caused by *Treponema pallidum.*

B. Describe the clinical course of this disease (3 marks)

Clinical Course of Syphilis

- *See* Figure 7.1.1.

C. Discuss the laboratory diagnosis of the disease. (5 marks)

Specimen Collection

- *Primary syphilis:* Exudate from chancre and blood for serology
- *Secondary, latent:* Exudate from skin lesions, blood for serology
- *Tertiary syphilis:* CSF and blood for serology

Microscopy

- *Dark-field microscopy:* Motile spiral rods seen
- Direct fluorescent antibody test

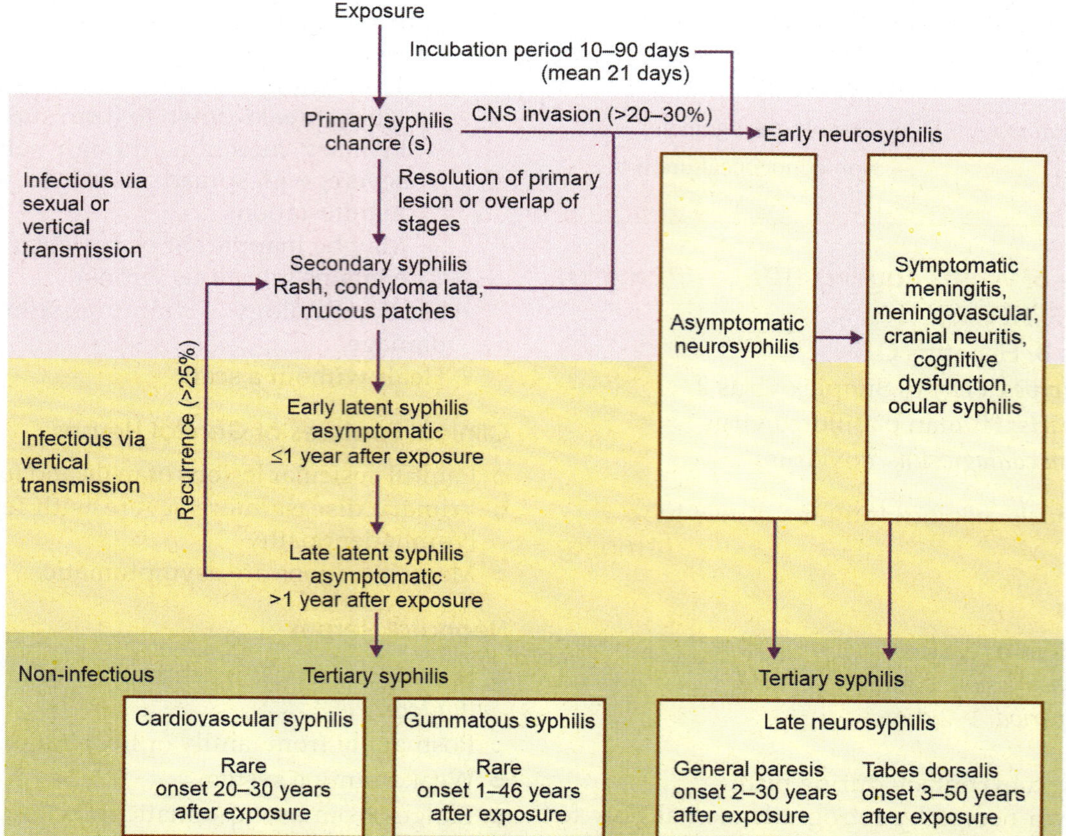

Fig. 7.1.1: Clinical course of syphilis

- Silver impregnation methods (Fontana for smears, Levaditi for tissue sections)

Serological Diagnosis

- 3 types of antibodies produced:
  1. Nonspecific anticardiolipin antibody (reagin)
  2. Group specific antibody against group specific antigen (Reiter's protein)
  3. Type specific antibody against Nichol's antigen.
- Tests are:
  1. *Non Treponemal tests (STS)*
     i. VDRL
     ii. RPR
  2. *Treponemal tests*
     i. Fluorescent treponemal antibody absorption test (FTA-Abs)
     ii. Treponema pallidum haemagglutination assay (TPHA)
     iii. Treponema pallidum immobilisation (TPI)
  3. *Non-treponemal tests*
     - Standard test for syphilis
     - Cardiolipin antigen is used to detect non-specific reagin
     - Microscopic tests—VDRL, unheated serum reagin.
     - Macroscopic tests—RPR, toluidine red unheated serum test (TRUST)
     - Measures antilipid Abs formed by the host in response to lipids released from damaged host cells early in infection.

VDRL Test

- Microflocculation test done for the serodiagnosis of syphilis
- Uses cardiolipin antigen and detects anticardiolipin antibody
- *Principle:*
  - VDRL test uses cardiolipin lecithin-coated cholesterol particles. Inactivated patient's serum or CSF and VDRL Ag emulsion are mixed and rotated for 8 min at 180 rpm. If reagin is present in the patient's serum, VDRL particles flocculate. Flocculation is read microscopically (10x). Reactive tests are quantitated.

No clumps	*Non-reactive*
• Small clumps	• Weakly reactive
• Medium and large clumps	• Reactive

- In Quantitative Testing—Report the titre in terms of the highest dilution that produces a reactive (not weakly reactive) result
- Reporting, e.g. reactive 4 dilution
- *Advantages:*
  1. Simple
  2. Screening test
  3. Highly sensitive
  4. Indicates active disease
  5. Ab titre falls after treatment.
  6. Diagnosis of neurosyphilis and congenital syphilis
- *Disadvantages.*
  1. Shelf life of Ag is only 24 hours
  2. Non-reactive in late syphilis
  3. Biological false positive reactions
  4. Prozone reactions

Rapid Plasma Reagin Test (RPR)

- RPR antigen
- Choline chloride—to block serum inhibitors
- EDTA—stabilizes Ag—6 months (4–10°C)
- Carbon particles—to read the results.
- When serum contains reagin antibodies, flocculation occurs with clumping of carbon particles of RPR Ag—black clumps against white background. Clumping is read macroscopically.
- *Advantages*
  1. Screening test.
  2. Heat inactivation not required as Ag contains choline chloride.
  3. Plasma or unheated serum can be used.
  4. Ag—ready to use form. 6 months (4–10°C).
  5. C-particles added to the Ag enables test reactivities to be read macroscopically.
- *Disadvantage:*
  1. CSF cannot be used.

Specific Tests

1. *Treponema Pallidum Immobilisation (TPI)*
   - Test serum is incubated with complement and Nicol's strain of *Treponema pallidum.*
   - If antibodies are present, treponemes are immobilised when examined under DGI.
2. *FTA –ABS.*
   - Indirect IF test. Smear of killed treponemes on a slide.
   - Serum is added followed by fluorescent dye labelled antiglobulin.
   - Observed under fluorescent microscope.
   - Specific, first serological test to be positive in 3–4 weeks.
3. *TPHA (Treponema Pallidum Haemagglutination).*
   - Patient's diluted serum + sheep or avian RBC'S sensitised with the Nicol's strain in wells of microtitre plate.
   - If antibodies are present, sensitised cells agglutinate, settle—mat pattern in bottom.
   - Nonspecific cross-reacting Abs in the patient's serum (commensal treponemes) are removed by extract of Reiter's treponemes contained in the diluent.

- Screened from initial dilution of 1:80 up to even 5120
- *Advantage:* Simple and kits are available

Serology at Different Stages of Syphilis

- *Primary syphilis:* Antibodies appear 1–4 weeks after chancre. FTA-ABS detects antibodies first (85–100%) followed a week later by VDRL/RPR (70–80%) and TPHA (65–85%) Microscopy is 50–80% sensitive
- *Secondary syphilis:* All serological test are positive.
- *Latent syphilis:* Reactivity of VDRL, RPR decreases
- *Late syphilis:* VDRL—RPR: R, NR or WR. Specific tests remain positive for years.
- *To evaluate treatment:* VDRL is done at 1st, 3rd month then at 6th and 12th month

D. How will you diagnose congenital infections caused by this organism? (1 mark)

- Recommended screening at the first prenatal visit for all women and at 32–36 weeks gestation for women who are at risk.
- Testing of mother's serum
- Testing cord blood or the infant's serum
- Parallel testing of mother's and infant's serum
- *Parallel VDRL:* Neonatal serum shows higher titre than maternal serum
- *Serial VDRL:* Every month up to 6 months (baby). Passively transferred antibodies reduce in titre by 3 months.
- A nontreponemal serologic test must be confirmed by a treponemal serologic test (IgM FTA-Abs test).

---

3. 32-year-old male patient presents with purulent discharge from his urethra. He gave history of sexual exposure in the past month. His genital examination revealed a reddened urethral meatus with a thick purulent discharge. Gram smear of the urethral discharge shows pus cells with intracellular gram-negative diplococci. No other lesions/lymphadenopathy was observed.

A. What is the probable diagnosis and aetiological agent? (1 mark)

Probable Diagnosis

- Gonorrhoea

Aetiological Agent

- *Neisseria gonorrhoeae*

B. Discuss the pathogenesis of this infection. (4 marks)

Source of Infection

- Human with symptomatic or asymptomatic infection

Mode of Transmission

- Sexual contact with infected individual
- To infants through infected mother

Incubation Period

- 2–8 days

Virulence Factors

1. **Pili**
   - Pili are hair-like appendages that enhance the attachment to the host cells and resistance to phagocytosis.
2. **POR (Protein I)**
   - Extends through the gonococcal cell membrane.
   - It occurs in trimers to form pores in the surface through which nutrients enter the cell.
   - Each gonococcal strain expresses only 1 type of Por but the Por of different strains are antigenically different.
3. **OPA (Protein II)**
   - This protein functions in the adhesion of gonococci within the colonies and in attachment of gonococci to the host cells.
4. **RMP (Protein III)**
   - Reduction modifiable protein and it associates with Por in the formation of pores in the cell surface.
5. **Lipooligosaccharide**
   - It is associated with the cell wall of gonococci.
   - Endotoxin is responsible for toxicity.
   - Gonococci make LOS similar to human cell membrane glycosphingolipids (molecular mimicry).

Sequence of Events

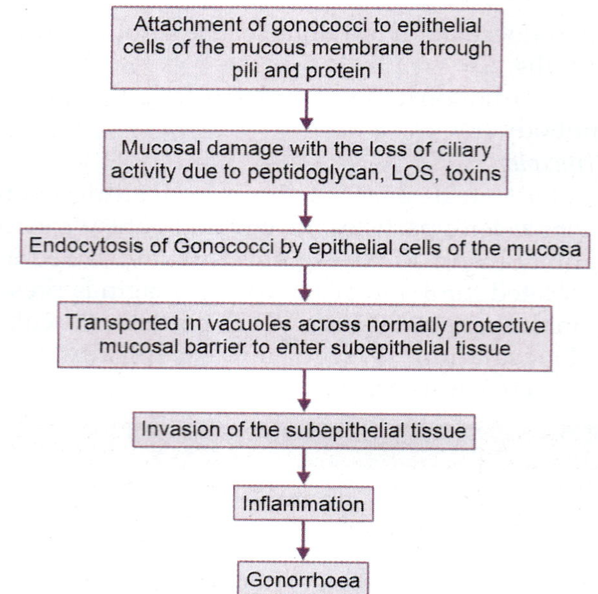

C. Discuss the clinical features of this infection. (3 marks)

- Infection may be symptomatic or asymptomatic.
- Symptomatic infections may be uncomplicated or complicated.

Gonorrhoea

- Acute pyogenic infection of the columnar and transitional epithelium of the various mucous membranes.
- In men:
  - Acute urethritis with yellow purulent discharge and dysuria
  - Untreated cases—prostatitis, eepididymitis
  - The infection may spread to periurethral tissues causing abscesses and multiple discharging sinuses (water can perineum).
- In women:
  - Increased vaginal discharge
  - Burning or frequency of urination
  - Menstrual abnormalities
  - Fever and pain
  - Coexisting *C. trachomatis, T. vaginalis*
  - Asymptomatic carriage of gonococci is common in women
- In neonates:
  - Infected mother may transmit *Gonococcus* to their babies at birth.
  - Conjunctiva is the major site (Gonococcal ophthalmia neonatorum).
- In prepubertal girls—(columnar epithelium).
  - Vulvovaginitis.
- Others.
  - Anorectal gonorrhoea in male and female
  - Pharyngeal infection.

D. Discuss the laboratory diagnosis of Gonorrhoea. (5 marks)

Specimen Collection

In Male

- Urethral discharge, urine
- Rectal swabs and pharyngeal swabs
- Chronic cases—discharge collected after prostatic massage, morning drop secretion.

In Female

- Urethral discharge
- Cervical swabs
- Rectal cultures

In Disseminated Gonococcal infection

- Blood cultures from male and female
- Endocervical and rectal swabs female
- Urethral cultures from male
- Biopsies from the skin lesions
- Aspirate from the joints

Specimen Transport

- *Media:* Transgrow and Jembec system—flat bottle with MNYC and partial CO_2

Identification

Gram's Stain

- Intracellular gram-negative kidney-shaped diplococci with adjacent sides concave with pus cells.
- 95% sensitive and 100% specific for the diagnosis of gonococcal urethritis in symptomatic male.

Fluorescent Antibody Technique for Identification

- Increases the sensitivity and specificity.

Culture

- *Nonselective:* Chocolate agar
- *Selective:* Thayer martin medium (chocolate agar with isovitale X, colistin, nystatin, vancomycin)
- Incubated at 35–37°C for 72 hours in 3–7% CO_2.
- *Colony morphology:* Small greyish white, convex, translucent, shiny colonies with smooth or irregular borders

Biochemical Reactions

- *Oxidase test:* Positive
- *Carbohydrate fermentation tests in Cysteine Trypticase soy agar:* Gonococci utilise glucose only with acid

Rapid Methods

- Serological and immuno serological identification
- Particle agglutination
- Fluorescent monoclonal antibody test for culture confirmation

Molecular Methods

- Probe assay chemiluminescence enhanced (PACE).

E. What is the treatment and prevention of this infection? (2 marks)

Treatment

- Initially Penicillin—Now resistance due to enzyme giving rise to PPNG—penicillinase-producing *Neisseria gonorrhoeae*
- Quinolone resistance, tetracycline resistance reported
- Ceftriaxone used now

Prevention

- Early diagnosis and treatment of cases
- Sex education and use of barrier methods like condoms.
- Contact tracing and treatment.

SHORT ESSAYS

1. Mention the bacteria causing anaerobic vaginosis. Describe in brief about Amsel's criteria of anaerobic bacterial vaginosis (1+4 marks)

Bacteria Causing Anaerobic Vaginosis

1. *Gardnerella vaginalis*
2. *Bacteroides* spp
3. *Peptococcus* spp
4. *Eubacterium* spp

Amsel's Criteria of Anaerobic Bacterial Vaginosis

- Four parameters used to determine the presence or absence of BV.
- These are:
  - Thin, white, yellow, homogenous discharge
  - Clue cells on wet mount microscopy
  - A vaginal fluid pH of over 4.5 when placing the discharge on litmus paper
  - Release fishy odor after adding 10% potassium hydroxide (KOH) solution to wet mount—also known as "whiff test"
- Three of the four above criteria must be present to confirm the diagnosis

2. Give examples of the parasites causing STDs. Describe the pathogenesis, clinical features, diagnosis, and treatment of vaginitis caused by flagellated protozoan. (1+1+1+1+1 marks)

Parasites Causing STDs

- *Vaginitis/NGU/balanitis: Trichomonas vaginalis*
- *Gay bowel syndrome: Entamoeba histolytica*

Flagellate Protozoan Causing Vaginitis—*Trichomonas vaginalis*

- A pear-shaped organism with a central nucleus and four anterior flagella
- It has an undulating membrane that extends about two-thirds of its length
- It exists only as a trophozoite.

Pathogenesis

- Transmitted by sexual contact
- Primary locations of the organism are the vagina and the prostate
- Found only in human
- Infection is in sexually active women in their thirties. Asymptomatic infections are common in both men and women.

Clinical Features

- *In women:* a watery, foul-smelling, greenish vaginal discharge accompanied by itching and burning occurs.
- *In men:* usually asymptomatic, but about 10% of infected men have urethritis.

Laboratory Diagnosis

- Wet mount of vaginal discharge, the pear-shaped trophozoites have a typical jerky motion.
- Nucleic acid amplification tests (NAATs) are often used because they are highly specific and sensitive.

Treatment

- Tinidazole or metronidazole for both partners to prevent reinfection.
- Maintenance of the low pH of the vagina is helpful.
- No prophylactic drug or vaccine is available.

3. Discuss in brief about the specimen collection in gonorrhoea. (3+2 marks)

Specimen Collection

In Men

- Urethral discharge, urine
- Rectal swabs and pharyngeal swabs
- Chronic cases—discharge collected after prostatic massage, morning drop secretion.

In Women

- *Endocervical swab in women:* Not vaginal
- Bartholin secretions

In Neonates

- Eye discharge

In Disseminated cases

- Blood, synovial fluid

In Homosexuals

- Rectal swab, pharyngeal swab.

4. Mention the causative agent of Lymphogranuloma venereum. Describe in brief the pathogenesis, clinical features of Lymphogranuloma venereum. (1+2+2 marks)

Causative Agent

- *Chlamydia trachomatis* L1, L2, L3.

Pathogenesis

Source of Infection

- Infected patients, asymptomatic carriers.

Mode of Transmission

- Sexually transmitted.

Incubation Period

- 3 days to 5 weeks

Sequence of Events

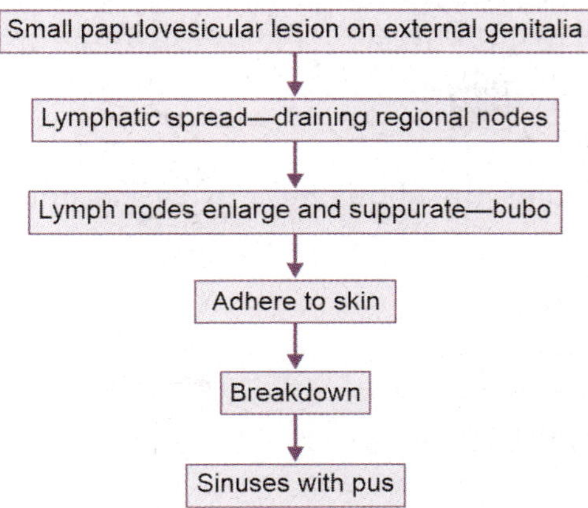

Clinical Features

- Transient genital ulcer
- Followed by the appearance of tender inguinal and/or femoral lymphadenopathy (most commonly unilateral) with a characteristic "groove sign" formed by swollen, matted lymph nodes developing along the course of the inguinal ligament.
- Untreated, the infection may lead to long-term complications, such as deep tissue abscess formation, strictures, fissures, and chronic pain.

5. List the aetiological agent of genital warts. Discuss the various types of this aetiological agent and their clinical significance and diagnosis. (2+3 marks)

Aetiological Agent of Genital Warts

- Human papilloma virus (HPV)

Types of HPV

1. *Skin warts:* HPV 2, 4, 27, 57
2. *Plantar warts:* HPV 1
3. *Laryngeal papillomas in children:* HPV 6 and HPV 11
4. *Genital warts (condyloma acuminata):* HPV 6 and HPV 11
5. *Carcinoma of uterine cervix, penis, anus, larynx, oesophagus:* HPV 16 and HPV 18, 30, 31, 33, 45 (high risk).

Clinical Significance

- Transmission by skin to skin contact and by genital contact.
- Infect squamous epithelial cells and induce within those cells a characteristic cytoplasmic vacuole. These vacuolated cells are called koilocytes.
- Most warts are benign; however, HPV infection is associated with carcinoma of cervix and penis.
- Both CMI and humoral immunity are involved in the regression of warts. Immunosuppressed have more extensive warts.

Laboratory Diagnosis

- *Cytology:* Pap smear, HPE of biopsies. Presence of koilocytes in the lesions indicate HPV infection
- PCR, DNA hybridisation test for the presence of viral DNA.

SHORT ANSWERS

1. Compare and contrast hard chancre and soft chancre. (3 marks)

Syphilitic/hard/ Hunterian chancre (Treponema pallidum)	*Chancroid/soft sore (Haemophilus ducreyi)*
• Painless ulcer	• Painful and tender ulcer
• Well circumscribed, indurated, regular margins	• Non-indurated, irregular margin
• Usually, single ulcer	• Multiple ulcers common • Autoinoculation lesions
• Local lymph nodes swollen, discrete, rubbery, non-tender	• Local lymph nodes enlarged, painful and tender

2. Describe in brief the clinical features of the disease caused by molluscum contagiosum. (1+2 marks)

Molluscum Contagiosum Virus (MCV)

- Member of the poxvirus family

Clinical Features

- Lesion.
  - Small (2–5 mm), flesh-coloured papule on the skin or mucous membrane that is painless, nonpruritic, and not inflamed.
  - Characteristic cup-shaped (umbilicated) crater with a white core.
  - Composed of hyperplastic epithelial cells within which a cytoplasmic inclusion body can be seen. The inclusion body contains progeny MCV.
  - Can be large and numerous in patients with reduced cellular immunity. In immunocompetent patients, the lesions are self-limited but may last for months.

3. Mention six bacterial examples causing UTIs. (3 marks)

1. *Escherichia coli*
2. *Klebsiella pneumoniae*
3. *Proteus mirabilis*
4. *Pseudomonas aeruginosa*
5. *Enterococcus faecalis*
6. *Staphylococcus saprophyticus*

4. Mention the causative agents of non-gonococcal Urethritis. (3 marks)

I. Bacteria

1. *Chlamydia trachomatis*
2. *Ureaplasma urealyticum*
3. *Mycoplasma hominis*
4. *Gardnerella vaginalis*
5. *Acinetobacter lwoffii*

II. Fungi

1. *Candida albicans*

III. Protozoa

1. *Trichomonas vaginalis*

IV. Virus

1. Herpes virus
2. Cytomegalovirus

5. A 22-year-old lady presents to the OBG OPD with h/o curdy white vaginal discharge and itching. Wet mount of the vaginal discharge shows yeast like budding cells. Discuss the pathogenesis and diagnosis of this infection. (2+2 marks)

Candidal Vulvovaginitis

- Caused by inflammatory changes in the vaginal and vulvar epithelium secondary to infection with *Candida* species, most commonly *Candida albicans*.
- *Candida* is part of the normal flora in many women and is often asymptomatic.
- Therefore, *Candidal* vulvovaginitis requires both the presence of candida in the vagina/vulva as well as the symptoms of irritation, itching, dysuria, or inflammation.

Aetiology

- *C. albicans* (in about 90% of cases) and *Candida glabrata*.

Risk Factors

- Estrogen use, elevated endogenous estrogens (from pregnancy or obesity), diabetes mellitus, immunosuppression and broad-spectrum antibiotic use.

Pathogenesis

- *Candida* species superficially penetrate the mucosal lining of the vagina and cause an inflammatory response. The dominant inflammatory cells are typically polymorphonuclear cells and macrophages.

Clinical Features

- Discharge, which is typically thick and adherent, or with excoriations, "external" dysuria, vaginal itching, vaginal burning, dyspareunia, or swelling.

Diagnosis

- *Vaginal swab:* Wet mount, Gram's stain
- Gram stain of the vaginal swab shows the presence of gram-positive yeast like budding cells with pseudohyphae.
- Culture on Sabouraud dextrose agar.
- *Identification of species:* Germ tube test, chlamydospore formation test

7.2 DESCRIBE THE AETIOPATHOGENESIS AND DESCRIBE THE LABORATORY DIAGNOSIS OF STD ADD A NOTE ON PREVENTIVE MEASURES

LONG ESSAY

1. Discuss in brief about venereal diseases under the following headings.

A. Definition (1 mark)

- Venereal diseases are infections which are transmitted through sexual contact, urogenital contact.

B. Classification with examples, based on clinical presentation. (2 marks)

Genital ulcers	• Syphilis • Genital herpes • Chancroid • Lymphogranuloma venereum • Donovanosis
Urethral discharge	• Gonorrhoea • Non-gonococcal urethritis (NGU)
Vaginal discharge	• Vulvovaginal candidiasis • Bacterial vaginosis • *Trichomonas vaginitis*
Genital warts	• *Condyloma acuminata*

Contd.

C. Pathogenesis, clinical features of syphilis. (5 marks)

Pathogenesis

- *Source:* Infected person
- *Mode of Infection:* Sexual contact, mother to fetus, blood transfusions in early stages (rare)
- *Incubation period:* 10–90 days

- *Virulence factors:*
  1. *OMP:* Adherence
  2. *Hyaluronidase:* Perivascular infiltration
  3. *Fibronectin:* Prevents phagocytosis
  4. Tissue destruction and lesions due to host's immune response (immunopathology)
  5. No important toxins

Clinical Features (Fig. 7.2.1)

D. Mention the preventive strategies for STDs. (2 marks)

- **Prevention:**
  - Early diagnosis and treatment of cases.
  - Sex education and use of barrier methods like condoms to prevent STDs.
  - Contact tracing of the primary case and treatment.

SHORT ESSAY

1. List the non-syphilitic causes of genital ulcers. Discuss the clinical presentation and diagnosis of STIs causing genital ulcers. (1+4 marks)

Non-syphilitic Causes of Genital Ulcers

1. *Herpes genitalis.*
2. Chancroid.
3. Lymphogranuloma venereum.
4. Donovanosis.

STIs Causing Genital Ulcers

See Table 7.2.1

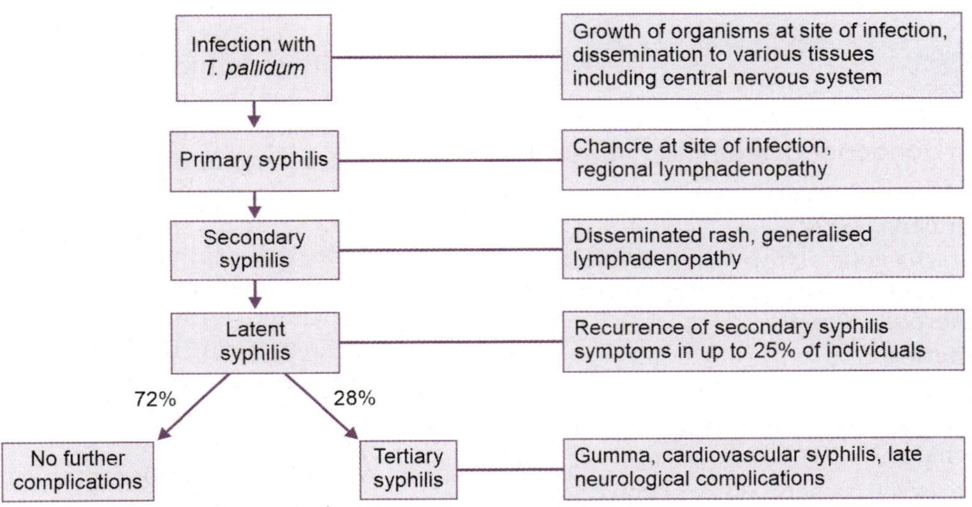

Fig. 7.2.1: Clinical features of syphilis

Table 7.2.1 Clinical presentation and diagnosis of genital ulcers

Infection	*Clinical Presentation*	*Diagnosis*
Herpes simplex virus infection	• Multiple vesicular lesions that rupture and become painful, shallow ulcers • Fever and lymphadenopathy in primary infections	• *Definitive:* herpes simplex virus identified on culture or PCR of ulcer scraping or vesicle fluid • *Presumptive:* typical lesions with positive Tzanck smear of ulcer scraping • 4-fold increase in antibody titer (in a first-time infection)
Syphilis (primary)	• Single, painless, well-demarcated ulcer (chancre) with a clean base and indurated border • Mild or minimally tender inguinal lympha denopathy	• *Treponema pallidum* identified on darkfield microscopy or direct fluorescent antibody testing of a chancre or lymph node aspirate *or* • Positive result on VDRL/RPR that is confirmed with a positive result on serologic treponemal testing (i.e., fluorescent treponemal antibody absorption or *T. pallidum* passive agglutination)
Chancroid	• Nonindurated, painful with serpiginous border and friable base; covered with a necrotic, often purulent exudate Tender, suppurative, unilateral inguinal lymphadenopathy or adenitis	• Gram stain suggestive of *Haemophilus ducreyi* (gram-negative, slender rod or coccobacillus in a "school of fish" pattern) • Definitive: *H. ducreyi* identified on culture

Contd.

Table 7.2.1 Clinical presentation and diagnosis of genital ulcers

Infection	Clinical Presentation	Diagnosis
Donovanosis	• Painless beefy red ulcer	• Giemsa stain • *Klebsiella granulomatis:* Donovan's bodies
Lympho-granuloma venereum	• Small papulovesicular lesion on external genitalia • Bubo which breaks down to form sinuses	a. Microscopy: not very useful. Inclusion bodies can be stained with Castaneda, Machiavelli, Gimenez stains b. Direct IF c. Ag detection d. Culture: McCoy cell culture/Yolk sac inoculation- difficult to isolate e. Serology i. CFT- Group-specific antibodies: titres: 1:64: Dis adv: False-positive ii. Microimmunoflorescence test: Type-specific antibodies: Titre: 1: 512 iii. NAAT: PCR

SHORT ANSWERS

1. Describe Non gonococcal Urethritis (3 marks)

- Sexually transmitted disease.
- Causative organisms.
  - *Chlamydia trachomatis, Ureaplasma urealyticum, Trichomonas vaginalis*, Group B *Streptococcus, G. vaginalis*, anaerobes, yeasts.
- Clinical presentation.
  - Male with NSU where no gonococcal cause can be found, have thinner, more mucoid purulent urethral discharge.
  - Female with NSU present with asymptomatic urethritis, cervicitis.
- Treatment.
  - Tetracycline for 3 weeks or erythromycin.

2. A 29-year-old woman presents with itching and burning pain of vagina. O/E, white discharge is apparent. On Sabourad's dextrose agar colonies are present. She also gives a h/o antibiotic consumption for sinus infection. What is the probable condition? Explain the diagnostic workup in this case. (1+2 marks)

Probable Condition

- Vulvovaginal candidiasis.

Diagnosis of Vulvovaginal Candidiasis

- Vulvovaginal candidiasis was diagnosed if one of the following criteria was fulfilled.
  1. Wet-mount and/or Gram's stain preparation with budding yeasts, pseudohyphae, and/or hyphal forms.
  2. Positive culture (>100 CFU/ml suspension) and negative microscopic examination results associated with one sign or symptom (thick, white vaginal discharge with no odor, vulvar and vaginal pruritus, burning, or dyspareunia); and.
  3. A positive culture result (>100 CFU/ml suspension) and a negative microscopic examination associated with one of the following clinical findings during the physical examination: vulvar and vaginal erythema, edema, fissures, or a thick, white vaginal discharge adhering to the vaginal walls.
  4. A negative microscopy result together with a small number of yeasts (<100 CFU/ml suspension) was considered to indicate *Candida* colonisation rather than infection.

3. Mention the genital lesions due to HSV. Add a note on importance of Tzanck smear. (2+1 marks)

Genital Lesions due to HSV

- Usually, multiple vesicular lesions that rupture and become painful, shallow ulcers constitutional symptoms, lymphadenopathy in first-time infections.

Importance of Tzanck Smear

- For viral infections, samples should be taken from a fresh vesicle.
- The vesicle should be unroofed, or the crust removed, and the base scraped with a scalpel or the edge of a spatula.
- Tzanck smear can be stained by a variety of methods, most commonly by Giemsa stain. Other stains used are haematoxylin and eosin, Wright, methylene blue, Papanicolaou and toluidine blue.

Findings in Herpes Simplex infection

- Characteristic multinucleated syncytial giant cells and acantholytic cells
- The cells appear as if they have been inflated (ballooning degeneration) and sometimes may grow tremendously, 60–80 m in diameter.
- Intranuclear inclusion bodies surrounded by subtle clear halo are characteristic of herpetic infection but are often difficult to find.

7.3 DESCRIBE THE AETIOPATHOGENESIS, CLINICAL FEATURES, APPROPRIATE METHOD OF SPECIMEN COLLECTION AND DISCUSS THE LABORATORY DIAGNOSIS OF UTI

LONG ESSAY

1. A 21-year-old female student visited OBG specialist with chief complaints of burning micturition and increased frequency of micturition. Urine sample is collected and sent for complete microscopic examination, culture, and AST. Urinalysis of a clean-catch urine sample was notable for >50 WBC/HPF, 3–10 RBC/HPF, and 3+ bacteria. Urine culture was subsequently positive for >100,000 CFU/ml of lactose fermenting gram-negative bacilli. Answer the following questions related to the case/condition.

A. Probable diagnosis of the case and mention the bacterial aetiology of the above condition. (2 marks)

Probable Diagnosis

- Lower urinary tract infection.

Bacterial Aetiology of the above condition

- Coliform bacilli.
  1. *E. coli.*
  2. *Klebsiella spp.*

B. Classification of UTI. (2 marks)

Based on the Aetiology

I. Bacteria

1. **Community acquired**
   - i. *Escherichia coli*
   - ii. *Staphylococcus saprophyticus*, *Proteus* spp
   - iii. *Enterococcus* spp
2. **Hospital acquired**
   - i. *E. coli*
   - ii. *Pseudomonas* spp
   - iii. *Serratia* spp
   - iv. *Staphylococcus aureus*
   - v. *Proteus* spp

II. Virus

1. *Adenovirus*
2. *Hantavirus*

III. Fungus

1. *Candida* spp

IV. Parasite

1. *Trichomonas vaginalis*
2. *Schistosoma haematobium*

Based on Anatomical Site

I. **Lower**
   1. Urethra
   2. Bladder

II. **Upper**
   1. Kidney
   2. Ureter

Based on the settings in which UTI occurs

I. Community
II. Nosocomial

C. Pathogenesis, clinical features of UTI. (3 marks)

Pathogenesis

Source of Infection

- Endogenous
- Exogenous

Mode of Infection

- Ascending
- Descending (haematogenous)

Host Factors

1. **Protective mechanisms**
   - Micturition, prostatic secretions, inhibitors of bacterial adherence, normal flora, vesicourethral valve
2. **Risk factors.**
   - *Gender:* female, incomplete bladder emptying, foreign bodies, obstruction, reduced host defenses, anatomical structure, instrumentation, surgery

Virulence Factors

1. Adhesion factors (*P. fimbriae* in uropathogenic *E coli*)
2. Capsule
3. Enzymes

4. Hemolysin
5. Lipopolysaccharide

Sequence of Events

1. **Ascending route**
   - Colonisation of urethra especially by *Coliform bacilli.*
   - Uroepithelium penetration in the bladder followed by multiplication of bacteria
   - *Ascends to Kidney:* Pyelonephritis
2. **Descending route**
   - It is by haematogenous seeding of bacteria in kidney following haematogenous spread, e.g. *Staphylococcus aureus.*

Clinical Features

- *Cystitis/urethritis:* Dysuria, urgency, frequency
- *Pyelonephritis:* Dysuria, urgency, frequency along with fever, vomiting, abdominal pain
- Prostatitis
- Asymptomatic bacteriuria

D. Discuss the laboratory diagnosis of UTI. (2 marks)

Specimen Collection

1. Clean catch midstream urine sample
2. Supra-pubic aspiration
3. *Catheterisation:* Urine aspirated from the catheter tube after clamping distally and disinfecting

Transportation

- Urine must be collected in sterile, wide mouthed, leak proof container
- Transported immediately
- In case of delay, it can be refrigerated at 4°C for 2 hours.

Methods

- *Macroscopy:* Turbidity, Blood, pH
- *Wet mount preparation:* Pus cells, RBCs, bacteria, epithelial cells
- *Culture:* Mac Conkey agar and CLED agar plates—Semi-quantitative method—Interpreted by colony forming units per ml of urine
- *Significant bacteriuria:* $>10^5$ CFU/ml → Diagnostic of UTI
- 10^3 CFU/ml suprapubic aspiration single organism also is significant.
- Antimicrobial susceptibility testing
- Screening tests
- Griess nitrite test
- Catalase test
- Triphenyl tetrazolium chloride (TTC)
- Gram's stain of urine
- Dip slide culture method

E. Significant bacteriuria and asymptomatic bacteriuria. (2 marks)

Significant Bacteriuria

- Presence of $>10^5$ CFU/ml of bacteria in a clean catch midstream sample of urine (Kass concept).
- A means of differentiating between contamination in the voided specimen and true urinary infection.

Asymptomatic Bacteriuria

- Presence of bacteria in the properly collected urine of a patient with no signs or symptoms of a urinary tract infection.
- Screening for asymptomatic bacteriuria is done in pregnancy and patients undergoing urologic procedures.

SHORT ESSAYS

1. 22-year-old female presents to OPD with complaints of vaginal discharge and dysuria. Wet mount examination of the vaginal swab reveals pear-shaped trophozoite of this flagellate.

A. What is the probable diagnosis?

B. Mention the parasites causing UTI.

C. Discuss in brief the pathological aspects and diagnosis of genitourinary infections due to genital flagellates. (1+2+2 marks)

A. Diagnosis

- Trichomoniasis caused by *Trichomonas vaginalis*

B. Parasites Causing UTI

1. *Trichomonas vaginalis*
2. *Schistosoma hematobium*

C. Pathogenesis of Trichomoniasis

- *Source:* Resides in the lumen of the urogenital tract
- *Virulence factors*
  - Proteases: Adherence to epithelium
  - Lactic acid: Reduces pH, which is cytotoxic to epithelial cells
  - Releases cytotoxic proteins that destroy the epithelial lining

Diagnosis of Trichomoniasis

- *Specimen collection:* Vaginal discharge (women), urethral discharge, prostatic fluid, early morning first voided urine (men)

- *Wet mount:* Pear shaped trophozoites of *Trichomonas vaginalis* with twitching motility seen (Fig. 7.3.1)

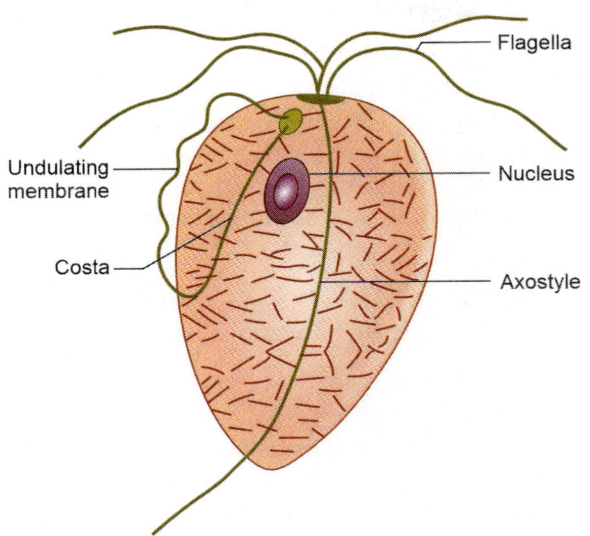

Fig. 7.3.1: Trophozoite of *Trichomonas vaginalis*

2. Enumerate the fungi causing UTI in sexually active young females. Discuss in brief the pathogenesis and microscopic morphology of the causative agent. (1+2+2 marks)

Fungi Causing UTI

1. *Candida albicans.*
2. *Non-albicans Candida.*

Pathogenesis of UTI due to *Candida* spp

Mode of Infection

- *Candida* species enter the upper urinary tract from the bloodstream (antegrade infection) or ascend the urinary tract from a focus of candidal colonisation at or near the urethra (retrograde infection).

Virulence Factors

- Adherence, dimorphism, phenotypic switching, hydrolytic enzymes, biofilm formation, and evasion of the immune response.

Host Factors

- Catheters, diabetes mellitus, immunosuppression.

Microscopic Morphology

1. *KOH mount:* Shows yeast cells with pseudo-hyphae.
2. *Gram's stain:* Gram-positive oval yeast like budding cells with pseudo-hyphae.

3. Discuss the clinical manifestations, complications, and laboratory diagnosis of *Schistosoma haematobium*. (2+1+2 marks)

Schistosoma haematobium

Clinical Manifestations

Acute Schistosomiasis

- *Cercarial dermatitis:* Itching and pruritic papular lesion in the skin within 24 hours by the invasion of cercariae
- Fever, malaise, right upper quadrant pain are the symptoms of serum sickness like illness.

Chronic Schistosomiasis

- Painless terminal haematuria dysuria and frequent urination.

Complications

1. Hydroureter
2. Hydronephrosis
3. Secondary microbial infection
4. Frequent UTI by *Salmonella*
5. Urinary bladder carcinoma

Laboratory Diagnosis

Parasitic Diagnosis

- *Specimen Collection:* Urine, aspiration obtained by cystoscopy
- *Urine:* Collected between 10 am and 2 pm, examined after centrifugation or membrane filtration. Presence of terminal spined eggs of *S. haematobium*
- *Urine egg count* in 24 hr collection to quantitate the severity of the infection (>50 eggs/10 ml is heavy infection).
- *Egg viability test* to assess the effectiveness of treatment. Done by mixing urine with distilled water and observe for hatching miracidium.

Sero Diagnosis

- Detection of antibodies—IHA, Indirect IF, ELISA, RIA. Diagnosis of infection in prepatent period, chronic and ectopic cases.
- Detection of antigen—in serum, urine by CIEP, ELISA, RIA. Helps to detect acute infection and of prognostic value.

Histological Diagnosis

- Detection of parasitic eggs in the biopsy specimens.

Other Tests

- Eosinophilia, haematuria, proteinuria.

4. A 23-year-old female presented with signs of cystitis. Clean catch midstream urine sample was sent for examination. Gram smear from the clean catch mid-stream urine is provided.

Culture: *Escherichia coli* >100000 CFU/ml

Antibiotic Sensitivity Report

Antibiotic	S/R
Ampicillin	R
Amikacin	S
Cefotaxime	S
Cefuroxime	S
Ciprofloxacin	S
Norfloxacin	S
Cotrimoxazole	S
Nitrofurantoin	S
Imipenem	S
Piperacillin tazobactam	S
S: Sensitive, R: Resistant	

A. What is significant bacteriuria and mention its clinical significance (1 mark)

- Presence of $>10^5$ CFU/ml of bacteria in clean-catch midstream sample of urine is called significant bacteriuria. It signifies true urinary tract infection and differentiates it from contamination (Kass concept).

B. What is the drug of choice in this case? (1 mark)

- Norfloxacin, or co-trimoxazole, or nitrofurantoin.

C. What are the methods of collecting urine specimen for culture? (1 mark)

- Clean catch midstream urine in a sterile screw capped container. In unconscious patients or patients with neurological bladder: suprapubic aspiration, urine from catheter.

D. What are the common aetiological agents of community acquired UTI? (1 mark)

- *Escherichia coli, Klebsiella* spp., *Enterococcus* spp.,.

CHAPTER 8

Zoonotic Diseases and Miscellaneous

MI 8.1 ENUMERATE THE MICROBIAL AGENTS AND THEIR VECTORS CAUSING ZOONOTIC DISEASES. DESCRIBE THE MORPHOLOGY, MODE OF TRANSMISSION, PATHOGENESIS AND DISCUSS THE CLINICAL COURSE, LABORATORY DIAGNOSIS AND PREVENTION

LONG ESSAYS

1. Define zoonoses. Classify zoonoses with examples from each category. Describe in detail about human anthrax under the following headings. (1 + 2 marks)

Zoonoses—Definition

- Infections in which non-human vertebrates are the reservoir of infections and humans are involved only incidentally.

Classification of Zoonoses

1. *Anthropozoonoses:* Infections transmitted from animals to man, e.g. rabies.
2. *Zooanthroponoses:* Infections transmitted from man to animals, e.g. influenza A.
3. *Amphixenoses:* Infections maintained in both animals and man and may be transmitted bidirectional, e.g. influenza.

A. Mode of transmission of anthrax. (1 mark)

- By contact with infected animals or inhalation of spores from hair and wool of animals—occupational exposure.

B. Different clinical forms of anthrax. (3 marks)

1. **Cutaneous Anthrax (Hide Porter's Disease)**
   - A typical skin lesion presents as painless ulcer with black eschar, e.g. malignant pustule—most common and self-limiting
2. **Pulmonary Anthrax (Wool Sorter's Disease)**
   - Rare and fatal.
   - Develops with nonspecific influenza like illness.
   - Rapid progression to haemorrhagic mediastinitis, bloody pleural effusions, septic shock, and death.
   - Characteristic chest X-ray findings with mediastinal widening
   - Complications such as haemorrhagic mediastinitis and haemorrhagic meningitis may be seen.
3. **Gastrointestinal Anthrax**
   - Vomiting, abdominal pain, and bloody diarrhoea.

C. Brief note on laboratory diagnosis and preventive measures. (3 marks)

Laboratory Diagnosis

Specimen Collection

- Pus, swab or tissue, exudate, sputum, blood, CSF, gastric aspirate depending on site of involvement.

Direct Demonstration

- *Gram's stain:* Large, gram-positive rods in chains
- *Mc Faydean's reaction:* With polychrome methylene blue stain shows amorphous purple capsule surrounding the blue bacilli
- *Direct IF:* Detects capsular antigen

Culture

- *Blood agar:* Dry, wrinkled, non-haemolytic colonies (comet tail appearance)
- *Nutrient agar:* Medusa head appearance of colonies
- *Gelatin stab agar:* Inverted fir tree appearance
- *Selective media*
  - PLET (Polymyxin, lysozyme, EDTA and thallous acetate) medium
  - Solid media with penicillin: String of pearl

Antibody Detection

- ELISA (Acute and convalescent sera)

Molecular Method

- PCR using specific primers

Prevention

General Prophylaxis

- Disposal of animal carcasses by deep burial in lime pits/burning
- Decontamination by autoclaving the animal products
- Use of protective clothes and gloves while handling infectious material

Specific Prophylaxis

- *Ciprofloxacin:* In case of outbreaks
- *Vaccine:* Cell free (Biothrax), 6 doses over 18 months and booster dose annually
- *Immunoglobulin's:* Monoclonal antibody against protective antigen.

---

2. An eight-year-old child was attacked by some stray dogs while playing on the street outside his house. O/E at ED, multiple bite marks with gaping wound were noticed on the left forearm. The doctor cleaned the wound and gave an injection and prescribed multiple injections on regular intervals.

A. What is your diagnosis (1 mark)

- This is a case of dog bit, rabies.

B. Mode of transmission, pathogenesis, clinical features of this condition. (4 marks)

Rabies

Mode of Transmission

- Bite of rabid animal such as dogs, bats, skunks. It is present in the saliva of the infected animal.
- Aerosols of infected bats
- Corneal transplants of infected patients (rare)

Pathogenesis

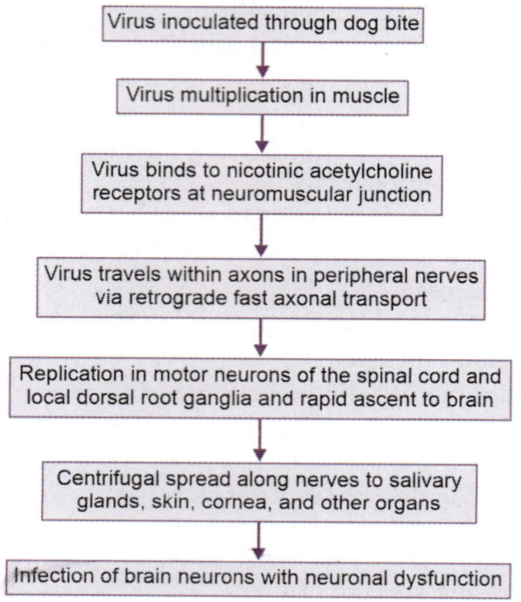

Clinical Features

- Incubation period ranges from 10 days to 16 weeks.
- **Prodromal Stage**
  - Lasts for 2–10 days.
  - The patients exhibit nonspecific symptoms such as fever, anorexia, and paresthesia at the site of bite.
- **Furious Rabies (Encephalitic)**
  - Seen in 80% cases
  - Last for 2–7 days
  - Hyperexcitability is followed by lucid state, autonomic disturbances such as increased salivation, lacrimation, sweating, arrhythmias and priapism
  - Hydrophobia, i.e. painful spasm of respiratory, laryngeal muscles
- **Dumb Rabies (Paralytic)**
  - Seen in 20% cases
  - Flaccid paralysis
  - Quadriparesis
- **Coma and Death**
  - Within 15 days of onset
  - Death is almost certain

C. Laboratory methods available for diagnosis of this case. (2 marks)

Lab Diagnosis

Specimen Collection

- Hair follicles from nape of neck, corneal smear, saliva, spinal fluid, brain tissue.

Antemortem Diagnosis

1. **Direct immunofluorescence test (DFA)**
   - Detects specific antigens by fluorescent antibody staining.
   - High sensitivity and specificity and considered gold standard test.
2. **Virus isolation**
   - Cell lines such as mouse neuroblastoma and brain hamster kidney
   - Viral growth is detected by direct IF test using specific antiserum.
3. **Antibody detection**
   - Detection of CSF antibody is more significant than serum antibodies.
   - Methods are:
     1. Mouse neutralisation test (MNT)
     2. Rapid fluorescent focus inhibition test (RFFIT)
     3. Indirect fluorescent assay (IFA)
4. **Virus RNA detection**
   - By Reverse transcriptase PCR

Post-mortem Diagnosis

- Intracytoplasmic inclusion body called Negri body in hippocampus or cerebellum is pathognomonic feature found in rabies using H and E stain or Seller's stain.

D. Add a note on immunoprophylaxis required for the child. (3 marks)

- Post-exposure prophylaxis (PEP) is the immediate treatment of a bite victim after rabies exposure.
- This prevents virus entry into the central nervous system and imminent death.
- PEP consists of:
  - After a suspected exposure extensive washing with soap and water along with local treatment of the bite wound or scratch as soon as possible. Suturing should be avoided as it promotes the spread of virus.
  - A course of potent and effective rabies vaccine on days 0, 3, 7, 14, 28 in previously unvaccinated and 0 and 3 in previously vaccinated.
  - Rabies immunoglobulin (RIG), if unvaccinated.
- *Types of Vaccines.*
  1. Purified chick embryo cell vaccine (PCEC)
  2. Purified vero cell (PVC)
  3. Human diploid cell vaccine (HDC)
- *Route of administration:* Either Intramuscular/ Intradermal
- *Site:* Anterolateral aspect of thigh in a child (Adults: Deltoid muscle)
- *Dose:* 0.1ml for intradermal or entire vial for intramuscular
- *Schedule.*
  - Intradermal regimen: (2–2-2): 2 sites on days 0, 3, 7.
  - Intramuscular regimen: 1 site on days 0, 3, 7.
- *Rabies Immunoglobulin—Human rabies immunoglobulin (20IU):*
  - Administered as soon as possible not beyond 7 days
  - Given in and around the wound
  - Neutralises the virus at the site of wound

3. Ortho-myxo viruses exhibit rapid rate of mutations due to the presence of special proteins on their surface. Swine flu virus is a classic example. Describe in detail about human influenza and swine flu under the following headings.

A. Mention the surface antigens/proteins of ortho-myxo virus and the role of this virus in antigenic variations. (2 marks)

Surface Antigens/Proteins of Ortho-myxo Virus

- The two major antigens are the haemagglutinin (16 HA) and the neuraminidase (9NA) as surface spikes.
- Viral proteins.
  - *8 structural:* PB1, PB2, PA, NP, HA, NA, M1, M2.
  - *2 Nonstructural:* NS1, NS2.
- The virus is enveloped with a helical nucleocapsid and single-stranded, segmented RNA of negative polarity.
- RNA polymerase in virion

Role of Ortho-myxo Virus in Antigenic Variations

- *Antigenic shift* results due to genetic re-assortment of RNA segments which accounts for the epidemics or pandemics of influenza caused by influenza A virus. Occurs less frequently for every 10–20 years.
- *Antigenic drift* due to point mutations. Seen in Influenza A and B. It results in outbreaks and minor periodic epidemic. Occurs periodically every 2–3 years.

B. Distinguish between Three Different Types of Influenza (2 marks)

Feature	*Influenza A*	*Influenza B*	*Influenza C*
Epide-micity	Epidemics and pandemic	Non-pandemic	Non-epidemic
Host	Humans and animals	Humans	Humans
Severity	Severe	Non-severe	Mild-infections
Examples	H1N1, H5N1, H3N2	B (Victoria)	Not of public health importance

C. Write in brief the pathogenesis of Influenza. (2 marks)

Mode of Transmission

- Inhalation of respiratory droplets.
- Contact of fomites or surfaces contaminated with respiratory droplets.

Sequence of Events

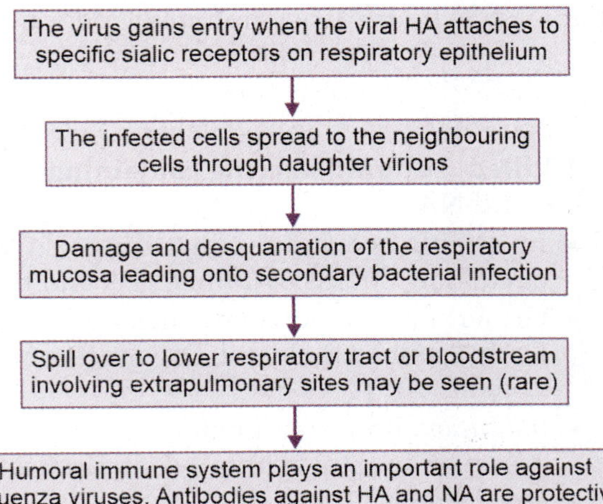

D. Laboratory diagnosis, preventive measures of Influenza. (4 marks)

Laboratory Diagnosis

Specimen Collection

- Nasopharyngeal swab or BAL. Nasal aspirate.

Transport Media

- Viral transport media (VTM)—can be stored at 4°C for 4 days and thereafter –70°C.

Direct Immunofluorescence Test

- Virus antigen detection using fluorescence tagged antibody.

Virus Cultivation

- Embryonated egg (amniotic cavity) and primary monkey kidney cell line.
- Viral growth-detected by haemadsorption or haemagglutination test.

Molecular Methods

- *RT PCR:* Highly sensitive, specific and results obtained in a day
- *Real time PCR:* Gold standard, highly sensitive and specific and quantitative, results available within 2–3 hours
- *Biofire film array respiratory panel:* Detects around 20 respiratory pathogens which includes influenza A, influenza A/H1, influenza A/H3, influenza A/H1–2009, Influenza B

Preventive Measures

General Prophylaxis

- Hand hygiene.
- Isolation.
- Precautions for droplet transmission to be considered by HCW
- *Work restriction:* CDC recommends home isolation for at least 24 hours of asymptomatic period

Specific Prophylaxis

- Two types of vaccines are available:
  1. **A killed (subunit) vaccine containing purified HA and NA**
     - Injectable vaccine containing currently circulating strains of influenza A and B virus.
     - Grown in embryonated chick egg or Madin Darby canine kidney cell lines or recombinant vaccine
     - *Indication:* Routine annual vaccination for age group >6 months without contraindications.
     - *Dose:* Single.
  2. **A live vaccine containing a temperature-sensitive mutant of influenza virus.**
     - The virus replicates and induces secretory IgA in cool nasal passages, but not in warm lower respiratory tract.
     - Its trivalent vaccine containing circulating strains of influenza A and B virus.
     - *Indication:* Healthy individuals of age 2–49 years.
     - *Dose:* Single
     - Not recommended for high-risk groups, pregnancy, immunocompromised.

Chemoprophylaxis

- Oseltamivir in those individuals who are unvaccinated.

---

4. A 28-year-old pregnant female exposed to cat bite at her home. She used to rare cats and always in close contact with the animals at her home. Few days after exposure, CT scan revealed some malformation in the developing foetus. OBG specialist and radiologist advised her that there might be chances of miscarriage. Serology report is reactive for IgG, IgM antibodies of a protozoan parasite. With this brief history discuss the following questions related to the case.

A. Probable diagnosis in this case and morphological forms of the protozoan parasite. (1 mark)

Probable Diagnosis

- Toxoplasmosis

Morphological Forms of the Protozoan Parasite

1. Trophozoite
2. Cyst form

B. Life cycle of this aetiological agent. (3 marks)

- *Aetiological agent: Toxoplasma gondii*
- *Definite host:* Cat
- *Intermediate host:* Human
- *Infective stage:* Oocysts
- *Diagnostic stage:* Tissue cysts
- *Life cycle:*

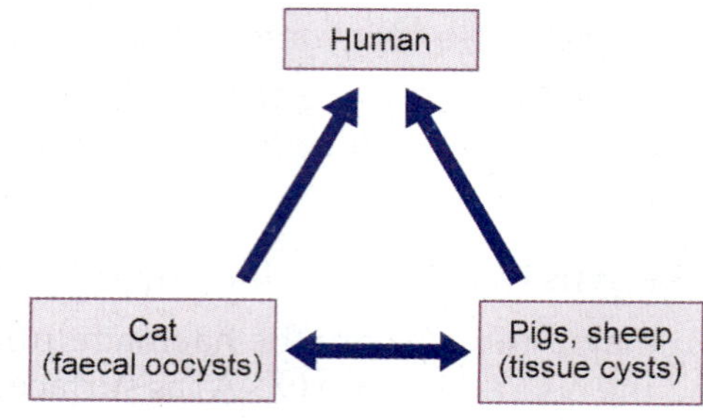

- Both oocytes and tissue cysts transform into tachyzoites shortly after ingestion.
- Tachyzoites localize in neural and muscle tissue and develop into tissue cyst bradyzoites.
- If a pregnant woman becomes infected, tachyzoites can infect the faetus via the bloodstream.

C. Pathogenesis, clinical features of this condition. (4 marks)

Pathogenesis

Mode of Transmission

- Toxoplasmosis is transmitted by ingestion of cysts present in uncooked meat or food contaminated with cat faeces.
- Transplacental transmission from the mother to foetus.

Sequence of Events

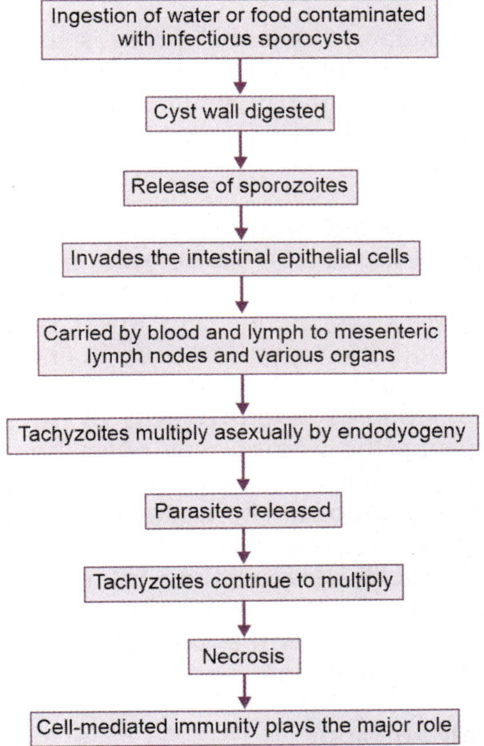

Clinical Features

- Asymptomatic.
- *In immunocompetent:* Fever, headache, malaise, cervical lymphadenopathy
- *In immunocompromised:* Encephalitis presenting with altered mental status, seizures, sensory abnormalities, cerebellar involvement or with focal neurological deficits, pulmonary infections and chorioretinitis seen in patients with HIV
- *Congenital toxoplasmosis:* Chorioretinitis, hydrocephalus, intracranial calcifications

D. Brief account on serological diagnosis and preventive measures of this disease. (2 marks)

Serological Diagnosis

Specimen Collection

- Blood, tissue biopsy

Serology

- Various methods such as capture ELISA, immunofluorescence assays.
- *Sabin Feldman dye test*—considered as gold standard test for antibody detection, usually done at reference lab
- Acute infection:
  - IgM antibodies appear within 1–2 weeks of infection, congenital infection.
  - IgG antibodies—A fourfold rise in titre.
  - Low IgG avidity test.
- Past/remote infection (>6 months)—IgG is raised.

Preventive Measures

- Cook meat thoroughly to kill the cysts.
- Hand hygiene recommended for people handling cats.

---

5. Describe in brief the life cycle, pathogenesis, clinical features and lab diagnosis of dog tape worm. (3+3+1+3 marks)

Life Cycle of Dog Tape Worm

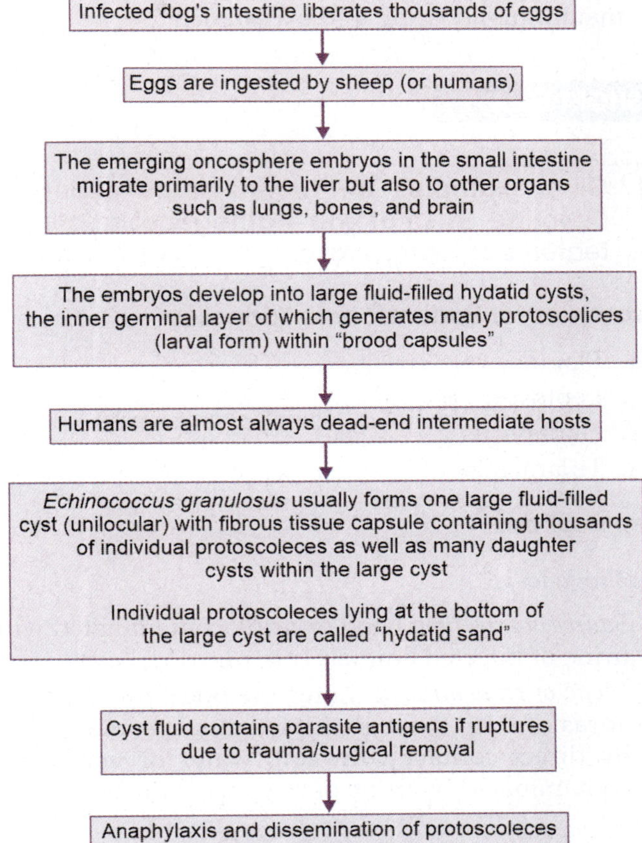

Clinical Features

- Asymptomatic in most cases.
- *Hydatid disease:* Liver—hepatomegaly or lung involvement
- Focal neurological deficits or shock.

Lab Diagnosis

Hydatid Fluid Microscopy

- Wet mount examination—to demonstrates protoscolices and brood capsule
- Histological examination—cyst reveals pericyst, ectocyst and endocyst layers of hydatid cyst

Casoni's Skin Test

- Immediate skin hypersensitivity reaction

Antibody Presence

- Indicates past infection, used for seroepidemiology.
- *Screening:* IHA, CIEP, ELISA
- *Confirmation:* Western blot
- *Detection of antigen:* Indicates recent infection

Radiology

- *USG, MRI, and X-ray:* To locate the size, exact location, and extension of the cysts
- *Water lily sign in USG:* Due to collapsed cyst (floating membrane) floating in the abdomen

SHORT ESSAYS

1. Give examples for rodent-borne zoonoses. Describe in brief the pathogenesis, clinical features of leptospirosis. (1+2+2 marks)

Examples for Rodent-borne Zoonoses

1. Plague
2. Leptospirosis
3. Hantavirus
4. Tularaemia

Leptospirosis

Pathogenesis

- *Source of infection:* Food or drink contaminated with urine of infected animals (rat, pig, dog, cow)
- *Mode of transmission:* Enter the body through skin abrasions or through intact mucous membrane by direct contact with soil, water or vegetation contaminated by urine of infected animals.
- *Sequence of events.*
  - Two phases: an initial bacteremic phase followed by immunopathologic phase with meningitis.
  - No toxins or virulence factors known.

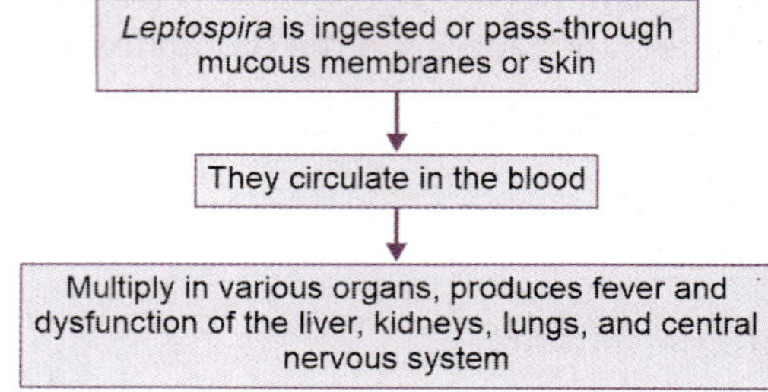

Clinical Features

- The illness is primarily **biphasic,** with fever, chills, intense headache, and conjunctival suffusion (diffuse reddening of the conjunctivae) appearing early in the disease, followed by a short period of resolution of the symptoms when the organisms are cleared from the blood.
- The secondary, "immune," phase is characterized by the features of aseptic meningitis and, in severe cases, jaundice and uraemia, acute renal failure, respiratory failure, haemorrhagic manifestations (Weil's disease).

2. A 28-year-old woman visits her physician complaining of a flu-like illness of slow, insidious onset. Her symptoms include fever, malaise, anorexia, headache, and lower back pain. Last week, the fever had risen during the day, only to break at night, with shaking chills. The patient denies sexual activity or travel. Upon enquiring, the woman only consumes organic foods and only consumes unpasteurised dairy products because she believes they are safer than pasteurised products. Gram-negative coccobacilli were cultured from the patient's blood. What is the most likely aetiology and infection? What is the pathogenesis and lab diagnosis for this infection? (1+2+2 marks)

Most Likely Aetiology

- *Brucella melitensis.*

Infection

- Brucellosis (Undulant fever).

Pathogenesis

Mode of Transmission

- The organism is transmitted to humans via consumption of contaminated, unpasteurised milk or by contact with infected farm animals.

Sequence of Events

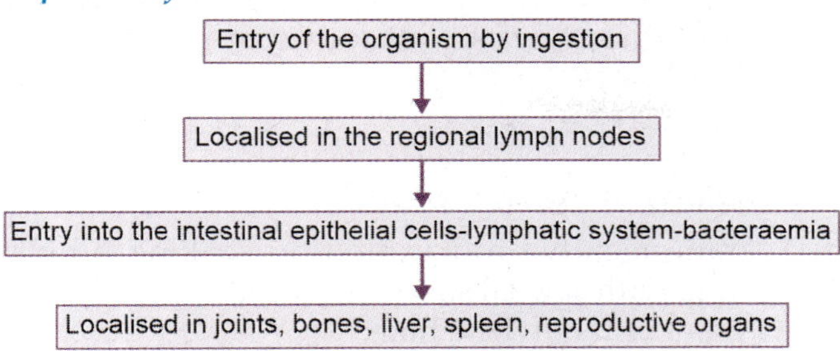

Lab Diagnosis

Specimen Collection

- Body fluids (blood, CSF, bone marrow, synovial fluid, etc.)
- Tissue biopsy.

Microscopy

- *Gram stain:* Gram-negative cocco bacilli

Culture

- *Culture media used:* Serum dextrose broth, tryptone soya broth, trypticase soy broth
- Two phase system 'Castaneda' in which both solid and liquid media are contained in the same bottle.
- *On blood agar:* Tiny transparent colonies

Biochemical Identification

- *Catalase test:* Positive
- *Oxidase test:* Positive
- *Urease test:* Positive
- *H2S production:* They reduce nitrate to nitrite.

Serological Test

1. **Standard Agglutination Test**
   - *Principle:* It is a tube agglutination test in which equal volume of serial dilution of the patient's serum and the standardized strain of *B. abortus* are mixed and incubated at 37°C for 24 hours.
   - A titre 160 and above is taken as significant in human beings.
   - Rising titre or titre that declines after appropriate antibiotic treatment, indicates recent active infection.
2. **Mercaptoethanol Agglutination Test**
   - The test is used to increase the specificity of the reaction where IgG only is observed, which is important in patients with a more persistent infection.
3. **ELISA**
   - Measures the level of IgG, IgM, IgA, a fourfold rise in titre is considered significant.

Molecular Method

- PCR.

3. Classify Cestodes. Describe in brief the life cycle of Pork Tapeworm. Add a note on neurological complications of Pork Tapeworm. (1+2+2 marks)

Classification of Cestodes

I. **Cyclophyllidean Cestodes**
   1. *Taenia saginata* (Beef tapeworm).
   2. *Taenia solium* (Pork tapeworm).
   3. *Diphyllobothrium latum* (Fish tapeworm).
   4. *Hymenolepis nana* (Dwarf tapeworm).
   5. *Dipylidium caninum* (Dog tapeworm).
   6. *Taenia saginata* (Beef tapeworm).
   7. *Taenia solium* (Pork tapeworm).

II. **Pseudophyllidean Cestodes**
   1. *Sparganum spp.*

Life Cycle of Pork Tapeworm

- *Infective stage:* Eggs of *Taenia solium*
- *Diagnostic stage:* Proglottids
- *Mode of transmission:* Ingestion of food contaminated with taenia eggs
- *Life cycle* (Fig. 8.1.1).

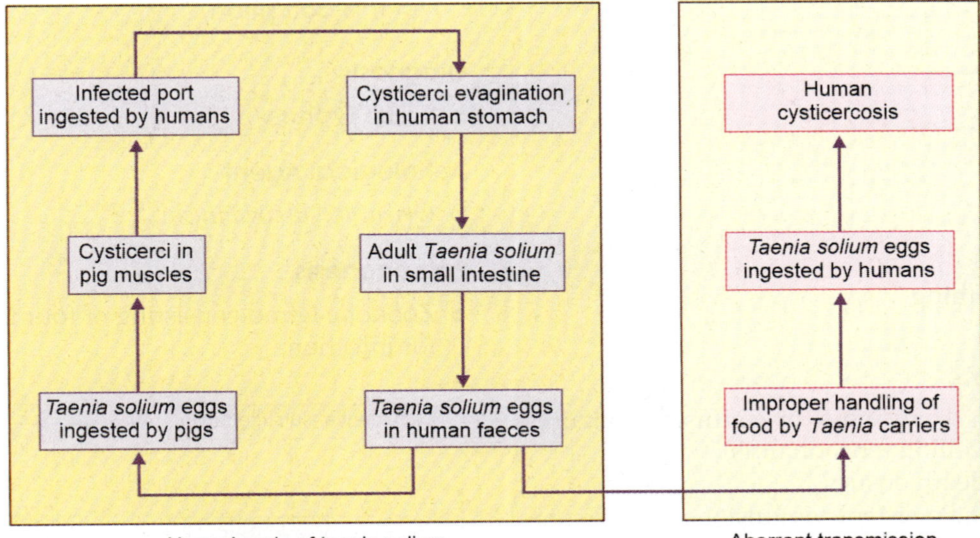

Fig. 8.1.1: Life cycle of Taenia solium

Neurological Complications (Neurocysticercosis)

1. Hydrocephalus
2. Raised Intracranial pressure and hypertension presents with headache, vertigo, and vomiting
3. Chronic meningitis
4. Focal neurological deficits
5. Psychological disorders and dementia
6. Cerebral arteritis
7. Involvement of ventricles—poor prognosis.

4. Give examples for zoonotic members of paramyxo viridae. Describe in brief about the mode of transmission, clinical features of a zoonotic disease which caused massive outbreak in 2018 in Kerala of India. (1+4 marks)

Examples for Zoonotic Members of Paramyxo viridae

1. Hendra virus
2. New castle disease virus (NDV)
3. Nipah virus.

Massive Outbreak in 2018 in Kerala of India

- Nipah virus outbreak was seen in Calicut, Kerala.

Nipah Virus Outbreak

Mode of Transmission

- Direct contact with infected animals, such as bats or pigs, or their body fluids (such as blood, urine, or saliva).
- Ingestion of food products that have been contaminated by body fluids of infected animals (such as palm sap or fruit contaminated by an infected bat).
- Close contact with infected persons (person to person).

Clinical Features

Initial Symptoms

- Fever
- Headache
- Cough
- Sore throat
- Difficulty breathing
- Vomiting

Severe Symptoms

- Disorientation, drowsiness, or confusion, seizures, coma, brain swelling (encephalitis).
- 40–70% cases death ensues
- *Long term effects:* Persistent convulsions and personality changes

5. Describe the morphology of *Yersinia pestis*. Enumerate the clinical forms of plague. Add a brief note on each of the clinical forms of plague. (1+1+3 marks)

Morphology of *Yersinia pestis*

- A gram-negative rod exhibiting striking bipolar staining with special stains such as Wright, Giemsa, Wayson, or methylene blue.

Clinical Forms of Plague

1. Bubonic plague
2. Pneumonic plague
3. Septicaemic plague

Bubonic Plague

- After an incubation period of 2–7 days, there is high fever and painful lymphadenopathy (buboes) in the areas involving the neck, groin, or axillae.

Pneumonic Plague

- Results from direct inhalation of organism into the lung
- Patients often have a fulminant presentation with chest pain, cough, haemoptysis, and severe respiratory distress.

Septicaemic Plague

- Begins with vomiting and diarrhoaea.
- Later, DIC leads to hypotension, altered mental status, and renal and cardiac failure.

6. A 40-year-old farmer presented to emergency department with 3-day history of fever headache with non-pruritic rash on face, extremities, and eschar on the right leg. Identify the aetiological diagnosis and briefly discuss the pathogenesis in this condition. (1+4 marks)

Diagnosis

- Scrub typhus.

Aetiological Agent

- *Orientia tsutsugamushi.*

Pathogenesis

- Zoonotic tetrad consisting of four factors favourable for infection.

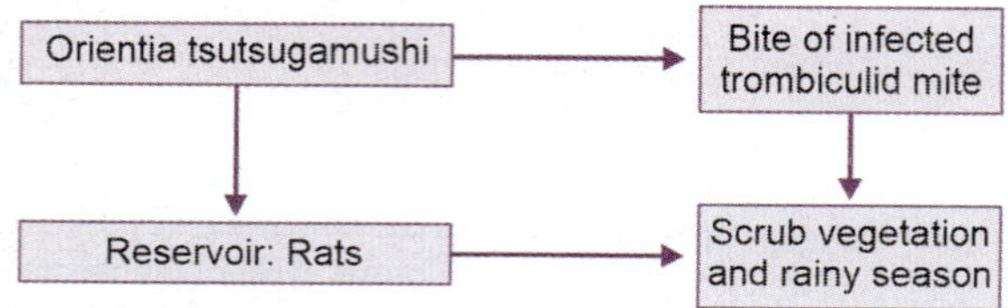

7. An 18-year-old boy was brought to the hospital with fever and altered sensorium. O/E, BP was 90/60 mmHg, rash all over the body sparing palms and soles. On enquiry, he was found to have been exposed to body lice. Similar rash was seen among his hostel mates.

A. What is the most probable diagnosis? (1 mark)

- Epidemic typhus caused by *Rickettsia prowazekii*.

B. Classify the other agents in the family along with mode of transmission and disease produced. (1+4 marks)

Typhus Group

Organism	Vector	Mode of transmission	Disease
Rickettsia prowazekii	Louse	• Infected louse faeces rubbed into the bite wound. • Human-to-human transmission by louse	• Epidemic typhus
Rickettsia typhi	Flea	• Infected flea faeces rubbed into the bite wound	• Endemic typhus
Orientia tsu-tsugamushi	Mite	• Bite of infected mite	• Scrub typhus

Spotted Fever Group

Organism	Vector	Mode of transmission	Disease
Rickettsia rickettsii	Ticks	• Bite of the infected vector	• Rocky mounted spotted fever
Rickettsia akari	Mite	• Bite of the infected vector	• Rickettsial pox

SHORT ANSWERS

1. Mention the clinical forms of brucellosis. Add a brief note on serological tests used to eliminate the blocking antibodies in the diagnosis of brucellosis. (1+2 marks)

Clinical Forms of Brucellosis

1. *Undulant fever:* Fever with intermittent remissions
2. *Triad:* Fever, arthralgia, hepatosplenomegaly
3. *Musculoskeletal:* Vertebral and septic osteoarthritis
4. *CNS:* Meningitis/meningoencephalitis
5. *Genitourinary:* Epididymo-orchitis, prostatitis, salpingitis and pyelonephritis

Serological Tests Used

Standard Agglutination Test (SAT)

- It is the gold standard serological assay for diagnosis.
- It is a tube agglutination test in which equal volume of serial dilution of the patient's serum and the standardized strain of *B. abortus* are mixed and looked for agglutination and clearing of serum.

ELISA

- Measures the level of IgG, IgM, IgA in acute, chronic and neurobrucellosis.

2. Give three examples for zoonotic viral diseases and their vectors/source of transmission. (3 marks)

Zoonotic viral disease	Vector/source of transmission
• Rabies	• Dog
• Influenza A	• Birds
• Kyasanur forest disease	• Monkeys/ticks

3. List three zoonotic parasite diseases along with their vector/source of transmission. (3 marks)

Disease	Vector/source
• Toxoplasmosis	• Cats
• Echinococcosis	• Dog/sheep
• Toxocariasis	• Dog/ cat

4. A farmer from a nearby village in Gujarat developed fever, chills, myalgia and jaundice. His renal function tests were also deranged. On evaluation, his serum was positive for IgM antibodies by ELISA. What is the most probable disease and aetiological agent? What is the source of infection and mode of transmission in this infection? (3 marks).

Most Probable Disease

- Leptospirosis

Aetiological Agent

- *Leptospira interrogans*

Source of Infection and Mode of Transmission

- Food or drink contaminated with urine of infected animal (rat, cow, dogs, pigs).

5. An obligate intracellular pathogen grows in the nucleus and cytoplasm and is transmitted to humans by ticks. What type of rash is a typical symptom of this disease? Justify your answer. What is the recommended therapy? (3 marks)

Type of Rash

- Macular rash

Justification

- Rocky mountain spotted fever is caused by *Rickettsia rickettsia*. The rash caused by this bacterium spreads centripetally from the palms of the hands and soles of the feet to the trunk.

Recommended Therapy

- Doxycycline

6. A pig farmer visits a nearby clinic with c/o abdominal pain and diarrhoea followed by muscle aches. A muscle biopsy was done which showed larvae in pain. What is the most likely disease and aetiological agent? Mention the mode of transmission. (3 marks)

Most Probable Disease

- Trichinellosis

Aetiological Agent

- *Trichinella spiralis*

Mode of Transmission

- Humans are infected by ingesting raw or undercooked meat containing larvae encysted in the muscle.

7. Weil Felix test is a heterophile agglutination test. Statement is true or false? Justify your answer. (3 marks)

Statement is

- True.

Justification

- Weil Felix test is done for diagnosis of rickettsial infections.
- Antibodies against rickettsial antigens are detected by using cross reacting *Proteus* antigens.
- Interpretation of Weil Felix.

Disease	*OX 19*	*OX 2*	*OX K*
Scrub typhus	–	–	+ + +
Typhus group	+ + +	+/-	–
Spotted fever group	+ +	+ +	–

- Heterophile agglutination test is a test in which antibody produced against one antigen reacts with that of the other antigen of different species which share similar epitopes.
- Examples of other heterophile agglutination tests:
  1. Paul-Bunnell tests
  2. Cold agglutination test and
  3. *Streptococcus* MG test

8. Toxin and capsule are key virulence factors in hide porter's disease. Statement is true or false? Justify your answer. (3 marks)

Statement is

- True

Justification

- Anthrax toxin, a tripartite toxin has three components:
  1. *Edema factor:* It is an active component acts as adenylyl cyclase and increases cAMP—oedema and other clinical manifestations seen in this condition.
  2. *Protective factor:* It binds to the host receptor and facilitates the entry of other components into the host cell.
  3. *Lethal factor:* Causes cell death.
- Anthrax capsule
  - It is a polypeptide capsule (polyglutamate).
  - Plasmid coded.
  - It inhibits complement mediated phagocytosis.

MI 8.2 DESCRIBE THE AETIOPATHOGENESIS OF OPPORTUNISTIC INFECTIONS (OI) AND DISCUSS THE FACTORS CONTRIBUTING THE OCCURRENCE OF OPPORTUNISTIC INFECTIONS AND THE LABORATORY DIAGNOSIS

LONG ESSAY

1. Define opportunistic infections. Discuss in detail about opportunistic infections under the following headings.

Definition of Opportunistic Infections

- Opportunistic infections are infections which occur or are more severe in individuals with weakened immunity.

A. Classify opportunistic infections with examples under each category. (3 marks)

Bacterial	• Tuberculosis: *M. tuberculosis* • Disseminated infections: *Mycobacterium avium intracellulare* complex • Shigellosis: *Shigella* spp.
Parasitic	• Opportunistic diarrhoea: *Cryptosporidium, Isospora belli, Cyclospora* • Toxoplasmosis: *Toxoplasma gondii* • Strongyloidiasis: *Strongyloides stercoralis*
Fungal	• Systemic candidiasis: *Candida albicans* and many other *Candida* species • Cryptococcosis: *Cryptococcus neoformans* • Aspergillosis: *Aspergillus fumigatus* and other *Aspergillus* species • Hyalohyphomycosis: Penicilliosis, species of *Fusarium, Paecilomyces, Trichosporon* • Mucormycosis (Zygomycosis): *Rhizopus* • *Pneumocystis* pneumonia: *Pneumocystis jirovecii* • Penicilliosis: *Penicillium marneffei*
Viral	• Herpes simplex virus • Kaposi sarcoma: Human herpes virus 8 • Cytomegalovirus

B. Mention the opportunistic microbes causing diarrhoea. (2 marks)

Bacterial	• *Salmonella* • *Shigella*
Parasitic	• *Cryptosporidium parvum* • *Isospora belli* • *Giardia lamblia*
Virus	• Cytomegalovirus

C. Describe in detail the laboratory diagnosis of candidiasis. (4 marks)

Specimen Collection

- Pus, swab, urine, CSF

Microscopy

- On Gram's stain, reveals gram-positive oval budding yeasts and pseudo hyphae.
- Presence of yeasts only, indicates colonisation.
- On Sabourad's agar: Pasty cream colonies

Other Methods

- Germ tube formation and production of chlamydospores are tests which identifies *C. albicans* from all other species of *Candida.*
- CHROMagar and carbohydrate assimilation test for species identification.

Serologic Tests

- Not useful

Molecular Diagnosis

- PCR

SHORT ESSAYS

1. Give four examples for opportunistic fungi causing respiratory tract infections. Describe in brief the pathogenesis, investigations for interstitial cell pneumonia. (1+4 marks)

Examples for Opportunistic Fungi Causing Respiratory Tract Infections

1. *Pneumocystis jirovecii*
2. *Aspergillus* species
3. *Mucor* spp.
4. *Cryptococcus neoformans*

Interstitial Cell Pneumonia

Pathogenesis

Aetiological Agent

- *Pneumocystis jirovecii*
- *Pneumocystis* exists in cyst found in the environment and human tissues whereas trophozoite forms found in human tissue.

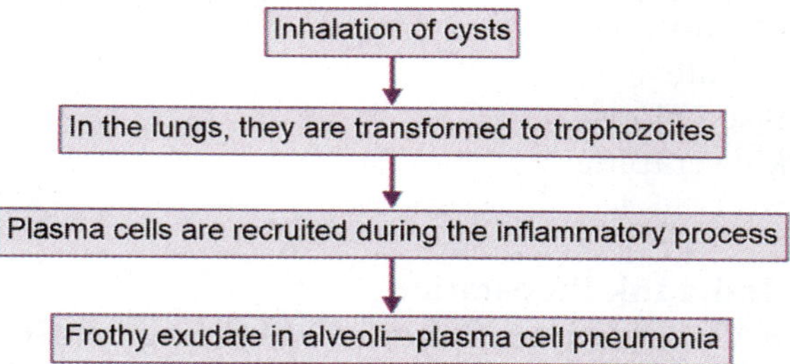

Investigation/Lab Diagnosis

Specimen Collection

- BAL
- Bronchial brushings
- Induced sputum
- Transbronchial or open lung biopsy

Microscopy

1. ***Toluidine blue:*** Blue coloured cysts seen
2. ***Gomori's Methenamine Silver (GMS):*** Cysts resembling black coloured crushed ping-pong balls against green background
3. ***Immunofluorescence:*** Direct immunofluorescent antibody on BAL specimen

Culture

- Not cultivable.

Serological Assays

- Not available.

PCR

- For detection of specific genes of *P. jirovecii*—Gold standard.

Radiological Examination

- Bilateral diffuse infiltrates, ground glass opacities.
- At early stage, atypical lesions such as nodular densities and cavity may also be seen.

2. Mention two examples for the microbes causing CNS infections in immunocompromised. Describe in brief the laboratory diagnosis of opportunistic pathogens causing CNS infections. (1 + 4 marks)

Microbes Causing CNS Infections in Immunocompromised

1. *Cryptococcus neoformans*
2. *Toxoplasma gondii*

Laboratory Diagnosis of Opportunistic Pathogens Causing CNS Infections for *Cryptococcus neoformans*

Specimen Collection

- CSF
- Sputum
- Exudate
- Tissue biopsy
- Skin scrapings

Microscopy

1. **India Ink Preparation**
   - Observation: Spherical budding yeast cells surrounded by wide capsule and dark background
2. **Gram's Stain**
   - Gram positive spherical budding yeast cells.
3. **Other Stains**
   - Mucicarmine stain, Grocott's methenamine silver stain, periodic acid schiff stain → spherical budding yeast cells seen.

Culture

- Plain Sabourad's dextrose agar
- *Colony morphology:* Colonies are mucoid, smooth, and cream in colour.

Biochemical Identification

- *Phenol oxidase test (using caffeic acid agar):* Gives brown to black coloured colonies (melanin production)
- *Urease test:* Positive
- *Carbohydrate assimilation test:* Assimilation of inositol and nitrate.

Serology

- *Antigen detection:* For the demonstration of cryptococcal capsular polysaccharide antigen in CSF

Lab Diagnosis of Toxoplasmosis

Specimen Collection

- Blood, tissue biopsy.

Microscopy

- Giemsa-stained smears shows presence of crescentic tachyzoites
- Cysts may be observed in the tissue

Culture

- The organism can be grown in cell culture. inoculation into mice confirms the diagnosis.

Serology

- Various methods such as capture ELISA, Immunofluorescence assays
- *Sabin Feldman dye test*—considered as gold standard test for antibody detection, usually done at reference lab
- Acute infection
  - IgM antibodies appear within 1–2 weeks of infection, congenital infection.
  - IgG antibodies—A fourfold rise in titre.
  - Low IgG avidity test.
- Past/remote infection (>6 months)—IgG is raised.

3. A 40-year-old man with asthma presents to his physician with cough, fever, and low blood oxygen saturation. Chest X-ray shows presence of small, well-demarcated spheres. Bronchoalveolar lavage was cultured on KOH mount revealed distinctive septate fungal hyphae. What is the most likely infection and its aetiological agent? Explain the mode of transmission, pathogenesis and laboratory work-up for this case. (1 + 1 + 1 + 2 marks)

Most Likely Infection

- Bronchopulmonary aspergillosis.

Aetiological Agent

- *Aspergillus* spp.

Bronchopulmonary Aspergillosis

Sources

- Dust, soil, decomposing organic matter

Mode of Transmission

- Inhalation of spores

Pathogenesis

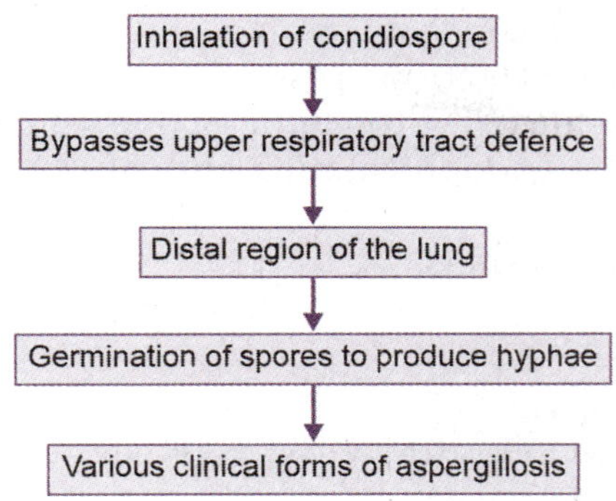

Laboratory Work-up

Specimen Collection

- BAL, sputum, tissue.

Microscopy

- *KOH mount:* Septate hyphae with acute angle branching. Invasion distinguishes disease from colonisation.

Culture

- On Sabourad's agar
- Colony morphology

Aspergillus species	Macroscopic features	Microscopic features
A. fumigatus	• Smoky green, velvety to powdery	• Conidia arise only in upper third of conical shaped vesicle • Phialides single row
A. flavus	• Yellow to green velvety	• Conidia arise from upper two third of globular shaped vesicle • Phialides two rows
A. niger	• Black powdery	• Conidia arise from upper two third of globular shaped vesicle • Phialides two rows • Black conidia

Serologic Tests

- Antigen detection.
  - *β-d Glucan antigen assay:* Raised in invasive aspergillosis.
  - *Galactomannan antigen:* ELISA for early diagnosis.

4. Evaluate the virulence factors, aetiopathogenesis, clinical presentation and treatment of those organisms in relation to burn wound infection. (5 marks)

Organisms in Relation to Burn Wound Infection

1. *Pseudomonas aeruginosa*
2. *Staphylococcus aureus*
3. *S pyogenes, Enterococci,* and other streptococci. (Table 8.2.1)

Table 8.2.1 Characteristics of brun wound infection

Virulence factors	Aetiopathogenesis	Clinical presentation	Treatment
Pseudomonas aeruginosa	• Abnormalities in the antibacterial activities of neutrophils • Deficiencies in serum opsonins • Virulence factors of the organism—production of elastase, protease, and exotoxin	• Burn wound, producing a foul, green-pigmented discharge, and necrosis • Skin lesions (ecthyma gangrenosum) that are pathognomonic of *P. aeruginosa* septicemia	• Combination therapy—Beta lactams antibiotics with Aminoglycosides such as gentamycin or tobramycin
Staphylococcus aureus	• Abnormality of the antibacterial function of neutrophils	• Destroys granulation tissue, invading and causing septicaemia	• Cloxacillin or nafcillin or clindamycin
S pyogenes* and other *Streptococci, Enterococci	• Infects healthy granulation tissue, freshly grated wounds, resulting in destruction of the graft	• Burn wound infections • Septicaemia	• Penicillin is the drug of choice for treatment, and erythromycin or vancomycin can be used for penicillin-allergic patients for group A streptococci • Enterococci—Beta lactams antibiotics with aminoglycosides

5. Give two examples for oral infections in immunocompromised. Add a note on laboratory diagnosis of these infections. (2+3 marks)

Oral Infections in Immunocompromised

1. Oral thrush
2. Herpes simplex virus infection

Laboratory Diagnosis of Oral Thrush

- The lesion can be diagnosed clinically.
- *Microscopic Examination:* Gram's stain of tissue reveals gram-positive oval budding yeast cells and pseudo hyphae. If only yeasts are found, indicates colonisation.
- *Culture:* Sabourad's agar—pasty cream colonies
- *Other tests:* Germ tube formation and production of chlamydospores tests identifies *C. albicans* from other species of *Candida*
- CHROMagar and carbohydrate assimilation test for species identification.
- Serologic tests not useful.

Laboratory Diagnosis of Herpes Simplex Virus

- *Specimen:* Swab from base of lesion
- *Microscopy:* Tzanck smear using Giemsa or Wright's stain of cells from the base of the vesicle reveals multinucleated giant cells with intranuclear inclusions. These giant cells are not specific for HSV-1.
- *Culture:* Virus cultivation: In Mc Coy cell lines, within 2–3 days cytopathic effects of diffuse ballooning and rounding of cell lines along with Cowdry type A inclusion bodies can be observed
- *Molecular method:* HSV DNA detection by PCR or real-time PCR
- *Serology:* Antibody detection by ELISA or indirect IF in 4–7 days which detects antibodies to glycoprotein

6. Explain in brief the characteristic features, clinical manifestations and lab diagnosis of talaromycosis (formerly known as penicilliosis). (1+2+2 marks)

Talaromycosis (Penicilliosis)

- Caused by *T. marneffei*

Characteristic Features

- Thermally dimorphic fungus.
- Opportunistic infection in HIV infected patients.
- Bamboo rats are the reservoirs of infection.

Clinical Manifestations

- Fever, general discomfort, weight loss, Cough.
- Swollen lymph nodes.
- Difficulty breathing.
- Hepatosplenomegaly.
- Diarrhoea.
- Abdominal pain.
- Systemic infection resembling disseminated histoplasmosis- prosthetic valve endocarditis, peritonitis, endophthalmitis, and infections at other sites.
- Warty skin lesions.

Lab Diagnosis

- **Microscopy.**
  - Oval or elliptical yeast cells showing central septation.
  - Mycelial form—hyaline thin septate hyphae, vesicles are absent, and with brush border appearance of conidia.
- **Culture.**
  - *Sabouraud dextrose agar*—yeast like colonies at 37°C and mold form with brick red pigment at 25°C.

SHORT ANSWERS

1. Give three examples for opportunistic protozoan parasites causing diarrhoea. Add a brief note on clinical manifestations due to protozoan parasites. (2+3 marks)

Opportunistic Protozoan Parasites Causing Diarrhoea

a. *Cryptosporidium parvum.*
b. *Cyclospora cayetanensis.*
c. *Isospora belli.*

Organism	*Clinical manifestations*
Cryptosporidium parvum	• *Cryptosporidium parvum* completes stages of life cycle in a single host. • Human infection is by ingestion of the oocyst • Inhabits the small intestine, intracellular protozoa
	• *Incubation period:* 3–6 days • *Source:* Faeces of domestic animals • *Mode of transmission:* ingestion of contaminated water with cysts • Self-limited diarrhoea in immunocompetent (6%) • Life threatening diarrhoea in immunocompromised (24%)
Isospora belli	• *Habitat:* Small intestine of humans—jejunum and distal duodenum • Diarrhoea, weight loss
Cyclospora cayetanensis	• *Habitat:* Small intestine • Diarrhoea, weight loss

2. Enumerate the microorganisms causing burn wound infections. (3 marks)

- The most important pathogens in burn wounds are:
  1. *Pseudomonas aeruginosa* and other gram-negative rods
  2. *Staphylococcus aureus*
  3. *Streptococcus pyogenes*
  4. Other streptococci, enterococci.

3. A patient on immunosuppressive drugs, presents at the emergency department with pneumonia. The patient c/o chest pain, coughing, and fever gradual in onset. Sputum samples revealed long filamentous gram-positive bacilli which were also acid fast. What is the most likely infection and aetiology? What are clinical manifestations caused by this pathogen? (3 marks)

Most Likely Infection

- Nocardiosis

Aetiology

- *Nocardia asteroids*

Clinical Manifestations

- Brain abscess
- Pulmonary abscess
- Cutaneous skin infections such as mycetoma
- Disseminated infections

MT 8.3 DESCRIBE THE ROLE OF ONCOGENIC VIRUSES IN THE EVOLUTION OF VIRUS-ASSOCIATED MALIGNANCY

LONG ESSAY

1. Mention the viruses causing cancer in humans. (1 mark)

Viruses Causing Cancer in Humans

1. Hepatitis B virus—Hepatocellular carcinoma
2. Hepatitis C virus—Hepatocellular carcinoma
3. Epstein–Barr virus—Burkitt's lymphoma
4. Human herpes virus 8—Kaposi sarcoma
5. Human T cell Lymphotrophic virus
6. Human papilloma virus—Cervical carcinoma

Discuss in detail about viral oncogenesis under the following headings:

A. Tenets (Properties) of Viral Oncogenesis. (3 marks)

1. Viruses are known to cause cancer in animals and humans.
2. Tumor viruses can establish persistent infection in natural host.
3. Host factors are important elements in virus-induced tumour genesis.
4. Viruses are occasionaly complete carcinogens.
5. Infections caused by viruses are more common than virus-induced tumour formation.
6. Long latent period usually intervenes between initial viral infection and tumour development.
7. These directly or indirectly acts as carcinogens.
8. Oncogenic viruses regulate growth control pathways in cells.
9. The mechanism of viral carcinogenesis can be studied in animal models.
10. Viral markers usually exist in tumour cells.
11. Association of one virus may be with more than one type of tumour.

B. Define Transformation and Oncogenes. (2 marks)

Transformation

- Viral transformation is the change in growth, phenotype, or indefinite reproduction of cells caused by the introduction of inheritable change.

Oncogenes

- Genes that promote autonomous cell growth in cancer cells.
- They are derived by mutations in proto-oncogenes.

C. Discuss in brief about tumour suppressor genes with suitable examples and mechanism of viral oncogenesis. (2+2 marks)

- These genes encode proteins that inhibit cellular proliferation by regulating the cell cycle, e.g. RB gene-involved retinoblastoma; carcinoma of breast, bladder, and lung
- P53.
  - Promotes apoptosis of cells whose DNA has been damaged or contain activated cellular oncogenes.
  - Involved in carcinoma of breast, colon, and lung, astrocytoma.

Mechanism of Viral Oncogenesis

1. Cellular oncogenes have acquired mutations that cause them to escape regulatory control and overproduce altered proteins, e.g. myc-transcription factor—Burkitt`s lymphoma.

2. Direct or indirect.
   - Direct oncogenic mechanism

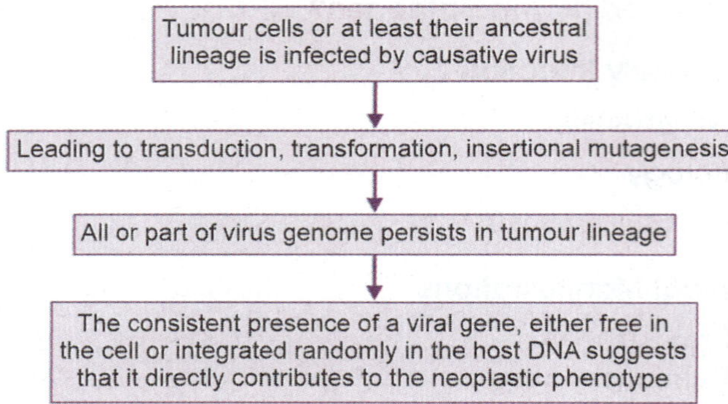

- Indirect oncogenic mechanism.
  - Tumour arise in response to virus infections of other cells, the nature of the response taking several forms—immunosuppression, tissue regeneration in uninfected cells, production of growth factors.

SHORT ESSAYS

1. Give two examples for DNA viruses causing cancer in humans. Add a note on pathogenesis, laboratory diagnosis of HCC. (1+4 marks)

Examples for DNA Viruses Causing Cancer in Humans

1. *Hepatitis B virus:* Hepatocellular carcinoma
2. *Epstein Barr virus:* Burkitt's lymphoma

Hepatocellular Carcinoma (HCC)

Pathogenesis

Reservoir of the Infection

1. Humans are the only reservoir of infection.
2. Can be spread either from carriers or from cases.

High Risk Groups

1. Physicians
2. Surgeons
3. Recipients of blood transfusion
4. Prostitutes
5. Drug abusers
6. Infants of HBV carrier mothers
7. Immunocompromised patients
8. Health care and laboratory personnel

Modes of Transmission

- Parenteral route
- Perinatal transmission
- Sexual transmission

Mechanism

- Chronicity in infection—proliferation of hepatocytes during regenerative process (uncontrolled regeneration)
- Block in cell apoptosis due to activation of NF-kB pathway which in turn leads to accumulation of mutations.
- HBx gene—activates cellular and viral genes.
- Deletion of tumour suppressor genes due to integration of viral genes with host cells –insertional mutagenesis

Laboratory Diagnosis

Specimen Collection

- Blood, serum.

Complete Blood Count

- Low hemoglobin, Thrombocytopenia

Electrolyte's Level

- Hyponatremia

Liver Function Tests

- SGPT and SGOT enzymes increased
- Serum bilirubin raised

Coagulations Studies

- PTT, INR → Prolonged

Alfa Fetoprotein

- Increased

Radiology: CT, MRI

- Focal nodule enhancement

2. A woman comes for her yearly routine check-up and a Pap smear. The gynaec notices anogenital warts. She counsels about safe sex practices. What is the probable infection and its pathogen? Describe in brief about the malignancy caused by this agent. Add a note on Pap smear and prophylaxis available. (1+2+3 marks)

Probable Infection

- Benign warts

Pathogen

- Human papilloma virus (HPV)

Malignancy Associated with HPV

1. Benign warts
2. Epidermodysplasia verruciformis
3. Cervical carcinoma
4. Laryngeal papillomas
5. Oesophageal carcinomas

Pap Smear

- A screening test for detection of precancerous or cancer cells in cervix
- Cervical or anal scrapings for microscopy and H and E staining
- Women of age 30 and older can consider Pap testing every five years

Specific Prophylaxis

1. **HPV vaccine**
   - For all adolescent girls and boys (11–12 years) and in 20's.
   - *Route:* IM
   - *Dose:* 2 doses
2. **Subunit vaccine**
   - Consists of virus-like particles composed of HPV L1 proteins produced by DNA recombinant technology.
   - *Route:* IM
   - *Dose:* 2 doses
3. **Nine valent vaccine.**
   - Containing serotypes 16, 18, 31, 33, 45, 52, 58
   - *Route:* IM
   - *Dose:* 2 doses
   - Long lasting protection.
4. **Quadrivalent vaccine.**
   - Contain serotypes 6, 11, 16, 18
   - *Route:* IM
   - *Dose:* 2 doses
5. **Bivalent**
   - Contain high risk serotypes 16 and 18
   - *Route:* IM
   - *Dose:* 2 doses

MI 8.4 DESCRIBE THE AETIOLOGICAL AGENTS OF EMERGING INFECTIOUS DISEASES. DISCUSS THE CLINICAL COURSE AND DIAGNOSIS

LONG ESSAYS

1. A patient presenting with fever, cough, and pneumonia with a h/o travel to another country. Discuss in detail about emerging infectious diseases under the following headings.

A. Define emerging infectious diseases with examples. (1+2 marks)

Definition

- A *newly emerging disease* is a disease that has never been recognised before and emerged or increased in past two decades and could increase in near future.

Examples

1. COVID-19 pandemic due to SARS CoV2
2. Influenza A
3. Nipah virus
4. *Candida auris*

B. Pathogenesis, clinical manifestations of this infection. (4 marks)

Pathogenesis

Incubation Period: 2–15 days

Transmission through Bats or Dromedary Camels

- Understudied and poorly understood
- Immune evasion to overcome innate immune response—inhibiting recognition, delaying interferon induction, dampening interferon-stimulated gene expression
- Leads to efficient viral replication, results in cell damage through direct virus-induced cytolysis or immunopathology via dysregulated pro-inflammatory cytokine induction
- T-cell deficiency or combined T- and B-cell deficiencies associated with persistent infections and lack of virus clearance
- Inadequate antibody response is associated with poor clinical outcome.

Clinical Manifestations

- *Primary cases:* Older patients with co-morbidities - diabetes mellitus (most common), chronic renal disease, HTN, chronic cardiac disease, chronic pulmonary disease, smoking and obesity.
- *Secondary cases:* Young patients and heathcare workers (HCWs) and patients sharing contaminated equipment with improper barrier control
- *Nonspecific symptoms:* Fever, chills, rigors, sore throat, cough, dyspnoea, malaise
- *Symptoms of respiratory tract infection:* Rhinorrhoea, sputum production, wheezing
- Rapid clinical deterioration due to development of respiratory failure
- *Extrapulmonary manifestations:* Acute renal impairment was most striking; others—hepatic dysfunction, pericarditis, arrhythmias, hypotension, haematological abnormalities
- *Complications:* Bacterial, viral, fungal coinfections, VAP, septic shock, delirium, stillbirth, respiratory failure with acute respiratory distress syndrome (ARDS) and multi-organ dysfunction.

C. Laboratory diagnosis useful in diagnosis of this condition. (2 marks)

WHO Criteria for a Lab-confirmed Case

- A positive RT-PCR result for at least two different specific targets on the MERS-CoV genome, or
- One positive RT-PCR result for a specific target on the MERS-CoV genome and an additional different RT-PCR product sequenced, confirming identity to known sequences of MERS-CoV.

Specimen Collection

- *Upper respiratory tract specimens:* Nasopharyngeal aspirates or swabs, oropharyngeal swabs.
- *Extra-pulmonary specimens:* Urine, faeces, blood and/or tissues.
- Under strict compliance with standard precautions along with additional measures like N95 respirators.

Transport Media

- Viral transport media at 4°C

Serology

- Antigen detection by immunochromatographic test

Viral Culture

- Monkey kidney cell lines or vero cell–syncytium formation.

Molecular Tests

- Nucleic acid amplification test

D. Prevention and control of emerging viral infectious diseases. (1 marks)

In the Community Settings

- Identify and isolate all zoonotic reservoirs and infected humans from non-immune persons.
- Avoid contact with environments soiled with animal body fluids, tissues, faeces.
- Avoid consumption of unpasteurised camel milk.
- Restrict air travel for lab-confirmed cases.
- Compliance with infection control measures and standard precautions should be applied.
- Air-borne precautions for aerosols generating procedures.

2. An 18-year-old boy with h/o of fever, petechiae like rash of 2-day duration. Lab investigations revealed low platelet count and positive NS1 antigen test.

A. What is the probable diagnosis? (1 mark)

- Dengue

B. Pathogenesis, clinical manifestations, and complications. (3+2+1 marks)

Pathogenesis (Fig. 8.4.1)

- Virus spreads from the initial infection site to regional lymph nodes, liver, and spleen.
- Virus enters host cells by receptor-mediated endocytosis.
- Due to already present antibody to different serotype of the dengue virus.
  - Previous infection with different serotype.
  - Passively transferred maternal antibody (in children).
- Secondary infection with dengue type 2 following a type 1 infection—particular risk factor for severe disease.
- Neutralising antibodies.
  - Protective.
  - Against infective serotype (lifelong) and against other serotypes (lasts for some time)
- Non-neutralising antibodies:
  - Lasts lifelong
  - Heterotypic (produced against other serotypes, not against infective serotype)
  - In secondary infection, instead of neutralising the second serotype, Abs protect the virus from immune system by inhibiting the bystander B cell activation (antibody-dependent enhancement).

Clinical Manifestations (Figs 8.4.1 and 8.4.2)

- *Dengue fever:* mild flu-like illness upon first exposure, rash, fever, headache, retro-orbital pain, nausea, vomiting, muscle, and joint pain
- *Dengue haemorrhagic fever:* Fever, hepatomegaly, thrombocytopenia, spontaneous bleeding from nose, skin, mouth, and gums. Positive tourniquet test
- *Dengue shock syndrome:* Rapid weak pulse, cold clammy skin, restlessness

Complications

1. Internal bleeding
2. Organ damage
3. Blood pressure can drop—causing shock

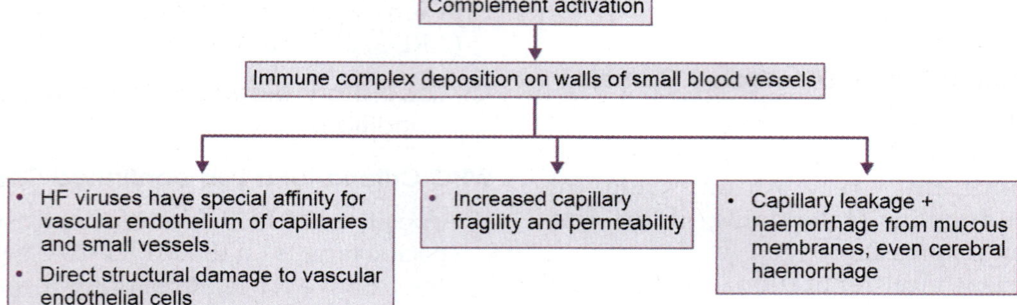

Fig. 8.4.1: Pathogenesis of dengue virus

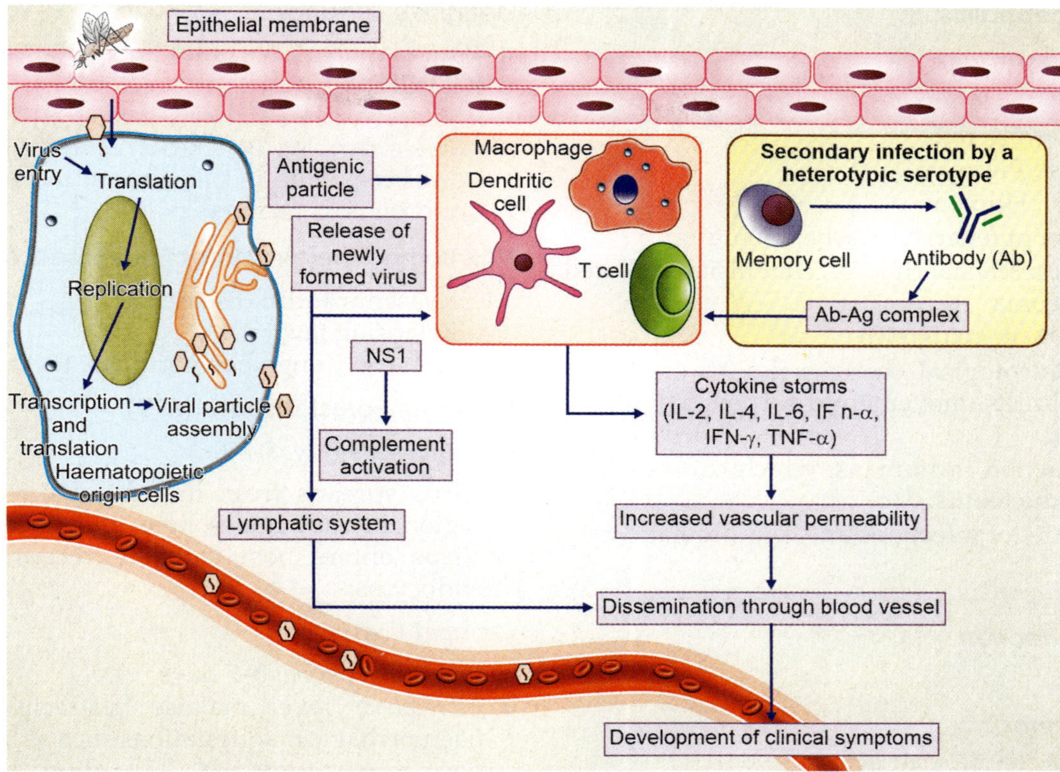

Fig. 8.4.2: Pathogenesis and manifestations of dengue fever

4. Death
5. During pregnancy—pre-term birth, low birth weight or foetal distress

C. Laboratory diagnosis. Advantages and disadvantages of rapid diagnostic tests. (3+1+1 marks)

Laboratory Diagnosis

Specimen Collection

- Blood or serum.

Serology

- *Viral antigen detection in tissue specimens:* Immunohistochemistry
- NS1 antigen detection in blood—useful in first 4–5 days of infection—ICT or ELISA
- Antibody detection of IgM antibodies and a rise in titre- ELISA—In primary infection
- IgG antibodies—Secondary infections
- Neutralisation tests are available but cumbersome to conduct.

Culture

- Isolation of virus
  - In adult mice
  - Cell culture—C6/36 for research purpose

Molecular Methods

- **RT-PCR:** for detection of viral nucleic acid and in dengue, to determine serotype also

Rapid Diagnostic Tests

Advantages	• Detects NS1 Antigen or IgM or IgG • Detects antigen in the first week • Rapid
Disadvantage	• Antibody detections have poor sensitivity and specificity compared to ELISA

D. Prevention and control measures for this disease. (2 marks)

- Vaccines are under trial
- Mosquito control measures
  - Use insect repellents
  - Proper clothing and bed nets
  - Window screens and other barriers
  - Use of periodic insecticide sprays

SHORT ESSAYS

1. Give two examples for emerging infectious diseases transmitted by mosquito vectors. Discuss in brief the clinical manifestations and lab diagnosis of Japanese encephalitis. (1+4 marks)

Emerging Infectious Diseases Transmitted by Mosquito Vectors

1. Dengue
2. Chikungunya

Japanese Encephalitis

Clinical Manifestations

- *Vector:* Culex mosquito
- *Reservoir:* Herons, pigs
- *Amplifier host:* Pigs
- *Dead end host:* Humans
- Abrupt onset of fever, headache, vomiting.
- *After 1–6 days:* Nuchal rigidity, convulsions, altered sensorium, coma
- Mortality 50% in epidemics
- Residual neurological changes in 50% survivors (seizures, paresis, movement disorders, or mental retardation).
- *In utero* infection in humans, which can result in abortion of the foetus.
- Large majority of infections are asymptomatic.

Laboratory Diagnosis

Specimen Collection

- Blood, CSF

Tentative Diagnosis

- *Antibody titre:* HI, IFA, ELISA
- JE-specific IgM in serum or CSF

Definitive Diagnosis

- *Virus isolation:* CSF, brain (mosquito cell lines)
- RT-PCR

2. Give examples for tick-borne emerging infectious diseases. Write in brief about the pathogenesis and clinical features of KFD. (1+4 marks)

Tick Borne Emerging Infectious Diseases

1. Kyasanur forest disease (KFD)
2. Relapsing fever
3. Crimean Congo haemorrhagic fever

Kyasanur Forest Disease (KFD)

Pathogenesis (Fig. 8.4.3)

- Virus spreads from the initial infection site to regional lymph nodes, liver, and spleen
- Virus enters host cells by receptor mediated endocytosis

Clinical Features

- *Incubation period:* 3–7 days
- *First phase:* fever, malaise, headache followed by haemorrhagic manifestations such as bleeding from nose, throat, gums and GI bleeding
- *Second phase:* Meningoencephalitis

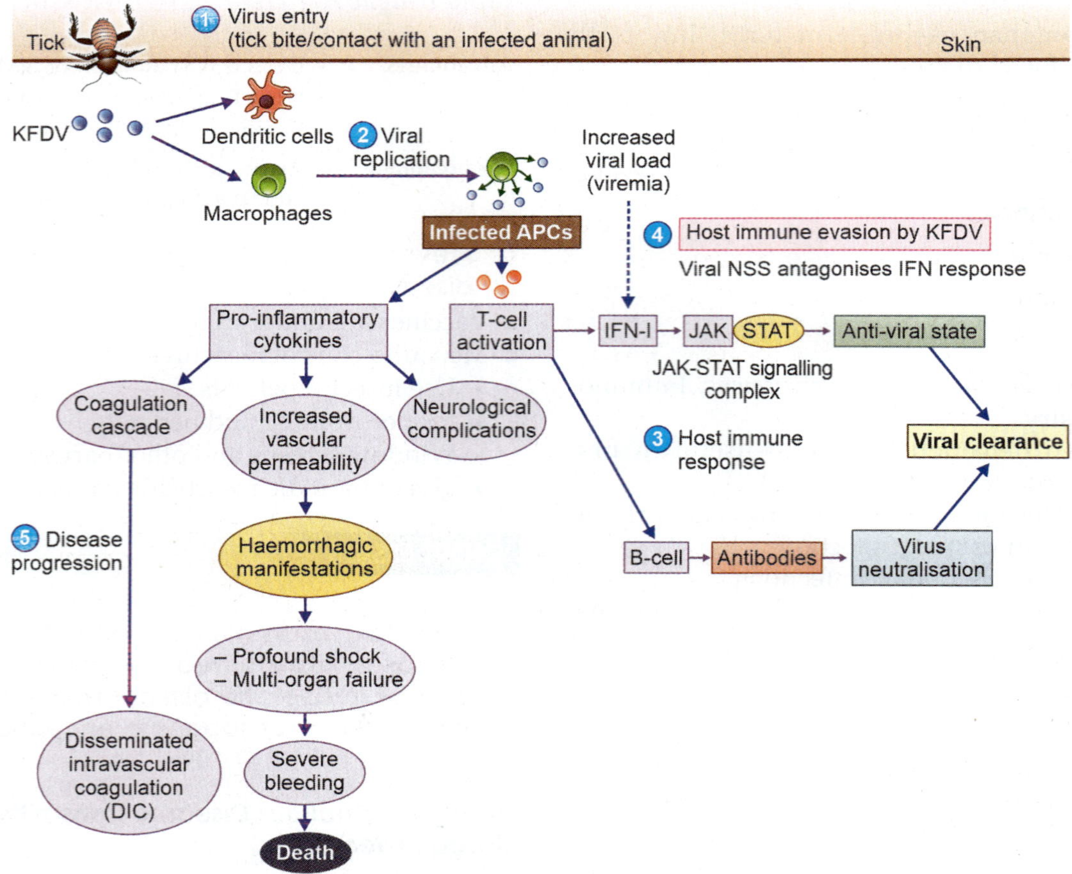

Fig. 8.4.3: Pathogenesis of Kyasanur forest disease

3. Give two examples for emerging infectious diseases of bacterial origin. Describe in brief about the pathogenesis and clinical features of leptospirosis. (1+4 marks)

Emerging Infectious Diseases of Bacterial Origin

1. Cholera
2. Plague

Leptospirosis

Pathogenesis

Mode of Transmission

- Ingestion or exposure to, contaminated water or food.

Leptospira interrogans	
Leptospira serogroup	• *Animal host*
L. canicola	• Dogs
L. icterohaemorrhagica	• Rats

Sequence of Events

- The infection can be acquired by swimming, working, or playing in contaminated water.

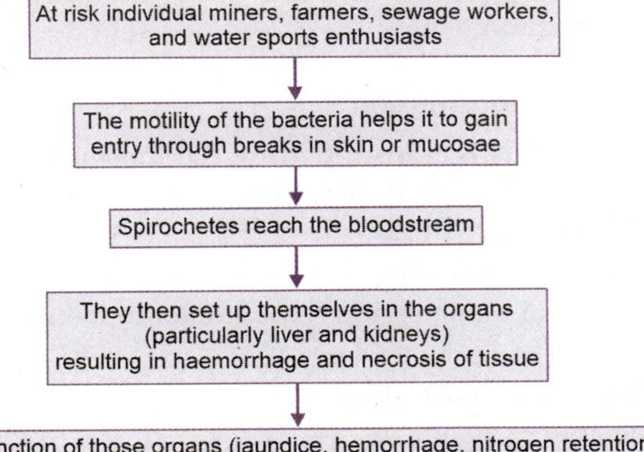

Clinical Features

- Onset of fever after 2 weeks of infection
- 90% of cases resolve with no complications (incubation period: 1–2 weeks)
- Anicteric and icteric phase
- *Spirochetes invades mainly 3 organs:* Liver, kidneys and CNS
- Jaundice, haemorrhage, necrosis of liver
- Uremia with bacteriuria—kidney
- Aseptic meningitis, scleral and conjunctival haemorrhage—CNS
- Severe form with haemorrhagic complications—Weil's disease

4. Give 4 examples for emerging infectious diseases. Discuss the factors responsible for evolution of such diseases. (2+3 marks)

Emerging Infectious Diseases

1. Avian influenza
2. Influenza A
3. Dengue
4. Kyasanur forest disease

Factors Responsible for Emergence/Re-Emergence

1. Variations in global population, demographics, and distribution
2. Human behaviour change
3. *Environmental and land use change:* Global warming, Deforestation, Land development, Natural disasters
4. Interruption in public health system and bioterrorism
5. Air travel
6. Microbial evolution
7. Enhanced pathogen detection

5. A man is found critically ill in his home with fever, hypotension, and bleeding onto his skin and mucous membranes. He was brought to a local hospital by his family, where he died later. A virus was isolated from the patient autopsy. The hospital and the patient's family were quarantined. What is the most likely infection and its aetiology? Add a note on mode of transmission and clinical presentation seen in this infection. (1+2+2 marks)

Most Likely Infection

- Ebola or viral haemorrhagic fever

Aetiological Agent

- Ebola virus.

Mode of Transmission

- Reservoir is unknown.
  - Bats, rodents implicated.
  - Monkeys—not considered (they die too rapidly)
- Human infections—highly communicable to human contacts
- Direct contact with blood and body fluids (maximum biologic containment conditions)
- Nosocomial transmission
  - Reuse of needles and syringes
  - Exposure to infectious tissues, excretions, and hospital wastes (Barrier nursing)
- Aerosol transmission
  - From infected primates

Clinical Presentation

- Most severe haemorrhagic fever
- *Incubation period:* 4–10 days
- Abrupt onset of fever, chills, malaise, and myalgia.
- Hemorrhage manifestations (bleeding from nose, gums, anus, and bruising) and DIC
- Loss of consciousness, massive internal bleeding, death around day 7–11

6. Describe the mode of transmission, clinical features and lab diagnosis along with preventive measures in yellow fever. (1+2+2+1 marks)

Mode of Transmission

- Yellow fever virus is transmitted by mosquito *Aedes aegypti.*
- It is restricted to Africa, Central and South America and the Caribbean.

Clinical Features

- Severe haemorrhagic fever.
- *Incubation period:* 3–6 days
- The clinical manifestations can range from mild to severe signs.
- Severe yellow fever begins abruptly with fever, chills, severe headache, lumbosacral pain, generalised myalgia, anorexia, nausea and vomiting, and minor gingival haemorrhages. A period of remission may occur for 24 hours followed by an increase in the severity of symptoms.
- Hepatocellular jaundice, renal failure, including acute tubular necrosis and shock.
- Death usually occurs on day 7–10.

Lab Diagnosis

Specimen Collection

- Blood

Microscopy

- *Histopathology:* Postmortem changes—mid-zonal changes and acidophilic inclusion bodies called Councilman bodies seen in the liver

Serology

- IgM specific antibody detection after 1 week of infection

Molecular Method

- Reverse transcriptase PCR

Preventive Measures

- Live attenuated 17D yellow fever vaccine
- Control of arthropod vectors—insecticides, attention to breeding sites
- Reduced exposure—insect repellents, mosquito nets

SHORT ANSWERS

1. Give three examples for viral emerging infectious diseases. Mention their major modes of transmission. (3 marks)

Viral emerging infectious disease	*Major modes of transmission*
Influenza A	• Contact and droplet from infected source
COVID-19	• Contact and droplet from infected source
MeRS CoV	• Infected bats or dromedary camels

2. Describe the mode of transmission, clinical manifestations and lab diagnosis in Zika virus infection. (1+1+1 marks)

Mode of Transmission

- The virus is transmitted by the mosquito vectors *Aedes aegypti* or *A. albopictus*
- Sexual intercourse
- Blood transfusion
- Vertical transmission from mother to foetus.

Clinical Manifestations

- Mild fever, a maculopapular rash, arthralgia, myalgia, and conjunctivitis
- Guillain–Barré syndrome
- Congenital Zika syndrome—microcephaly, ocular abnormalities, craniofacial disproportion, spasticity, and seizures

Lab Diagnosis

- *Specimen:* Serum, saliva, or urine
- *Serology:* IgM antibody detection after 1st week of infection
- *Molecular method:* Reverse transcriptase PCR.

MI 8.5 DEFINE HEALTHCARE-ASSOCIATED INFECTIONS (HAI) AND ENUMERATE THE TYPES. DISCUSS THE FACTORS THAT CONTRIBUTE TO THE DEVELOPMENT OF HAI AND THEIR METHODS OF PREVENTION

LONG ESSAY

1. **Define and classify Healthcare-associated Infections (HAI). Mention the common etiological agents of healthcare associated infections. Discuss in detail about the predisposing factors for HAI. Add a note on methods available for the prevention and control of HAI.**

(1+2+2+3+2 marks)

Definition

- Healthcare-associated infection is generally defined as any infection acquired while in the hospital, occurring 48 hours or more after admission and up to 48 hours after discharge.

Classification, Common Aetiological Agents, Predisposing Factors, Prevention and Control

See Table 8.5.1.

SHORT ESSAYS

1. **What is MRSA? Mention the types of MRSA. Discuss in brief the role of MRSA in outbreak of HAI. Add a note on infection control practices available for its prevention in a hospital**

(2+2+1 marks)

Definition

- Methicillin resistant *S. aureus* is a type of *S. aureus* that is resistant to currently available beta lactam antibiotics, anti-staphylococcal penicillins (e.g. methicillin, oxacillin, nafcillin) and cephalosporins.

Types of MRSA

1. Community-acquired MRSA.
2. Hospital-acquired MRSA.

Table 8.5.1 Characteristics of healthcare-associated infections

Type of HAI	*Most common organisms*	*Risk factors*	*Prevention and control*
Catheter-associated urinary tract infection (CAUTI)	• *E. coli* • Other coliforms • Enterococci • *P. aeruginosa* • *Candida*	• Catheter insertion • Instrumentation • Long duration • Latex catheters > Silicon catheters = more risk • Female sex • Catheter insertion technique not appropriate • Underlying patient conditions	• Aseptic technique during insertion • Reduced duration of catheterisation • Maintain closed drainage
Ventilator-associated pneumonia (VAP)	• *Acinetobacter* • Enterobacteriaceae • *P. aeruginosa* • *S. pneumoniae* • *S. aureus*	• Presence of endotracheal tube causes a direct Breach of the natural defense • Micro-aspiration • Improper asepsis • Failed subglottic aspiration • Underlying patient conditions	• Handwashing • Aseptic techniques • Early removal of endotracheal tubes • Head-end elevation
Surgical site infection	• *Saureus* • *P. aeruginosa* • *Coliforms* • Enterococci	• Colonisation • Presence of foreign body • Reduced blood supply • Devitalised tissue • Underlying patient conditions	• Meticulous technique • Preoperative care • Hand washing • Surveillance (Follow-up)
Catheter-related bloodstream infections (CRBSI)	• Coagulase-negative • *Staphylococcus aureus* • Coliformes • Enterococci • Group B streptococci • *Candida*	• IV devise relate or from unknown source • Long duration catheters • Femoral site > Subclavian/Jugular line • Multi lumen • Improper insertion technique • Underlying patient conditions	• Handwashing • Aseptic precautions • IV device care • Early diagnosis and treatment • Closed system

Outbreaks of MRSA

- Can occur in hospitals as well as community

Risk Factors

- Close contact with individuals with MRSA carriers.
- Poor hygiene
- Contaminated items
- Strains express mecA gene
- Multidrug resistant organisms

Sources

- Healthcare personnel
- Patient environment
- Equipment
- Detection by using cefoxitin disc or oxacillin MIC-based method.
- PCR detection of mec A gene.
- Latex agglutination test—PBP2a.

Infection Control Practices

- Screening of MRSA carriers in HCW during an outbreak
- Treatment of carriers –topical mupirocin for nasal carriers, chlorhexidine body bath
- Contact precautions to be taken are:
  - Hand hygiene
  - Gloves and gown
  - Single use equipment used or period disinfections of items after use
  - Cohort the patient
  - Patient room should be frequently cleaned and disinfected.

---

2. Discuss in brief the methods available to prevent the spread of N-COVID-19 infection in a hospital. Mention the measures required to prevent the spread of N-COVID-19 from hospitalised patients to healthcare personnel.

(3+2 marks)

- The N-COVID 19 can be transmitted by contact of objects or individuals infected with COVID 19 or droplet while conducting aerosol generating procedures (AGP) on an infected individual.

IPC at Healthcare Facility

- Hand hygiene using soap and water or hand rub (as per WHO 5 moments of hand hygiene).
- *Personal Protective Equipment (PPE):* HCW while giving care to infected persons—Surgical mask or N95 if conducting AGP, gloves, gown, face shield
- *In non-COVID area:* Surgical mask should be worn appropriately during working hours
- Universal masking by staff working at the hospital is mandatory.

The measures required to prevent the spread of N-COVID 19 from hospitalised patients to healthcare personnel

- *Environmental cleaning:* Floor and surfaces- detergent followed by disinfectant for cleaning
- Cleaning of equipment such stethoscope, BP cuff using 70% alcohol.
- Cleaning of high touch surfaces such as floor railings, doorknobs, lift buttons, bed rails, trolleys with alcohol.
- Terminal disinfection after discharge/transfer/death of a patient.
- *Respiratory and cough etiquette:* Cough /sneeze into one`s elbow, hand hygiene
- *Biomedical waste management:* must be carried out as per BMW 2016 guidelines. Additional precautions of doubling bagging of COVID 19 waste
- *Laundry:* Should be washed at 60–90ºC followed by soaking in 1% sodium hypochlorite for 30 min

---

3. Discuss in brief about Antibiotic Policy in a tertiary care hospital and its importance in minimising the outbreak of HAI. (2+3 marks)

- An antibiotic policy is an evidence Based anti-microbial treatment guidelines framed-based on existing microbial flora and their resistance to antibiotics, drafted by Hospital Infection Control Committee.
- The antibiotic policy is reviewed every year or earlier if necessary.

Aim of Antibiotic Policy

- ↓ morbidity and mortality due to antimicrobial-resistant infection
- Preserve the efficacy of antimicrobial agents in treatment
- Prevention of communicable diseases
- Identifying source and controlling of outbreaks in a hospital by targeted surveillance

Its Importance in Minimizing the Outbreak of HAI Healthcare-associated infection surveillance.

- To monitor trends, incidence and distribution of nosocomial infection, prevalence rate, attack rate.
- To identify need for new prevention programme and evaluate the impact of preventive measure and control of the outbreak.

---

4. Discuss the transmission-based precautions and recommended precautions with examples.

(4+1 marks)

See Table 8.5.2

- Hand hygiene must be done for all types of precautions
- Single use or reprocessed of equipment's for patient use

Table 8.5.2 Characteristics of transmission-based precautions

Type of transmission-based precautions	*Isolation/ cohorting*	*Gloves**	*Apron/gown*	*Mask*	*Visitors*
Standard	• No	• As required*	• If soiling likely	• As required	• No additional measures
Contact	• Essential	• Essential	• Essential	• As required	• Same as for HCW
Droplet	• Essential	• As required*	• If soiling likely	• Surgical mask	• Restricted precautions, same as for HCW
Airborne	• Essential (negative pressure)	• As required*	• If soiling likely	• N95 respirator	• Restricted precautions, same as for HCW

**Gloves used when chances of exposure to blood or body fluids*

- Contact precautions, e.g. MRSA infections in hospitals
- Droplet precautions, e.g. COVID-19
- Air-borne precautions, e.g. tuberculosis

5. A patient on follows up visited the hospital after 20 days of surgery with complaints of pus discharge from the operated wound site. Give two examples of common aetiological agent causing surgical Site Infections (SSI). Discuss the preventive measures to be followed for SSI. (2 +3 marks)

Common Aetiological Agent Causing Surgical Site Infections (SSI)

1. *S. aureus.*
2. *Pseudomonas species.*

Preventive Measures for SSI

1. Preoperative bathing using soap and water.
2. Hair removal should be avoided and if necessary, hair clippers must be used.
3. For MRSA carriers, Mupirocin ointment must be used for decolonisation.
4. Intra operative surgical antibiotic prophylaxis should be given 1–2 hours prior to incision. For surgeries beyond 4 hours second dose of antibiotic must be initiated.
5. Scrubbing is an important step.
6. Surgical site preparation: Alcohol-based chlorhexidine antisepsis must be done.
7. Normothermia, blood glucose levels <200 mg/dl, O_2 saturation maintenance, adequate fluids should be appropriately maintained.

MI 8.6 DESCRIBE THE BASICS OF INFECTION CONTROL

SHORT ESSAYS

1. Describe in detail about hospital infection control methods under the following headings.

A. Expand HICC. Mention the members constituting the HICC team. (1+2 marks)

Expansion of HICC

- Hospital Infection Control Committee.

Members in the HICC team

- Hospital director
- Infection control officer—Microbiologist or physician
- The infection control practitioner (often a nurse with special training)
- The hospital epidemiologist (usually an infectious disease physician)
- The members of the committee would also include representatives of all the major specialties, housekeeping, CSSD, and hospital administration.

B. Discuss in detail about infection control policy in a tertiary care hospital. (3 marks)

Infection Control Policy

1. To review and approve a yearly programme for activity, surveillance, and prevention.
2. To review and provide input into investigation of an outbreak/epidemic.
3. To review and epidemiological surveillance data and identify areas for intervention.
4. To assess and promote improved practices at all levels of health facility.
5. To review risk associated with new technologies and monitor infectious risk of new devices and products, prior to their approval for use.
6. To ensure appropriate staff training in infection control and safety.

7. To communicate and cooperate with other departments of hospitals with common interests such as pharmacy and therapeutics, or antimicrobial use committee, blood transfusion committee, health and safety committee.

2. Explain in detail about Biomedical Waste Management in a tertiary care hospital (5 marks)

- Waste generated during the diagnosis, treatment or immunisation of human beings or animals or in research activities pertaining there to or in the production of testing biological.
- Segregation in colour coded bags at the site of generation.

Colour of the Bag/ Container	*Used for*	*Examples*
Yellow bag	• Infectious non plastic waste	• Mask, linen
Red bag	• Infectious plastic waste	• Gloves, catheters
White puncture proof container	• Metal sharps	• Scalpels, needles
Blue puncture and leak proof container	• Implants, Glass	• Implants, broken glass vials

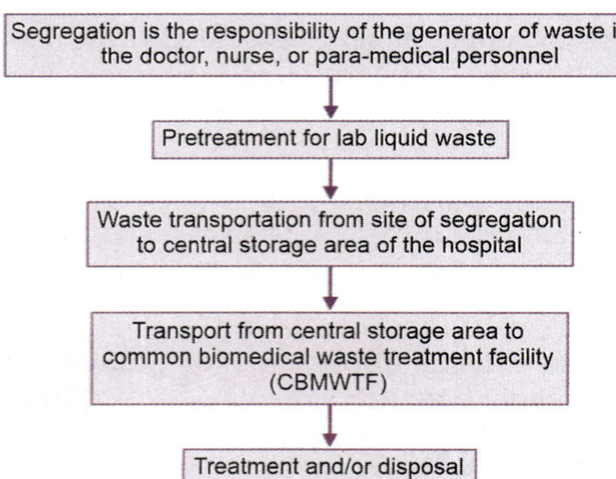

3. A HCW accidently pricked by a needle when the patient's blood was being drawn for investigations. What are the recommended steps advised to be followed by the HCW? (5 marks)

- The following steps are recommended.
  1. Provide immediate care to the exposure site.
  2. Wash the site of injury as soon as possible under running water and allow free flow of blood.
  3. Flush splashes to the nose, mouth, or skin with water.
  4. Irrigate eyes with clean water or saline.
  5. Report the exposure to the CMO/infection control team.
- Management of the needle wound.

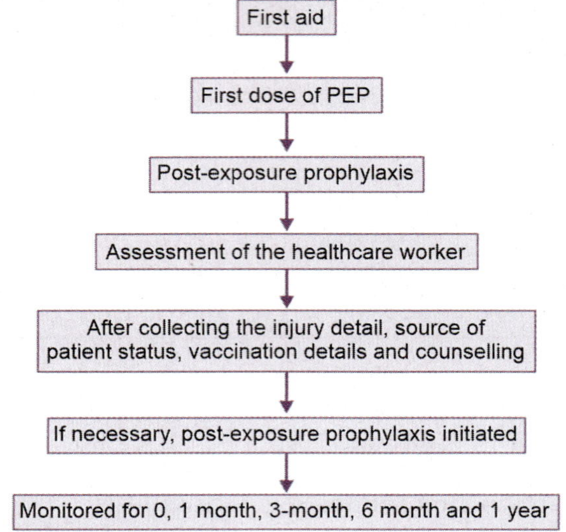

Preferred Ragimen for PEP

- Adolescent and adults: Tenofir (300 mg) + Lamivudine (300 mg) + Dolutegravir (300 mg)
- Children (2–6 years): Zidovudine + Lamivudine + Dolutegravir
- Children (>6 years old): Zidovudine + Lamivudine + Lopinavir/Ritonavir
- The first dose of PEP should be administered immediately (preferably within 2 hours)

SHORT ANSWERS

1. List the components of standard precautions in the healthcare set-up. (3 marks)

1. Hand hygiene.
2. Personal Protective Equipment (PPE).
3. Respiratory hygiene and cough etiquette.
4. Environmental cleaning.
5. Linen handling.
6. Biomedical waste management.
7. Safe handling of sharps.

2. A microbiology lab technician while conducting her daily serological assays drops a glass tube filled with patient`s blood. What are the measures to be followed during a blood spill? (3 marks)

- The following steps are to be followed during a blood spill.
  1. Preparation and Safety—Cordon the area of spill using wet floor sign board and wear the required PPE such as gloves, apron, mask, goggles.
  2. Place absorbent material such as tissue paper on spill.

3. Apply disinfectant—1% Sodium hypochlorite allow sufficient contact time: 15–30 minutes.
4. Clean up the spill—Use cardboard or forceps to pick the glass pieces.
5. Dispose of contaminated materials in appropriate colour coded bag.
6. Disinfect spill area again.
7. Clean the equipment or floor.
8. Remove personal protective equipment and discard in appropriate colour coded bag.
9. Wash Your Hands.
10. Report the spill, fill out an incident report.

MI 8.7 DEMONSTRATE INFECTION CONTROL PRACTICES AND USE OF PERSONAL PROTECTIVE EQUIPMENT (PPE)

SHORT ESSAYS

1. A nurse was drawing blood from an admitted patient in the ward. There was an accidental blood spill while drawing blood. She opened the spillage kit and wore disposable gloves, mask, goggles, and plastic cover for shoes. She covered the total spillage area with 1% freshly prepared sodium hypochlorite, covered it with absorbent paper/material and left it undisturbed for 20 minutes. She then mopped it with cotton wool or absorbent paper.

A. List the different biomedical waste generated during the above-mentioned procedure? (1 mark)

1. Gloves.
2. Goggles.
3. Plastic cover for shoes.
4. Mask.
5. Absorbent paper.

B. Mention the appropriate colour-coded bag indicated for their disposal (1 mark)

1. *Gloves, Goggles, Plastic cover for shoes:* Red.
2. *Absorbent paper/cotton, Mask:* Yellow.

C. What do you mean by biomedical waste? (1 mark)

- Bio-medical waste means any waste, which is generated during the diagnosis, treatment or immunisation of human beings or animals or in research activities or in the production or testing of biologicals in a healthcare set-up.

D. Enumerate the different methods of biomedical waste disposal. (2 marks)

See Table 8.7.1

2. A specimen needs to be collected from a patient suspected to suffer from infection with H1N1. As an intern in the fever clinic, you are expected to collect the appropriate specimen for diagnosing H1N1.

A. What is the appropriate specimen to be collected? (1 mark)

- Nasopharyngeal swab specimens should be collected using swabs with a synthetic tip (e.g., polyester or Dacron).

B. Choose the appropriate PPE. (2 marks)

1. Masks (N-95).
2. Gloves.

Table 8.7.1 Different categories of biomedical waste disposal

Category	Type of waste	Method of disposal
Yellow	• Human and animal anatomical waste • Soiled waste • Microbiology and other clinical laboratory waste • Discarded/expired medicines • Chemical waste	• Incineration or plasma pyrolysis at >1200▯ or deep burial • In the absence of the above facilities combination of autoclaving/microwaving/hydroclaving and shredding • Chemical liquid waste shall be pre-treated in separate effluent treatment system before mixing with other wastewater
Red	• Contaminated plastic waste (recyclable)	• Combination of autoclaving/microwaving/ hydroclaving and shredding
White (leak proof Puncture proof container)	• Waste sharps including metals	• Combination of autoclaving or dry heat sterilisation and shredding
Blue	• Glassware • Metallic body implants	• Autoclaving/microwaving/hydroclaving or disinfection by Sodium Hypochlorite solution followed by washing with detergent prior to sending it for recycling

3. Protective eye wear (goggles)
4. Face shield
5. Boot or shoe covers
6. Protective clothing (gown or apron)

C. Demonstrate the right sequence of donning and doffing for the procedure. (2 marks)

Sequence of Donning

- Hand hygiene → Gown → Mask → Goggles → Hood cap → Hand hygiene → Gloves.

Sequence of Doffing

- Hand hygiene → Gloves → Hand hygiene → Hood cap → Hand hygiene → Gown → Hand hygiene → Goggles, Mask → Hand hygiene → Gloves → Hand hygiene.

3. A nurse in the ICU records BP in one patient and notes it in the case sheet. She then moves to the next patient for drawing blood.

A. How many times does she need to perform Hand hygiene? (1 mark)

1. Before recording BP
2. After recording BP/before drawing blood
3. After drawing blood.

B. Demonstrate the steps of hand hygiene. (2 marks)

Steps of Hand Hygiene

1. Wet hands with water.
2. Apply enough soap to cover all hand surfaces.
3. Rub hands to palm.
4. Right palm over left dorsum with interfaced fingers and vice versa.
5. Palm to palm with fingers interlaced.
6. Backs of fingers to opposing palms with fingers interlocked.
7. Rotational rubbing of left thumb clasped in right palm and vice versa.
8. Rotational rubbing, backwards and forwards with clasped fingers of right hand in left palm and vice versa.
9. Rinse hands with water.
10. Dry hands thoroughly with a single use towel.
11. Use towel to turn off faucet.
12. Your hands are now safe.

C. What is the difference between handwash and hand rub? (1 mark)

Feature	*Handwash*	*Hand rub*
Method	• Washing hands with soap and water is the best way	• Cleaning hands by use of alcohol-based hand sanitizer
Action	• Removes germs and chemicals from your hands	• Works by killing germs on your hands,
Disadvantage	–	• Does not kill all types of germs or removes harmful chemicals

D. Enumerate the 5 moments of hand hygiene. (1 mark)

1. *Moment 1:* Before touching a patient.
2. *Moment 2:* Before a procedure.
3. *Moment 3:* After a procedure or body fluid exposure risk.
4. *Moment 4:* After touching a patient.
5. *Moment 5:* After touching a patient's surroundings.

MI 8.8 DESCRIBE THE METHODS USED AND SIGNIFICANCE OF ASSESSING MICROBIAL CONTAMINATION OF FOOD, WATER AND AIR

LONG ESSAYS

1. Name the bacterial agents causing water contamination and enumerate the diseases caused by them. Discuss in brief the methods available for the detection of bacterial agents in water. Mention their merits and demerits. (2+2+4+2 marks)

Bacterial Agents Causing Water Contamination

Microorganisms	*Water-borne pathogen and diseases*
Bacterial	• *V. cholera*—Cholera, • *S. typhi, S. paratyphi*—Typhoid, • *Shigella spp, Yersinia enterocolitica, Campylobacter jejunum*—Dysentery • *Diarrhoeagenic E. coli*—Diarrhoea

Methods for Bacteriological Analysis of Water

1. **Presumptive coliform count (multiple tube method):**
   - Here measured volume of water samples are added to tube containing MacConkey purple broth with durham tubes.

Quality of drinking water supply	*Most probable number (MPN) 100 ml of water coliform count/ml*	*E. coli count/100 ml*
Excellent	0	0
Satisfactory	1–3	0
Intermediate/ Suspicious	4–9	0
Unsatisfactory	>10	≥1

- It must be incubated for 48 hours.
- Positive test indicate.
  - Change in colour of medium from purple to yellow.
  - Gas collection in Durham tube.
- Merits and Demerits.
  1. It is of inadequate value by itself, but provides information about the amount and type of organic matter in the water which may be useful in indicating the efficiency of the processes used for water treatment.
  2. Affordable.
  3. Appropriate in areas where large scale production of food and drink takes place.

2. **Differential coliform count (Eijkman method):**
   - Here by subculturing the positive tubes on to the lactose containing medium.
   - This test is done to confirm that coliform bacilli detected in the test are thermotolerant *E. coli*.
3. **Membrane filtration method:**
   - In this method, a measured volume of the water sample is filtered through a membrane of pore size, then the membrane is placed on to the selective medium and incubated, then the number of colonies grown in media must be calculated for CFU/100 ml of water.
   - *Merits:*
     1. To test dialysis water
     2. For testing clean water
     3. For testing large volume of water
   - *Demerits:*
     1. Unsuitable for turbid water
     2. Expensive compared to multiple tube method.

2. Enumerate the bacterial agents causing food poisoning based on pathogenic mechanism. Discuss in brief the methods available for the detection of bacterial agents causing food contamination. (5+5 marks)

Bacterial Agents Causing Food Poisoning Based on Pathogenic Mechanism

Pathogenic mechanism	*Major symptoms*	*Examples of aetiologic agents*
Pre-formed toxin	• Vomiting	• *Staphylococcus aureus,* • *Bacillus cereus (short IP)* • *Clostridium botulinum*
Toxin production in vivo (non-inflammatory)	• Watery diarrhoea • No fever • No faecal leukocytes	• *Clostridium perfringens* • *Bacillus cereus (long IP)* • *Infant botulism* • *ETEC* • *Vibrio cholerae O1 or O139* • *Vibrio cholerae non O1*
Tissue invasion and cytotoxin (inflammatory)	• Dysentery, fever • Faecal leucocytes	• *Campylobacter jejuni* • *Salmonella enteritidis* • *Shigella spp* • *EIEC* • *Vibrio parahaemolyticus*
Tissue invasion with access to bloodstream	• Systemic symptoms, fever	• *Salmonella typhi* • *Yersinia enterocolitica*

Methods Available for the Detection of Bacterial Agents Causing Food Contamination

Appropriate Specimen Collection

- Faeces, vomitus, rectal swabs, serum and blood.
- Leftover food (10 g food in 90 ml of sterile diluent).
- Cultures from food preparation environment
- Cultures from food handlers

Transport

- Under refrigeration in Cary–Blair or other suitable transport medium.
- Remnants of food in sterile container in icepack
- Stool specimens refrigerated till processed.
- Swabs are not suitable for toxin detection.

Macroscopic Examination

- *Of food:* To look for evidence of spoilage
- *Of stool:* To see if watery or mucoid/bloody

Microscopic Examination

- Wet mount of faeces
- Methylene blue staining
- Gram's staining of faeces/homogenised, centrifuged food deposit

Culture

- Samples inoculated into several media for maximal yield like MacConkey, XLD, TCBS, SS agar, etc.
- Choice of media is arbitrary
- Enrichment broths to enhance recovery

Toxin Detection

- Antigen: Antibody precipitation reactions in gel
- Reverse passive latex agglutination
- Ligated rabbit ileal loop test
- Tissue culture tests
- ELISA, DNA probes, RIA.

SHORT ANSWERS

1. Enumerate the bacteria causing water-borne diseases. (3 marks)

Water-borne Pathogens

See Table 8.8.1.

2. Define "MPN" (Most Probable Number). Mention its significance. (2+1 marks)

Most Probable Number

- The total number of tubes giving positive reaction is analysed with the McCrady statistical table to determine the most probable number of coliform count present per 100 ml of water. This is presumptive coliform count.

Significance

- The count measures the quality of water whether satisfactory, excellent, or unsatisfactory for use.

3. Mention the methods available for detection of bacterial count in operation theatre before fumigation and after fumigation. Mention their merits and demerits. (2+1 marks)

Methods for Monitoring Air Quality in OT

Method	Advantages	Disadvantages
Passive/ settle plate method	• Simple	• Cannot measure small particles suspended in air • Cannot quantify the volume of air sampled • It cannot measure fungal spores
Active/slit sampler method	• Can quantify the volume of air sampled • Useful in OT, transplant units	• Cannot measure when concentration of microorganisms is high
Air particle counter	• Detects air-borne particles containing micro-organisms	• Expensive

4. Enumerate the indications of environmental sampling in a healthcare set-up. (3 marks)

Indications for Environmental Sampling

1. For research as a part of epidemiological surveillance or outbreak investigation
2. After new construction or renovation of buildings
3. After fogging
4. For initial period of evaluation of change in infection control practices
5. Routine periodic surveillance not recommended.

5. Enumerate the indicator organisms of faecal pollution. (3 marks)

Microorganisms	Interpretation (Presence in Water Indicates)
Coliform (other than *E. coli*)	• Remote contamination with either fecal (presumptive) or soil and vegetation
Faecal (thermotolerant) *E. coli*	• Confirms recent fecal contamination of water • Most sensitive indicator.
Faecal streptococci	• Confirms remote fecal pollution
Clostridium perfringens	• Remote contamination

Table 8.8.1 Waster-born pathogens

Bacteria	Viruses	Protozoa	Helminths
Shigella spp. *Vibrio cholerae* *Salmonella typhi,* *Salmonella paratyphi* *Campylobacter*	• Rotavirus • Enteroviruses	• *Entamoeba histolytica* • *Giardia lamblia* • *Cryptosporidium*	• *Schistosoma haematobium* • *Dracunculus medinensis*

6. Mention the bacterial agents which cause disease in humans through infected air/ contaminated air. (3 marks)

Droplet transmission	*Air-borne*
Streptococcus pyogenes *Neisseria meningitides* *Corynebacterium diphtheria* *Haemophilus influenza* type B *Bordetella pertussis* *Yersinia pestis (pneumonic plague)* *Mycoplasma pneumoniae*	*Mycobacterium tuberculosis*

7. Enumerate the bacterial agents causing food poisoning based on incubation period. (3 marks)

Incubation period	*Examples*
1–6 hours	• *S. aureus* • *B. cereus* (emetic type)
8–16 hours	• *Cl. Perfringens* • *B. cereus* (diarrhoeal form)
>16 hours	• *V. cholera* • *V. parahaemolyticus* • ETEC • EHEC • *Salmonella* spp. • *Shigella* spp. • *C. jejuni*

MI 8.11 DEMONSTRATE RESPECT FOR PATIENT SAMPLES SENT TO THE LABORATORY FOR PERFORMANCE OF LABORATORY TESTS IN THE DETECTION OF MICROBIAL AGENTS CAUSING INFECTIOUS DISEASES

SHORT ANSWERS

1. A mid-stream urine sample collected from a 22-year-old patient have burning micturition was received in the microbiology laboratory after 48 hours for culture and sensitivity. What is inappropriate in this case scenario?.

- Delay in arrival of sample.
- Sample must be transported immediately without delay or can be stored in refrigerator for 2–4 hours only.

2. Tissue obtained from OT after resection of appendix by a surgeon was sent in formalin for routine culture and sensitivity. What is inappropriate in this case scenario?

- Rejection due improper method of collection.
- Tissue should be stored in normal saline or distilled water for routine culture and sensitivity.
- Essential Information required for sample collection:
  1. Appropriate sample—Type, volume/amount, collection method, preservatives, type of containers, transport and storage.
  2. Labelling appropriately.
  3. Clinical details on sample requisition form.
  4. Informed consent for specific samples.

MI 8.12 DISCUSS CONFIDENTIALITY PERTAINING TO PATIENT IDENTITY IN LABORATORY RESULTS
MI 8.14 DEMONSTRATE CONFIDENTIALITY PERTAINING TO PATIENT IDENTITY IN LABORATORY RESULTS

SHORT ANSWERS

1. A pregnant lady in her first trimester visits the hospital for her routine antenatal check-up, following which her HIV test report was reactive. Her office colleague came to collect the report. Can the report be released to her colleague? Give reason.

- The HIV report cannot be handed over to a third party including her close relatives and employers without patients consent.

Reason

- Confidentiality urges you to keep a secret by which we mean knowledge or information that a person has the right or obligation to conceal.
- For example, if the family of a person who has had an HIV test demands that you give thern the result, you must not tell them you must keep the result confidential unless your client gives you permission to tell their family.

2. A 55-year-old male businessman was diagnosed to have lung cancer. On investigation and examination, the doctor suggested that resection of the tumour was the best available treatment. But it was hard for the patient to know that he had cancer and was not willing for the surgery. Which element comes into picture with regards to the patient and treating doctor?

- In this scenario, it is the patient's autonomy either to refuse or accept the treatment.

- *Autonomy:* Ultimate decision or responsibility lies with the patient
- May be for diagnosis, treatment—agreeing or denial.
- Medical practitioner or bystander cannot influence the patient's decision.
- Exceptions.
  - Mental incapacity should be in patients' interest.
  - Among small children, parents can decide.
- For the doctor paternalism prevails, paternalism is based on the Latin word *pater* ("father").
- Action or decision done in the assumed interest of a person without informed consent.
- Medical practitioner does this as ethical binding to do good.
- Family member due to the relationship/bond shared.

3. An 18-year-old is posted for emergency surgery. A set of investigations were conducted for the patient before being posted to the OT. The consultant explained about the procedure and asked to sign the informed consent. What is informed consent? Why should we take informed consent and its indications? What is the component of informed consent?.

Informed Consent

- Informed consent is a process of education of competent patient about the risks, benefits, and alternatives of the procedure.

Informed Consent is Required Because

- Legal obligations
- Ethical requirement

Indications

1. Before any procedures
2. Before HIV testing
3. Before anaesthesia
4. Clinical trials

Components

1. Nature of the procedure
2. Risk and benefit of the procedure
3. Reasonable alternatives
4. Risk of not taking the treatment
5. Assessment of patient's understanding

Note

- Below 18 years consent should be sought from parents.

MI 8.13 CHOOSE THE APPROPRIATE LABORATORY TEST IN THE DIAGNOSIS OF THE INFECTIOUS DISEASE
MI 8.15 CHOOSE AND INTERPRET THE RESULTS OF THE LABORATORY TESTS USED IN DIAGNOSIS OF THE INFECTIOUS DISEASES

SHORT ESSAYS

1. Pregnant lady is diagnosed with Rubella in the 8th week of pregnancy. What is the risk to the developing foetus? Justify the answer with clinical presentation and diagnosis of this syndrome. (1+2+3 marks)

Risk to the Developing Foetus

- Effect of maternal infection depends on the stage of foetal development and mother's immune status.
  - Preconception: Minimal risk.
  - 0–12 weeks: 80–90%: Congenital rubella syndrome, spontaneous abortion occurs in 20% of cases.
  - 13–16 weeks: Deafness and retinopathy 15%.
  - After 16 weeks: Normal development, slight risk of deafness, retinopathy.

Clinical Features of Congenital Rubella Syndrome

- *Category A:* Cataracts/congenital glaucoma, congenital heart disease (most commonly patent ductus arteriosus or peripheral pulmonary artery stenosis), hearing impairment, pigmentary retinopathy
- *Category B:* Purpura, hepatosplenomegaly, jaundice, microcephaly, developmental delay, meningoencephalitis, radiolucent bone disease

Diagnosis

Mother

- *IgM +:* Primary infection
- *IgM + IgG+:* Avidity test (low: primary; high: past infection)
- *IgM–, IgG +:* Immune

Baby

- *Prenatal:* IgM in foetal blood (6 weeks)
- Post-natal.
  - Urine +/– CSF for rubella virus PCR.
  - White blood cells (infant blood) for rubella PCR.
  - Serum (infant blood) for rubella IgM.

2. 32-year-old pregnant lady in her 30th week of pregnancy got an ultrasound examination that revealed foetus with Intrauterine Growth retardation, hydrocephalus, and calcifications in the brain. Umbilical blood was cultured, and crescent shaped trophozoites were grown. What is the probable diagnosis in the foetus? Discuss the clinical presentation and diagnosis of this condition. (1+2+3 marks)

Probable Diagnosis

- This is a scenario of congenital toxoplasmosis.

Clinical Presentation

- Classical triad of chorioretinitis, hydrocephalus, and intracranial calcifications.
- Stillbirth, psychomotor disturbance, and microcephaly.
- Ocular involvement:
  - At 2nd–3rd decade when the cysts ruptures.
  - Bilateral chorioretinitis with visual impairment, blurred vision, scotoma, photophobia, strabismus, and glaucoma.

Diagnosis

Antenatal

- Ultrasonography of foetus at 20–24 weeks of gestation and repeated every 2–4 weeks.
- *PCR and/or isolation:* Amniotic fluid sample

Postnatal

- Isolation of the parasite from amniotic fluid, placenta, and cord leucocyte.
- *IgM and IgG:* Newborn and maternal sera: IgG or IgM by IFA or ELISA
- IgG titre of more than or equal to 1,000 in neonate, indicates possible diagnosis which should be followed by IgM testing.
- IgM titre of neonate more than or equal to 1:4 after 2 weeks of age indicates probable diagnosis and guides the clinicians to initiate treatment to the neonate

SHORT ANSWER

1. Discuss the clinical features and diagnosis of Cytomegalic inclusion disease. (2+2 marks)

Cytomegalic Inclusion Disease

Clinical Features

- Jaundice (62%)
- Petechiae (58%)
- Hepatosplenomegaly (50%)
- IUGR (33%); Preterm (25%)
- Microcephaly (21%)
- Chorioretinitis (12%)
- Fatal outcome (4%)

Diagnosis

Maternal

- Serology IgG and IgM. CMV specific IgM can persist up to 18 months and is present in 10% recurrent cases.
- Presence of both IgG and IgM are presumptive evidence of primary infection. Paired specimen needed if seroconversion from negative to positive not documented.

Antenatal

- *Amniotic fluid:* Virus culture, PCR for viral DNA
- *Fetal blood:* CMV specific IgM, culture, LFT's, PCR
- *Ultrasound:* Ascites and hydrops, microcephaly, IUGR, ventriculomegaly, intracerebral calcification.

In Neonates

- Urine culture for CMV (must be in first two weeks of life to confirm congenital infection).
- Cord or infant blood for CMV PCR.
- Serology of blood or urine. IgM persist for 8 months.
- Head ultrasound.
- *Long-term:* Serial audiology and developmental assessment, head circumference, ophthalmology.

MI 8.16 DESCRIBE THE NATIONAL HEALTH PROGRAMMES IN THE PREVENTION OF COMMON INFECTIOUS DISEASE

NATIONAL HEALTH PROGRAMMES

- Launched by the central government for control/eradication of communicable diseases, improvement of environment sanitation, raising the standard of nutrition, control of population and improving rural health.
- International agencies like WHO, UNICEF, UNFPA, World Bank and also a number of foreign agencies like SIDA, DANIDA, NORAD, and USAID have been providing technical and material assistance in the implementation of these.

List of National Health Programmes

1. National Vector Borne Disease Control Programme (NVBDCP)
   - Malaria, Filariasis, Kala-azar, Japanese encephalitis, Dengue, Chikungunya
2. National Leprosy Eradication Programme (NLEP)

3. National Tuberculosis Elimination Programme (NTEP)
4. National AIDS Control Programme
5. Integrated Disease Surveillance Programme (IDSP)
6. Programme for Prevention and Control of Leptospirosis
7. Pulse Polio Programme
8. National Viral Hepatitis Control Programme
9. National Rabies Control Programme
10. National Programme for Containment of Anti-Microbial Resistance.

1. National Vector-borne Disease Control Programme (NVBDCP)

- Reducing mortality on account of malaria, dengue and JE by half.
- Elimination of Kala-azar by 2010.
- Elimination of lymphatic filariasis by year 2015.

i. National Anti-malaria programme (NAMP)
- Early case detection and prompt treatment.
- Vector control by indoor residual insecticide spray, Long-lasting Insecticidal Nets (LLINs), use of larvivorous fish, anti-larval measures Health education and community participation.
- Strengthening of referral services, epidemic preparedness, and rapid response.

ii. National Filaria Control Programme (NFCP)
- Launched in 1955.
- *Control measures:*
  - Assessing the extent of problem of filariasis
  - Treating diagnosed cases with DEC
  - Controlling the disease through anti-larva and anti-parasite measures
  - Annual Mass Drugs Administration
  - Activities for community awareness

iii. Kala-azar Programme
- An organised centrally sponsored Control Programme launched in endemic areas in 1990–91.
- Government of India provided kala-azar medicines, insecticides and technical support implemented by state governments.
- Vector control.
- Early Diagnosis and Complete treatment.
- Information Education Communication.
- Capacity Building.

iv. Dengue Fever Control Programme
- The National Dengue Prevention and Control Programme were first initiated by the Department of Health (DOH) in 1993.
- 2016: Dengue Notifiable Infection.
- Vector control.
- Early Diagnosis and Complete treatment.

v. Chikungunya Control Programme
- During 2006 there was huge outbreak of Chikungunya in India.
- Symptomatic and supportive treatment is provided to patients.

2. National Leprosy Eradication Programme

- Decentralisation and Institutional Development.
- Strengthening Delivery system (case detection in endemic area and campaign for hot spots).
- Disability Prevention, Care and Rehabilitation.
- IEC activities to reduce social stigma.
- Training of staff of General Health Services.
- India achieved elimination of leprosy in December 2005.

3. National Tuberculosis Elimination Programme (NTEP)

- Renamed in 2020 (previously RNTCP).
- National Strategic plan (2020–2025): elimination of TB Burden with zero deaths and Disease by 2025
- Objectives of the programme.
  - i. To reduce the incidence of and mortality due to TB.
  - ii. To prevent further emergence of drug resistance and effectively manage drug-resistant TB cases.
  - iii. To improve outcomes among HIV-infected TB patients.
  - iv. Early case detection, Quality assured sputum examination and DOT therapy services.

4. National Aids Control Programme

- Established in 1992 under NACO.
- Comprehensive programme for prevention and control of HIV/AIDS in India.
  - Scaling up coverage of targeted interventions in High-risk groups.
  - Scaling up of interventions among other vulnerable populations.
  - Expanding IEC services for (a) general population and (b) high risk groups with a focus on behavior change.
  - Comprehensive Care, Support and Treatment.
  - Strengthening institutional capacities.
  - Strategic Information Management Systems (SIMS).
- National Strategic plan for HIV /AIDS and STI (2017–24).
  - For ending the AIDS epidemic by 2030.

5. Integrated Disease Surveillance Programme (IDSP)

- Integration and decentralisation of surveillance activities through establishment of surveillance units at Centre, State and District level.
- Human Resource Development—Training of State Surveillance Officers, District Surveillance Officers, Rapid Response Team, and other Medical and Paramedical staff on principles of disease surveillance.

- Use of Information Communication Technology for collection, collation, compilation, analysis, and dissemination of data.
- Strengthening of public health laboratories.
- Inter sectoral Co-ordination for zoonotic diseases.

6. Programme for Prevention and Control of Leptospirosis

- The **objective** of the programme is to reduce the morbidity and mortality due to leptospirosis in Humans.
- The strategies of Programme for Prevention and Control of Leptospirosis includes.
  1. Development of trained manpower.
  2. Strengthening the surveillance of Leptospirosis in humans.
  3. Strengthen diagnostic laboratory in programme states.
  4. Create awareness regarding timely detection and appropriate treatment of patients.
  5. Advocacy for strengthening of patient management facilities in programme states.
  6. Strengthening Inter-Sectoral Coordination at state and district level for outbreak detection, prevention, and control of leptospirosis.

7. Pulse Polio Programme

- Pulse polio eradication: Pulse Polio Initiative was started with an objective of achieving hundred per cent coverage under Oral Polio Vaccine.
- Children in the age group of 0–5 years administered polio drops during National and Sub-national immunisation rounds (in high-risk areas) every year.
- The last polio case in the country was reported from Howrah district of West Bengal with date of onset 13th January 2011. Thereafter no polio case has been reported in the country (25th May 2012).
- WHO on 24th February 2012 removed India from the list of countries with active endemic wild polio virus transmission.

8. National Viral Hepatitis Control Programme

- National Viral Hepatitis Control Programme has been launched by Ministry of Health and Family Welfare, Government of India on the occasion of the World Hepatitis Day, 28th July 2018.
- integrated initiative for the prevention and control of viral hepatitis in India to achieve Sustainable Development Goal (SDG) 3.3 which aims to ending viral hepatitis by 2030.
- Achieve reduction in infected population, morbidity and mortality associated with Hepatitis viruses.
- Hepatitis A, B, C, D and E, from prevention, detection, and treatment to mapping treatment outcomes.

9. National Rabies Control Programme.

- Was approved on 03.10.2013 .
- Objectives:
  - i. Training of Healthcare professionals on appropriate Animal bite management and Rabies Post-exposure Prophylaxis.
  - ii. Advocacy for states to adopt and implement Intradermal route of Post-exposure prophylaxis for Animal bite Victims and Pre-exposure prophylaxis for high-risk categories.
  - iii. Strengthen Human Rabies Surveillance System.
  - iv. Strengthening of Regional Laboratories under NRCP for Rabies Diagnosis.
  - v. Creating awareness in the community through Advocacy and Communication and Social Mobilisation.

10. National Programme for containment of Anti-microbial Resistance

- This programme was launched under the aegis of the National Centre for Disease Control (NCDC).
- The objectives of this programme are establishing a laboratory AMR surveillance system of 30 Network laboratories generating quality data on AMR for pathogens of public health importance.
- Activities carried out in this programme.
  - i. AMR surveillance
  - ii. National treatment guidelines
  - iii. **Infection Prevention and Control guidelines and surveillance of healthcare associated infections**
  - iv. **IEC activities**
  - v. Review meetings, trainings, and workshops.
  - vi. Strengthening laboratory capacity for AMR detection.

Multiple Choice Questions

MI 1.1

1. **Bacteria which grow best at temperatures below 20°C are termed as:**
   A. Mesophilic
   B. Psychrophilic
   C. Thermophilic
   D. Microaerophilic
2. **The following structure in *C. neoformans* is demonstrated using negative staining:**
   A. Bacterial spore
   B. Bacterial flagella
   C. Bacterial capsule
   D. Bacterial fimbriae
3. **Which of the following statement is true in the case of endotoxins?**
   A. Highly antigenic
   B. Proteins in nature
   C. Heat stable
   D. Action is often enzymatic
4. **Craigie's tube method, inoculation into semi-solid medium is used to demonstrate which one of the following bacterial appendages?**
   A. Flagella
   B. Ribosomes
   C. Mesosomes
   D. Fimbriae

MI 1.2

5. **----% of H_2SO_4 used to demonstrate the bacilli from slit skin smears?**
   A. 1%
   B. 3%
   C. 25%
   D. 5%

MI 1.3

6. **Most common causative agent of lobar pneumonia is?**
   A. *Staphylococcus aureus*
   B. *Streptococcus pyogenes*
   C. *Streptococcus pneumoniae*
   D. *Haemophilus influenza*

MI 1.4

7. **Who introduced Sterilisation techniques and the development of steam steriliser, autoclave?**
   A. Sir Louis Pasteur
   B. Sir Robert Koch
   C. Sir Paul Ehrlich
   D. Sir Edward Jenner

MI 1.5

8. **Heart-lung machines are best disinfected by:**
   A. Iso-propyl alcohol
   B. ETO
   C. Glutaraldehyde
   D. Formalin
9. **Cystoscopes, bronchoscopes, endoscopes are best disinfected by:**
   A. Formaldehyde
   B. Glutaraldehyde
   C. ETO
   D. Hydrogen peroxide

MI 1.6

10. **Drug of choice for MRSA infections in a hospital**
    A. Ofloxacin
    B. Ciprofloxacin
    C. Vancomycin
    D. Polymyxin-B

MI 1.7

11. **Which of the following statements is true about hapten?**
    A. It induces brisk immune response
    B. It needs carrier to induce immune response
    C. It is a T-independent antigen
    D. It has no association with MHC

1. B 2. C 3. C 4. A 5. D 6. C 7. A 8. B 9. B 10. C 11. B

12. Which of the following best denotes classical complement pathway activation in immune-inflammatory condition?

A. C2, C4 and C3 decreased
B. C2, and C4 normal, C3 is decreased
C. C3 normal and C2 C4 decreased
D. C2, C4, C3 all are elevated

13. Immune cells which are considered as bridges between innate and acquired immunity:

A. Marginal zone B cells
B. Dendritic cells
C. C3, C4 components of complement
D. Mast cells

14. Rare subtype of T cells:

A. Cytotoxic T cells
B. Suppressor T cells
C. T regulatory cells
D. T-helper cells

15. Which of the following cell types are the most potent activators of T-cell?

A. Bell cells
B. Follicular dendritic cells
C. Mature dendritic cells
D. Macrophages

16. Antigen presentation pathway by MHC class-1 molecule include:

A. Cytosolic pathway
B. Endocytic pathway
C. Lectin pathway
D. Classical pathway

MI 1.8

17. Role of cromolyn sodium as a drug of choice in the treatment of anaphylaxis/type-1 hypersensitivity?

A. Blocks Ca^{+2} influx into mast cells
B. Blocks Cl^{-} influx
C. Blocks cAMP levels
D. Inhibits H1 receptors

MI 1.9

18. Conjugate vaccine are available for the prevention of invasive disease caused by all of the following bacteria *except*:

A. *H. influenzae*
B. *Strep pneumoniae*
C. *Neisseria meningitidis* (Group-C)
D. *Neisseria meningitidis* (Group-B)

19. Role of adjuvant in vaccine is:

A. Stimulation of toll like receptors
B. Increase both adaptive and innate immune response
C. Activate both B and T lymphocyte
D. All the above

MI 1.10

20. Adenosinedeaminase deficiency is seen in the following:

A. Common variable immunodeficiency
B. Severe combined immunodeficiency
C. Chronic granulomatous disease
D. Nezelof syndrome

21. Salivary protein which prevents transmission of human immunodeficiency virus via saliva is:

A. Sialoperoxidase
B. Secretory IgA
C. Salivary leukocyte proteinase inhibitor
D. Histidine rich proteins

22. Drug-induced haemolytic anemia is a classic example of:

A. Type II hypersensitivity
B. Type III reaction
C. Type IV hypersensitivity
D. Type I hypersensitivity

MI 1.11

23. A woman with infertility receives an ovary transplant from her sister who is an identical twin. What type of graft is it?

A. Xenograft
B. Autograft
C. Allograft
D. Isograft

24. Neonatal thymectomy leads to:

A. Decreased size of germinal centre
B. Decreased size of para-cortical areas
C. Increased antibody marrow production by B cells
D. Increased bone marrow production of lymphocytes

25. Type of immunological response in transplant rejection is:

A. Type I
B. Type II
C. Type III
D. Type IV

12. A 13. B 14. C 15. C 16. A 17. A 18. D 19. D 20. B 21. C 22. A 23. D 24. B 25. D

MI 2.1

26. True statement regarding "Streptolysin-O" is:
A. Raised ASO Abs are used as markers for retrospective diagnosis of GAS infection
B. ASO titres are low in pyoderma
C. Streptolysin-O is O_2 labile
D. All are true

27. Group A carbohydrate of Str. pyogenes cross reacts with human:
A. Synovial fluid
B. Myocardium
C. Cardiac valves
D. Vascular intima

28. A patient of RHD developed infective endocarditis after dental extraction. Most likely organism causing this is:
A. *Streptococcus viridans*
B. *Streptococcus pneumoniae*
C. *Streptococcus pyogenes*
D. *Staph. aureus*

MI 2.2

29. Most common causative agent of native valve endocarditis:
A. Pneumococci
B. *S. aureus*
C. *Enterobacter*
D. *S. pyogenes*

30. Duke's criteria for infective endocarditis includes all, *except:*
A. Single positive blood culture for coxiella
B. Negative rheumatoid factor
C. Osler's nodes
D. Pyrexia >38°C

MI 2.3

31. A beta haemolytic bacterium is resistant to vancomycin, shows growth in 6.5% NaCl, is non-bile sensitive. It is likely to be:
A. *Streptococcus agalactiae*
B. *Streptococcus pneumoniae*
C. *Enterococcus*
D. *S. bovis*

32. Vegetations in Infective endocarditis includes the following, *except:*
A. Thrombocytes
B. Fibrin
C. RBCs
D. Micro-colonies of organisms

MI 2.4

33. Megaloblastic anemia is caused by:
A. *Diphyllobothrium latum*
B. *Schistosoma haematobium*
C. *Echinococcus granulosus*
D. *Taenia solium*

34. Type of anaemia caused by old world hook-worm:
A. Microcytic hypochromic
B. Aplastic
C. Haemolytic
D. None of the above

MI 2.5

35. Recrudescence is seen in which of the following combination of *Plasmodium* species?
A. Falciparum, ovale
B. Vivax, ovale
C. Falciparum, malariae
D. Falciparum, vivax

36. Merozoites in grape like clusters, ranging from 8–24 in number are seen in:
A. *P. vivax*
B. *P. ovale*
C. *P. falciparum*
D. *P. malariae*

37. All are true regarding filariasis *except:*
A. Ticks are the vectors.
B. Caused by *Wuchereria bancrofti*
C. Involves lymphatic system
D. DEC is used in treatment.

38. Infective stage of *P. falciparum* to primary host:
A. Merozoites
B. Sporozoites
C. Gametocytes
D. Cryptozoites

39. Infective stage of *Leishmania donovani* to humans:
A. Amastigote
B. Promastigote
C. Trypomastigote
D. Endomastigote

26. D 27. C 28. A 29. B 30. B 31. C 32. C 33. A 34. A 35. C 36. C 37. A 38. C 39. B

MI 2.6

40. All of the following are true about *Brugia malayi* *except:*

A. The intermediate host in the India is *Mansonia annulifera*
B. The tail tip is free from nuclei.
C. Adult worm is found in the lymphatic system.
D. Nuclei are blurred, so counting is different.

41. Following all are the complications of Falciparum Malaria, *except:*

A. Black fever
B. Tropical splenomegaly syndrome
C. Algid malaria
D. Black water fever

42. Infective stage of *Plasmodium* to the vertebrate host:

A. Tachyzoites
B. Sporozoites
C. Gametocytes
D. Cryptozoites

43. Infective stage of *Wuchereria bancrofti* to humans:

A. 1st stage larva
B. 3rd stage sheathed microfilaria
C. 5th stage sheathed microfilaria
D. 2nd stage sheathed microfilaria

MI 2.7

44. Following is the outstanding character of protozoan parasite causing diarrhoea in seropositive HIV cases:

A. Oocysts are acid fast.
B. Sporulated oocysts are the infective forms.
C. Diarrhoea is severe, watery.
D. All the above

45. env gene products includes all, *except:*

A. gp120
B. gp41
C. gp160
D. p24

46. *Pneumocystis jirovecii* causes the following infection in HIV seropositive cases:

A. Interstitial cell pneumonia
B. Pulmonary abscess
C. Chronic meningeal abscess
D. Bronchiolitis

47. Stage of "clinical latency" in HIV is:

A. Symptomatic HIV
B. Acute retroviral syndrome
C. Asymptomatic stage
D. Typical infective stage

48. HIV wasting syndrome is:

A. Slit disease
B. Slim disease
C. Slot disease
D. Angular slap syndrome

49. Uses of p24Ag detection includes all, *except:*

A. Diagnosis during window period
B. Monitoring the progression of HIV
C. To resolve western blot results
D. Confirmation of HIV in infants

50. 5th generation ELISA differentiates:

A. HIV-1 and HIV-2
B. Detects HIV-1 p24Ag
C. Detects only HIV-2
D. Both A and B

MI 3.1

51. Infective stage of *E. histolytica* to humans:

A. Sporulated oocyst
B. Tachyzoite
C. Matured tetranucleated cyst
D. Binucleated cyst

52. Protozoan parasite causing "fatty diarrhoea"

A. *Cryptosporidium*
B. *Isospora belli*
C. *Trichomonas*
D. *Giardia intestinalis*

53. Incubation period for food poisoning due to *S. aureus enterotoxin:*

A. >16 hrs
B. 1–6 hrs
C. 8–16 hrs
D. >24 hrs

54. All of the following are implicated in causing "Traveler's diarrhoea" *except:*

A. ETEC
B. *V. parahaemolyticus*
C. *Campylobacter jejuni*
D. *Giardia lamblia*

40. B 41. A 42. B 43. B 44. D 45. D 46. A 47. C 48. B 49. D 50. C 51. C 52. D 53. B 54. B

55. Site commonly affected in non-inflammatory watery diarrhoea:
A. Colon
B. Distal small bowel
C. Proximal small bowel
D. Both A and B

56. Following all are implicated in causing "inflammatory diarrhoea", *except:*
A. *Clostridium difficile*
B. *Yersinia enter colitica*
C. *Aeromonas hydrophila*
D. *Rota virus*

57. Poultry food, consumption of raw milk causes inflammatory diarrhoea due to:
A. *Campylobacter jejuni*
B. *V. Parahaemolyticus*
C. *V. cholerae*
D. All the above

58. Late Lactose fermenting species of *Shigella:*
A. *S. flexnerii*
B. *S. boydii*
C. *S. sonneii*
D. *S. dysentriae*

59. Anchovy sauce pus is associated with:
A. Bacillary dysentery
B. Giardia diarrhoea
C. Watery diarrhoea in cryptosporidiasis
D. Amoebic dysentery

60. Incubation period for diarrhoeal type of food poisoning due to *bacillus cereus*:
A. 1–6 hrs
B. 6–12 hrs
C. >24 hrs
D. 8–16 hrs

61. All the following are true statements regarding O139 Bengal strain of *V. cholerae*, *except:*
A. Isolated 1st in Chennai
B. Non-capsulated
C. Capsulated
D. Can cause extraintestinal manifestations

62. Indicators used in TCBS medium for the isolation of *V. cholerae:*
A. Methyl red
B. Bromo thymol blue
C. Phenol blue
D. Phenol red

63. Common serotypes of ETEC causing watery diarrhoea in infants and adults:
A. O6, O8, O25
B. O6, O8, O112
C. O25, O114, O124
D. O8, O112, O152

64. False statement regarding EIEC (Entero- invasive *E. coli*)
A. Causes ulceration of bowel
B. Sereny test is useful in detection
C. EIEC strains are non-motile
D. Causes diarrhoea without mucus, but with RBC

65. Undercooked ground beef is one of the sources causing diarrhoea due to:
A. EIEC
B. EHEC
C. ETEC
D. EAEC

MI 3.2

66. All the following species of Shigella ferment mannitol, *except:*
A. Flexneri
B. Boydii
C. Sonnei
D. Dysenteriae

67. Colonies of *Shigella* appear red without black centre on the following medium:
A. DCA
B. SS Agar
C. Hektoen enteric agar
D. XLD agar

68. All the following are opportunistic protozoan parasites causing severe diarrhoea in immuno compromised, *except:*
A. *Cryptosporidium*
B. *Isospora belli*
C. *Giardia intestinalis*
D. *Naegleria fowleri*

69. Stool microscopy in *Strongyloides stercoralis* causing diarrhoea in immuno compromised aims to detect:
A. Plano convex egg
B. Rhabditiform larva
C. Matured oocysts
D. Tetranucleated cyst

55. C 56. D 57. A 58. C 59. D 60. D 61. B 62. B 63. A 64. D 65. B 66. D 67. D 68. D 69. B

70. Electron microscopy of rotavirus causing gastroenteritis:
A. Cup like depression on the capsid
B. Star like spokes
C. Spokes around a wheel
D. Flower like lunar depressions

71. Tear drop shaped binucleated trophozoites on stool microscopy is the feature of:
A. *Giardia intestinalis*
B. *Trichuris trichiura*
C. *Entamoeba histolytica*
D. *Ascaris lumbricoides*

MI 3.3

72. Bacteria-mediated endocytosis with respect to enteric fever caused by *salmonella* is mediated by:
A. Type-I secretory system
B. Type-II secretory system
C. Type-III secretory system
D. Type-IV secretory system

73. Loss of flagella to demonstrate OH-O variation in *Salmonellae* can be achieved by:
A. Culturing on WBBS medium
B. Culturing on SS agar
C. Culturing on phenol agar
D. Culturing on XLD agar

74. Loss O Ag side chain from LPS in *Salmonella* leads to:
A. S-R variation
B. OH-O variation
C. Vi Ag variation
D. Both A and B

75. Faint, salmon coloured maculopapular rash on the chest and trunk in enteric fever are termed as:
A. Koplik's spots
B. Maroon spots
C. Crescent spots
D. Rose spots

76. Major signs related to enteric fever includes all, *except:*
A. Epistaxis
B. Splenomegaly
C. Hepatomegaly
D. Anorexia nervosa

77. Following all are true related to *S. paratyphi B, except:*
A. Citrate utilisation test: positive
B. Ferments xylose
C. Anerogenic
D. Produces abundant H2S

78. Serum for the detection of antibodies to Vi Ag is useful in the diagnosis of:
A. Enteric fever in 2nd week of illness
B. Diagnosis of carriers
C. Enteric fever in 3rd week of illness
D. Both B and C

79. True statement regarding MDR *S. typhi:*
A. Resistance to chloramphenicol, ampicillin +Co-trimoxazole
B. Resistance to nalidixic acid
C. Resistance to ceftriaxone
D. All are true

80. Parenteral Vi polysaccharide vaccine is derived from
A. *S. typhi* Ty2
B. *S. paratyphi* A Ty2
C. *S. paratyphi* B 2
D. *S. paratyphi* C Ty2

MI 3.4

81. Following species of *Salmonella* does not produce H2S:
A. Paratyphi A, typhi
B. Paratyphi A, choleraesuis
C. Typhi, paratyphi B
D. Cholerae suis, typhi

82. Most reliable clinical specimen/method for the diagnosis of enteric fever in 1st week of illness:
A. Stool, blood culture
B. Bone marrow aspirate/stool
C. Duodenal aspirate/stool
D. Blood culture/duodenal aspirates

83. Growth of *S. typhi* on XLD medium produces
A. Red colonies with black centre
B. Colourless colonies with black centre
C. Green colonies with black centre
D. Pale pink colonies with black centre

84. *S. typhi* when cultured on the following medium produces bluish-green colonies with black centre
A. DCA
B. XLD
C. Hektoen Enteric agar
D. WBBS

70. C 71. A 72. C 73. C 74. A 75. D 76. A 77. C 78. B 79. A 80. A 81. B 82. D 83. A 84. D

MI 3.5

85. A Widal test report of a 20-year-old college student interpreted as: Rise of TO and AH antibodies. It suggests:
A. Enteric fever due to *S. paratyphi* A
B. Enteric fever due to *S. typhi*
C. Enteric fever due to *S. paratyphi* B
D. Post-TAB vaccination

86. Rise of titres of all TH, AH, BH antibodies suggests
A. Post-TAB vaccination
B. Anamnestic response
C. Enteric fever due to *S. paratyphi* B
D. Both A and B

87. False statement regarding amino acid decarboxylation by salmonella
A. *S. typhi:* Decarboxylates lysine
B. *S. paratyphi* A: Decarboxylates ornithine
C. *S. paratyphi* B: Decarboxylates lysine, arginine, but not ornithine
D. *S. paratyphi* B: Decarboxylates lysine, arginine, ornithine

88. Highest dilution of the serum at which agglutination occurs is known as:
A. Endpoint
B. Titre
C. Prozone phenomenon
D. Lattice theory

89. Transient augment of titre in Enteric fever due to unrelated diseases like malaria in people with history of enteric fever is known as:
A. Prozone phenomenon
B. Blocking antibody
C. Anamnestic response
D. Lattice theory

90. Significant titre in many parts of India for H agglutination in relation to Widal test for enteric fever:
A. >1:100
B. >1:200
C. 1:80
D. <1:16

91. One of the following factors may lead to false-negatives in Widal test:
A. Widal test performed after 4th week
B. Prozone phenomenon
C. Patients on antibiotic treatment
D. All the above

92. *True* statement regarding O agglutination in Widal test:
A. Presence of chalky clumps
B. Presence of loose woolly clumps
C. Titre >1:200
D. Dreyer's tube is used for O agglutination.

93. Following all are true statements regarding non-typhoidal *Salmonella*, *except:*
A. Dairy products are the sources of food poisoning.
B. Zoonotic in transmission
C. Under cooked ground meat is one of the sources for food poisoning
D. All are true.

94. Canned foods like salads, meat are the sources of food poisoning due to:
A. *S. aureus*
B. *V. Parahaemolyticus*
C. *Clostridium botulinum*
D. *Bacillus cereus*

95. Food sources such as dried beans, vegetables, cereals are the sources of food poisoning due to
A. *B. cereus*
B. Non-typhoidal *Salmonella*
C. *V. cholerae*
D. ETEC

96. Incubation period for *Cl. perfringens* food poisoning associated with consumption of beef, poultry food
A. 1–6 hrs
B. 8–16 hrs
C. >16 hrs
D. > 24 hrs

97. Raw milk, poultry foods are the important sources of food poisoning due to:
A. *Campylobacter jejuni*
B. EHEC
C. ETEC
D. *Cl. botulinum*

98. Following are the enrichment media used for the inoculation of fecal specimens
A. SS broth
B. Selenite F broth
C. HEA agar
D. VR medium

85. A 86. A 87. C 88. B 89. C 90. B 91. D 92. A 93. D 94. C 95. A 96. B 97. A 98. B

99. Shellfish, water are the common food sources causing food poisoning due to:
A. *V. cholerae*
B. Non-typhoidal *Salmonella*
C. *Cl. Perfringens*
D. *C. jejuni*

100. Abdominal cramps, diarrhoea without vomiting/ rarely vomiting are the major symptoms of food poisoning due to
A. *B. cereus, Cl. Perfringens*
B. *V. cholerae, B. cereus*
C. *S. aureus* enterotoxin, *B. cereus*
D. ETEC, *S. aureus* enterotoxin

MI 3.6

101. True statement regarding *Helicobacter pylori:*
A. Motile with unipolar flagella
B. Curved, gram-negative bacilli
C. Sea gull shaped
D. All are true

102. Nobel prize winners who worked on *H. pylori* and its role in gastritis and peptic ulcer disease:
A. Robin warren and blumberg
B. Robin warren and barry marshall
C. Barry marshall and blumberg
D. Barry marshall and peter atkinson

103. Cytotoxin associated gene (*CagA*) encodes:
A. Type-IV secretory system
B. Type-II secretory system
C. Type-III secretory system
D. Type-I secretory system

104. True statement regarding *CagA* in *H. pylori:*
A. Modulates cytoskeleton rearrangements
B. Modulates proto-oncogenes expression
C. Modulates the release of pro-inflammatory cytokines
D. All are true.
E. Only A and C are true.

105. True statement regarding acute gastritis due to *H. pylori:*
A. Antral gastritis leads to duodenal ulcers
B. Pan gastritis results in adenocarcinoma
C. Peptic ulcer disease
D. All the above

106. Following all are invasive tests employed for the diagnosis of *H. pylori* associated clinical disease, *except:*
A. Biopsy urease test
B. Endoscopy guided biopsy
C. Coproantigen assay
D. Both A and B
E. B and C

107. In the diagnosis of *H. pylori* associated disease IgG antibody detection is useful for:
A. Screening after endoscopy
B. Sero-epidemiological study
C. To monitor treatment response
D. Screening of children

108. Culture media plates used for the isolation of *H. pylori* are incubated at 37°C under:
A. Microaerophilic condition
B. 50% Nitrogen, 5% O_2, 20% CO_2
C. 5% Nitrogen, 5% O_2, 10% CO_2
D. Only under anaerobic atmosphere

109. Colonisation of gastric mucosa by *H. pylori* is favored by:
A. *H. pylori* motility
B. Urease enzyme
C. Ure-I protein
D. All the above

110. Treatment for *H. pylori* infection is indicated for:
A. All asymptomatic colonizers
B. People with gastric ulcers
C. People with high grade B- cell carcinoma
D. Both A and C
E. Both B and C

MI 3.7

111. All the following combinations represent blood borne viral pathogens, *except:*
A. NANB hepatitis, HIV
B. HBV, NANB hepatitis
C. HEV, HCV
D. HBV, HDV

112. True statement regarding HBV
A. Belongs to Hepadnaviridae family
B. HBsAg 1st appears in the blood
C. Immuno fluorescence is useful to demonstrate HBcAg in liver cells
D. 1st discovered by blumberg
E. All are true.

113. BCP mutations in HBV genotype C are associated with:
A. Mutations in core promoter region
B. Increased risk of HCC
C. RNases activity
D. Both A and B

99. A 100. A 101. D 102. B 103. A 104. D 105. D 106. C 107. B 108. A 109. D 110. B 111. C 112. E 113. D

114. Select the wrong statement regarding HAV:
A. SsRNA, nonenveloped
B. Nonenveloped, ds DNA
C. Nonenveloped, icosahedral symmetry
D. Family picornaviridae

115. Select the true statement regarding HBV super carriers:
A. Have high levels of HBsAg, HBeAg but moderately infectious
B. Highly infectious, high levels of HBsAg, DNA polymerase
C. DNA polymerase is absent, but HBsAg is present.
D. HBsAg is absent, but DNA polymerase can be detected

116. Following is a true statement regarding HCV genotypes which vary in eepidemiological distribution:
A. Genotype 6 is common in Asia.
B. Genotype 4 is common in Asia, North Africa.
C. Genotypes 1, 3 prevalent in South Africa, but not in India
D. Both A and C are true.

117. Extrahepatic manifestations due to HCV includes:
A. Glomerulonephritis
B. Arthralgia
C. RF
D. Both A and B

118. 1st major epidemic of NANB enterically transmitted hepatitis was reported in:
A. Kolkata, 1995
B. Chennai, 1995
C. New Delhi, 1985
D. New Delhi, 1995
E. New Delhi, 2015

119. Presence of HBsAg with absence of other serological markers is suggestive of:
A. Chronic hepatitis
B. Liver cirrhosis
C. HCC
D. Incubation period

120. HDV is endemic among people with HBV and can be transmitted by:
A. Per- cutaneous route
B. Close direct contact
C. Surgical incisions
D. Blood and blood products

121. Which of the following is a polymerase inhibitor employed in the treatment of HCV infection?
A. Sofosbuvir
B. Ribavirin
C. Pegylated IFN-2
D. Simeprevir

122. True statement regarding "P" gene of HBV genome is:
A. Has DNA polymerase activity
B. Has reverse transcriptase activity
C. Codes for HBeAg
D. Both A and B are true.
E. B & C are true.

123. Anti-HBeAg presence signifies:
A. Decrease in viral replication activity
B. Highly infectious stage
C. Decreased infectivity
D. Both A and C

124. Protective antibody titre against HBV among Vaccinated people:
A. ≥5 mIu/ml
B. >3 mIu/ml
C. >10 mIu/ml
D. 3–7 mIu/ml

125. Age of administration of HBV vaccine under National Immunisation Schedule given along with DPT Vaccine
A. 6, 10, 12th week
B. 6, 8, 10th week
C. 6, 10, 14 weeks
D. 8, 10, 12th week

MI 3.8

126. Only marker of hepatitis B vaccination:
A. HBeAg
B. Anti-HBs
C. Anti-HBcAg
D. Both B and C

127. Site of administration of HBV vaccine in Infants:
A. Right deltoid region
B. Cubital fossa
C. Antero-lateral thigh
D. Left deltoid region

128. Gold standard method for the confirmation and determining HCV genotype and subtype:
A. RIBA
B. 5th generation ELISA
C. Real-time reverse transcriptase PCR
D. Ultra-bio rad

114. B 115. B 116. A 117. D 118. D 119. D 120. B 121. A 122. D 123. D 124. C 125. C 126. B 127. C 128. C

129. A test outcome for HCV interpreted as: HCV RNA detected and HCV Ab reactive. It indicates:
A. Current HCV infection
B. Presumptive HCV infection
C. No current HCV infection
D. HCV infection due to needle stick injury

130. Presence of IgM anti-HEV in serum indicates:
A. Recovery from the disease
B. Acute infection
C. Past infection
D. Both current and past infection

131. True statement regarding Chronic Inactive Hepatitis due to HBV (HBeAg negative):
A. Elevated ALT + moderate liver fibrosis
B. Elevated ALT + HBV DNA >2000 IU/ml
C. Decreased ALT + HBV DNA >2000 IU/ml
D. Both A and B

MI 4.1

132. Established species of *Clostridium* causing gas gangrene among the following combination:
A. *C. welchii, C. histolyticum*
B. *C. welchii, C. septicum*
C. *C. welchii, C. fallax*
D. *C. welchii, C. sporogenes*

133. Target haemolysis is exhibited by
A. *C. perfringens*
B. *C. tetani*
C. *C. botulinum*
D. *C. septicum*

134. 1st symptom in tetanus with increased masseter muscle tone is termed as:
A. Rigidity
B. Trismus
C. Tetanus synomata
D. Ocular tetanus

135. Primary Immunisation Schedule for tetanus in children according to NIP, India:
A. 1 dose of pentavalent vaccine (DPT, HBV, Hi-b)
B. 3 doses of pentavalent vaccine (DPT, HBV, Hi-b)
C. 2 doses of pentavalent vaccine (DPT, HBV, Hi-b)
D. 5 doses of pentavalent vaccine (DPT, HBV, Hi-b)

136. Floppy child syndrome is caused by:
A. *C. difficile*
B. *C. Novyi*
C. *C. botulinum*
D. *C. septicum*

137. Indiscriminate intake of antibiotics like ceftriaxone, clindamycin may lead to:
A. Pseudomembranous colitis
B. Gangrenous appendicitis
C. Pseudomembranous oesophagitis
D. None of the above

138. Lemierre's syndrome is caused by:
A. *Fusobacterium nucleatum*
B. *Fusobacterium necrophorum*
C. *Fusobacterium fusiforme*
D. *Prevotella*

139. Inflamed pharyngeal mucosa covered by greyish membrane resembling diphtheria caused by leptotrichia buccalis is:
A. Trench mouth
B. Gingival plaque
C. Ulcerative gingival stomatitis
D. A and C

140. Meleney's gangrene a rare infection of superficial fascia is caused by:
A. *Bacteroides*
B. *Fusobacterium*
C. *Peptostreptococcus*
D. *Eubacterium*

141. Motile, curved anaerobic Gram variable bacilli causing anaerobic vaginosis is:
A. *Actinomyces*
B. *Mobiluncus*
C. *Bacteroides*
D. *Fusobacterium*

142. Anaerobic bacterial infections are characterised by all the following, *except:*
A. Spreading gangrene with fascia involvement
B. Marked pyrexia
C. Toxaemia
D. Foul smelling pus

143. Toxin of *C. welchii* with lecithinase activity
A. Epsilon
B. Iota
C. Beta
D. Alpha

144. Anaerobic bacteria implicated in causing chronic suppurative otitis media is:
A. *Eubacterium*
B. *Peptostreptococcus*
C. *Bacteroides fragilis*
D. *Prevotella*

129. A 130. B 131. D 132. B 133. A 134. B 135. B 136. C 137. A 138. B 139. C 140. C 141. B 142. B 143. D 144. C

145. Common non-sporing anaerobic bacteria causing necrotising pneumonitis:

A. *Bacteroides fragilis*
B. *Peptostreptococcus*
C. *Actinomyces*
D. *Fusobacterium*

146. Non-sporing anaerobic bacteria causing anaerobic septic arthritis:

A. *Bacteroides*
B. *Fusobacterium*
C. *Lactobacillus*
D. *Porphyromonas*

147. Non-sporing anaerobic bacterial infection associated with cellulitis involving scrotum, abdominal wall, perineum is:

A. Gas gangrene
B. Meleney's gangrene
C. Fournier gangrene
D. None of the above

148. Colonies produced by *Prevotella melaninogenica* when exposed to UV light produces:

A. Pink fluorescence
B. Purple fluorescence
C. Black fluorescence
D. Red fluorescence

149. Anaerobic bacteria associated with endocarditis, pericarditis?

A. *Bacteroides fragilis*
B. *Lactobacillus*
C. *Fusobacterium*
D. All the above

150. *Porphyromonas gingivalis* is associated with

A. Root canal infections
B. Periodontal disease
C. Bacteraemia
D. All the above

MI 4.2

151. Most affected bones in osteomyelitis?

A. Clavicle, femur
B. Femur, scapula
C. Femur, humerus
D. Humerus, ulna

152. Bacteria most involved in causing osteomyelitis

A. *S. aureus, Escherichia coli*
B. Pneumococci, *Strep. Pyogenes*
C. Enterococci, pneumococci
D. *Strep. agalactiae*, pneumococci

153. Risk factors for septic arthritis/infectious arthritis includes

A. IV Drug use
B. Osteoarthritis
C. Rheumatoid Arthritis
D. All the above
E. Only A and C

MI 4.3

154. Painful, red, indurated, swollen lesion involving dermis with a raised border associated with pyrexia:

A. Pustule
B. Impetigo
C. Erysipelas
D. Pyomyositis

155. Following bacterial combinations are commonly associated with pyomyositis

A. *Strep. pyogenes, S. aureus*
B. *S. aureus, Bacillus anthracis*
C. Enterococci, *Klebsiella*
D. *E. coli, Klebsiella*

156. A fluid-filled lesion with abundant polymorphs, >0.5 cm in diameter is known as:

A. Pustule
B. Abscess
C. Vesicle
D. Plaque

157. Bacterial agents causing surgical site infections (clean wounds):

A. *S. aureus*, enterococci
B. CONS, *Candida*
C. *E. coli, Candida*
D. *Candida, S. aureus*

158. Flat, non-palpable, discolouration of skin <5 cm in size is termed as:

A. Nodule
B. Papule
C. Ulcer
D. Macule

159. Flesh eating bacteria causing "necrotising fasciitis":

A. *S. aureus*
B. *Enterococcus faecalis*
C. *Streptococcus pyogenes*
D. All the above

145. B 146. B 147. C 148. D 149. A 150. B 151. C 152. A 153. D 154. C 155. A 156. B 157. A 158. D 159. C

160. Chronic infection of obstructed sweat glands is:
A. Cellulitis
B. Hidradenitis
C. Scale
D. Myonecrosis

161. Mycetoma like condition with subcutaneous swelling, sinuses, discharge with granules is:
A. Psoas abscess
B. Pyomyositis
C. Botryomycosis
D. Hidradenitis suppurativa

162. Infection involving skin and subcutaneous tissues caused by *S. pyogenes* is:
A. Cellulitis
B. Erysipelas
C. Scarlet fever
D. Necrotising fasciitis

163. Most common site for erysipelas:
A. Conjunctiva
B. Scapular area
C. Malar area of face
D. Scapula

164. Cutaneous anthrax is also known as:
A. Wool Sorter's disease
B. Hide–Porter's disease
C. Malignant cellulitis
D. Necrotising dermatitis

MI 5.1

165. Member of streptococci causing pyogenic meningitis in neonates:
A. *S. pyogenes*
B. *S. agalactiae*
C. *S. dysgalactiae*
D. All the above

166. All the following are the aetiological agents of pyogenic meningitis, except
A. Pneumococci
B. *S. aureus*
C. HSV
D. *Klebsiella*

167. Principal virulence factor of meningococci in association with meningococcal meningitis:
A. LPS
B. OMP
C. Capsular polysaccharide
D. All the above

168. Chronic meningococcaemia is characterized by:
A. Petechial rash, arthralgia
B. Neck stiffness without vomiting
C. Pericarditis, fever
D. Mild arthralgia, absence of fever

169. CSF analysis in a case of meningococcal meningitis includes all, *except:*
A. Elevated CSF pressure, low protein levels
B. Low glucose levels, increased protein levels
C. Elevated CSF pressure, elevated protein levels
D. Elevated CSF pressure, low glucose levels

170. Recurrent lymphocytic meningitis caused by HSV is termed as:
A. Granuloma meningitis
B. Durck's granuloma
C. Mollaret's meningitis
D. GBS

171. CoxSackie group causing aseptic meningitis
A. All group B, A7 and A9
B. All group A, B3 and B4
C. All sub types of group A and B
D. Only group-A, but not group-B

172. Echo group of viruses cause all the following, *except:*
A. Aseptic meningitis
B. Encephalitis
C. Suppurative meningitis
D. Ocular disease

173. Term "Trojan horse" used to describe the movement of macrophages in CNS is associated with
A. Meningitis due to *Candida*
B. Cryptococcal meningitis
C. HSV meningitis
D. All the above

174. Cobweb coagulum when CSF is kept for prolonged time in a test tube at room temperature is characteristic of:
A. HSV meningitis
B. Enterovirus-72
C. Rhabdo viral meningitis
D. Tuberculous meningitis

175. Most common causative agent of pyogenic meningitis in children <2years of age with fever, cervical rigidity:
A. Hi-b
B. Meningococci
C. HSV
D. Enterovirus-72

160. B 161. C 162. A 163. C 164. B 165. B 166. C 167. C 168. A 169. A 170. C 171. A 172. C 173. B 174. D 175. A

176. Most common causative agent of pyogenic meningitis in 2–20 years age group

A. *Listeria monocytogenes*, meningococci
B. Pneumococci, Hi-b
C. Meningococci, Hi-b
D. HSV, pneumococci

177. Parasites commonly implicated in causing "aseptic meningitis":

A. *Naegleria*, hookworm
B. *Acanthamoeba*, *Trichinella*
C. *Naegleria*, *Toxoplasma*
D. *Toxoplasma*, *Trichuris*

178. Following all viruses are associated with "aseptic meningitis", *except:*

A. Polio, HSV
B. HSV, Echo
C. ECHO, VZV
D. RSV, SARS-CoV

179. Bacterial pathogens causing aseptic meningitis:

A. *Leptospira*, Hi-b
B. *Treponema pallidum*, *M. tuberculosis*
C. *Leptospira*, *Listeria*
D. *Listeria*, HSV

180. With respect to pathogenesis of pyogenic meningitis, most common route through which microbe enters subarachnoid space is by:

A. Choroid plexus
B. Pia mater
C. Nuclei of cerebellum
D. Cribriform plate

MI 5.2

181. Vector for the transmission of "Western equine encephalitis":

A. *Culex tritaenorhyncus*
B. *Culex tarsalis*
C. *Culex annulirostris*
D. *Sand fly*

182. Vector for the transmission of 'California encephalitis virus':

A. *Aedes aegypti*
B. *Aedes triseriatus*
C. *Culex*
D. Sand fly

183. In 2017 maximum cases of Japanese encephalitis in India were reported from

A. West Bengal
B. Uttar Pradesh
C. Chennai
D. Konkan coast

184. Inactivated vaccine against Japanese encephalitis is available in the form of

A. Beijing strain
B. SA 14–14-2
C. Nakayama strain
D. Both A and C

185. St. Louis Encephalitis is transmitted by:

A. Culex tritaenorhyncus
B. Mansonella pseudotitillans
C. Aedes aegypti
D. Aedes albopictus

186. All of the following are true regarding 'KFD', *except:*

A. Tick borne haemorrhagic fever
B. Causes meningoencephalitis
C. Endemic in Udupi, Chikmagalur of Karnataka
D. Transmitted by Culex tarsalis

187. Vector for the transmission of Chandipura virus:

A. Sand fly
B. *Mansonella pseudotitillans*
C. *Aedes albopictus*
D. Both A and C

188. *Ixodes persculatus* is the principal vector for the transmission of

A. Western Siberian encephalitis
B. Russian spring summer encephalitis
C. Central european encephalitis
D. Louping-Ill virus

189. Principal vector for the transmission of Central European encephalitis is:

A. *Ixodes ricinus*
B. *Ixodes persculatus*
C. *Ixodes cookie*
D. *Culex tarsalis*

190. Schedule for the administration of killed KFD vaccine:

A. 2 doses, 2 months gap, booster between 6–9 months
B. 1 dose, 2 months gap, booster 6–9 months
C. 2 doses, 1 month gap, booster 3–6 months
D. 3 doses, 3 months gap, booster 9–12 months

191. Diagnostic test used to detect 'E' gene in blood of Japanese encephalitis

A. MAC ELISA
B. Reverse transcriptase PCR
C. JE recombinant Ag assay
D. All the above

176. B 177. C 178. D 179. B 180. A 181. B 182. B 183. B 184. D 185. B 186. D 187. A 188. B 189. A 190. A 191. B

192. IgM Ab Capture assay (MAC ELISA) developed by IV, Pune for JE is based on:
A. One step sandwich ELISA
B. Two-step sandwich ELISA
C. Four-step sandwich ELISA
D. Three-step sandwich ELISA

193. Most common vector for the transmission of Japanese encephalitis in India:
A. *Culex tritaenorhyncus*
B. Sand fly
C. *Culex vishnui*
D. *Aedes aegypti*

194. *True* statement regarding SA 14–14-2 vaccine given against Japanese Encephalitis is:
A. It is live attenuated.
B. It is primarily a cell derived.
C. Given subcutaneously at left upper arm
D. All are true.
E. Except A, both B and C are true.

195. Sub-acute prodromal stage in JE lasts for:
A. 1–2 days
B. 1–6 hrs
C. 2–6 days
D. None of the above

196. Combined vaccine given against JE is:
A. Killed vaccine
B. Genetically engineered
C. Whole cell derived
D. Animal derived vaccine

197. Which of the following encephalitis group of viruses is endemic in Northern Australia, Papua New Guinea?
A. St. Louis encephalitis
B. Murray valley encephalitis
C. West nile virus
D. Rocio encephalitis virus

198. Lethal encephalitis in rodents and moderate illness in humans is caused by the following encephalitis virus confined to Africa is:
A. Semliki forest virus
B. Murray valley encephalitis
C. Rocio river virus
D. St. Louis encephalitis

199. Age group included for the administration of JE Vaccine under NIP, India:
A. Children of 3–5 years of age
B. Children of 5–15 years of age
C. Children of 1–15 years of age
D. Children of 10–12 years of age

200. Zoonotic paramyxoviruses causing encephalitis in humans:
A. Zika and Nipah
B. Hendra and Nipah
C. Hendra and RSSE
D. Nipah and St. Louis

201. In 2018, cluster of 18 Nipah virus cases were reported from the following state in India:
A. Allepey, Kerala
B. Udupi, Karnataka
C. Kasargod, Kerala
D. Calicut, Kerala

202. Protozoan parasite causing meningoencephalitis in immunocompromised hosts is:
A. *Taenia solium*
B. *Trichinella spiralis*
C. *Toxoplasma gondii*
D. *Leishmania donovani*

203. Amoebic meningoencephalitis is primarily caused by:
A. *Acanthamoeba*
B. *Naegleria fowleri*
C. *Trypanosoma brucei gambiense*
D. All the above

MI 5.3

204. Selective culture media for the isolation of meningococci from CSF specimen:
A. Levinthal's medium
B. Modified Thayer Martin medium
C. Tinsdale medium
D. Both A and B

205. Following all are the combinations of capsulated microbes causing meningitis/encephalitis in humans, *except*:
A. *Cryptococcus, Klebsiella*
B. *Escherichia coli, Cryptococcus*
C. Hi-b, pneumococci
D. *Treponema pallidum, Listeria*

206. Culture media for the isolation of *Cryptococcus* from CSF specimen:
A. Bird seed agar, Niger seed agar, chocolate agar
B. Chocolate agar, blood agar, bird seed agar
C. Niger seed agar, MacConkey, blood agar
D. Chocolate agar, Levinthal's medium, niger seed agar.

192. B 193. C 194. D 195. C 196. B 197. B 198. A 199. C 200. B 201. D 202. C 203. B 204. B 205. D 206. A

MI6.1

207. A 12-year-old boy developed sore throat grayish pseudomembrane covering tonsils and pharynx. Probable causative agent is?

A. Gram-positive bacilli
B. Gram-negative bacilli
C. ss positive sense RNA viruses
D. A gram-negative catalase positive coccus arranged in cluster

208. Aetiological agent of primary atypical pneumonia:

A. Pneumococci
B. *Mycobacterium tuberculosis*
C. *Listeria*
D. *Mycoplasma pneumonia*

209. Common causative agent of 'pneumatocele' in neonates:

A. *S. pyogenes*
B. *S. aureus*
C. RSV
D. Pneumococci

210. Most common bacterial agent causing lobar pneumonia:

A. *S. pyogenes*
B. Pneumococci
C. *C. diphtheriae*
D. *M. tuberculosis*

211. Most common sites of respiratory diphtheria:

A. Tonsils, pharynx
B. Larynx, tongue
C. Nose, larynx
D. Alveoli

212. Woolsorter's disease is:

A. Cutaneous anthrax
B. Intestinal anthrax
C. Pulmonary anthrax
D. Malignant pustule

213. Hallmark of pneumonia due to SARS CoV-2:

A. Dry cough
B. Decreased V/Q ratio
C. High grade pyrexia with nasal congestion
D. All the above

214. Community acquired pneumonia with Co morbidity is caused by all the following, *except:*

A. Adenovirus
B. *H. influenzae*
C. Pneumococci
D. Both B and C
E. A and C

215. Grade 1 for ventilator associated pneumonia according to clinical pulmonary infection score

A. Non purulent tracheal aspirates
B. CXR: Diffuse opacity
C. Culture of tracheal aspirate: Pathogenic bacteria heavy growth
D. All the above

216. Following all are bacterial causative agents of bronchitis, *except:*

A. *B. pertussis*
B. *Mycoplasma pneumoniae*
C. *Chlamydophila pneumoniae*
D. *Listeria*

217. Symptoms of rhinovirus infection includes all, *except:*

A. Nasal obstruction
B. High grade pyrexia
C. Nasal discharge
D. Sore throat

218. Serotypes 1, 2, 3, 5 of adenovirus are associated with:

A. Pneumonia in children
B. URT in children
C. Shipyard eye in adults
D. All the above

219. 10–20% of cases of pneumonia in children are caused by the following serotypes of adenovirus;

A. 1, 2, 3, 5
B. 3, 7, 21
C. 8, 19, 37
D. 19, 23, 37

220. Common bacteria causing secondary infections in people with pneumonia due to influenza

A. *H. influenzae*
B. *Mycoplasma*
C. *M. tuberculosis*
D. *Legionella pneumophila*

221. Flu syndrome/uncomplicated influenza is characterised by:

A. Dry cough with high fever
B. Myalgia with productive cough
C. Dry cough without fever
D. Productive cough without fever

222. Following is the most common avian flu strain that has been endemic in the world for the last 15 years:

A. H1N1
B. H7N7
C. H5N1
D. H7N9

207. A 208. D 209. B 210. B 211. A 212. C 213. D 214. D 215. D 216. D 217. B 218. B 219. B 220. A 221. A 222. C

223. Most common presentation of all the serotypes of para-influenza viruses in humans:
A. Rhinitis, pharyngitis
B. Bronchiolitis, croup
C. Croup, rhinitis
D. Pharyngitis, croup

224. Prodromal stage of rubeola infection is characterised by:
A. Koplik's spots
B. Maculopapular rash
C. Rose spots
D. All the above

225. Most common causative agent of tracheo-bronchitis in 25–35% of infants is:
A. Nipah virus
B. Rubella
C. Rubeola
D. RSV

226. Prediction of prognosis in CAP can be monitored by:
A. CIPS score
B. Glasgow Coma Scale
C. CURB score
D. A and C

227. Parasite associated with 'endemic haemoptysis'
A. Liver fluke
B. *Paragonimus westermanii*
C. *Trypanosoma*
D. All the above

228. Salivary glands affected in mumps:
A. Submaxillary
B. Sublingual
C. Parotid
D. B and C

229. Viruses implicated in causing hospital- acquired pneumonia
A. VZV
B. Adenovirus
C. CMV
D. HSV

230. Nonproductive cough with scanty sputum is associated with:
A. Interstitial pneumonia: Pneumococci
B. Interstitial pneumonia: *S. aureus*
C. Interstitial pneumonia: Viral pneumonia
D. Interstitial pneumonia: Hi-b

231. Fungal ball is:
A. *Histoplasma* pneumonia
B. *Candida* pneumonia
C. *Pneumocystis* pneumonia
D. Aspergilloma

232. Following all are the manifestations of pulmonary aspergillosis, *except:*
A. Bronchial asthma
B. Angioinvasive aspergillosis
C. Extrinsic allergic alveolitis
D. Granulomatous sinusitis

233. Loeffler's pneumonia is associated with:
A. *Leishmania donovani*
B. Lung fluke
C. Human round worm
D. *Mansonella*

234. Hecht's pneumonia is a complication of:
A. RSV
B. Para influenza
C. Measles
D. Mumps

235. Walking pneumonia is caused by:
A. *M. tuberculosis*
B. Measles
C. *Mycoplasma pneumoniae*
D. *Legionella pneumophila*

236. Age of administration of rubella vaccine according to NIP, India:
A. 9–12 months, 16–24 months
B. 3–6 months, 16–24 months
C. 6–9 months, 12–18 months
D. 9–12 months, 24–36 months

237. Pontiac fever is caused by:
A. *Chlamydophila pneumophila*
B. *Mycoplasma pneumoniae*
C. *Legionella pneumophila*
D. *S. pneumoniae*
E. RSV

238. Pseudomembrane coat in faucial diphtheria is composed of all the following, *except:*
A. RBC
B. Inner band of fibrin with neutrophils
C. Bacteria
D. Lymphocytes

223. A 224. A 225. D 226. C 227. B 228. C 229. B 230. C 231. D 232. D 233. C 234. C 235. C 236. A 237. C 238. D

239. Following all are true regarding PCV-13 given against pneumococcal pneumonia, *except:*

A. Promotes herd immunity
B. Provides mucosal immunity
C. Effective against children <2 years age
D. Does not promote herd immunity

MI 6.2

240. Appropriate clinical sample for smear microscopy in a case of upper respiratory tract infection:

A. BAL
B. Tracheal aspirate
C. Induced sputum
D. Throat swab

241. Babes-Ernst granules in *C. diphtheriae* can be best demonstrated by:

A. Gram's stain
B. GMS stain
C. Albert's stain
D. India Ink preparation

242. Lanceolate shaped cocci on smear microscopy by Gram's stain with >25 polymorphs/LPF, scanty epithelial cells and growth of Carrom coin shaped colonies on blood agar with greenish discolouration indicates

A. *S. agalactiae*
B. *S. pyogenes*
C. Pneumococci
D. Viridans streptococci

243. Following all viruses are implicated in causing 'Rhinitis', except

A. Human meta pneumovirus
B. Adenovirus
C. RSV
D. *Moraxella*

244. Presence of exudates in a case of laryngitis may be due to

A. EBV infection
B. *S. pyogenes*
C. Adenovirus
D. Both A and B
E. Both B and C

245. Presence of a soft tissue above the vocal cords with edema of epiglottis in a child aged 3 years indicates

A. RSV infection
B. Hi-b infection
C. Para-influenza infection
D. CoxSackie-A virus infection

246. Gram's stain in a suspected case of diphtheria in a 5-year-old child demonstrates all the following properties of the aetiological agent, except

A. Shape of the bacteria
B. Polar bodies
C. Cuneiform arrangement
D. Both A and B
E. Both B and C

247. Most common viral aetiological agent of sore throat is

A. SARS Cov-2
B. RSV
C. Rhinovirus
D. Both A and C
E. Both A and B

248. Gram's stain of nasopharyngeal aspirate in a suspected case of whooping cough appears as

A. Cuneiform cells
B. Mercury drops
C. Bipolar metachromatic granules
D. Thumb print

MI 6.3

249. Decolouriser used in Z–N staining to demonstrate lower respiratory tract bacterial pathogens:

A. 5% H_2SO_4
B. 25% H_2SO_4
C. 1% HCl
D. 10% H_2SO_4

250. A good quality sputum sent for culture should contain:

A. Polymorphs: >25/Lpf, epithelial cells <5/Lpf
B. Polymorphs: <4/Lpf, epithelial cells >20/Lpf
C. Polymorphs: <5/lpf, epithelial cells >25/Lpf
D. Polymorphs: >15/Lpf, epithelial cells >20/Lpf

251. Following are demerits of smear microscopy for the detection of *M. tuberculosis*:

A. Smear microscopy is less sensitive than culture
B. Smear microscopy cannot determine viability of bacilli
C. Detection limit: 10^4 bacilli/ml of sputum
D. All are demerits

239. A 240. D 241. C 242. C 243. D 244. D 245. B 246. E 247. D 248. D 249. B 250. A 251. D

252. RNTCP grading for ZN-stained sputum smears is useful for:
A. Assessing disease severity
B. For monitoring the treatment
C. Assessing infectiousness of the patient
D. All the above
E. Only A and C

253. RNTCP grading of a sputum smear is interpreted as 2+, it indicates
A. >10 AFB/OIL
B. 1–10 AFB/OIL
C. 1–9 AFB/OIL
D. 10–99 AFB/OIL

254. Decolouriser used in Preston-Morrell's modification of Gram's staining:
A. Aniline-Xylol
B. Iodine-Acetone
C. Absolute alcohol
D. Methyl violet

MI 7.1

255. Gram-negative, actively motile bacilli causing UTI
A. *S. saprophyticus, Escherichia coli*
B. *Escherichia coli, Klebsiella*
C. *Klebsiella, Proteus*
D. *Escherichia coli, Pseudomonas aeruginosa*

256. Presence of classical symptoms of lower UTI with low bacterial count is a feature of:
A. Significant bacteriuria
B. Cystitis
C. Pyelonephritis
D. Acute urethral syndrome

257. Following all viruses are implicated in causing UTI, *except:*
A. HSV
B. CMV
C. Rotavirus
D. Adenovirus

258. Catalase-positive, oxidase positive, gram-negative actively motile bacilli causing UTI:
A. *Escherichia coli*
B. *Pseudomonas aeruginosa*
C. *Proteus*
D. *Citrobacter*

259. Parasite causing haematuria:
A. *Trichomonas vaginalis*
B. *Clonorchis sinensis*
C. *Schistosoma haematobium*
D. *Naegleria fowleri*

260. Collected urine specimen should be processed on
A. Mannitol salt agar
B. XLD agar
C. Tinsdale medium
D. CLED agar

261. Gram stained from the culture of a urine specimen collected from 22-year-old female revealed the presence of gram-positive cocci with spectacle shape in pairs. Most probable bacteria exhibiting such morphology is:
A. *S. saprophyticus*
B. *Proteus*
C. *Enterococcus*
D. Pneumococci

262. Following all are the host defense mechanisms against UTI, *except:*
A. Mucosal IgA
B. Long urethra
C. Cytokines secretion
D. Alkaline pH

263. Uro mucoid protein secreted by epithelial cells of kidney serving as anti-adherence factor by binding to type-I fimbriae of *E. coli*
A. Citroen protein
B. Cytoverdin
C. Tactile protein
D. Tamm–Horsfall protein

264. Following all are causative agents of non-specific urethritis, *except:*
A. Gonococci
B. *Chlamydia*
C. HSV
D. *Trichomonas vaginalis*

MI 7.2

265. Donovanosis is caused by:
A. *Leishmania donovani*
B. *H. ducreyi*
C. HPV
D. *Klebsiella granulomatis*

266. Absence of genital lesions with systemic manifestations are associated with
A. *Mobiluncus* species
B. *Klebsiella granulomatis*
C. HBV
D. *Haemophilus ducreyi*

252. D 253. B 254. B 255. D 256. D 257. C 258. B 259. C 260. D 261. C 262. D 263. D 264. A 265. D 266. C

267. Small painless papule with ulceration and hard in texture is a feature of:

A. Secondary syphilis
B. Primary syphilis
C. Latent syphilis
D. *Haemophilus ducreyi*

268. Water can perineum in gonorrhea is characterized by:

A. Abscess without sinus formation
B. Sinus formation without abscess
C. Abscess with sinus formation
D. A malignant pustule

269. Most common presentation of gonococcal infection in females:

A. Fitz–Hugh–Curtis syndrome
B. Acute urethritis
C. Mucopurulent cervicitis
D. Vulvovaginitis

270. Which stage of lymphogranuloma veneraum is characterised by enlarged Inguinal lymph nodes which are soft, tender?

A. 1st stage
B. 2nd stage
C. 3rd stage
D. 4th stage

271. *C. trachomatis* serovars causing lymphogranuloma veneraum?

A. L3, L4, L5
B. L1, L2, L3
C. L2, L4, L5
D. L4, L5, L6

272. Reiter's syndrome is characterized by:

A. Conjunctivitis, arthritis, cervicitis
B. Sinusitis, arthritis, cervicitis
C. Cervicitis without arthritis and conjunctivitis
D. Arthritis, conjunctivitis without cervicitis

273. Yaws is caused by:

A. *Treponema carateum*
B. *Treponema endemicum*
C. *Treponema pertenue*
D. *Treponema pallidum*

274. Late pigmented lesions in Pinta containing *Treponemes* are known as:

A. Pruritic macules
B. Dyschronic macules
C. Pintides
D. Mother yaw

MI 7.3

275. If delay is expected in processing urine sample, it can be preserved by adding

A. Calcium carbonate
B. Calcium hydroxide
C. Sodium bicarbonate
D. Boric acid

276. Urine becomes cloudy with offensive odour without any systemic manifestations in:

A. Symptomatic bacteriuria
B. Cystitis
C. Urethritis
D. Pyelonephritis

277. Gram-negative, actively motile bacilli causing UTI with seminal odour in cultures is:

A. *Acinetobacter*
B. *Enterobacter*
C. *Klebsiella*
D. *Proteus*

278. Griess test is used to detect

A. Sulphide-reducing bacteria
B. Phosphate-reducing bacteria
C. Nitrate-reducing bacteria
D. Iron-reducing bacteria

279. Inflammation of renal parenchyma, renal pelvis is known as:

A. Pyelonephritis
B. Cystitis
C. Acute urethral syndrome
D. B and C

280. Species of staphylococci causing UTI in sexually active young females:

A. Epidermidis
B. Haemolyticus
C. Saprophyticus
D. All the above

281. Gram-stained smear of urine sample revealed the presence of gram-positive spherical shaped budding cells. Most probable organism is:

A. *Curvularia*
B. *Fusarium*
C. *Enterococcus*
D. *Candida* species

267. B 268. C 269. C 270. B 271. B 272. C 273. C 274. B 275. D 276. B 277. D 278. C 279. A 280. C 281. D

MI 8.1

282. Rats, rice fields, rainy season are associated with the following zoonotic disease:

A. Plague
B. Brucellosis
C. Leptospirosis
D. Anthrax

283. All are true about *Bacillus anthracis*, except:

A. Capsule is present.
B. Bamboo stick appearance
C. Causes black eschar
D. Drumstick appearance

284. Which of the following is *not* a parasitic zoonotic disease?

A. Neurocysticercosis
B. Toxoplasmosis
C. Leishmaniasis
D. Filariasis

285. Which of the following is a zoonotic paramyxoviral disease 1st isolated in Australia in 1994?

A. Nipah virus
B. Zika virus
C. Hendra virus
D. Ebola virus

286. Mode of transmission of Hendra viral infection to humans:

A. Exposure to infected body fluids
B. Exposure to fruit bats
C. Ingestion of sap
D. All the above

287. Site of presence of Negri bodies in rabies infection:

A. Purkinje cells of cerebellum
B. Hippocampus
C. Thalamus
D. A and B

288. Histopathological changes in brain parenchyma of a patient infected with rabies includes all, *except:*

A. Babes nodules with glial cells
B. Negri bodies
C. Perivascular cuffing of lymphocytes
D. RBC plugging

289. Milk ring test is used for the diagnosis of:

A. Plague
B. Leptospirosis
C. Anthrax
D. Brucellosis

290. Burdon's method is used to demonstrate:

A. Capsule of *B. anthracis*
B. Spores of *B. anthracis*
C. Lipid granules of *B. anthracis*
D. Haemolytic colonies of *B. anthracis*

291. Seal finger/whale finger is associated with:

A. Erysipeloid
B. Whipple's disease
C. Leptospirosis
D. Plague

292. Violaceous swelling with severe pain without pus is characteristic of:

A. Human brucellosis
B. Bubonic plague
C. Septicaemic plague
D. Erysipelothrix

293. Erythema arthriticum epidemicum is:

A. Haverhill fever
B. California fever
C. Desert rheumatism
D. Tularaemia

294. Plague like disease of rodents and other small animals which causes ulceroglandular lesions in humans is:

A. Pasteurella disease
B. Tularaemia
C. Anthrax
D. None

295. Following are the special media for isolation of *Francisella tularensis*

A. BCG agar
B. HE agar
C. CHAB agar
D. A and C
E. B and C

296. Causative agent of cat scratch disease

A. *Bartonella quintana*
B. *Bartonella henselae*
C. *Bartonella bacilliformis*
D. *Brucella abortus*

282. C 283. D 284. D 285. C 286. A 287. D 288. D 289. D 290. C 291. A 292. D 293. A 294. B 295. D 296. B

297. Intracellular survival in Phagosomes and trafficking in *Brucella* is regulated by:
A. Type-II secretory system
B. Type-IV secretory system
C. Type-III secretory system
D. Type- I secretory system

298. Undulating fever caused by *Brucella* is also known as:
A. Mediterranean fever
B. Trench fever
C. Lemming's fever
D. Rat bite fever

299. Rose Bengal card test is useful for diagnosis of:
A. Anthrax in humans
B. Brucellosis in humans
C. Brucellosis in animals
D. Pneumonic plague

MI 8.2

300. Which of the following is a opportunistic fungi infection associated with plasma cell pneumonia?
A. *Aspergillus flavus*
B. *Pneumocystis jirovecii*
C. *Histoplasma capsulatum*
D. *Penicillium marneffei*

301. Opportunistic protozoan parasite causing meningo-encephalitis in humans is:
A. *Cryptosporidium*
B. *Isospora belli*
C. *Acanthamoeba*
D. *Toxoplasma*

302. Following all are opportunistic fungi, *except:*
A. *Cryptococcus, Aspergillus*
B. *Candida, Cryptococcus*
C. *Penicillium, Cryptococcus*
D. *Coccidioidis, Paracoccidioidis*

303. Kaposi sarcoma-associated herpes virus is:
A. HHV-6
B. HHV-3
C. HHV-8
D. HHV-7

304. Opportunistic bacterial agent causing aseptic meningitis in humans:
A. *Leptospira*
B. *M. tuberculosis*
C. *Staphylococci*
D. *Klebsiella*

305. Following group are opportunistic atypical mycobacteria:
A. *M. szulgai*
B. *M. marinum*
C. MAC complex
D. CMM complex

MI 8.3

306. Following all are oncogenic ssRNA viruses, *except:*
A. EBV
B. HCV
C. HIV
D. A and C

307. Naso-pharyngeal carcinoma is the malignancy associated with the following DNA virus
A. HIV
B. CMV
C. EBV
D. VZV

308. Which of the following are cellular counter parts of viral oncogenes in the normal host cells?
A. C-onc
B. Proto-oncogenes
C. V-oncogenes
D. None of the above

309. E7 inhibits the tumour suppressor gene RB by:
A. Stimulating p53
B. Inhibiting p21
C. Directly inhibiting RB gene
D. B and C

310. Events which occur before oncogenesis include:
A. Immunosuppression
B. Evading host immune response
C. Establishing persistent infections
D. All the above

MI 8.4

311. Which of the following paramyxoviral disease/ causative agent is included under top 8 emerging diseases according to WHO in 2015?
A. SARS CoV-2
B. Crimean Congo haemorrhagic fever
C. Nipah virus
D. Lassa fever

297. B 298. A 299. C 300. B 301. D 302. D 303. C 304. B 305. C 306. A 307. C 308. B 309. D 310. D 311. C

312. Killed Zika virus vaccine is evaluated by Bharat Biotech, Hyderabad which uses:
A. European strain of ZIKV
B. African strain of ZIKV
C. Indian strain of ZIKV
D. B and C

313. Focal cases of the emerging Crimean Congo haemorrhagic fever virus were reported from the following state in 2011 and 2013 in India:
A. Kerala
B. Maharashtra
C. Goa
D. Gujarat

314. Emerging ARBO viral fever endemic in Egypt, Sub-saharan Africa and transmitted by Aedes mosquito is:
A. Chandipura virus
B. Ganjam virus
C. Rift valley virus
D. Colourado tick fever virus

MI 8.5

315. Which of the following is *not* a "ESKAPE" pathogen?
A. *Proteus vulgaris*
B. *Pseudomonas aeruginosa*
C. *S. aureus*
D. *Klebsiella* species

316. A clinical nurse carrying a tube with suspected seropositive HCV blood collected from a 24-year-old healthcare worker. If there is sudden spillage, that spill area should be disinfected with
A. Phenol
B. Lysol
C. Hypochlorite
D. Alkali

317. NHSN stands for:
A. National Health Surveillance Norms
B. National Health Care Safety Network
C. National Health Standards Systems Network
D. National Hospital Standards Norms

318. SSI rate in a hospital can be calculated by:
A. No. of SSI/No. of surgeries done × 100
B. No. of surgeries/No. of SSI × 100
C. No. of surgeries/No. of complications × 100
D. No. of SSI in males/No. of complications × 100

319. Device criteria for stage-1 ventilator-associated condition in a 75-year-old male admitted in ICU:
A. Presence of mechanical ventilator for at least 2 weeks
B. Presence of mechanical ventilator for at least 3 calendar weeks
C. Presence of mechanical ventilator for at least 2 calendar days
D. None of the above

320. Decolonisation with mupirocin ointment should be done for the:
A. Nasal carriers of respiratory viral infection
B. Nasal carriers of diphtheria
C. Nasal carriers of pneumococcal pneumonia
D. Nasal carriers of MRSA

321. A 25-year-old pregnant female is in ICU for 6 days. She developed fever after the insertion of urinary catheter for >3 days. Urine sent to the lab and culture reported as *Klebsiella* species with a colony count >10^5 CFU/ml. Surveillance diagnosis is:
A. Community-acquired UTI
B. Hospital-acquired CAUTI
C. Community-acquired CAUTI
D. Pregnancy-induced PUO

322. For infection related ventilator-associated complication (IVAC), VAC plus antibiotic criterion is:
A. New antibiotic started >1 day
B. New antibiotic started and continued >8 days
C. New antibiotic started and continued >4 days
D. New antibiotic started and continued >10 days

323. For possible ventilator-associated pneumonia, IVAC plus culture criterion depicts as:
A. Isolation of significant count of pneumonia pathogen from respiratory samples
B. Isolation of a rare respiratory pathogen from both respiratory and nonrespiratory samples
C. Isolation of any pathogen related to any disease of upper respiratory tract
D. None of the above

312. B 313. D 314. C 315. A 316. C 317. B 318. A 319. C 320. D 321. B 322. C 323. A

324. HICC stand for

A. Hospital Infection Coordinating Committee
B. Hospital Infection Control Committee
C. Hospital Infection Chain Committee
D. Hospital Information Coordinating Committee

MI 8.6

325. CSSD stands for:

A. Central Sanitaztion Supplying Department
B. Central Sterile Supplies Department
C. Central Sterile Storage Department
D. None of the above

326. Components of "Contact Precaution" include all, *except:*

A. Patient movement
B. Isolation
C. No requirement of PPE
D. Environmental cleaning

327. A colony in a highly populated city had a sudden surge of COVID positive cases in a apartment with 10 families. Select the *true* statement:

A. Entire colony should be considered as containment zone with lockdown for 2 weeks
B. Only the apartment should be considered as micro containment zone and families with positive cases should be isolated.
C. Immediate administration of remdesivir for all the families
D. Both B and C

328. Airborne transmission is possible with:

A. Varicella
B. SARS-CoV2
C. Measles
D. All the above

329. All of the following are possible modes of transmission of COVID-19, *except:*

A. Close contact with a person returned from any country
B. Close contact with asymptomatic person with positive RT-PCR report in a COVID endemic community
C. Direct contact with respiratory secretions from a person in quarantine ward
D. All the above
E. B and C

330. All the following are the core members of HICC, *except:*

A. Forensic expert, physiologist
B. Nursing superintendent, epidemiologist
C. CSSD Head, epidemiologist
D. Microbiology faculty, in-charge of engineering department of a hospital

331. Risk factors for the development of hospital acquired Pneumonia includes all, *except:*

A. Endotracheal intubation
B. Aspiration of oro-pharyngeal flora
C. Staying in hospital for 6 hrs
D. Poor hand hygiene

332. Sequence of events in order in donning of PPE (Personal protective equipment):

A. Gown 1st, gloves, mask, goggles
B. Gloves, gown, mask, goggles
C. Gown 1st, mask, face shield, floves
D. Face shield, gown, mask, goggles

333. Sequence of events in doffing of PPE in order:

A. Gloves, gown, face shield, mask
B. Mask, face shield, gloves, gown
C. Gloves, face shield, gown, mask
D. Face shield, mask, gloves, gown

334. Functions of HICC includes all, *except:*

A. Antimicrobial stewardship
B. Educating health care personnel
C. Publication of research articles
D. Developing a system for controlling HAI

MI 8.7

335. HAI surveillance includes the following parameters:

A. CA-UTI surveillance
B. SSI surveillance
C. VAP surveillance
D. All the above
E. Only B and C

336. Selection of appropriate PPE is based on:

A. Risk level associated only with skin
B. Risk level associated with skin, mucous membrane, blood
C. Risk level associated with alcoholic, smoking patients
D. All the above

324. B 325. B 326. C 327. B 328. D 329. E 330. A 331. C 332. C 333. C 334. C 335. D 336. B

337. Total number of steps in "hand hygiene" according to WHO.

A. Four
B. Seven
C. Six
D. Five

MI 8.8

338. Indicator organism for remote contamination of water

A. Fecal streptococci
B. *Pseudomonas*
C. *Clostridium perfringens*
D. Bacteriophages

339. All the following are water borne viral pathogens, *except:*

A. Polio virus
B. Rota virus
C. HAV
D. HDV

340. Targeted air surveillance as recommended by CDC includes:

A. Investigation of an outbreak
B. To carry out research
C. For short-term evaluation of infection control practices
D. All the above

341. Recommended temperature in an orthopedic OT

A. 18–20°C
B. >24°C
C. <14°C
D. >35°C

342. Methylene blue reduction test is employed for:

A. Bacteriological examination of water
B. Bacteriological examination of air
C. Bacteriological examination of milk
D. Bacteriological examination of surfaces

343. Which of the following are diseases primarily of human origin, but transmitted by milk?

A. Brucellosis, cowpox
B. Shigellosis, typhoid fever
C. Q fever, brucellosis
D. Q fever, *M. bovis* TB

344. In ultra heat-treated milk, milk is exposed to:

A. 57–60°C, 15 seconds
B. 70°C, 15 seconds
C. 135°C, 1 second
D. 37°C, 1 second

MI 8.9

345. Most reliable and recommended clinical sample for the laboratory diagnosis of UTI in a female of 23 years age visiting an OPD:

A. Random urine sample
B. Catheter tube sample
C. Mid-stream sample
D. All the above

346. Quantity of blood to be collected for performing blood cultures in a child of 5 years of age with a suspected sepsis:

A. >7 ml/ bottle
B. 6 ml/ bottle
C. 1–3 ml/ bottle
D. 5 ml/ bottle

347. *True* statement regarding CSF sample collected from a 78 year-old female patient in a suspected case of pyogenic meningitis:

A. Collected by lumbar puncture
B. Gram's stain may or may not reveal pus cells.
C. Culture should be performed on enriched medium.
D. Sample should not be refrigerated.
E. All are true.
F. Only A and D are true

MI 8.10

348. Application of tourniquet and marking the vein are the vital steps in the collection of:

A. Pus sample for culture
B. Erythematous fluid from skin
C. Blood sample for culture
D. Slit skin smears for *M. leprae*

349. Ideal clinical specimen for the diagnosis of suspected lower respiratory tract infection in a 55-year-old chronic smoker

A. Throat swab
B. Naso-pharyngeal aspirate
C. BAL
D. A and C

MI 8.11

350. Informed patient consent is mandatory for:

A. HIV screening
B. COVID-19 screening
C. Performing a cesarean delivery
D. All the above
E. A and C

337. D 338. C 339. D 340. D 341. A 342. C 343. B 344. C 345. C 346. C 347. E 348. C 349. C 350. D

351. Clinical report, laboratory report confidentiality is essential for:

A. HBV management
B. Malaria management
C. EBV management
D. *Toxoplasma* management

352. 3Cs protocol in HIV does not include:

A. Care
B. Consent
C. Counselling
D. All the above

MI 8.13

353. Weil-Felix test is used for the diagnosis of:

A. Typhoid fever
B. Typhus fever
C. Glandular fever
D. Scarlet fever

354. All the following are heterophile tube agglutination tests, *except:*

A. Weil–Felix test
B. RA test
C. Paul–Bunnel test
D. Cold agglutination test

355. Blocking antibodies can be detected/eliminated by:

A. Preheating the serum
B. Coombs' test
C. Latex test
D. All the above
E. A and B

351. A 352. A 353. B 354. B 355. E

Fill in the Blanks

Fill in the Blanks

1. ________ and ________ are the examples of bacteria which deviate from Koch's postulates.
2. ________ was the name of the boy who was injected by cowpox vaccine by Sir Edward Jenner.
3. Intradermal injection of PPD into the flexor aspect of forearm is the best example for ________ type of hypersensitivity.
4. Fifth day disease in children is caused by ________ virus which is having ssDNA as genome.
5. Sach's buffered glycerol saline is a ________ medium for the maintenance of viability of *Shigella*.
6. Dental equipment, heart-lung machines were disinfected by ________.
7. Neufeld's Quellung reaction is the method used to demonstrate ________ structure of a bacterial cell.
8. ________ is the most advanced and complex classification of β-lactamases.
9. Secretion in bacteria refers to ________ of effector molecules, such as proteins, enzymes, toxins across the cell membrane from cytoplasm to its exterior.
10. Genes encoded in a ________ are expressed in a coordinated manner to begin or to initiate the virulence process.
11. Monoclonal antibodies are produced by hybridoma technology and were developed by ________ and ________.
12. C5 convertase in classical complement pathway is ________.
13. Skin contains few loose lymphocytes and specialised APCs in epidermis termed as ________.
14. Immunodeficiency disorder characterized by congenital aplasia of thymus is ________.
15. Cytoplasmic membrane antigen of *Streptococcus pyogenes* exhibits antigenic cross reactivity with ________.
16. Eighth day disease according to WHO is ________.
17. ________ is the vector for the transmission of kala-azar.
18. Anchovy-sauce pus is associated with ________ parasitic infection.
19. HHV-6 infects T cells by binding to ________ receptors.
20. ________ strain of Influenza caused severe Pandemic in 1918–1919.
21. Antigenic drift is a minor change occurring due to ________.
22. Capsule of *Haemophilus influenzae* is made up of ________.
23. Vietnam time-bomb disease is ________.
24. *Pseudomonas aeruginosa* causes Cellulitis which is characterized by ________.
25. Indole and nitrate reduction test can be tested together by adding few drops of H_2SO_4 to peptone water culture of *Vibrio*. This test is known as ________.
26. Germ tube test a specific test for *Candida albicans* is also known as ________.
27. Mycetoma like condition caused by certain pyogenic bacteria like *S. aureus* is known as ________.
28. Abundant, club-shaped macroconidia are seen in ________ without any microconidia.
29. Certain dermatophytes exhibit fluorescence under Wood's lamp examination which is due to the presence of ________in the cell wall.
30. ________are the infective stages of *Plasmodium* to the invertebrate host.
31. Infective stage of *Taenia solium* to humans is ________.
32. Non-bile-stained egg with segmented blastomeres is a feature of ________.
33. Serum sickness is a classic example of ________type of hypersensitivity.
34. Subcutaneous fungal infection which is also known as "Rose Gardner's disease" is ________.
35. Deep systemic mycotic infection affecting reticuloendothelial system is ________.
36. Toxin of *S. aureus* responsible for causing "staphylococcal-scalded skin syndrome" is ________.
37. Species of *Clostridium* exhibiting "target haemolysis" is ________.
38. Woolsorter's disease is ________.
39. Type of motility exhibited by *Listeria monocytogenes* is ________.
40. Inner band of peudomembrane produced by *C. diphtheriae* is composed of ________.
41. Gram-negative, non-motile bacilli which produces "Currant jelly" like sputum is ________.
42. Cataract, deafness and congenital anomalies are the triad of features caused by ________.
43. "Shipyard eye" is caused by ________.
44. Oncogenic DNA virus causing glandular fever is ________.
45. People on prolonged steroid therapy as a part of COVID-19 treatment may be exposed to ________ sub cutaneous fungal infection.

46. Species of *Clostridium* causing "pseudomembranous colitis" is ________.
47. Pseudohaemoptysis caused by *Serratia marcescens* is due to ________ pigment which diffuses completely into the culture medium.
48. Gram-negative, actively motile bacilli producing H2S in TSI commonly isolated from urine samples is ________.
49. Live attenuated viral vaccine given for children after attaining 9th month is ________.
50. Zoonotic members of paramyxoviruses are ________.
51. Infective form of fasciola hepatica to the definitive host is ________.
52. Pork round worm is ________.
53. Aetiological agent of Lemierre's syndrome is ________.
54. Nonsporing anaerobe causing dental root canal infections is ________.
55. In primary pulmonary TB, calcified primary complex is known as ________.
56. In a hard tubercle, central zone is composed of ________.
57. Photochromogen which causes "fish tank granuloma" is ________.
58. Hansen's bacilli appear as cigar bundle bacilli present inside the lipid-laden macrophages termed as ________.
59. Heterophile Agglutination test in which nonmotile strains of proteus are used is ________.
60. Staining method/ stain which demonstrates the typical "safety pin" appearance of *Yersinia pestis* is ________.
61. ________ refers to a transient rise of titre due to unrelated infections like dengue fever in a person who have had prior "enteric fever".
62. Twitching motility is exhibited by ________ bacteria due to contractions of fimbriae.
63. Intracellular pathogen infecting RES transmitted by infected milk is ________.
64. Coproantigen assay for the diagnosis of *Helicobacter pylori* is useful for ________.
65. Painless papule which becomes a "beefy red ulcer" is a feature of ________.
66. Reagent used in Whiff test for mixing the vaginal secretions is ________.
67. Immunoglobulin which participates in allergic reactions like "anaphylaxis" is ________.
68. HLA allele associated with the disease rheumatoid arthritis is ________.
69. National Salmonella Reference Centre is located at ________.
70. Species of *Vibrio* which exhibits motility due to peritrichous flagella, but does not show darting motility is ________.
71. Carrion's disease is caused by ________.
72. Trench fever or 5 days fever is caused by ________.
73. In the disease "trachoma", follicles rupture during acute infection to leave shallow pits known as ________.
74. Conjunctivitis, arthritis, urethritis with muco-cutaneous lesions is known as ________.
75. Most common sites of Negri bodies are ________ and ________.
76. Opportunistic fungal infection in AIDS patients caused by *Pneumocystis jirovecii* is ________.
77. Rotavac a live attenuated vaccine given against rota viral diarrhoea contains ________ strain.
78. Non-A Non-B post-transfusion hepatitis virus belongs to the family ________.
79. Genotypes of HEV which are more virulent are ________.
80. At present the 1st choice of treatment of HBV infection is ________.
81. Extrahepatic manifestations like mixed cryo-globulinemia due to HCV is due to ________.
82. Gram variables are produced during ________ phase of bacterial growth curve.
83. Selective media for the isolation of *S. aureus* from faeces, swabs from carriers ________.
84. Pneumovax 23 which is a 23 valent pneumococcal polysaccharide vaccine promotes ________.
85. Gram-positive oval cocci with typical spectacle shape is ________.
86. Incubation period for "emetic type of food poisoning" due to *Bacillus cereus* is ________.
87. Brownie nose appearance in chikungunya fever is known as ________.
88. Vector for the transmission of western equine encephalitis (WEE) is ________.
89. Three confirmed cases of Zika viral infection in 2017 in India were reported from ________.
90. Vector for the transmission of "Kyasanur forest disease" is ________.
91. Recurrent lymphocytic meningitis caused by HSV is known as ________.
92. Fatty degeneration of liver following excess intake of aspirin is known as ________.
93. In zoster infection most common nerve involved is ________.
94. *In vitro* replication of CMV in human fibroblast cell lines produces ________ type of cytopathic effects.
95. Sereny test is useful for the detection of ________ type of diarrhoeagenic *Escherichia coli*.
96. Undercooked ground beef is one of the sources for transmission of ________ type of diarrhoeagenic *Escherichia coli*.
97. Bilateral knee effusions seen in late congenital syphilis are known as ________.
98. *Treponema pallidum* exhibits typical rotation movement around its longitudinal axis and is described as ________ motility.

99. Acute ulcerative gingivostomatitis is known as ________.
100. Aetiological agent of endemic typhus is________.
101. Louse-borne typhus is caused by ________.
102. Failure of AICD (apoptosis via fas-fas ligand) is observed in patients suffering with ________ a type of multisystem connective tissue disorder.
103. Radioallegrosorbent test is useful to quantify the serum level of ________.
104. ________phenomenon is useful to demonstrate anaphylaxis *in vivo* by injecting allergen into the Guinea pigs.
105. Macrophages of placenta are known as ________.
106. Dendritic cells carry high level of ________ and co stimulatory B7 molecules.
107. Cold sterilisation is achieved by ________rays to sterilize disposable rubber, plastic syringes.
108. High level disinfectant used to disinfect haemodialyzers is ________.
109. Efficacy of plasma sterilisation is tested by using ________.
110. Shaggy, thin-walled cavities in the lungs of neonates caused by *S. aureus* is termed as ________.
111. Swimming pool conjunctivitis in adults is caused by ________serovars of *Chlamydia trachomatis.*
112. Intranuclear inclusions seen in yellow fever virus are known as ________.
113. Reservoir hosts for "Ebola virus" ________.
114. Type of genome in Rota virus ________.
115. HBsAg earlier known as ________.
116. Infective stage of *Ascaris lumbricoides* to humans ________.
117. Bile stained, barrel-shaped egg, with bi-polar mucous plugs is a feature of ________.
118. Non-human species of hookworm causes ________.
119. Black water fever is a complication of ________.
120. Species of *Plasmodium* exhibiting "relapse form of malaria" is ________.
121. Hypoglycaemia in falciparum malaria is common following treatment with ________.
122. Infective stage of *Leishmania donovani* to humans ________.
123. Infective stage of *Trypanosoma brucei gambiense* to humans ________.
124. Phage-mediated gene transfer in bacteria is known as ________.
125. Self-transmissible plasmids are termed as ________.
126. Southern blotting technique is useful to detect / interpret ________.
127. Conjugation method of gene transfer in bacteria was first demonstrated by ________ and ________.
128. Luria and Delbruck developed fluctuation test to demonstrate ________type of mutations
129. Sum of idiotopes on an Ig molecule constitutes its ________.
130. Heterophile agglutination test used for the diagnosis of pneumonia due to *Mycoplasma* is ________.
131. Theory which postulates that tumour cells arise frequently in our body and are recognised as foreign is ________.
132. Protozoan flagellate causing non-gonococcal urethritis is ________.
133. Serogrouping of *Neisseria meningitidis* is based on ________.
134. National Institute of Cholera and Enteric Diseases is located at ________.
135. Pittsburgh pneumonia agent is ________.
136. Pan gastritis due to *H. pylori* may predispose to ________.
137. *Francisella tularensis* causing "tularaemia" is included under ________ agent of Bio terrorism.
138. Haverhill fever is caused by ________.
139. Catalase +, gram-negative actively motile bacilli, producing greenish diffusible pigment is ________.
140. Albert's stain is used to demonstrate ________ of *Corynebacterium diphtheriae.*
141. Leifson's method is used to demonstrate ________ of bacteria.
142. Type of motility exhibited by *Proteus* on blood agar ________.
143. Biological indicators used as sterilisation controls for hot air oven ________.
144. Mobile genetic elements are ________.
145. Presence of rash in skin folds in a child with scarlet fever is termed as ________.
146. Polypeptide capsule of bacillus anthracis can be demonstrated by ________ reaction.
147. Route of administration of BCG vaccine is ________.
148. Nontypical mycobacteria which behaves as scoto chromogen at 37°C and photo chromogen at 25°C is ________.
149. Aetiological agent of "Whipple's disease" is ________
150. "Desert rheumatism" a systemic fungal disease is caused by ________.
151. Noncultivable fungus causing large friable nasal polyps is ________.
152. Histopathological findings of chromoblastomycosis with characteristic brown thick-walled cells are known as ________.
153. Neurotropic phaeoid fungi producing typical brain abscess affecting frontal lobe is ________.
154. A specific lectin receptor present in skin and mucosal surfaces binding to HIV-1, but does not mediate cell entry is ________.
155. Non-structural gene found in HIV-2 and SIV, closely related to Vpr ________.
156. 5th generation ELISA distinguishes between HIV-1 and HIV-2 antibodies and also detects ________.
157. Neural vaccine for rabies derived from infected sheep brain and inactivated with phenol is ________.

158. Fixed viruses are propagated in rabbits by ________ method.
159. According to National Immunisation Schedule IPV is given at ________ and ________ weeks of age along with OPV.
160. An outbreak of vaccine-induced "paralytic poliomyelitis" which occurred in America in 1955 is known as ________.
161. Recrudescence of paralysis of polio viral infection and muscle wasting observed in individuals after 20–40 years of paralytic poliomyelitis attack is known as ________.
162. Infective stage of *Taenia saginata* to humans is ________.
163. Infective stage of *Plasmodium* to intermediate hosts ________.
164. African eye worm is ________.
165. River Blindness is caused by ________.
166. Infective stage of *Cryptosporidium parvum* to humans is ________.
167. Giant intestinal fluke is ________.
168. Infective form of human lung fluke is ________.
169. Infective form of *Wucheraria bancrofti* to humans is ________
170. "Walking pneumonia" is caused by ________.
171. Examination method used to measure the number of bacteria carrying particles in given volume of air ________.
172. Faecal coliforms in water can be determined by ________ test.
173. According to ablett classification of tetanus severity, respiratory rate if > 30 breaths/ min with rigidity and short spasms suggest ________.
174. Incubation period for ETEC associated watery diarrhoea is ________.
175. *Salmonella typhi* produces ________ type of growth on XLD agar.
176. Shigellae are lactose and sucrose non fermenters, except ________ which ferments them slowly.
177. Significant bacteriuria according to Kass concept ________.
178. Pertussis component acts as ________ and enhances the immunogenicity of TT and DT.
179. Site of administration of DPT vaccine ________.
180. Koplik's spots are the characteristic of ________ stage of measles.
181. Father of modern microbiology is ________.
182. *Enterococcus* species produces black coloured colonies when cultured on ________.
183. Relapse forms of malaria caused by *P. vivax* is due to ________.
184. Property of "satellitism" is exhibited by ________.
185. *Vibrio cholerae* produces yellow-coloured colonies on TCBS medium due to ________.
186. Teratogenic member of "Herpesviridae" family causing fetal deaths is ________.
187. Silicon rubber materials are sterilised by ________
188. Moist heat method of sterilisation below 100°C used to sterilize LJ medium is ________.
189. Mode of transmission of HAV is ________.
190. Anaerobic culture media most commonly used for the detection of *Cl. tetani* in OT surveillance is ________.
191. Nonbile stained, plano convex egg with a tadpole like larva is a feature of ________.
192. New world hook worm is ________.
193. Dwarf tapeworm is ________.
194. Vector for the transmission of "Chagas disease" is ________.
195. Unarmed tapeworm is ________.
196. Dog tapeworm is ________.
197. Cataract, deafness and cardiac anomalies are the features of ________ member of togaviridae family.
198. Protozoan parasite causing "Espundia" is ________.
199. Yellow fever vaccine is prepared from ________ strain of yellow fever virus
200. Generation time of *Mycobacterium tuberculosis* is ________.
201. Bacteria attain maximum size at the end of ________.
202. Aetiological agent of "Lyme disease" is ________.
203. Tertiary stage of syphilis affects ________ part of central nervous system.
204. Member of Enterobacteriaceae producing diffusible magenta colour pigment is ________.
205. Reagent used to perform catalase test is ________.
206. Modification of PCR used for syndrome approach is ________.
207. Modification of PCR used to detect "RNA" is ________.
208. Ability of a test to identify all the "true-positives" is known as ________.
209. Highest dilution of the serum that shows an observable reaction with the antigen in a test is known as ________.
210. Cytokine which is not secreted by TH-2 cells is ________.
211. Primary function of bradykinin, a 2nd mediator of type-I hypersensitivity ________.
212. Toxin of *S. aureus* which exhibits "hot-cold" phenomenon is ________.
213. Quartan malaria is caused by ________.
214. Rose spots which appear on the trunk, fade out with pressure are the characteristic of ________.
215. Burkitt's lymphoma is caused by ________ member of Herpesviridae.
216. Vector used to carry the genetic material of the spike protein of SARS-CoV-2 into human cells in covishield vaccine is ________.
217. Alternative adjuvant used by Bharath BioTech in the preparation of Covaxin which stimulates Th-1 type of immunity in the human is ________.
218. Location of "naive cells" ________.

219. Large granular lymphocytes which constitute 10–15% of peripheral blood lymphocytes are________.
220. Immunological reason for "disseminated *Neisseria* infections" ________.
221. Surface markers of TC cells ________.
222. For category C, other wounds recommended immunisation schedule for the prevention of tetanus after injury ________.
223. Bacterial infection affecting fingers leading to "seal finger" form is ________.
224. Nonfermenting, oxidase negative, motile bacilli which is a saprophyte in rhizosphere and resistant to all β-lactam antibiotics is ________.
225. 100 days fever is ________.
226. Toxin of *Bordetella pertussis* which cause damage to the cilia of respiratory epithelial cells ________.
227. Acellular pertussis vaccine is available as ________ and can be given safely after 5-6 years for a child.
228. "Milk ring test" is useful for the diagnosis of ________ in animals.
229. Vector for "Trypanosoma *brucei gambiense*" is ________.
230. Kovac's reagent is added in________test for placing a gram-negative bacillus in Enterobacteriaceae.
231. Reagent used in string test to demonstrate the unique property of *Vibrio cholerae* is ________.
232. To differentiate *Vibrio* from the related genera *Aeromonas* and *Plesiomonas* ________tests are useful
233. "Strauss reaction" in guinea pigs is used for ________
234. Granzymes induce cell death by apoptosis by ________.
235. With respect to structure of thymus concentric layers of degenerating epithelial cells are known as ________.
236. Type of paralysis induced by polio virus in an infected child is ________.
237. Bornholm Disease is caused by ________.
238. Coagulase-negative staphylococci causing severe UTI in sexually active young females is ________.
239. Mode of transmission of polio virus is ________.
240. Infection caused by Enterovirus-70 is ________.
241. Oral and pharyngeal lesions caused by Coxsackie A16 with rashes on palms, sole is ________
242. Vector for the transmission of "Chandipura virus" is ________.
243. *Aedes triseriatus* is the vector for the transmission of ________virus.
244. Nairo viral fever which is endemic in West Africa , but cases were observed in Gujarat , India in 2013 is ________.
245. Hepatitis G virus belongs to the genus ________.
246. 1st major epidemic of HEV was reported from ________ due to contamination of drinking water due to Yamuna river floods.
247. Consumption of sea foods like molluscs , crustaceans leads to dysentery due to ________.
248. Protozoan parasite exhibiting falling leaf like motility is ________.
249. Prediction of prognosis of "community-acquired pneumonia" in an adult can be done by ________ score.
250. Direct ELISA is used for the detection of ________.
251. Some serotypes of "pneumococci" exhibit ________ which may contribute to the development of antibiotic resistance
252. In patients with lepromatous leprosy, ________ immunity is very low
253. Most common type of pneumonia caused by *Nocardia* with sub-acute cough, thick purulent sputum is ________.
254. *Actinomyces* produces ________type of colonies on solid media.
255. Lumpy jaw is ________.
256. Rainbow agar is used for the isolation of ________ strains of *Escherichia coli.*
257. Genome is segmented in to 8 equal pieces in ________ virus
258. Salivary glands commonly affected in mumps infection ________.
259. *Shingles* is ________.
260. ORF virus is included in the family ________.
261. Loeffler's serum slope is sterilised by ________.
262. Zaire, Sudan and Reston are the strains of ________ virus.
263. Normal gap between dose-1 and dose -2 for COVAXIN vaccine for N-COVID-19 is ________.
264. Shipping fever is caused by ________.
265. Strain of diphtheria used for toxin preparation is ________.
266. P-K reaction is associated with ________type of hypersensitivity.
267. Major application of HLA typing is employed in ________.
268. ________stain is used to demonstrate *Treponemes* in tissue sections
269. ________stain is used to demonstrate *Treponemes* for smears made from exudates.
270. Verruga peruana is a late manifestation of ________.
271. Metabolically inactive form and infectious form in the life cycle of "Chlamydiae" is ________.
272. Detection of amplification products of real time PCR uses ________dye to stain any nucleic acid non-specifically.
273. DNA polymerase used for LAMP assay is derived from ________.
274. In MALDI-TOF , TOF represents ________.
275. Reagent used in PPA test for the identification of tribe Proteae members is ________.
276. Nobel Prize along with Sir Kary B Mullis for the development of PCR was shared by ________in 1993 in the field of chemistry.

277. Healthy carriers refers to ________who develop into carriers without suffering from overt disease
278. Exotoxin–A of *Pseudomonas aeruginosa* inhibits protein synthesis by inhibiting ________.
279. Deficiency of factor H leading to deregulation of alternative pathway results in ________disease.
280. Macrophages of "lymphoid follicles" are known as ________.
281. Most common site where β-lactamases are located contributing to antibiotic resistance is ________.
282. *Diphtheroids* differ from *C. diphtheriae* in the absence of characteristic ________granules.
283. Improperly canned vegetables, smoked fish are the important sources for food poisoning due to ________.
284. Exfoliatin causing scalded skin syndrome in young children cleaves ________in desmosomes leading to separation of epidermis at granular cell layer.
285. ________streptococci are the most common cause for "SABE" leading to severe vegetations.
286. ________enzyme is known as "spreading factor" in *Streptococcus pyogenes* leading to cellulitis.
287. When cultured on ________media *Escherichia coli* produces characteristic green sheen colonies.
288. Destruction of virus infected cells, tumour cells , graft rejection are the functions of ________.
289. Autosomal recessive immunodeficiency disease due to IgE deficiency is ________.
290. Defect in chemotaxis and neutrophil mobility leads to ________immuno deficiency disease.
291. *Legionella micdadei* is termed as ________.
292. HACEK group of bacterium exhibiting "twitching mobility" is ________.
293. In cold chain refrigerated vaccines are stored at ________.
294. Polio, measles vaccines are stored at ________zone of cold chain.
295. Site of attachment of *Fasciolopsis buski* in man is ________.
296. Colour of the eggs of Lung fluke ________.
297. Application of DDT in 1948 for the destruction of mosquitoes causing malaria was explained by ________.
298. Presence of circum sporozoite protein is the major virulence factor of ________causing black water fever.
299. ________are not stained in fluorescent microscopy used to demonstrate malarial parasite.
300. Arrangement of *H. ducreyi* in microscope is described as ________.
301. *Elizabethkingia meningosepticum* produces ________ pigment.
302. *Burkholderia pseudomallei* produces wrinkled purple colonies on ________medium.
303. Johne's *Bacillus* is ________.
304. A web-based solution for monitoring of TB patients is ________.
305. Microbiological waste should be segregated into ________bags/bins.
306. According to biomedical waste rule 1998 and 2016 blue coloured puncture proof box or bin is used for the disposal of ________.
307. Hand wash should be performed for a minimum of ________seconds.
308. Large volume of blood spillage should be disinfected with ________.
309. Isolation rooms for a positive COVID patient should be maintained with ________as a precaution to prevent the spread of air-borne transmission.
310. Fungus which is commonly known as "lid lifter" is ________.
311. ________stains the carminophilic cell wall of *Cryptococcus neoformans*.
312. Alcian blue stain is used to demonstrate ________ structure of *Cryptococcus neoformans*.
313. ________virus causes slow progressive fatal haemorrhagic pneumonia of sheep
314. Neurotropic virus causing neuropsychiatric disorders in horses, sheep in certain areas of germany is ________.
315. *Mansonia pseudotitillans* is the vector for transmission of ________.
316. Indian state which accounted for maximum number of cases of Chikungunya in 2017 is ________.
317. India has been declared as polio-free country since ________.
318. Country which is still considered as endemic for polio viral infection along with Pakistan and Nigeria is ________.
319. Paramyxovirus group which causes severe Bronchiolitis in children <1 year of age is ________.
320. Avian flu strain which caused a severe outbreak in China in 2013 is ________.
321. Reye's syndrome is associated with acute encephalopathy in children due to intake of ________.
322. With respect to classical triad of congenital rubella syndrome, ocular defects are characterized by ________.
323. Mutation type which results in blockade of HIV entry into the cells is ________.
324. Nucleoprotein complex in HIV replication comprising linear dsDNA, gag matrix protein, accessory vpr protein, viral integrase is known ________.
325. Anchoring transmembrane pedicles in HIV envelope is formed by ________.
326. Matrix or shell antigen is constituted by ________in HIV.
327. Breteau index is the ratio between number of containers showing breeding of *Aedes aegypti* larvae to that of ________.

328. Complication associated with the administration of equine rabies immunoglobulin is ________.
329. Furious rabies is also known as ________.
330. Covaxin, India's 1st indigenous vaccine against COVID has proven to neutralise ________variant 1st isolated in UK along with good efficacy against delta variants in India and other countries.
331. Technology employed in preparing "Moderna vaccine"for COVID-19 is ________.
332. Holder method and flash process are the subtypes of ________method of sterilisation.
333. Heart-lung machines are disinfected by ________.
334. Parasite implicated in causing "non-gonococcal urethritis" is ________.
335. Bacteria exhibiting "bamboo stick appearance" under microscope on Gram's staining is ________.
336. L-forms are cell wall deficient forms discovered by Klieneberger while studying ________bacteria.
337. Bacteria which grow in the presence of low O_2 tension of 5–10% are known as ________.
338. In bacteria like *Pseudomonas* glucose is converted to KDPG (keto-deoxy-phospho gluconate) which is further converted to Pyruvate. The pathway is known as ________.
339. Bacteria which require higher amount of CO_2 of 5–10% for their growth are known as ________.
340. Inspissation is also known as ________.
341. Cystoscopes, endoscopes are best disinfected by ________.
342. Tonometer biprisms, soft contact lenses are best disinfected by ________.
343. According to Spaulding's classification surgical instruments, cardiac, urinary catheters are included under ________.
344. ECG electrodes, crutches, stethoscopes are included under ________according to Spaulding's classification of medical devices.
345. Sulfhydryl group containing reducing substance in RCM broth is ________.
346. Indicator used in Simmon's citrate medium is ________.
347. In TSI medium glucose, sucrose, lactose are incorporated in the ratio of ________.
348. Indicator of H2S production in TSI medium ________
349. Enzyme responsible for DNA unwinding during DNA replication in bacteria ________.
350. Enzyme which reduces the tension generated by rapid unwinding by removing the super twists during DNA replication is ________.
351. Ceftobiprole belongs to ________.
352. Enhancement of virulence in a microbe is known as ________.
353. Perforins are produced by ________.
354. Cutaneous anthrax is described as ________.
355. California fever is ________.
356. Gilchrist's disease is ________.
357. Cysts of *P. jirovecii* resemble crushed Ping-pong balls on performing ________ staining.
358. Hyaline septate hyphae with round microconidia, sickle-shaped large macroconidia and chlamydospores are the characters of ________.
359. Dermatophyte infection of the non-hairy skin of the body is ________.
360. Dermatophyte infection of the palmar aspects of hands is ________.
361. Dermatophyte infecting skin and nail but not hair is ________.
362. ________gene in HBV genome can activate the transcription of cellular and viral genes.
363. MERS-CoV infection is more likely to infect the people who have high exposure to ________.
364. Source of infection for Marburg virus is ________.
365. Most common subtype of HIV found globally is ________.
366. According to revised NACO guidelines 2017, ART should be started in all patients if the CD4T cell count is below or ________.
367. Certificate for yellow fever vaccine is valid for ________.
368. State with highest prevalence of Japanese B encephalitis in India is ________.
369. E1-A226V mutation is noticed in ________.
370. Pigs are the amplifier hosts for ________Arbo viral flavi virus.
371. People coming from endemic area of yellow fever without immunisation should be in quarantine centre in airport for ________.
372. After a travel to endemic area of Zika virus or with symptoms of Zika virus , sexual restriction should be followed upto ________.
373. Most common serotypes of Coxsackie A virus causing aseptic meningitis ________.
374. Jeryl–Lynn strain is used for the preparation of ________vaccine.
375. Type specific antigens (A, B, C) of influenza viruses are present on ________viral constituent.
376. Decolourizer used in Preston and Morrell's modification of Gram's staining is ________.
377. Slicing is a step in specimen preparation of ________ microscopy method.
378. Site of respiration in prokaryotes ________.
379. Concentration of sulphuric acid required to demonstrate *Nocardia* species ________.
380. Concentration of sulphuric acid required to demonstrate bacterial spore ________.
381. Acid–fast staining was first developed by ________.
382. Sterilisation by gamma rays is known as ________.
383. Approximate pH of thioglycolate broth is ________.
384. Commonly used enrichment media for *Vibrio cholerae* is ________.

385. ________culture method is useful for bacteriophage typing.
386. Culture method used to demonstrate motility using semisolid agar is ________.
387. Automated equipment which evacuates air from Jar and replaces by H_2 gas from a cylinder is ________.
388. Removal of residual O_2 from McIntosh and Filde's anaerobic jar is achieved by ________.
389. Freeze-drying method of preservation of microorganisms is also known as ________.
390. Siderophore production is a classic example of ________type of plasmids.
391. F-plasmids contain________which code for the expression of sex pili that help in bacterial conjugation.
392. Replica plating method was 1st explained by ________.
393. ________refers to the substitution of a purine for a pyrimidine.
394. 2nd mutation in a different gene that reverts the phenotypic effects of an already existing mutation is known as ________.
395. ________ type of mutation converts the mutant nucleotide sequence back to the wild type sequence.
396. Pearly white umblicated lesions are characteristic of ________.

ANSWERS FOR FILL UP THE BLANKS

1. *Treponema pallidum, M. leprae*
2. James Phipps
3. Delayed /Type 4
4. Parvovirus B19
5. Transport
6. Ethylene oxide gas
7. Capsule
8. Bush Jacoby Medeiros classification
9. Translocation
10. Pathogenicity island
11. Kohler and Milstein
12. C14b2a3b
13. Langerhans cells
14. DiGeorge syndrome
15. Glomerular vascular intima
16. Neonatal tetanus
17. Sand fly
18. *Entamoeba histolytica*
19. CD46
20. H_1N_1 (Spanish flu)
21. Point mutations
22. Polyribosyl ribitol phosphate [PRP]
23. Melioidosis
24. Blue green pus
25. Cholera red reaction
26. Reynolds Braude phenomenon
27. Botryomycosis
28. Epidermophyton
29. Pteridine pigment
30. Gametocytes
31. *Cysticercus cellulosae*
32. *Ancylostoma duodenale*
33. Type-3
34. Sporotrichosis
35. Histoplasmosis
36. Exfoliative toxin
37. *Cl. perfringens*
38. Pulmonary anthrax
39. Tumbling motility
40. Fibrin
41. *Klebsiella pneumoniae*
42. Rubella
43. Adenovirus
44. EBV
45. Mucormycosis
46. *Cl. difficile*
47. Prodigiosin
48. *Proteus* pp
49. MMR
50. Hendra and Nipah virus
51. Metacercaria larva
52. *Trichinella spiralis*
53. *Fusobacterium necrophorum*
54. *Porphyromonas endodontalis*
55. Ranke complex
56. Activated macrophages
57. *M. marinum*
58. Virchow's lepra cells
59. Weil–Felix reaction
60. Wayson stain
61. Anamnestic response
62. *Eikenella corrodens*
63. Brucella
64. Screening of children
65. Donovanosis or granuloma inguinale
66. 10% KOH
67. IgE
68. DR-4
69. Central Research Institute, Kasauli
70. *Vibrio parahaemolyticus*
71. *Bartonella bacilliformis*
72. *Bartonella quintana*
73. Herbert's pits
74. Reiter's syndrome
75. Neurons of cerebellum and hippocampus
76. Plasma cell pneumonia or interstitial cell pneumonia
77. 116E (Gap[10] strain)

78. Flaviviridae
79. Genotypes 1 and 2
80. Tenofovir
81. Deposition of Immune complexes
82. Stationary
83. Mannitol salt agar
84. Herd immunity
85. Enterococci
86. 1–6 hrs
87. Chick sign
88. Culex tarsalis
89. Gujarat
90. *Haemophysalis spinigera*
91. Mollaret's meningitis
92. Reye's syndrome
93. Ophthalmic branch of trigeminal nerve
94. Owl's eye
95. Entero invasive
96. EHEC
97. Clutton's joints
98. Corkscrew
99. Vincent's angina (trench mouth)
100. *Rickettsia typhi*
101. *Rickettsia prowazekii*
102. SLE (systemic lupus erythematosus)
103. Allergen specific IgE
104. Theobald smith phenomenon
105. Hofbauer cells
106. MHC Class 2
107. Ionising rays
108. Peracetic acid
109. *Geobacillus stearothermophilus*
110. Pneumatocele
111. D – K
112. Torres bodies
113. Fruit bats
114. Segmented dsRNA
115. Australia Ag
116. Matured embryonated egg
117. *Trichuris trichura* (whipworm)
118. Cutaneous larva migrans
119. *Plasmodium falciparum*
120. *Plasmodium vivax*
121. *Quinine*
122. Promastigote in midgut
123. Metacyclic trypo mastigotes
124. Transduction
125. Conjugative plasmids
126. DNA
127. Lederberg and tatum
128. Spontaneous
129. Idiotypes
130. Cold agglutination test
131. Immunosurveillance theory
132. *Trichomonas vaginalis*
133. Capsular polysaccharide
134. Kolkata
135. *Legionella micdadei*
136. Adenocarcinoma of stomach
137. Category A
138. *Streptobacillus moniliformis*
139. *Pseudomonas aeruginosa*
140. *Metachromatic granules*
141. Flagella
142. Swarming
143. Spores of *Bacillus atrophaeus*
144. Transposons
145. Pastia's lines
146. Mc Fadyean's
147. Intradermal
148. *Mycobacterium szulgai*
149. *Tropheryma whippeli*
150. *Coccidioidis immitis*
151. *Rhinosporidium seeberi*
152. Sclerotic bodies/Medlar bodies
153. *Cladophialophora bantiana*
154. DC – sign (Dendritic cell specific lectin receptor)
155. Vpx
156. HIV -1 P24Ag
157. Semple vaccine
158. Serial brain-to-brain passage
159. 6th and 14th
160. Cutter incident
161. Post-polio muscle atrophy syndrome
162. *Cysticercus bovis*
163. Sporozoite
164. Loa loa
165. *Onchocerca volvulus*
166. Matured sporulated oocyst
167. Fasciolopsis buski
168. Metacercaria
169. 3rd stage sheeted microfilaria
170. *Mycoplasma pneumoniae*
171. Slit sampler method
172. Eijkman
173. Grade – 2 (moderate)
174. >16 hrs
175. Red colonies with black centre
176. *Sh. sonnei*
177. >10^5 CFU/ML
178. Adjuvant
179. Anterolateral aspect of thigh
180. Prodromal
181. Robert Koch
182. Bile Aesculin agar
183. Hypnozoites
184. *Haemophilus influenzae*
185. Sucrose fermentation

186. CMV
187. ETO
188. Inspissation
189. Faecooral route
190. RCM broth
191. Enterobius vermicularis
192. *Necator americanus*
193. *Hymanolepis nana*
194. Reduviid bug (Triatoma infestans)
195. *Taenia saginata*
196. *Echinococcus granulosus*
197. Rubella/German measles
198. *L. braziliensis*
199. 17D strain
200. 15 – 20 hrs
201. Lag phase
202. *Borrelia burgdorferi*
203. Dorsal columns
204. *Serratia marcescens*
205. 3% H_2O_2
206. Multiplex PCR
207. Reverse transcriptase PCR
208. Sensitivity
209. Antibody titre
210. IL – 2
211. Increased vascular permeability
212. Hemolysin
213. *P. malariae*
214. Enteric fever/typhoid fever
215. EBV
216. Adenovirus
217. Algel-IMDG (Imidazoquinolone)
218. Lymphoid organs
219. NK cells
220. Deficiency of membrane attacking complex (C5–C9)
221. CD3, CD8
222. Toxoid 1 dose + HTIG
223. Erysipeloid
224. *Stenotrophomonas maltophila*
225. Whooping cough
226. Tracheal cytotoxin
227. aP
228. Brucellosis
229. Tse – tse fly
230. Indole production test
231. 0.5% sodium deoxycholate
232. Amino acid decarboxylation tests
233. *Burkholderia mallei*
234. Caspase pathway
235. Hassall's corpuscles
236. Flaccid muscle
237. Coxsackie – B
238. *Staphylococcus saprophyticus*
239. Faeco-oral route
240. Acute haemorrhagic conjunctions
241. Hand foot mouth disease (HFMD)
242. Sand fly
243. California encephalitis virus
244. Crimean Congo haemorrhagic fever
245. Pegi virus
246. New Delhi
247. *V. parahaemolyticus*
248. *Giardia lamblia*
249. CURB
250. Antigen
251. Capsule switching
252. CMI
253. Lobar pneumonia
254. Spidery molar teeth
255. Cervico facial actinomycosis
256. 0157
257. Influenza-A (Orthomyxoviruses)
258. Parotid
259. Zoster (reactivation of varicella)
260. Poxviridae
261. Inspissation
262. Ebola
263. 28–38 days
264. Para-influenza type-IV
265. Park Williams-8
266. Type-I
267. Forensic science and graft compatibility testing
268. Levaditi stain
269. Fontana stain
270. *Bartonella bacilliformis* infection
271. Elementary body
272. SYBR green dye
273. *Geobacillus stearothermophilus*
274. Time of flight
275. 10% ferric chloride
276. Michael smith
277. Sub-clinical cases
278. Elongation factor-2 (EF-2)
279. Immune-complex diseases and pyogenic infections
280. Tangible body, macrophages
281. Plasmids
282. Metachromatic granules/volutin granules
283. *Clostridium botulinum*
284. Desmoglein-1
285. Viridans streptococci (*Streptococcus sanguis*)
286. Hyaluronidase
287. Eosin methylene blue agar
288. Natural killer cells (NK)
289. Ataxia-telangiectasia
290. Lazy-leukocyte syndrome
291. Pittsburgh pneumonia agent
292. *Eikenella corrodens*

293. +2 and + 8°C
294. Freezer compartment
295. Mucosa of duodenum and jejunum of man
296. Reddish brown
297. Herman Muller
298. *Plasmodium falciparum*
299. WBC (leucocytes)
300. School of fish or railroad track appearance
301. Yellow non-diffusible pigment
302. Ashdown's medium
303. *Mycobacterium paratuberculosis*
304. Nikshay
305. Yellow bags
306. Glassware
307. 40 seconds
308. 1% Sodium hypochlorite
309. Negative pressure
310. *Rhizopus*
311. Mucicarmine
312. Capsule
313. Maedi virus
314. Scrapie
315. St. Louis encephalitis virus
316. Karnataka
317. March 2014
318. Afghanistan
319. Respiratory syncytial virus (RSV)
320. H5N1
321. Aspirin/acetyl salicylate
322. Salt and pepper retinopathy
323. Mutation in CCR5/delta 32 mutation
324. Pre-integration complex
325. Glycoprotein 41(gp-41)
326. P18
327. Number of houses surveyed
328. Serum sickness
329. Encephalitic rabies
330. AY 4.2
331. mRNA
332. Pasteurisation
333. Ethylene oxide gas (ETO)
334. *Trichomonas vaginalis*
335. *Bacillus anthracis*
336. *Streptobacillus moniliformis*
337. Microaerophilic bacteria
338. Entner-Doudoroff pathway
339. Capnophilic
340. Fractional sterilisation
341. Glutaraldehyde
342. Hydrogen peroxide (H_2O_2)
343. Critical devices
344. Non-critical devices
345. Glutathione
346. Bromothymol blue
347. 1:10:10
348. Ferric salts
349. Helicase
350. Topo-isomerase
351. 5th generation cephalosporin
352. Exaltation
353. Cytotoxic T lymphocytes
354. Woolsorter's disease
355. Coccidioidomycosis
356. Blastomycosis
357. Gomori's methanamine silver staining (GMS)
358. *Fusarium*
359. *Tinea corporis*
360. *Tinea manum*
361. Epidermophyton
362. X-gene
363. Camels
364. African green monkeys
365. HIV-1 subtype-C
366. Irrespective of CD4 count
367. 10 years
368. Uttar Pradesh
369. Chikungunya fever
370. Japanese B encephalitis
371. 6 days
372. 6 months for males, 8 weeks for females
373. A7 and A9
374. Mumps vaccine
375. Nucleo capsid
376. Iodine-acetone
377. Transmission electron microscope
378. Mesosomes
379. 1%
380. 0.25–0.5%
381. Sir Paul Ehrlich
382. Cold sterilisation/ionising radiation
383. 7.2
384. Alkaline peptone water
385. Lawn culture method
386. Stab culture method
387. Anoxomat
388. Palladium catalyst
389. Lyophilisation
390. Virulence plasmids
391. Tra A genes
392. Lederberg
393. Transversion
394. Suppressor mutation
395. True reversion
396. Molluscum contagiosum